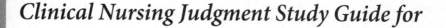

Clinical Nursing Judgment Study Guide for

Medical-Surgical Nursing
Patient-Centered Collaborative Care

Eighth Edition

Donna D. Ignatavicius, MS, RN, ANEF
Speaker and Curriculum Consultant for
Academic Nursing Programs
Founder, Boot Camp for Nurse
Educators
President, DI Associates, Inc.
Placitas, New Mexico

M. Linda Workman, PhD, RN, FAAN
Senior Volunteer Faculty
College of Nursing
University of Cincinnati
Cincinnati, Ohio;
Formerly Gertrude Perkins Oliva
Professor of Oncology
Frances Payne Bolton School of Nursing
Case Western Reserve University
Cleveland, Ohio

Clinical Nursing Judgment Study Guide prepared by:

Linda A. LaCharity, PhD, RN
Retired Accelerated Program Director
and Assistant Professor
College of Nursing
University of Cincinnati
Cincinnati, Ohio

Candice K. Kumagai, RN, MSN
Former Instructor in Clinical Nursing
School of Nursing
University of Texas at Austin
Austin, Texas

ELSEVIER

ELSEVIER

3251 Riverport Lane
St. Louis, Missouri 63043

CLINICAL NURSING JUDGMENT STUDY GUIDE FOR
MEDICAL-SURGICAL NURSING: PATIENT-CENTERED
COLLABORATIVE CARE, EIGHTH EDITION

ISBN: 978-0-323-22231-0

Executive Content Strategist: Lee Henderson
Traditional Content Development Manager: Billie Sharp
Associate Content Development Specialist: Samantha Taylor
Publishing Services Manager: Debbie Vogel
Project Manager: Brandi Flagg

Printed in the United States of America

Last digit is the print number: 9 8 7 6 5 4 3 2 1

V011

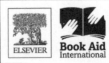

Reviewers

Margaret-Ann Carno, PhD, MBA, RN, CPNP, D,ABSM, FAAN
Associate Professor of Clinical Nursing and Pediatrics
School of Nursing
University of Rochester
Rochester, New York

Diane Daddario, MSN, ACNS-BC, RN, BC, CMSRN
Adjunct Faculty
School of Nursing
Pennsylvania State University
University Park, Pennsylvania

LaWanda Herron, PhD, MSA, MSN, FNP-BC
Director of Nursing
Holmes Community College
Grenada, Mississippi

Jamie Lynn Jones, MSN, RN, CNE
Assistant Professor
University of Arkansas at Little Rock
Little Rock, Arkansas

Tamara M. Kear, PhD, RN, CNS, CNN
Assistant Professor of Nursing
College of Nursing
Villanova University
Villanova, Pennsylvania

Jason Mott, PhD, RN
Instructor of Nursing
Bellin College
Green Bay, Wisconsin

Denise A. Sevigny, MSN, RN, CNE
Associate Professor
Sentara College of Health Sciences
Chesapeake, Virginia

Preface

The *Clinical Nursing Judgment Study Guide for Medical-Surgical Nursing: Patient-Centered Collaborative Care, 8th* Edition is a companion publication for Ignatavicius & Workman's *Medical-Surgical Nursing: Patient-Centered Collaborative Care, 8th* Edition. This Study Guide, written by experts in the fields of adult medical-surgical nursing and nursing education, will help to ensure mastery of the textbook content and help you learn about collaborative practice in the care of the adult medical-surgical patient.

The 8th Edition has been carefully revised and updated for an increased emphasis on clinical decision-making. An introductory "pre-chapter" includes concrete study tips to help you make the most of your individual learning style.

The overall organization of the *Clinical Nursing Judgment Study Guide for Medical-Surgical Nursing* directly corresponds to the unit/chapter name and number in the textbook so that you or your instructor can readily select the corresponding learning exercises in the Study Guide. Chapters are focused on:

- **Study/Review Questions** which are designed to encourage prioritizing, clinical decision-making, and application of the steps of the nursing process. Questions have been updated to focus on the question formats of the NCLEX examination, and emphasize the NCLEX priorities of delegation, management of care, and pharmacology.

Answers to the Study/Review Questions are provided in the back of the Study Guide. Case Studies and answ guidelines for the Case Studies are available on the Evolve website at http://evolve.elsevier.com/Iggy/ in the "Prepare for Class" folder. Each chapter's Case Studies can also be downloaded and completed as a word p cessing file, if preferred.

The *Clinical Nursing Judgment Study Guide for Medical-Surgical Nursing* is a practical tool to help you pr for classroom examinations and standardized tests, as well as a review for clinical practice. This improv mat will help you review and apply medical-surgical content and help you prepare for the NCLEX Exa tion.

Student Tips for Clinical Application of Textbook Material

There are many challenges in nursing programs. One of the critical tasks is to embrace the transition of obtaining information and then applying nursing knowledge at the bedside.

Medical-Surgical Nursing: Patient-Centered Collaborative Care (8th Ed.), *Clinical Nursing Judgment Study Guide for Medical-Surgical Nursing: Patient-Centered Collaborative Care* (8th Ed.), and the Case Studies-Interactive folder on Evolve are a few important resources that you should use as you work towards your goal of becoming a great nurse. Below are some suggestions for organizing your clinical day and using and incorporating material from your core textbook, Study Guide, and Case Studies on Evolve. This model of a "clinical day" is divided into three sections and includes suggestions for work and learning habits that can be useful throughout your nursing career.

BEFORE CARE BEGINS

In most nursing programs, students are required to do some preparation before initiating the nurse-patient relationship. Although this preparation may seem arduous and time-consuming, it will increase your confidence and your ability to function smoothly when caring for real patients. It is likely that you will have limited time to devote to the preparation, so let's focus your efforts into four areas.

- Making a clinical tool kit
- Focusing on patient chart data
- Using the medical diagnosis to plan and anticipate collaborative care
- Identifying specific strategies to ensure safety

1. Making a clinical tool kit

You should create a clinical tool kit as soon as possible. Do not wait until the night before (or worse, the morning of) your clinical day to gather items that you will need at the bedside when caring for a patient. The following list includes some typical items that can be used. However, you will need to adapt the tool kit to the unit where you are assigned or for a specific patient. For example, in Chapter 41 (p. 843) of your core textbook, there is an example of the Glasgow Coma Scale (GSC). Consider the types of patient conditions where you would need a copy of the GSC in order to perform the necessary assessment. Another example, for patients who require an assessment of sensation in the extremities, you may need to add a paper clip or a cotton-tip applicator to your kit [see Chapter 51 of your core textbook (p. 842), Assessment of Neurovascular Status in Patients with Musculoskeletal Injury].

Sample List for Clinical Tool Kit

- Copy of your objectives for the day to share with nurse/instructor
- ID badge (student or hospital as required)
- Instructor's cell phone number or contact information
- Computer access code/password (often assigned during orientation)
- All assignments required by instructor (e.g., care plan, drug research, etc.)
- Extra copies of your time-management tool
- Blank paper or report form
- Drug reference (book or electronic)
- Stethoscope
- Calculator

- Black pen, red pen, highlighter
- Penlight
- Pill cutter
- Bandage scissors
- Energy snack

Adapted from Kumagai, C. (2013), Susan C. deWit's *Clinical Quick Reference for Medical-Surgical Nursing Concepts & Practice* (2nd ed.) p. 50. Philadelphia: Saunders. https://evolve.elsevier.com/ Evolve Resources for *Medical-Surgical Nursing*, (2nd ed.).

2. Focusing on patient chart data

Chart information never replaces the firsthand information obtained from the patient or hands-on physical assessment, but in order to prepare, students generally start by looking at the patient's chart. This is usually done the evening before the clinical experience. For legal reasons, instructors may ask you not to meet, question, or assess the patient during the evening because this initiates the nurse-patient relationship and you would be obligated to intervene if something happened (e.g., initiate CPR).

The patient chart includes information that is vital for continuity of care and complete legal documentation; however, the amount of data can be overwhelming, especially if you have a limited amount of time and are seeking information specific to your learning objectives. Below is a guideline to help you focus on the most relevant information.

Sample list of data to collect from the patient's chart

Data Source	*Minimal* information needed to prepare for clinical	If you have extra time
Face sheet	Patient's initials, age, gender	Occupation, marital status
Health care provider order sheets	Current medications, treatments, procedures	Review all past orders since admission
Health care provider history and physical	Admitting diagnosis and summary of problems	Review past admissions to compare to the current admission
Health care provider or multidisciplinary progress notes		Status of current problems; future plans
Nurses' admission sheet	Allergies, prosthetics	Total biopsychosocial health review
Nurses' notes	Review past 24 hours	Review all nurses' notes for trends and charting style
Flow sheets	Review vital signs, I&O, neuro checks for past 24 hours	Review all data for trends
Nursing care plan or needs list	Current problems, interventions, goals	Review all revisions of plan since admission
Laboratory reports	Note abnormal results	Review all reports for trends
Radiology reports		Review reports
Operative reports	Date and type of procedure	Review abnormalities, problems encountered
Kardex*	Treatments, procedures, activity, diet, IV fluids; all details needed to care for patient during shift*	
Medication administration record (MAR)*	Types of medications, frequency, dose; also PRN medications	

*The Kardex and MAR are daily tools that are usually not kept with the hardcopy charts. Ask for help in locating these items on the clinical unit. In computerized systems, ask for help in locating these on the drop-down menus.

*Hardcopy and electronic Kardexes and MARs can be out of date, or contain errors and discrepancies. Refer to the health care provider's orders for the definitive answers (e.g., health care provider writes new orders and transcription is pending).

Adapted from Kumagai, C. (2013), Susan C. deWit's *Clinical Quick Reference for Medical-Surgical Nursing Concepts & Practice* (2nd ed.) p. 50. Philadelphia: Saunders. https://evolve.elsevier.com/ Evolve Resources for *Medical-Surgical Nursing*, (2nd ed.).

You should plan on spending at least 30-45 minutes to do this initial chart review. As you are reading the patient's chart, you should be formulating questions about the patient data. Next, decide where to get the answers. Primary nurse? Instructor? Textbooks? Internet? For example, let's say that you are assigned to care for a 58-year-old woman who was admitted for probable thrombophlebitis. Her chief complaint is pain and edema in the right calf. The chart indicates that the patient is receiving intravenous heparin and oral warfarin (Coumadin). What question(s) would you want to ask the primary nurse or the instructor? Any questions that relate to the patient's current status are best directed towards the primary nurse. For example, how is the patient responding to the medication? How are the symptoms of pain and edema compared to previously? Questions for the instructor are likely to be related to performance. For example, "What are my responsibilities related to intravenous heparin?" Answers to questions about pathophysiology can be obtained by using your core textbook or approved Internet sites. For example, what are the risk factors for developing DVT? (See Chapter 36, p. 729 in your core textbook for discussion of venous thrombosis and DVT. For additional critical thinking questions about this type of patient, see Case Study: The Patient with Deep Vein Thrombosis on the Evolve site. For NCLEX-style questions related to this type of patient, see Chapter 36, question 98, p. 274 and question 121, p. 277 of the Study Guide.)

There is a great deal of variation in how students are permitted to obtain and use patient data for purposes of writing papers or completing homework assignments. Various institutions even within the same city may have different interpretations of the Health Insurance Portability and Accountability Act (HIPAA). For example, some facilities may allow students to make computer printouts or Xerox copies of information, such as medications lists, if the patient's name, room number, health care provider's name, or any other information that could be used to identify the patient is completely removed. In other circumstances, students may be permitted to look at data and make handwritten notes. Please remember to exercise extreme caution in handling information from the patient's chart or electronic medical record because HIPAA violations can have serious consequences for you, your instructor, and your nursing program. Ask your instructor for specific advice about how to handle the chart data and be sure to follow the guidelines specific to your clinical facilities. **Patient identifying information should never be associated with any data that you use for your clinical preparation or written assignments.**

3. Using the medical diagnosis to plan and anticipate collaborative care

You can use the medical diagnosis to plan and anticipate collaborative care. For example, a 74-year-old patient is admitted for pulmonary edema secondary to heart failure. Based on the medical diagnosis, what signs and symptoms is the patient likely to display? What types of medications or treatments would you anticipate that the health care provider will prescribe for this condition? Which laboratory values do you need to follow up on? Which interdisciplinary team members are likely to be involved in the care of this patient? What patient teaching should you perform? (See Chapter 35, p. 681 in your core textbook for information about caring for patients with heart failure. For additional critical thinking questions about this type of patient, see Case Study: The Patient with Heart Failure on the Evolve site. For NCLEX-style questions related to this type of patient, see Chapter 35, questions 1-42, pp. 253-258 in the Study Guide.)

4. Identifying specific strategies to ensure safety

a.   If you take steps to ensure your patient's safety your instructor will approve, you will feel more confident and relaxed and your patient will be safe at the end of the day. For example, review the core textbook Chapter 35 for information about the care of a patient with heart failure and pulmonary edema. The discussion on heart failure has many "Nursing Safety Priority" boxes, Chapter 35, pp. 678-691. Throughout the book, these yellow boxes alert you to dangerous signs and symptoms, as well as interventions that you should take for various disorders and patient conditions.

b.   Become aware of high-alert drugs that are prescribed for your patients and know the nursing responsibilities related to these medications. For example, look at Case Study: The Patient with Deep Vein Thrombosis found on the Evolve site. Can you identify the high-alert drug(s) that are included in the scenario? (For additional information about high-alert drugs, see http://www.ismp.org.)

c. Be aware of specific conditions that increase risk for injury for your patients. For example, if you are caring for an older patient, you may also want to review the best practice box of "Assessing Risk Factors and Preventing Falls in Older Adults" (Chapter 2, p. 21). For NCLEX-style questions related to falls in older adults, see Chapter 2, questions 6-7, p. 4 and question 19, p. 5 of the Study Guide. Another example is polypharmacy, which is common among older patients and increases risk for injury. (See Case Study: Medication Use in Older Adults on the Evolve site. For NCLEX-style questions related to medication use in older adults, see Chapter 2, questions 10 and 11, p. 4 of Study Guide.)

d. Another strategy would be to brainstorm with classmates to identify other interventions to ensure safety, such as instructing the patient to ask for help, proper use of side rails, call bells/lights, frequent offers to assist with toileting, and encouraging the use of assistive devices.

CARING FOR THE PATIENT DURING THE CLINICAL EXPERIENCE

Going into the clinical setting, caring for patients, and performing in front of an instructor cause most students to feel stressed or anxious. This is a normal response and recall that mild anxiety is likely to improve your performance. You can create a plan with some structure that will help you move forward, even if you feel nervous. Creating this structure is divided into four sections:

- Listening to report
- Organizing your clinical day
- Using nursing concepts and clinical judgment review
- What if I don't know what to do? Knowing when and how to get help

1. Listening to report

Remember, it is your responsibility to be ready to take report at the beginning of the shift. You must take notes during the report. How you take notes may be affected by your personal style, the assigned unit, or specific instructions from your clinical instructor. A common-sense approach for taking notes is to adapt the personal style that you use while listening to a lecture. Another approach would be to observe how the nurses on your unit take notes. For example, some nurses will use one sheet of paper that is divided into four or more sections so that data for all assigned patients is on one sheet of paper. Other nurses have designed report forms and will use one page per patient keeping all pages together in a three-ring binder or on a clipboard. Other units have electronic MARs; nurses print out a hardcopy MAR for each assigned patient and staple them together for daily use. A red pen or highlighter can be used for important information or for timed tasks that you must remember to do later during the shift. Choose a form that seems to work for you and then consistently use that method during the semester. Currently, most nurses rely on paper and pen, but in the future personal electronic devices may be more common.

A good report lasts about 2-3 minutes per patient and is well organized with important points emphasized. SBAR or SBAR-R (Situation, Background, Assessment, Recommendations–Response) described in Chapter 1, p. 5 of your core textbook is a recommended method to organize and improve communication between staff members. (See Study Guide Chapter 1, question 12, p. 2 for NCLEX-style question related to SBAR.) A list of information that is included in a typical hand-off or change of shift report is shown below.

Sample list of what to include in report

- Patient's name, gender, and age
- Admitting medical diagnosis and/or recent surgeries or procedures

- Relevant conditions (e.g., LUQ surgical incision with dressing dry/intact)
- Changes in condition or risks (e.g., dizziness with fluctuating BP; at risk for falls)
- Immediately pending procedures, labs, treatments, or surgery (e.g., call to OR this am) or those needing follow-up (e.g., CBC drawn, call provider with results ASAP)
- Presence of equipment (e.g., SCDs, NG tubes, chest tube)
- Last BM, voiding status, special dietary considerations
- Rate and type of IV fluids and appearance of IV site
- Last PRN medication and effects (e.g., had morphine 1 hour ago with complete relief)
- New orders and status of orders (e.g., provider changed antibiotic to gentamicin; pharmacy notified to send drug)
- Specific patient or family concerns (e.g., would like to see social worker this afternoon)

Adapted from Kumagai, C. (2013), Susan C. deWit's *Clinical Quick Reference for Medical-Surgical Nursing Concepts & Practice* (2nd ed.) p. 50. Philadelphia: Saunders. https://evolve.elsevier.com/ Evolve Resources for *Medical-Surgical Nursing*, (2nd ed.).

Listening to a good report is easy; however, listening to a rambling and disorganized report is a problem, particularly for students or new nurses. There are several strategies to use if you are listening to a report that is disorganized. First, based on the clinical preparation that you did during the evening, you can anticipate what should be reported and listen for and write down key information.

Second, prioritize information needs. What information is critical to get from the off-going nurse before report is over? Change in status must be reported by the off-going nurse. For example, if your patient is a confused 98-year-old female, is her confusion new-onset or is this the patient's baseline behavior? Knowing about pending procedures or the need to follow up is also important information to get from the off-going nurse. Likewise, if information was exchanged verbally between nurse-patient or nurse-health care provider, it may not be in the written record. For example, did the health care provider say when he/she would be in to see the patient? Conversely, you can figure out some information even if the reporter forgets (e.g., patient's name, age, and gender or presence of equipment), so this type of information would have lower priority to obtain during report.

Third, asking questions is always a useful strategy. It can alert the speaker to gaps in the report. Also as a student or a novice nurse, you should pose questions that tap into the expertise of experienced nurses, such as "What is the most important issue for this patient? Which patient [of these five] needs attention first? What should I be watching for?"

2. Organizing your clinical day

Organization is a learned skill that takes practice. Planning is essential and below is a sample of how tasks are linked to a specific time of day. However, prioritization and flexibility are also essential. For example, a patient's status can suddenly change. Review the Case Study: The Patient Receiving Intravenous Therapy on the Evolve site and then think about or discuss with a classmate how a change in patient status could affect the timed plan that is listed below.

- 06:30 Arrive 15-30 minutes early; check your personal equipment; review charts.
- 06:45 Quickly check patients (ABCs); reassure patients that you will be in after report.
- 07:00 Listen to report; mentally prioritize (e. g., who is the sickest, which procedure cannot wait, etc.); clarify priorities with off-going nurse.
- Review Kardex and medication administration record (MAR); make notations on time-management sheet for meds and treatments. (Refer to orders if there are any discrepancies among shift report, Kardex, or MAR.)
- 07:30 Assess all patients; make notes as you work; attend to most critical patients; formulate critical thinking questions based on your assessment.
- 08:00 Check blood sugar results; give early am meds (e.g., 08:00 am insulin) or PRN meds if appropriate.

- 08:30 Assist patients who need help with breakfast and morning hygiene care. (May be delegated according to agency policy and preference of your instructor.)
- 09:00 Document assessments.
- 10:00 Give routine am meds and document (as you work, remind patients about ambulating; using spirometers; teach about meds; reassess IV sites and fluids).
- 10:30 Check and follow up on lab results. Catch up on documentation (e.g., medication teaching, calling provider, etc.); assist with or delegate ambulation as appropriate. Formulate critical thinking questions about laboratory results or tasks that you have delegated.
- 11:00 Go to lunch.
- 11:30 Assist patients who need help with lunch; use therapeutic communication. Formulate critical thinking questions about the patients' psychosocial needs.
- 12:00 Give routine medications and document; reassess patients as you work (e.g., IV sites and fluids, equipment in place and functioning).
- 12:30 Catch up on documentation (e.g., update assessments as appropriate).
- 12:45 Daily procedures (e.g., dressing changes, tracheostomy care).
- 2:00 Give routine medications and document. Do end-of-shift assessment, total I&O, hang new IV fluids if needed, complete documentation.
- 3:00 Give report, remember to thank nurses and unlicensed assistive personnel (UAPs), and attend postconference.

Adapted from Kumagai, C. (2013), Susan C. deWit's *Clinical Quick Reference for Medical-Surgical Nursing Concepts & Practice* (2nd ed.) pp. 52-53. Philadelphia: Saunders. https://evolve.elsevier.com/ Evolve Resources for *Medical-Surgical Nursing*, (2nd ed.).

Nurses and nursing students rarely "run out of things to do," but sometimes it may seem as though you have done all the planned tasks. Consider these six options.

- Is/are my patient(s) safe and resting comfortably?
- Is/are my patient(s)' environment clean and comfortable?
- Do(es) my patient(s) need any teaching or reinforcement of information?
- Do(es) my patient(s) have psychosocial needs that I have overlooked?
- Would my overall understanding of the patient(s) be improved by an in-depth chart review?
- Do nurses, UAPs, or classmates need my help? (Note to student: Helpful students are fondly remembered by nurses and UAPs and their good recommendations can help you get a job after you graduate.)

3. Using nursing concepts and clinical judgment review

Medical-Surgical Nursing: Patient-Centered Collaborative Care, 8th Ed. has included a feature at the end of many of the chapters called Nursing Concepts and Clinical Judgment Review. For example, look at Chapter 16, p. 272, and you will see that information contained under the headings of "Notice, Respond, Interpret, and Reflect" apply to any patient with a wound. Use Nursing Concepts and Clinical Judgment Review in the various chapters whenever it applies to your patients' conditions. You can also use the model of "Notice, Respond, Interpret, and Reflect" when studying with a classmate to expand your mental database of conditions. For example, select one example of the Nursing Concepts and Clinical Judgment Review in the core textbook, such as Chapter 57, p. 1190, "Impaired digestion and inadequate nutrition as a result of inflammatory problem" and quiz each other about "Notice, Respond, Interpret, and Reflect" and then check your answers against the textbook. Next, select a condition that you or a classmate observed during a clinical experience, such as "Hypoglycemia as a result of imbalance between nutritional intake and antidiabetic medication" and quiz each other about "Notice, Respond, Interpret, and Reflect," and then check your answers against the core textbook section on hypoglycemia (See Chapter 64, "Preventing Hypoglycemia," p. 1330 of the textbook). With practice and experience, you can use this model of nursing concept review to build your knowledge of concepts that will apply to a wide variety of patients' conditions.

4. "What if I don't know what to do?" Knowing when and how to get help

You are not supposed to know what to do in every situation (remember you are a student), but the most important thing is to know when and how to call for help and whom to call. Talk to your instructor about your concerns beforehand and use orientation or clinical prep time to learn about location and use of phones, call bells/lights, and emergency alert systems. Know how to locate and contact the instructor, charge nurse, primary nurse, pharmacist, and your classmates. (Classmates are often the most comforting resource if you have a nonemergent question or issue.)

An activity that you can do with a classmate, instructor, or by yourself is go into an empty patient room and play "worst-case scenario." Look at the empty room and think about different patient scenarios: elderly patient crawls over side rail and is found on the floor, patient lying supine in bed who has sudden and severe respiratory distress, patient sitting in chair has a grand mal seizure, or patient has a wound dehiscence with gushing blood while taking a shower. What you would do first? What immediate actions would you do to ensure safety? Who and how would you call for help? Where and how you would obtain the necessary equipment? This activity helps increase your confidence, improves your critical thinking, and helps orient you to the clinical environment.

AFTER THE CLINICAL DAY IS OVER

Although it is tempting to go home and collapse after a long hard day in the clinical setting, participation in these three activities will enhance the learning that occurred during your clinical experience.

- Review your performance at the end of the day.
- Cite at least two things that you will look up in your core textbook.
- Use concept mapping to visualize the linkage of patient data, care, and outcomes.

1. Review your performance at the end of the day.

If your instructor is agreeable, postconference is the ideal opportunity to review the clinical experience. First, practice giving report using the SBAR format to your classmates during postconference. Classmates can give you feedback on your report style. Next, share your success stories, cite at least two things that you did well, and two areas that need improvement. If postconference time is not available, then you can make a personal journal or have informal meetings with classmates.

2. Cite at least two things that you will look up in your textbook.

Looking things up is an important habit that should continue throughout your nursing career. Being able to link textbook information to a real patient experience will help you retain the information long after the patient is discharged and you have graduated. Knowledge + Experience = Clinical Expertise.

3. Use concept mapping to create visual linkage of patient data, care, and outcomes.

Concept mapping is a method of linking the numerous bits of information that you have collected into a whole picture. Many instructors use concept mapping as a comprehensive assignment that reflects understanding of the total biopsychosocial care of the patient. Your core textbook contains many examples. See Concept Map: Diabetes Mellitus—Type 2 (Chapter 64) or Concept Map: End-Stage Kidney Disease (Chapter 68). Also consult the index under "concept map" for additional examples.

Generally, concept mapping is built around a medical diagnosis, but you can also use a diagnostic procedure or a symptom as the central concept. Emergency department (ED) nurses or nurses who work in clinics frequently care for patients who have no official medical diagnosis, because the health care provider is in the process of determining the diagnosis. For example, the patient presents with an abrupt change of mental status. "Change of mental status" is the central concept and the ED nurse would have to think about all potential causes (Can you think of several possible causes?) and obtain history and seek signs and symptoms to help determine the cause. Nurses must be able to quickly recognize a serious symptom and intervene accordingly. For example, what would the nurse do if change of mental status is caused by hypoglycemia? (See Chapter 64, p. 1336 of the textbook, Critical Rescue for Hypoglycemia.)

If you are having trouble with concept mapping, try this easy exercise. Select a process that is very familiar to you, such as making and drinking a cup of coffee. Now write down everything you know about making and drinking coffee. As you write, notice that certain thoughts about coffee can be grouped together; for example, the equipment you need or the steps in making the coffee. Other thoughts are linked by arrows; for example, the smell may trigger a memory or drinking the coffee may be linked to a physical response, such as alertness or feeling jittery. You may have personal rituals associated with making or drinking coffee that make your concept map unique to your own preferences. At the end of the exercise, your paper should be full of categories and arrows showing linkage. This concept map is a depiction of how your brain actually thinks about making and drinking coffee. Now try to make a concept map related to your last patient by using the same process of building categories and drawing arrows to make linkage.

In summary, *Medical-Surgical Nursing: Patient-Centered Collaborative Care* (8th Ed.), *Clinical Nursing Judgment Study Guide for Medical-Surgical Nursing: Patient-Centered Collaborative Care* (8th Ed.), and learning material on the Evolve site are resources you can use to meet your clinical objectives and support your transition from being a great nursing student to being a great nurse! Good luck and best wishes as you progress through your nursing program.

Contents

1 CHAPTER

Introduction to Medical-Surgical Nursing Practice

1. The Institute of Medicine report *To Err Is Human* highlighted the need to improve patient safety. Which national organization requires its accredited agencies to meet specific national patient safety goals?
   a. National Hospital Council
   b. *Healthy People 2020*
   c. National Patient Safety Foundation
   d. The Joint Commission

2. What is the purpose of the Rapid Response Team (RRT)?
   a. Provide Code Blue teams in case of simultaneous emergencies
   b. Enable the nurse to recognize changes in patient status before an acute emergency
   c. Replace immediate consultation with the physician or medical resident
   d. Provide teams of staff already familiar with the patient's medical diagnosis

3. In addition to providing care with skill in techniques and procedures, what must the medical-surgical nurse also be prepared to utilize when caring for the patient? *(Select all that apply.)*
   a. Teaching
   b. Patient advocacy
   c. Spiritual counseling and support
   d. Rehabilitation strategies and methods
   e. Administrative scheduling and budgeting
   f. Coordination of care

4. Which health care workers are likely to be members of a Rapid Response Team (RRT)? *(Select all that apply.)*
   a. Critical care nurse
   b. Respiratory therapist
   c. Intensivist
   d. Pharmacist
   e. Medical resident

5. Which is the best way for the nurse to assess the patient's learning after teaching?
   a. Have the patient write a summary of the points covered.
   b. Ask the patient to repeat the information back.
   c. Quiz the patient on relevant points in the instruction.
   d. Repeat the important points to the patient.

6. Which type of evidence is rated highest on a level of evidence scale?
   a. Well-designed case control with cohort studies
   b. Randomized trials of small descriptive studies
   c. Well-designed controlled trials without randomization
   d. Systematic review or meta-analysis of all randomized controlled trials

7. Which is the best use of information from electronic sources, such as websites or e-mail, for retrieving data for the evidence-based practice process?
   a. Being sure to include links to articles so the reader can follow up on subsequent results
   b. Evaluating the information for credibility and reliability before putting it to use
   c. Using only university-related sources to ensure the most current results
   d. Assessing the number of hits the sources have on a search engine to determine popularity

8. Which action exemplifies the goal of case management in an acute care setting?
   a. Making sure the patient's dietary choices meet prescribed nutritional needs
   b. Scheduling home visits after discharge and monitoring patient progress
   c. Monitoring the patient's vital signs and noting trends of elevations
   d. Reviewing the patient's hospital bill for accuracy and any excessive charges

9. Which actions best demonstrate a collaborative nursing function? *(Select all that apply.)*
   a. Requesting the assistance of another staff member to turn a patient
   b. Administering medications as prescribed by the health care provider
   c. Maintaining patient confidentiality by not notifying the family members of a change in the patient's condition
   d. Making a referral to the case manager to assist with discharge planning
   e. Ensuring clear communication with other health care providers

10. Which is an example of a skill needed to develop the Institute of Medicine/Quality and Safety Education for Nurses (IOM/QSEN) patient-centered care competency?
    a. Recognize personally held attitudes about working with different ethnic, cultural, and social backgrounds.
    b. Demonstrate comprehensive understanding of the concepts of pain and suffering, including physiologic models of pain and comfort.
    c. Provide patient-centered care with sensitivity and respect for the diversity of human experience.
    d. Explore ethical and legal implications of patient-centered care.

11. Treating all patients equally and fairly is an example of which ethical principle?
    a. Social justice
    b. Fidelity
    c. Autonomy
    d. Beneficence

12. When using the SBAR (Situation, Background, Assessment, Recommendation) method of communication, the nurse would include which information in the B section?
    a. Recommend fingerstick glucose monitoring
    b. Patient states he feels dizzy and light-headed
    c. Admission diagnosis is new-onset type 2 diabetes
    d. Blood pressure 130/90 mm Hg, heart rate 89 beats per minute

13. Which tasks should the nurse delegate to UAP (unlicensed assistive personnel)? *(Select all that apply.)*
    a. Turn patient every 2 hours.
    b. Teach patient to cough and deep-breathe.
    c. Feed patient breakfast and lunch.
    d. Assist patient with morning care.
    e. Take and record patient vital signs.

14. Which occurrence does the Joint Commission's National Patient Safety Goals designate as a high-risk issue?
    a. Health care workers' exposure to infectious diseases in the workplace
    b. Violating privacy considerations of patients' confidential information
    c. Administering medication that is not familiar to the nurse
    d. Failure to review patients' food allergies before serving meals

2 CHAPTER

Common Health Problems of Older Adults

1. Which statements about the health of older adults in the United States are true? *(Select all that apply.)*
   a. The fastest-growing group is between 85-99 years of age.
   b. Only 5% of older adults are in nursing homes.
   c. Older adults are at risk for poor nutrition.
   d. Older adults 85-95 years old are often wrongly referred to as the "frail elderly."
   e. Men live longer than women in the old-old subgroup.

2. The nurse is caring for an older adult patient. What are the best interventions to help reduce relocation stress in this patient? *(Select all that apply.)*
   a. Explain all procedures to the patient before they occur.
   b. Reorient the patient frequently to location.
   c. Allow the patient adequate time for rest, and encourage family and friends to keep their visits to a minimum.
   d. Provide ample opportunity and time for the patient to participate in decision making.
   e. Arrange for familiar keepsakes to be at the patient's bedside.

3. Which statements would be included in an educational program on wellness behaviors for the older adult? *(Select all that apply.)*
   a. Allow at least 10-15 minutes of sun exposure 2-3 times weekly.
   b. Take one aspirin twice a day.
   c. Obtain a yearly influenza vaccination.
   d. Create a hazard-free environment to prevent falls.
   e. Increased dietary needs include calcium and vitamins A, D, and C.
   f. Reduce dietary intake of complex carbohydrates and fiber.
   g. Drink 6-8 glasses of water per day to prevent dehydration.

4. Which statement about how nutrition is affected in older adults is true?
   a. Changes in smell and taste can result in decreased use of sugar.
   b. Older adults need increased calorie intake to maintain ideal body weight.
   c. Loneliness and boredom may impact the older adult's incentive to eat.
   d. Obesity is the most common nutritional problem in nursing homes.

5. What are the direct benefits of exercise? *(Select all that apply.)*
   a. Decreases depression symptoms
   b. Reduces muscle strength
   c. Improves sleep apnea
   d. Increases mobility
   e. Decreases risk of heart disease
   f. Reduces or maintains body weight

6. Which assessment findings in the older adult indicate an increased risk for falls? *(Select all that apply.)*
   a. Increased mobility
   b. Macular degeneration
   c. Postural instability
   d. Full joint range of motion (ROM)
   e. Peripheral neuropathy

7. The nurse is caring for the confused older patient who is at risk for falls. Which interventions should the nurse implement to ensure patient safety? *(Select all that apply.)*
   a. Remind the patient to use ambulatory devices as needed.
   b. Instruct the patient to limit activity as much as possible.
   c. Provide appropriate lighting in the patient's environment.
   d. Make sure the patient's eyeglasses are functional, and routine eye examinations have been performed.
   e. Implement facility-specific fall protocols.

8. The patient requires physical restraints. Which interventions must the nurse perform for this patient? *(Select all that apply.)*
   a. Check the patient every 30-60 minutes.
   b. Release the restraints at least every 4 hours.
   c. Turn on the television to provide distraction.
   d. Place the patient in an area for careful observation.
   e. Decrease communication with the patient.

9. Which type of psychoactive drug requires the most careful monitoring by the nurse because of the drug's potential for causing confusion and incontinence?
   a. Tricyclic antidepressants
   b. Antipsychotics
   c. Antianxiety agents
   d. Sedative-hypnotics

10. Which factors must the nurse acknowledge and include in discharge education for the older adult about medication administration? *(Select all that apply.)*
    a. Suggest a simple type of reminder to take daily medications.
    b. Ensure that medication labels have large print to assist patients with identification.
    c. Request easy-open caps for medication bottles and ensure that they remain out of reach of visiting children.
    d. Instruct patients that use of herbal supplements without consulting the health care provider is acceptable.
    e. Provide a complete list of the patient's regularly taken over-the-counter medications to health care providers.

11. Which physiologic changes must the nurse teach an older adult who is taking medication to be aware of? *(Select all that apply.)*
    a. Oral drugs will be ineffective because of an age-related increase in GI motility.
    b. There may be an alteration in the ratio of adipose tissue to lean body mass, which may affect the distribution of a drug.
    c. Decreased function of the liver may alter the metabolism of certain drugs.
    d. Altered kidney function may affect excretion, causing increased plasma concentrations of drugs.
    e. Most older adults will not have any significant physiologic alterations.

12. Which interventions are effective in helping to reorient the older adult who is suffering from delirium? *(Select all that apply.)*
    a. Talk to the patient using a calm voice.
    b. Restrict visitors during periods of agitation.
    c. Remove personal items and store them safely.
    d. Apply wrist restraints to keep the patient from endangering him- or herself.
    e. Provide calming music.

13. Which symptoms of depression in older adults should be carefully evaluated by the health care provider? *(Select all that apply.)*
    a. Early morning insomnia
    b. Reluctance to participate in social activities
    c. Reminiscing about the past
    d. Normalization of appetite and intake
    e. Excessive daytime sleeping

14. In planning care for the older adult with dementia, the nurse identifies which intervention as the first priority goal of care?
    a. Prevent cognitive decline.
    b. Reorient on a regular basis.
    c. Prevent injury.
    d. Assist with ambulation.

15. Which statements regarding elder abuse are true? *(Select all that apply.)*
    a. The abuser is often a close family member or caregiver.
    b. Only physically dependent older adults are vulnerable to elder abuse.
    c. Elder neglect is categorized as a type of elder abuse.
    d. Elder abuse includes misuse of patients' money or property.
    e. There is a need for mandatory reporting laws for suspected elder abuse.

16. On assessment of a newly admitted older patient, the nurse notes cigarette burns on the lower abdomen. Which term best describes this finding?
    a. Neglect
    b. Physical abuse
    c. Elder abuse
    d. Mistreatment

17. The patient is both confused and agitated. Which action is most important at this time?
    a. Place the patient in a quiet supervised area.
    b. Check the patient every 2 hours.
    c. Sedate the patient using IV medication.
    d. Turn on the television to keep the patient's attention.

18. Which task should the nurse delegate to unlicensed assistive personnel (UAP) when caring for an older adult?
    a. Instruct the patient to drink at least 2 liters of fluids each day.
    b. Assess the patient's skin every 2 hours during repositioning.
    c. Assist the patient with feeding at mealtimes.
    d. Teach the patient to use incentive spirometry every hour while awake.

19. Which factors place the older adult at increased risk for a fall? *(Select all that apply.)*
    a. Age >90 years
    b. Urinary continence
    c. Corrected visual impairment
    d. Postural instability
    e. Impaired communication

20. What are signs indicating that the older adult is experiencing dementia or delirium? *(Select all that apply.)*
    a. Temporary, acute confusion
    b. Progressive loss of cognitive function
    c. Agitation and combative behavior
    d. Complaints of weakness or dizziness
    e. Sudden onset of apathy and withdrawn behavior

3

CHAPTER

Assessment and Care of Patients with Pain

1. The nurse is working at a walk-in clinic and has just interviewed several patients. Which patient represents the most common reason for seeking medical care?
   a. Has a family history of cardiac disease
   b. Has a personal history of chronic pain
   c. Has annual appointment for cancer screening
   d. Has a desire to lose weight and improve health

2. Which factors affect pain and its management? *(Select all that apply.)*
   a. Age
   b. Disease process
   c. Gender
   d. Sociocultural background
   e. Absence of physiologic response
   f. Genetics

3. The patient reports that he has chronic lower back pain that is not relieved by the prescribed medication and that the primary care provider is unwilling to prescribe anything stronger. Who should the nurse consult first?
   a. Pharmacist
   b. Physical therapist
   c. Pain resource nurse
   d. An alternate health care provider

4. Which patient has the highest risk for inadequate pain management?
   a. 56-year-old man who had major abdominal surgery for a stab wound
   b. 78-year-old woman who was transferred to a nursing home after hip surgery
   c. 10-year-old child who had a tonsillectomy and his parents can't speak English
   d. 24-year-old postpartum woman with a history of drug abuse

5. The nurse is taking a health history of a patient who has persistent pain related to interstitial cystitis. How does the nurse categorize this pain?
   a. Acute pain
   b. Chronic pain
   c. Chronic noncancer pain
   d. Somatic pain

6. A patient with chronic leg pain reports pain level at 7/10, so the nurse administers a prn medication. Which observation best suggests that the goal of therapy is being met?
   a. Patient appears relaxed while talking with family members.
   b. Pulse, blood pressure, and respirations are not elevated.
   c. Patient ambulates independently down the hall without distress.
   d. Patient asks for additional food between lunch and dinner.

7. Despite the nurse's best efforts, the patient's wife continuously asks the nurse to reassess her husband's pain and to give him additional medication. What is the best rationale for using the concept of "self-report"?
   a. The wife's behavior indicates that she is overly anxious.
   b. The concerns of the wife make accurate pain assessment very difficult.
   c. The health care provider needs to be contacted for a dosage increase.
   d. The patient is the only one who can describe his experience of pain.

8. Which patient is most likely to report pain that would be considered acute?
   a. Has a history of peripheral vascular disease, foot is suddenly cold and blue
   b. Has a history of diabetic neuropathy, reports burning sensation in lower leg
   c. Has a history of old ankle fracture, reports recent diagnosis of osteoarthritis
   d. Has a history of osteosarcoma in the femur with tumor growth and expansion

9. In assessing pain in an older adult patient, what is a major barrier to accurate assessment?
   a. Many older adults are reluctant to report pain.
   b. Pain perception increases with age.
   c. Pain scales are inaccurate for older adults.
   d. Most older adults have some cognitive impairment.

10. The nurse is caring for a patient on the first postoperative day. The patient denies pain, but his blood pressure and pulse are elevated and he is diaphoretic and anxious. What should the nurse do first?
    a. Believe and document the patient's self-report of "denies pain."
    b. Call the health care provider and report the vital signs, diaphoresis, and anxiety.
    c. Assess the patient for postoperative complications or barriers to reporting pain.
    d. Ask a family member if the patient would typically be stoic during pain or discomfort.

11. A patient reports a deep, poorly localized, cramping type of pain. These assessment findings indicate which type of pain?
    a. Somatic
    b. Psychosomatic
    c. Neuropathic
    d. Visceral

12. The nurse knows that acute pain serves a biologic purpose. How does the nurse apply this knowledge in caring for a patient with a history of cardiac problems, who now reports severe chest pain?
    a. Immediately administers supplemental oxygen
    b. Reassures that acute pain is usually temporary
    c. Assesses for anxiety, restlessness, or apprehension
    d. Obtains an order for prn pain medication

13. A patient with rheumatoid arthritis reports having chronic pain for years with an exacerbation that started in the morning. Which observation indicates the patient has a physiologic adaptation to pain?
    a. Pupils are dilated.
    b. Breathing is shallow.
    c. Pulse rate is 70/min.
    d. Temperature is 98.6° F.

14. The nurse is caring for several patients who will receive pain medication. Which patient is most likely to receive around-the-clock oral opioids?
    a. Patient with fibromyalgia
    b. Patient with chronic cancer pain
    c. Patient with Crohn's disease
    d. Patient who had a stroke

15. A patient reports a constant "achy" type of pain after abdominal surgery. This is an indication of which type of pain?
    a. Somatic
    b. Visceral
    c. Neuropathic
    d. Psychosomatic

16. Nociception involves the normal function of physiologic systems and four processes. When the nurse suggests listening to music as a distraction, which process is the target of the intervention?
    a. Transduction
    b. Transmission
    c. Sensory perception
    d. Modulation

17. Which patient is having pain that is unlikely to respond to first-line analgesics?
    a. 62-year-old woman who fractured her wrist
    b. 70-year-old woman with postherpetic neuralgia
    c. 50-year-old man with a recently inserted chest tube
    d. 45-year-old man who sustained burns to the hands

18. Which behavior exemplifies the nurse's primary role in assessing and managing the patient's pain?
    a. Administers pain medication as ordered if pain is sufficient to warrant therapy.
    b. Listens to the patient's self-report and forms an opinion about the veracity of the description.
    c. Observes for concurrent verbal reports and nonverbal signs to substantiate presence of pain.
    d. Listens to and accepts the self-report of pain and assesses patient's preferences and values.

19. What are physiologic responses that indicate a patient is experiencing pain? *(Select all that apply.)*
    a. Diaphoresis
    b. Restlessness
    c. Bradycardia
    d. Hypotension
    e. Bradypnea

20. What is the best type of pain scale to use for patients who have language barriers or reading problems, or for children?
    a. 0 to 10 numeric rating scale
    b. FACES (smile to frown)
    c. Verbal description scales
    d. Pasero opioid-induced sedation scale

21. The nurse asks the patient, "Sir, where is your pain?" The patient repeatedly responds, "It hurts all over." What is the best rationale for taking the extra time to help the patient to identify specific areas that hurt?
    a. Documentation is incomplete as a legal document if the nurse charts "hurts all over."
    b. Formulating an achievable therapeutic goal is very difficult for a vague complaint.
    c. The health care provider cannot prescribe appropriate medication for relief of generalized pain.
    d. Differentiating between painful and nonpainful areas helps the patient understand the origin.

22. Which therapy is the first-line choice for severe acute pain?
    a. Opioids
    b. Nonsteroidal antiinflammatory drugs (NSAIDs)
    c. Adjuvants
    d. Cutaneous stimulation

23. The nurse is assessing an elderly patient who has "pain all over." Which strategy would the nurse use to help the patient identify which areas of the body are painful?
    a. Start with gentle palpation on the abdomen and chest.
    b. Focus on the hand and fingers of one extremity.
    c. Direct the patient to find one area that does not hurt.
    d. Provide examples and comparisons of severe pain.

24. The nurse monitors for gastric irritation, signs of bleeding, and bruising as side effects of which pain medications? *(Select all that apply.)*
    a. Aspirin (nonopioid analgesic, NSAID)
    b. Acetaminophen (nonopioid analgesic)
    c. Ibuprofen (nonopioid analgesic, NSAID)
    d. Morphine (opioid analgesic)
    e. Demerol (opioid analgesic)

25. The nursing student is using the Wong-Baker FACES pain rating scale to assess the pain of a 4-year-old child. The nurse would intervene if the student performed which action?
    a. Points to the smiling face and tells the child that this face has "no pain"
    b. Tells the child that FACES helps nurses understand how he is feeling.
    c. Points to the tearful face and tells the child that the picture means "worst pain."
    d. Observes the child's facial expression and matches it to a face on the scale.

26. The nurse is assessing the patient for pain or discomfort. Which is the best question to use to elicit the quality of the pain?
    a. "So you are not having any pain or discomfort, right?"
    b. "Would you describe the pain as sharp?"
    c. "Choose two or three words to describe your pain."
    d. "How would you describe your pain?"

27. A patient with chronic bone pain as a result of rheumatoid arthritis may be prescribed which agents? *(Select all that apply.)*
    a. Aspirin
    b. COX-2 inhibitor such as celecoxib (Celebrex)
    c. Opioid such as morphine
    d. Acetaminophen (Tylenol)
    e. NSAID such as ibuprofen (Motrin, Advil)

28. The nurse is assisting a surgical patient with pain management. Which outcome statement best demonstrates that the short-term functional goal is being met 45 minutes after receiving pain medication?
    a. Patient reports that the pain level is 4/10.
    b. Patient ambulates in hallway with physical therapist.
    c. Patient declines a prn anxiolytic medication.
    d. Patient does not demonstrate facial grimacing.

29. The patient reports a vivid childhood memory of having severe pain during and after a dental procedure. The patient confides a reluctance to visit the dentist even for routine cleanings. What should the nurse do?
    a. Refer the patient for psychological counseling before seeking dental care.
    b. Obtain an order for antianxiety medication and suggest relaxation techniques.
    c. Suggest talking to a dentist about current pain management techniques.
    d. Advise patient that past fears should not interfere with good health practices.

30. The nurse is interviewing a patient who frequently comes to the clinic to obtain medication for chronic back pain. The patient states, "I know you guys think I am faking, but I hurt and I am really sick of your attitude." What is the best response?
    a. "Sir, tell me about your pain and how it is affecting your life."
    b. "Sir, you can speak to a pain specialist if you would prefer."
    c. "Sir, I see you are frustrated, but you are unfairly judging me."
    d. "Sir, we are trying our best, let's just continue the interview."

31. Which nursing action indicates that the nurse is performing the first step of McCaffery and Pasero's Hierarchy of Pain Measures?
    a. Premedicates before a dressing change
    b. Uses a standard pain assessment tool
    c. Compares vital signs before and after pain medication
    d. Starts with a low dose and observes for behavioral changes

32. Which are advantages of the patient-controlled analgesia (PCA) method of medication administration? *(Select all that apply.)*
    a. It allows for a predetermined bolus.
    b. It maintains a constant level of pain relief.
    c. It diminishes patient anxiety by allowing the patient control over administration.
    d. It eliminates the need for repeated injections.
    e. The patient needs no education for effectiveness.

33. The nurse is assessing a patient with severe dementia who resides in a long-term care facility. A score of 8 is obtained by using the Pain Assessment in Advanced Dementia Scale. Based on assessment findings, which action will the nurse take?
    a. Speak calmly to the patient and explain that repositioning will make him more comfortable.
    b. Gently reassure the patient and continue routine observation for discomfort or pain.
    c. Assess the patient for the source of the pain and immediately inform the health care provider.
    d. Contact the family and ask how the patient would typically respond to discomfort.

34. The home health nurse is visiting a 73-year-old diabetic patient who was recently discharged after surgery. While reviewing a list of the patient's medications, the nurse sees that there are several different classes of analgesics listed. Which action is the nurse most likely to take?
    a. Assesses patient's understanding of the multimodal treatment plan and ability to comply
    b. Contacts the health care provider to discontinue medications that contribute to polypharmacy
    c. Emphasizes that medications with more side effects are the last choice for pain
    d. Advises the patient not to take any NSAIDs because of irritation of gastric mucosa

35. Which drugs can cause adverse effects, particularly in an older adult, because of an accumulation of toxic metabolites? *(Select all that apply.)*
    a. Ibuprofen (Advil, Motrin)
    b. Morphine
    c. Meperidine (Demerol)
    d. Acetaminophen (Tylenol)
    e. Codeine

36. The nurse is giving discharge instructions about multimodal analgesia to a daughter who will care for her elderly father at home while he recovers from surgery. The daughter suggests that the single best medication should be recommended for convenience and to save money. What is the best response?
    a. "The doctor always prescribes this combination of medications as the best therapy."
    b. "Elderly people frequently do better with fewer medications; let me call the doctor."
    c. "Just see how it goes for your dad. It is likely that you can gradually decrease the medication."
    d. "Combining different analgesics gives greater relief with lower doses and fewer side effects."

37. For early postoperative pain or pain that is severe and escalating, what is the preferred route?
    a. Oral
    b. Intravenous
    c. Intranasal
    d. Subcutaneous

38. The postanesthesia care unit reports to the nurse in the medical-surgical unit that the patient received 2 mg of intravenous morphine with relief. When is the patient likely to be transitioned to oral analgesics?
    a. Upon arrival to the medical-surgical unit
    b. When the health care provider writes postoperative orders
    c. When the patient is able to tolerate oral intake
    d. When the intravenous access is discontinued

39. A patient is prescribed morphine sulfate, an opioid analgesic, for pain. Which nursing interventions decrease the risk of constipation? *(Select all that apply.)*
    a. Give foods low in bulk and roughage.
    b. Instruct the patient to increase water consumption.
    c. Administer a stool softener every morning.
    d. Change the dose of the opioid.
    e. Encourage activity.

40. A new inexperienced nurse sees that the patient is receiving around-the-clock medication, but also has orders for prn analgesic every 4-6 hours as needed. How will the new nurse determine when a prn dose is given?
    a. Administer a dose every 6 hours to ensure adequate relief.
    b. Call the health care provider and ask for specific parameters for prn dosing.
    c. Look at the medication administration record to see what the previous nurse gave.
    d. Assess the patient for breakthrough pain and anticipate painful procedures.

41. Which statements are true regarding the side effects of respiratory depression as a result of administering an opioid analgesic? *(Select all that apply.)*
    a. Respiratory depression develops when opioid tolerance occurs.
    b. Respiratory depression is less of a problem in the older adult.
    c. The drug used to reverse respiratory depression is naloxone (Narcan).
    d. A one-time dose of naloxone (Narcan) is all that is needed to reverse the effects of the opioid.
    e. Sedation will occur before opioid-induced respiratory depression.

42. Which patient is least likely to be a good candidate for PCA?
    a. 32-year-old male with severe burns and a history of drug abuse
    b. 16-year-old male with multiple injuries sustained during an accident
    c. 34-year-old female with functional blindness who had abdominal surgery
    d. 25-year-old female with intermittent lucidity after a severe head injury

43. The nurse is assessing a patient who is receiving pain medication via a PCA device. The patient is very drowsy and difficult to arouse. What should the nurse do first?
    a. Wake the patient and tell him to stop pushing the button so frequently.
    b. Stay with the patient and discontinue the basal rate.
    c. Let the patient sleep, but increase the frequency of assessment.
    d. Obtain an order for exclusive use of non-opioid medication.

44. What is the drug category of choice for the treatment of mild to moderate bone pain?
    a. NSAIDs
    b. Opioids
    c. Anticonvulsants
    d. Antianxiety agents

45. The nurse is caring for a patient who has an epidural catheter for pain management. Which information is appropriate in the care of this patient?
    a. Pain assessments are performed less frequently if epidural catheters are used for pain management.
    b. Morphine and hydromorphone (Dilaudid) may be used, with a local anesthetic such as bupivacaine.
    c. Epidural catheters are used exclusively to deliver single bolus doses during surgical procedures.
    d. The patient will be confined to bed during the therapy because of lower extremity weakness.

46. The patient has a history of rheumatoid arthritis and is also being treated for acute pain from a hip fracture. Which medication is likely to be prescribed to reduce the pain and discomfort caused by inflammation?
    a. Morphine (MS Contin)
    b. Acetaminophen (Tylenol)
    c. Ibuprofen (Motrin)
    d. Bupivacaine (Marcaine)

47. The nurse is reviewing the patient's medication list and sees that acetaminophen (Tylenol) and celecoxib (Celebrex) are scheduled to be administered at the same time. What should the nurse do?
    a. Call the health care provider for an order to stagger the administration of these two pain medications.
    b. Ask the patient which one he prefers to take; administer the preferred drug and assess for relief.
    c. Give the acetaminophen (Tylenol) because it is less likely to cause gastric irritation and bleeding.
    d. Administer the medications as ordered, because they can be given together without ill effects.

48. Acetaminophen (Tylenol) is the first-line medication for which patient?
    a. Needs relief from pain related to osteoarthritis
    b. Has chronic pain and discomfort due to rheumatoid arthritis
    c. Experiences burning and tingling in legs due to diabetes
    d. Has intermittent abdominal cramping due to Crohn's disease

49. Which nonpharmacologic therapies stimulate the skin and subcutaneous tissues to produce pain relief? *(Select all that apply.)*
    a. Massage
    b. Imagery
    c. Vibration
    d. Heat application
    e. Therapeutic touch

50. A patient using a transcutaneous electrical nerve stimulation (TENS) unit asks the nurse how it works to decrease pain. What is the best response?
    a. "It delivers an electric shock to relieve muscle tension."
    b. "Low-voltage electrical currents are delivered to the painful area."
    c. "Endorphins are blocked, which inhibits pain transmission."
    d. "The nerves causing pain will swell, raising the pain threshold."

51. Which statement about the strategy of distraction is true?
    a. Distraction is most effective for acute pain relief.
    b. Distraction directly influences the cause of pain.
    c. Distraction is tried when medication is ineffective.
    d. Distraction alters the perception of pain.

52. The nurse is teaching a patient about acupuncture as an alternative therapy for pain relief. Which statement by the patient indicates the nurse's teaching was effective?
    a. "Acupuncture is used for pain control and anesthetic purposes."
    b. "Acupuncture is commonly used to relieve pain and inflammation."
    c. "A local anesthetic is injected which decreases pain perception."
    d. "Needles are inserted into the body to temporarily deaden the nerve."

53. The nurse is reviewing the medication list for a patient who had open heart surgery. The nurse is likely to query the prescription for which medication, because prostaglandin inhibition is associated with adverse cardiovascular effects?
    a. Duloxetine (Cymbalta)
    b. Acetaminophen (Tylenol)
    c. Naproxen (Naprosyn)
    d. Morphine (MS Contin)

54. The patient reports that he has been taking hydrocodone (Vicodin) as prescribed by his provider and uses over-the-counter acetaminophen (Tylenol) whenever he needs additional pain relief. Which laboratory test indicates that the patient is having adverse effects because of the additive effects of these two medications?
    a. Decreased clotting times
    b. Decreased hematocrit
    c. Elevated white blood cell count
    d. Elevated liver enzymes

55. The patient with chronic cancer pain has been taking oral morphine for several months. The health care provider suggests a very low dose of nalbuphine (Nubain) for relief of opioid induced pruritus. The nurse recognizes that frequent assessment is required for:
    a. higher risk for respiratory depression.
    b. severe pain or withdrawal symptoms.
    c. hemodynamic adverse effects.
    d. bleeding and increased clotting time.

56. A patient develops a physical dependence after taking an opioid as prescribed for postsurgical pain. What is the recommended approach for dealing with the dependence?
    a. Immediate discontinuation of the opioid
    b. Administering an antagonist, such as naloxone (Narcan)
    c. Gradual reduction of the opioid as pain decreases
    d. Referral to a substance specialist for treatment

57. In applying the concept of titration, which route is likely to have the shortest intervals between the increases in dosage?
    a. Transdermal
    b. Oral
    c. Intravenous
    d. Intramuscular

58. A patient with chronic cancer pain has been taking opioids for several months and now reports needing increasing doses to achieve pain relief. What is the most likely rationale that explains the need for increasing amounts of medication for this patient?
    a. Patient is addicted to opioids.
    b. Disease is progressing.
    c. A different opioid is needed.
    d. Patient has developed a tolerance for opioids.

59. A modified-release opioid is ordered for a patient who is currently NPO (nothing by mouth) and receiving nutrition and fluids through a small-bore nasogastric (NG) tube. What should the nurse do?
    a. Crush the medication and mix it with water to instill through the NG tube.
    b. Contact the health care provider for an order to administer the medication rectally.
    c. Have the patient swallow the medication with a very small amount of water.
    d. Hold the medication and document that the patient is NPO for foods and fluids.

60. Which assessment would the nurse perform to determine if a patient would be an appropriate candidate for using imagery as a distraction therapy?
    a. Determine if touch and physical proximity are culturally acceptable.
    b. Ensure that the patient can speak, read, and write English.
    c. Assess environmental factors that contribute to discomfort or annoyance.
    d. Confirm that the patient can follow a logical and sustained conversation.

4 CHAPTER

Genetic and Genomic Concepts for Medical-Surgical Nursing

1. What are autosomes?
   a. The chromosomes not involved in gender determination
   b. The organized arrangement of chromosomes in one cell
   c. The proteins needed to generate chromosome pairs
   d. Structures composed of two Xs as the sex chromosomes

2. Which statement best reflects the correct actions of the health care professional who is providing genetic counseling?
   a. "This test will tell us everything about you!"
   b. "We are going to perform this testing because you asked for it and it won't affect your family in any way."
   c. "The results of this genetic testing will be sent to your health insurance carrier immediately."
   d. "I'm here to provide information so that you can make an informed decision about genetic testing."

3. When assessing for genetic risks, which factors indicate that a patient may have an increased genetic risk for a disease or disorder? (Select all that apply.)
   a. A close family member has an identified genetic problem.
   b. A patient tells you that he was exposed to a carcinogenic substance during a war.
   c. A patient has been diagnosed with two different types of cancer.
   d. A patient's sister had breast cancer at age 24.
   e. A patient's father was diagnosed with rheumatic fever at 10 years of age.

4. Which disorders have a genetic pattern of inheritance? (Select all that apply.)
   a. Malignant hyperthermia
   b. Gallstones
   c. Cystic fibrosis
   d. Acute lymphocytic leukemia
   e. Polycystic kidney disease
   f. Sickle cell disease

5. What is the smallest functional unit of deoxyribonucleic acid (DNA)?
   a. Chromosome
   b. Allele
   c. Nucleotide
   d. Gene

6. A newborn infant inherits a blood type A allele from his mother and a blood type B allele from his father. What type of blood will the infant have?
   a. Type A
   b. Type B
   c. Type AB
   d. Type O

7. A child has two identical alleles for pointed ears. Which term best describes the child's likelihood of developing pointed ears?
   a. The child is homozygous and will develop pointed ears.
   b. The child is heterozygous and may develop pointed ears.
   c. The child has dominant alleles and will develop pointed ears.
   d. The child has codominant alleles and may develop pointed ears.

8. A person's hair is curly. Which statement is true about this person's alleles for hair type?
   a. The person must have two identical alleles for curly hair.
   b. The person may have one allele for curly hair and one allele for straight hair.
   c. The person's parents must both have the phenotype of curly hair.
   d. The person must have two recessive alleles for curly hair.

9. A person's genetic sequencing for a specific protein has a variation or mutation. Which statements express what may happen to that person? *(Select all that apply.)*
   a. Function of the protein may be reduced.
   b. Function of the protein may be the same.
   c. Function of the protein may be eliminated.
   d. Function of the protein may be enhanced.
   e. Function of the protein may be completely different.

10. The patient is of Chinese heritage. Which heritage-based precaution is essential when the health care provider prescribes warfarin (Coumadin) for this patient?
    a. Teach the patient to use a soft-bristled toothbrush.
    b. Assess the patient for signs of abnormal bleeding every shift.
    c. Instruct the unlicensed assistive personnel (UAP) to avoid the use of a regular razor during morning care.
    d. Monitor the patient's INR (International Normalized Ratio) more frequently.

11. Which criteria are used to determine if inheritance is autosomal-dominant (AD)? *(Select all that apply.)*
    a. The trait appears in every other generation.
    b. The risk for the affected person to pass the trait to a child is 50% with each pregnancy.
    c. Unaffected people do not have affected children.
    d. The trait is found equally in males and females.
    e. For the trait to be expressed, both alleles must be dominant.

12. The patient has the gene for Huntington disease (HD). What is her risk for developing this disease?
    a. The HD gene has low penetrance and the patient is unlikely to develop the disease.
    b. The patient must have two genes for HD for the disease to develop.
    c. The HD gene is autosomal-dominant; patient has a moderate risk for developing the disease.
    d. The HD gene has high penetrance and the patient's risk is almost 100%.

13. Which statement about autosomal-recessive patterns of inheritance is accurate?
    a. The trait appears in every generation.
    b. The children of two affected parents will always be affected.
    c. About 50% of a family will be affected by the trait.
    d. The trait is found more commonly in female than male family members.

14. Which statement about a sex-linked recessive pattern of inheritance is accurate?
    a. The trait cannot be passed down from mother to son.
    b. The incidence is much higher in females than males in a family.
    c. Female carriers have a 50% risk with each pregnancy of passing the gene to their children.
    d. Transmission of the trait is from mother to all daughters who will become carriers.

15. Which feature is "key" when a genetics counselor is providing a patient with genetics counseling?
    a. The counseling should be nondirective.
    b. The counselor provides information and advice to the patient.
    c. The counseling should be provided by an advanced-practice nurse.
    d. The counselor discusses risks, benefits, and suggestions for early diagnosis.

16. The patient desires genetic testing for the HD gene but does not want other members of his family to know the results. Which ethical issue would be violated if the patient's family was informed of these results?
    a. The right to know versus the right not to know
    b. Confidentiality
    c. Coercion
    d. Privacy

17. What is the role of the medical-surgical nurse in genetic testing? *(Select all that apply.)*
    a. Ensure that the patient's rights are respected.
    b. Provide complete information on the results of the testing.
    c. Refer the patient to a genetic counseling expert.
    d. Teach patients about the nature of genetics testing.
    e. Always be present when the patient receives genetics counseling.

18. For a patient with a genetic predisposition to develop type 2 diabetes mellitus, which factor increases the risk that the patient will be diagnosed with this disease?
    a. Patient lives sedentary lifestyle
    b. Grandfather with type 1 diabetes
    c. Mother with coronary artery disease
    d. Patient consumes high-fat diet

5 CHAPTER

Evidence-Based Practice in Medical-Surgical Nursing

1. Based on its definition, which example best exemplifies evidence-based practice (EBP)?
   a. Developing a plan of care for recognition of decubitus ulcers.
   b. Teaching a new orienting nurse to provide patients with information prior to procedures.
   c. Making a research-based change in the practice of fall prevention on a patient care unit.
   d. Providing guidance for delegated patient care tasks to be completed by unlicensed assistive personnel (UAP).

2. Which components are included in the process of EBP? *(Select all that apply.)*
   a. Evaluating outcomes
   b. Finding the best evidence to answer a clinical question
   c. Critically appraising and synthesizing the relevant evidence
   d. Developing recommendations to improve current practice
   e. Conducting quantitative research

3. On which levels do most clinically based "burning questions" need to be answered? *(Select all that apply.)*
   a. The individual patient level
   b. A small group of patients
   c. The level of the patient care unit
   d. An ecosystem level
   e. The organizational level

4. Which is the best example of a foreground question related to a clinical problem?
   a. What are the most frequently used analgesics for postoperative pain?
   b. What is the etiology of postoperative pain?
   c. What is the relationship between alternative therapies and relief of postoperative pain?
   d. What are pain theories that explain why postoperative pain occurs?

5. Which term best describes the research question: What is the experience of surviving breast cancer for middle-aged women?
   a. Quantitative
   b. Qualitative
   c. Mixed method
   d. Measurable phenomenon

6. Based on the PICO(T) format for clinically focused research questions, which portion of this question refers to the intervention element: Would "Cover your cold" signs in a cold prevention program decrease the number of colds for elementary school children more than for institutionalized adults during winter months?
   a. Elementary school children
   b. Institutionalized adults
   c. "Cover your cold" signs
   d. Decrease the number of colds

7. Which factors have been identified as barriers for nurses to participate in EBP? *(Select all that apply.)*
   a. Limited timeframe to participate
   b. Difficulty in accessing research materials
   c. Lack of adequate research methods
   d. Difficulty understanding research articles
   e. Lack of value for research in practice

8. The nurse is interested in discovering evidence-based assessment tools for determining if a patient is experiencing depression. Which database will best provide this information?
    a. Cochrane Library of Systematic Reviews
    b. Medline
    c. PsychINFO
    d. Cumulative Index to Nursing and Allied Health Literature

9. How does the Reavy and Tavernier Model of implementing EBP in the clinical setting see the role of the nurse researcher? *(Select all that apply.)*
    a. A role model
    b. Support in identifying areas for improvement
    c. An extra pair of hands for patient care
    d. A clinical expert ready with all of the answers
    e. An aid with literature review

6 CHAPTER

Rehabilitation Concepts for Chronic and Disabling Health Problems

1. Which problem is the leading cause of trauma and death in young and middle-aged adults?
   a. Stroke
   b. Cancer
   c. Arthritis
   d. Accidents

2. As a result of a car accident, an adult patient is unable to perform certain activities of daily living (ADLs), such as bathing, without assistance. This is an example of which concept listed below?
   a. Rehabilitation health problem
   b. Chronic health problem
   c. Disability health problem
   d. Accidental health problem

3. The rehabilitation (rehab) patient wears street clothes and makes decisions about how her day will be planned. Which type of rehab setting is this patient in? *(Select all that apply.)*
   a. Inpatient rehab center
   b. Short-term rehab
   c. Skilled nursing facility
   d. Acute care
   e. Long-term care facility

4. The patient needs help with self-feeding, bathing, and dressing himself. Which rehabilitation team member would best help him develop these skills?
   a. Physical therapist
   b. Rehabilitation nurse
   c. Rehabilitation case manager
   d. Occupational therapist

5. What best describes the primary goal of the rehabilitation team?
   a. To rely on a specific plan of care standardized to the medical diagnosis
   b. To identify and use one conceptual framework to serve as the sole model for the practice of rehabilitation nursing
   c. To restore and maintain the patient's function to the best extent possible
   d. To enable patients and their families to identify strategies to successfully meet short-term goals

6. What are the nurse's responsibilities regarding the skin care assessment of a rehabilitation patient? *(Select all that apply.)*
   a. Identification of actual or potential interruptions of skin integrity
   b. Keeping track of patient urination patterns and bowel movements
   c. Assessment of the skin for all patients under the nurse's care
   d. Education of the patient in how to inspect his or her own skin
   e. Thorough documentation of the integrity of the skin

7. Which factors does the nurse assess when implementing a position change schedule for an older adult? *(Select all that apply.)*
   a. Ability of the patient to change positions
   b. Condition of the patient's skin with each position change
   c. Presence of abnormal breath sounds
   d. Type of injury the patient sustained
   e. Age of the patient

8. Which priority gastrointestinal problem should the nurse plan to prevent with a rehab patient?
   a. Constipation
   b. Diarrhea
   c. Emaciation
   d. Electrolyte imbalance

9. A patient with decreased cardiac output is entering a rehabilitation program. What will the nurse expect to find during the assessment of this patient?
   a. Shortness of breath on activity
   b. Ability to ambulate without angina
   c. Feeling rested upon awakening from sleep
   d. Ability to move from sitting to standing position easily

10. A patient with musculoskeletal disability is entering a rehabilitation program. What does the nurse focus on first in assessing this patient?
    a. Family and cultural background
    b. Baseline hemoglobin and hematocrit measurements
    c. Habits of bowel elimination before illness
    d. Muscle strength, range of motion, and mobility

11. A patient with a neurogenic bladder is to be taught how to perform intermittent self-catheterization. Before beginning the teaching-learning sessions, what will the nurse assess in this patient first?
    a. Motor function of both upper extremities
    b. Type of neurogenic bladder the patient has
    c. Patient's gender
    d. Age of the patient

12. To maintain skin integrity of a patient in a rehabilitation unit, what does the nurse assess? *(Select all that apply.)*
    a. Sensation of the skin
    b. Placement of clear dressings over reddened areas
    c. Ability to move extremities
    d. Nutritional status
    e. Ability to change position as needed

13. Which statements correctly describe the Functional Independence Measure (FIM)? *(Select all that apply.)*
    a. It is a basic indicator of the severity of a disability.
    b. It tries to measure what a person should do, whatever the diagnosis or impairment.
    c. It tries to measure what a person actually does, whatever the diagnosis or impairment.
    d. The assessment may be performed by various health care disciplines.
    e. Categories for assessment are self-care, sphincter control, mobility and locomotion, communication, and cognition.
    f. Evaluations may be done at specified times during therapy to determine patient progress.

14. Which of the following are activities of daily living? *(Select all that apply.)*
    a. Bathing
    b. Using a telephone
    c. Dressing
    d. Ambulating
    e. Preparing food

15. What best describes the purpose of a vocational assessment for a patient in rehabilitation?
    a. Assist the patient to find meaningful training, education, or employment after discharge from a rehabilitation setting.
    b. Evaluate and retrain patients with deficits that distort consonant and vowel sound production.
    c. Identify resources to assist with patient injuries that cause deficits in cognition.
    d. Demonstrate improvements in physical, social, cognitive, and emotional functions.

16. The nurse reviews with a patient the results of manual muscle testing performed by physical therapy. What ability of the patient does this procedure determine?
    a. Body flexibility and muscle strength
    b. Range of motion and resistance against gravity
    c. Muscle strength and amount of pain on movement
    d. Voluntary versus involuntary muscle movement

17. While performing a psychosocial assessment on an older adult who is a newly admitted rehab patient, the nurse discovers that her only support system is a married son who lives 2500 miles away. Which priority complication must the nurse monitor for?
    a. Anxiety
    b. Fear
    c. Depression
    d. Panic

18. When assisting a patient with a cane to transfer or ambulate, what does the nurse instruct the patient to do?
    a. Lean the body weight backward.
    b. Use the weaker hand to assist.
    c. Lean the body weight toward the nurse.
    d. Use the strong hand to assist.

19. The nurse's facility follows a no-lift policy to prevent musculoskeletal injury to staff. Which methods for patient transfer can the nurse use? *(Select all that apply.)*
    a. Independent movement of the patient when he or she is able
    b. Mechanical full-body lift
    c. Following facility guidelines for safe patient transfer
    d. No transfers for patients who are unable to move independently
    e. Multiple staff assistance

20. A patient with impaired physical mobility must be monitored for which early potential complication?
    a. Pressure ulcers
    b. Renal calculi
    c. Osteoporosis
    d. Fractures

21. Which methods to prevent pressure ulcers resulting from immobility are best to teach patients and their significant others? *(Select all that apply.)*
    a. Change position often to relieve pressure on all bony prominences.
    b. Maintain good skin care by keeping the skin clean and dry.
    c. Inspect the skin at least once a day for problems such as reddened areas that do not fade readily.
    d. Use pressure-relieving devices as a substitute for changing position.
    e. Eat foods high in protein, carbohydrates, and vitamins for sufficient nutrition.

22. Which assistive-adaptive device would be recommended for a patient with a weak hand grasp?
    a. Gel pad
    b. Long-handled reacher
    c. Hook and loop fastener straps
    d. Buttonhook

23. When teaching a patient with hemiplegia about energy conservation techniques, which method does the nurse include?
    a. Using a walker instead of a cane
    b. Scheduling physical therapy immediately before eating
    c. Using a bedside commode
    d. Scheduling recreational activities in the afternoon or evening

24. Which statement is true about the use of mechanical pressure-relieving devices?
    a. They effectively eliminate the need to turn patients.
    b. Patients still require regular repositioning.
    c. They prevent pressure ulcers in debilitated patients.
    d. They have been shown to be ineffective in preventing pressure ulcers.

25. A patient has a lower motor neuron injury below T12. This injury results in which type of neurogenic bladder?
    a. Reflex or spastic
    b. Flaccid
    c. Uninhibited
    d. Inhibited

26. A patient with a flaccid bladder will have which urinary elimination problem?
    a. Incontinence and inability to empty the bladder completely
    b. Incontinence caused by inability to wait until on a commode or bedpan
    c. Urinary retention and dribbling because of overflow of urine
    d. Incontinence due to loss of sensation

27. Which statements are correct principles for performing an intermittent catheterization? *(Select all that apply.)*
    a. A catheter is inserted every few hours.
    b. It is usually performed after the Valsalva or Credé maneuver.
    c. A residual of less than 100-150 mL increases the interval between catheterization.
    d. The maximum time interval between catheterizations is 4 hours.
    e. The patient uses sterile technique at home.

28. Which medication would a patient with a mild overactive bladder most likely be given?
    a. Dantrolene sodium (Dantrium)
    b. Bethanechol chloride (Urecholine)
    c. Tolterodine (Detrol LA)
    d. Trimethoprim (Trimpex)

29. Which patient is most likely to have a flaccid bladder dysfunction?
    a. 28-year-old man with a crushed pelvis
    b. 54-year-old man with Guillain-Barré syndrome
    c. 18-year-old woman with a displaced cervical fracture
    d. 48-year-old woman who has multiple sclerosis

30. In which patients with constipation does the nurse avoid performing digital stimulation? *(Select all that apply.)*
    a. Patient with myocardial infarction who is starting cardiac rehabilitation
    b. Patient with chronic diarrhea resulting from radiation to the bowel
    c. Patient with bowel incontinence resulting from cognition deficit
    d. Patient with a spinal cord injury resulting from a diving accident
    e. Patient with a spinal cord injury resulting from a motor vehicle accident

31. Lower motor neuron disease or injury results in which bowel dysfunction?
    a. Flaccid bowel pattern
    b. Reflex (spastic) bowel pattern
    c. Uninhibited bowel pattern
    d. Inhibited bowel pattern

32. The older rehab patient also has a diagnosis of hypertension for which he is prescribed antihypertensive drugs. Before assisting this patient to rise from bed, which priority assessment should be completed by the nurse?
    a. Blood pressure in both arms
    b. Gait assessment
    c. Orthostatic vital signs
    d. Chest pain with activity

33. The unlicensed assistive personnel (UAP) is assisting a rehab patient with ADLs in the morning. What is the priority instruction the nurse should give the UAP?
    a. Encourage the patient to do as much self-care as possible.
    b. Bathe the patient but let him dress and feed himself.
    c. Let the patient inform you about the help he needs.
    d. Stress to the patient that his ADLs need to be completed as soon as possible.

34. In the long-term care setting, which are foci for the coordinated efforts of restorative nursing programs? *(Select all that apply.)*
    a. Dressing
    b. Passive range of motion
    c. Communication
    d. Nutrition
    e. Walking

35. What is the priority intervention for prevention of skin breakdown in bedfast patients?
    a. Place the patient on an air mattress.
    b. Use a draw sheet when moving the patient.
    c. Turn and reposition the patient every 2 hours.
    d. Massage all bony prominences at least once every shift.

36. Which description characterizes uninhibited bowel pattern dysfunction?
    a. Defecation occurring suddenly and without warning.
    b. Defecation occurring infrequently and in small amounts.
    c. Frequent defecation, urgency, and complaints of hard stool.
    d. Intermittent constipation and diarrhea.

7 CHAPTER

End-of-Life Care

1. Which are direct causes of death? *(Select all that apply.)*
   a. GI bleeding
   b. Heart failure
   c. Respiratory failure
   d. Shock
   e. Kidney failure

2. The terminally ill patient has an advance directive living will, which states that she does not want heroic measures such as cardiopulmonary resuscitation (CPR) and intubation. She also has a do not resuscitate order in her chart written by the provider. As the patient nears death, her daughter tells the hospice nurse that she wants everything possible done to save her mother's life. What is the nurse's best action?
   a. Call a code and bring the crash cart to the patient's bedside.
   b. Inform the health care provider of this change in the plan of care.
   c. Respect the patient's wishes and ask the chaplain to stay with the daughter.
   d. Inform the daughter that further interventions are futile.

3. Which statement regarding the approach to hospice/end-of-life care is correct?
   a. Hospice programs only include provision of care in the home.
   b. Admission to hospice is involuntary and directed by a health care provider's order.
   c. The focus is on facilitating quality of life just for the dying patient.
   d. An interdisciplinary team approach is used for the care of the patient and family.

4. A patient receiving nursing care in a home hospice program can expect which kind of care?
   a. The use of high-technology equipment such as ventilators until time of death.
   b. Around-the-clock skilled direct nursing patient care until time of death.
   c. Pain and symptom management that will achieve the best quality of life.
   d. Complete relief of only distressing physical symptoms.

5. To qualify for hospice benefits, a criterion for admission is that the patient's prognosis must be limited to what amount of time?
   a. 2 weeks or less
   b. 3 months or less
   c. 6 months or less
   d. 1 year or less

6. Which items are relevant to the concept of hospice? *(Select all that apply.)*
   a. Unit of care is the patient and family.
   b. Preferred location is the hospital setting.
   c. Interdisciplinary team approach is used.
   d. Focus is on alleviating pain and suffering.
   e. Hospice care does not hasten death.

7. Which characteristics apply to the concept of palliative care? *(Select all that apply.)*
   a. Patient must have less than a year to live.
   b. Care time is not limited to specific periods of time.
   c. Care focus is curative or may prolong life.
   d. Care is provided when curative treatments have been stopped.
   e. Patient can be in any stage of serious illness.

8. Which statements about the assessment of a terminally ill patient are true? *(Select all that apply.)*
   a. Assess only the patient; do not include the family's perception of the patient's symptoms.
   b. When the patient is unable to communicate, there is no need to assess symptoms of distress any longer.
   c. Assess patients who are unable to communicate distress by observing for objective signs of discomfort.
   d. Assess the patient for dyspnea, agitation, nausea, and vomiting only.
   e. Identify alternative methods to assess for symptoms of distress.
   f. The family can help identify patient habits and preferences, which may aid in the overall assessment.

9. Which symptom is most distressing and feared by terminally ill patients?
   a. Difficulty breathing
   b. Confusion
   c. Pain
   d. Loss of consciousness

10. The terminally ill patient is nearing death. His wife expresses concern that he has no appetite and eats very little. What is the nurse's best response to this concern?
    a. Teach the patient's wife about the risk of aspiration and explain that loss of appetite is normal when a patient nears death.
    b. Encourage the patient's wife to feed the patient as much as he will take to maintain adequate nutrition.
    c. Request that the health care provider order a dietary nutrition consult to include foods that the patient prefers.
    d. Keep fluids and finger foods at the bedside for easy access whenever the patient is hungry or thirsty.

11. The terminally ill patient who is near death has loud, wet respirations that are disturbing to the family. Which interventions by the nurse are appropriate at this time? *(Select all that apply.)*
    a. Position the patient on her side.
    b. Place a small towel under her mouth.
    c. Use oropharyngeal suctioning to remove the secretions.
    d. Administer an ordered anticholinergic drug to dry up the secretions.
    e. Teach family members how to use the suctioning device whenever needed.

12. Which intervention should be done when performing postmortem care?
    a. Place the head of the bed at 30 degrees.
    b. Remove pillows from under the head.
    c. Leave a Foley (indwelling) catheter in place in the bladder.
    d. Place pads under the hips and around the perineum.

13. Which interventions after a patient's death are appropriate to perform? *(Select all that apply.)*
    a. Remove the body to the morgue or funeral home immediately after death.
    b. Follow agency policies to remove all tubes and lines from the body.
    c. Make sure that the physician has completed and signed the death certificate.
    d. Provide privacy for the family and significant others with the deceased.
    e. Allow family and/or significant other to perform religious and cultural customs.

14. A hospice patient is deteriorating and the family is concerned about his restlessness and agitation. Which intervention is the nurse prepared to perform?
    a. Notify the primary health care provider and request orders for transfer to the hospital.
    b. Determine if the patient is in pain, provide analgesics, and make the patient as comfortable as possible.
    c. Initiate IV hydration to provide the patient with necessary fluids.
    d. Encourage the family to assist the patient to eat in order to gain energy.

15. The most common treatment of pain in a terminally ill patient is administration of which kind of therapy?
    a. Opioids
    b. Steroids
    c. Nonsteroidal antiinflammatory agents
    d. Radiation treatments

16. Which phrase correctly describes palliative care?
    a. Care for patients with a prognosis of 6 months or less
    b. Diagnoses and treatment for patients with a life-threatening illness
    c. Patient care with a focus on treatment of symptoms
    d. Patient education about relevant treatment alternatives

17. While caring for a patient of the orthodox Jewish faith who is dying, what cultural concept should the nurse keep in mind?
    a. Traditionally, Jewish cultures are male-dominated.
    b. Expression of grief is open, especially among women.
    c. An autopsy after death will not be permitted.
    d. Family members are likely to avoid visiting the terminally ill family member.

18. Which statements about pain management in a patient who is dying are true? *(Select all that apply.)*
    a. The patient's pain may come from many areas.
    b. Patients who are dying should discontinue long-acting opioids.
    c. Alternative therapies have been shown to be useful when integrated into a pain management plan of care.
    d. When using massage for patients with cancer, deep pressure is the preferred method.
    e. Aromatherapy, massage, music therapy, and therapeutic touch are a few alternative therapies that have been shown to be useful.

19. Which statements about caring for a patient with dyspnea are true? *(Select all that apply.)*
    a. Pharmacologic interventions should begin early in the course of dyspnea.
    b. Nonpharmacologic, alternative treatments may be used successfully in place of pharmacologic interventions.
    c. Dyspnea may be caused by the primary diagnosis or its treatments.
    d. Diagnostic testing must be used to determine the cause of dyspnea before beginning treatment.
    e. Oropharyngeal suctioning is appropriate for patients with loud, wet respirations nearing death.

20. Which action is an example of active euthanasia for a dying patient?
    a. Removal of a patient from a mechanical ventilator
    b. Discontinuing intravenous fluids
    c. Withdrawal of telemetry heart monitoring
    d. Administering a large dose of intravenous morphine

21. Which end-of-life interventions must the nurse be prepared to perform for a dying patient and his or her family? *(Select all that apply.)*
    a. Allow the family to verbalize fears and concerns about the impending loss of their loved one.
    b. Listen and acknowledge the legitimacy of the family's pain.
    c. Minimize the family's loss by using statements such as "Don't be upset."
    d. Assist the patient and family with reminiscence or storytelling.
    e. Work to determine the patient's and family's spiritual needs.

Concepts of Emergency Care and Trauma Nursing

1. Which emergency department (ED) patient represents an issue that has been addressed by the Core Measure Sets for the ED that are established by the Joint Commission?
   a. Patient has no health insurance and no steady source of income.
   b. Patient has waited 7 hours to be transferred to the medical-surgical unit.
   c. Patient has a history of falls and sustains a fall in the ED waiting room.
   d. Patient has respiratory arrest and requires emergency intubation.

2. The ED nurse is preparing a report on a patient being admitted for bacterial meningitis. Which points are included in the ED nurse's report to the medical-surgical nurse? *(Select all that apply.)*
   a. "Patient reports severe headache with high fever that started 4 days ago."
   b. "Patient currently alert and oriented x 2; speech clear, but rambling."
   c. "Patient is divorced and currently does not have any health insurance."
   d. "IV normal saline into left anterior forearm; received first dose of IV ceftriaxone (Rocephin) at 0700."
   e. "Lumbar puncture results are pending, but meningococcal meningitis is suspected."
   f. "Received 1000 mg acetaminophen (Tylenol) (for pain (9/10) and fever 103° F at 0400; pain continues (7/10), temperature now 100.9° F."

3. The ED nurse is attempting to transfer a patient to the medical-surgical unit. When the receiving nurse answers the phone, he says, "You people always dump these admissions on us during shift change." Which response by the ED nurse represents the best attempt at respectful negotiation and collaboration?
   a. "I am sorry. I realize you are busy, but we are busy too."
   b. "When would you be willing to take our patients?"
   c. "I apologize for the timing. I will call back in 30 minutes."
   d. "I apologize. We just received the bed assignment."

4. The nurse is interviewing a psychiatric patient who has been verbally aggressive for the past several hours according to the family. The family states, "He won't hurt anybody." However, the patient is pacing and appears suspicious and angry. Which strategy does the nurse use to conduct the interview?
   a. Sit at eye level with the patient in a quiet, secluded room.
   b. Conduct the interview standing near the door in a quiet room.
   c. Bring the entire family in and have everyone sit in comfortable chairs.
   d. Have the security guard stand by the patient during the interview.

5. The nurse is working alone in triage. It is a busy night and the waiting room is full of people who are restless and unhappy about having to wait. Which situation warrants the nurse to activate the panic button under the triage desk?
   a. The line for patients waiting to be triaged becomes overwhelmingly long.
   b. EMS calls to announce they are en route with a patient in full arrest.
   c. Several patients in the waiting room start to complain very loudly.
   d. A person walks in and starts threatening the registration staff with a weapon.

6. The ED nurse is caring for a patient who was found in an alley with no identification and no known family. The nurse must give medication to the patient. What is the correct procedure?
   a. Emergent conditions prevent identification, so the nurse gives the medication as ordered.
   b. The patient is designated as John Doe and the nurse uses two unique identifiers.
   c. The nurse validates the order with another nurse and both verify that the patient is unidentified.
   d. The nurse gives the medication and identification is made as soon as possible.

7. The nurse is using the SBAR method to give a handoff report to the nurse who will assume care of the patient. What would the nurse say first?
   a. "CAT scan results are negative and neurology consult is pending."
   b. "Mr. S. has a history of high blood pressure, but stopped taking medication 3 months ago."
   c. "Current vital signs: temperature 98.6° F, pulse 80/min, respiratory rate 16/min and blood pressure 160/80."
   d. "Mr. S. is a 65-year-old male who came to the ED for a severe headache."

8. An older adult is in the ED for over 48 hours awaiting transfer to an inpatient bed. The charge nurse delegates turning the patient every 2 hours to the unlicensed assistive personnel (UAP) for Risk for impaired skin integrity. The ED is busy; the patient is not turned and begins to develop a pressure ulcer. What does the charge nurse do to prevent a recurrence of this type of problem for future patients? (*Select all that apply.*)
   a. Nothing; in the overall priorities of the ED, the situation is inevitable.
   b. Make anecdotal notes and counsel all the involved UAPs.
   c. Delegate the duty of turning and repositioning to the physical therapist.
   d. File an incident report and seek resolution at the systems level.
   e. Reeducate staff on the need to turn patients at risk for skin breakdown.

9. An older couple on vacation comes to the ED. The man appears to be having a stroke and is unable to speak clearly or coherently. His wife is very distraught and states, "He has many allergies and takes many medications, but I can't remember anything right now!" What should the nurse do first to quickly obtain drug and allergy information?
   a. Call the patient's family health care provider for a phone report about his drugs and allergies.
   b. Remind the wife to keep a list of the patient's drugs and allergies in her purse.
   c. Call the pharmacy where the patient obtains his medications.
   d. Check for a medical alert bracelet and help the wife to look in the patient's suitcase.

10. A patient is brought to the ED by friends who report "he probably overdosed on downers." The patient has a decreased level of consciousness and a decreased gag reflex; his face and chest are covered with emesis; he demonstrates spontaneous sonorous respirations; and pulse oximetry is 87% on room air. What type of airway management does the nurse expect this patient to receive?
    a. Supplemental oxygen per nasal cannula at 4-6 L/min
    b. Bag-valve-mask and 100% oxygen to assist with ventilatory effort
    c. Nonrebreather mask with high-flow oxygen
    d. Endotracheal intubation with initial high-concentration oxygen

11. The ED nurse is caring for several patients, all of whom are currently lying on stretchers either pending discharge or awaiting transfer to a hospital bed. Which patients have the greatest risk for falls? *(Select all that apply.)*
    a. Patient with chronic pain who received 10 mg PO oxycodone for myalgia
    b. Opioid-naive teenager with a fracture who received 3 mg IV morphine for pain
    c. Middle-aged woman with severe vomiting and frequent watery stools for 3 days
    d. Child with a fever of 102° F, crying, with an ear infection
    e. Older adult patient with acute dementia secondary to infection

12. For which circumstance would the use of Standard Precautions be adequate to ensure the safety of the nurse, staff, and other patients?
    a. Performing hygienic care for a patient with copious watery diarrhea
    b. Assisting with intubation of a patient with symptoms of tuberculosis
    c. Initiating a peripheral intravenous access attached to a saline lock
    d. Assessing a child with a fever and rash and known exposure to chickenpox

13. A patient is brought to the ED by the family because he has verbally threatened others and attempted to stab the neighbor's dog. What does the nurse do in order to ensure the safety of the patient and others? *(Select all that apply.)*
    a. Search the patient's belongings and secure personal effects.
    b. Instruct the patient's family to stay with him and call for help as necessary.
    c. Remove dangerous equipment from the room, such as sharps containers or portable instruments.
    d. Escort the patient to the waiting area where he can readily be observed by the triage nurse.
    e. Use a metal detector to search for objects that could be used as weapons.
    f. Instruct nursing students to avoid wearing a stethoscope around their necks.

14. For which patients would the nurse advocate for a social services consult? *(Select all that apply.)*
    a. Toddler who bumped her head on a table; observation for 24 hours is required.
    b. Homeless woman who will be discharged with a splint to the lower leg and crutches.
    c. Woman who was punched and beaten by her husband and sustained a broken jaw.
    d. Man who drove himself to the ED for a dressing change of an infected wound on his back.
    e. Preteen admitted for vaginal bleeding and sexually transmitted infection.

15. Which function represents an appropriate referral to the case manager?
    a. Check with the admissions office to get a count of available intensive care beds.
    b. Contact the peripherally inserted central catheter (PICC) nurse, because the patient has bad veins.
    c. Investigate whether the patient is abusing and overusing ED services.
    d. Follow the patient into the community setting and evaluate the home environment.

16. Three people who came to the ED with a patient have become verbally argumentative and threatening towards each other. Which actions does the ED nurse take to ensure staff safety? *(Select all that apply.)*
    a. Ask the individuals to sit down and offer them coffee.
    b. Follow the hospital's security plan.
    c. Attempt to deescalate the situation.
    d. Quietly ask the individuals to leave.
    e. Identify potential escape routes.

17. The nurse is evaluating the lower extremities of several patients. Which description represents the least serious physical presentation?
    a. Pain in calf; lower leg is swollen and red.
    b. Progressively increasing pain; distal portion is cool and bluish.
    c. Decreased sensation; lower leg has widespread brownish discoloration.
    d. Tight sensation in ankle; skin appears tight, shiny, and edematous.

18. A parent brings her 2-year-old child to the ED, stating, "She fell and bumped her head and forearm." Which behavior by the child causes the nurse the least concern during the initial triage interview?
    a. Crying and reaching for the parent as the nurse approaches
    b. Alert and still, quietly watching as the nurse approaches
    c. Asleep, limp, with even and unlabored respirations
    d. Crying loudly and inconsolably since she was brought in

19. The ED trauma team is preparing to receive a motor vehicle crash victim with severe chest trauma with coughing of blood and a crush injury to the right leg. What type of personal protective equipment (PPE) does the nurse assigned to be the recorder put on?
    a. No PPE is necessary because the nurse is only recording and not giving direct care
    b. Gloves
    c. Gown, gloves, eye protection, face mask, a cap, and shoe covers
    d. The patient situation must first be assessed before determining what PPE to wear

20. The nurse is working in the ED with an emergency health care provider, but the provider is currently involved in the care of several critical patients. The ED nurse must initiate care for patients under interdisciplinary and medical protocols. Which intervention is the least likely to be covered by a standing protocol?
    a. Give 50% dextrose IV push for low blood sugar.
    b. Obtain an arterial blood gas and start oxygen therapy.
    c. Ventilate with bag-valve-mask at 100% oxygen and intubate.
    d. Start a peripheral IV with normal saline at 125 mL/hour.

21. Several patients have been waiting for more than 36 hours to be transferred to an inpatient room because the census is high during flu season. The ED staff is attempting to meet basic health needs in these difficult circumstances. Which need is the priority?
    a. Helping the patients with hygiene
    b. Making sure that patients are fed
    c. Informing patients about admission status
    d. Ensuring safety of environment and care

22. Which patient should be triaged as emergent (E)?
    a. 56-year-old man with severe unilateral back pain and previous history of kidney stones
    b. 23-year-old woman with severe abdominal pain; positive home pregnancy test; BP 80/40 mm Hg
    c. 6-year-old with a temperature of 101° F and flulike symptoms
    d. 10-year-old girl with vomiting, diarrhea, and abdominal pain onset 4 hours after eating fish

23. Which patient should be triaged as urgent (U)?
    a. 44-year-old man with a dislocated elbow
    b. 35-year-old man with chest pain and diaphoresis
    c. 85-year-old man with new onset of confusion; BP grossly elevated compared to his usual
    d. 65-year-old woman with redness and swelling on the forearm associated with a bee sting

24. The nurse is trying to prepare an intravenous antibiotic medication for a patient, but the ED is very busy, chaotic, and noisy and the nurse is continuously interrupted. What should the nurse do first?
    a. Ask the charge nurse to administer the antibiotic medication or send additional help.
    b. Prioritize the urgency of the medication in relation to the urgency of the interruptions.
    c. Shut the door and proceed through the six rights of medication administration.
    d. Prepare the medication, while fielding the interruptions and delegating appropriately.

25. Because of the high risk for health care–acquired urinary tract infections, the nurse would question an order for a catheterized urine specimen for which patient?
    a. 78-year-old female transferred from a long-term care facility for urinary retention
    b. 25-year-old female with back pain and hematuria, currently menstruating
    c. 3-year-old with severe dehydration after prolonged diarrhea and vomiting
    d. 43-year-old multiple trauma patient with signs of hypovolemic shock

26. The nurse has administered pain medication to a patient who has a migraine headache. What instructions should be given to the UAP?
    a. Wait 45 minutes and then ask the patient how he feels and if the pain is relieved.
    b. When helping him to get out of bed, sit him up, dangle feet, then assist him to stand.
    c. Check the patient frequently to make sure he arouses and is not decompensating.
    d. Ask the patient if he has a ride home; if not, call a family member to make arrangements.

27. Which intervention would be addressed during the primary survey?
    a. Insert a urinary catheter.
    b. Establish patent airway.
    c. Stabilize a fracture.
    d. Insert a nasogastric tube.

28. What is the fastest way for the nurse to estimate the systolic blood pressure in a patient with multiple injuries, who has just been moved from the transport stretcher to the ED resuscitation stretcher?
    a. Palpate for presence of a radial pulse.
    b. Use the automated blood pressure cuff.
    c. Place the patient on a cardiac monitor.
    d. Check for the presence of capillary refill.

29. A patient comes to the ED after falling off a roof. He displays absent breath sounds over the left chest, severe respiratory distress, hypotension, jugular vein distention, and tracheal deviation. Based on these assessment findings, for which condition does the nurse anticipate the patient must receive immediate treatment?
    a. Tension pneumothorax
    b. Cardiac arrest
    c. Airway obstruction
    d. Multiple fractured ribs

30. The nurse is helping the health care provider treat a patient with a tension pneumothorax. What type of equipment does the nurse obtain to immediately alleviate this life-threatening condition?
    a. Large adult endotracheal tube
    b. Transvenous pacemaker insertion
    c. Chest tube insertion tray
    d. Tracheostomy tray

31. The nurse's next-door neighbor has sustained a deep laceration to the right upper arm and there is active bright-red bleeding. What does the nurse do to immediately control the bleeding? *(Select all that apply.)*
    a. Apply a tourniquet just above the laceration.
    b. Have the neighbor lie flat and elevate the arm.
    c. Apply direct pressure with a thick, dry towel.
    d. Apply sterile gauze and wrap the wound with an Ace bandage.
    e. Rinse the wound gently with tepid water and apply direct pressure with a towel.

32. A patient who sustained multiple injuries in a job site accident has a BP of 100/60 mm Hg and pulse of 120/min. Two large-bore IVs are established and IV fluid resuscitation is initiated. After receiving IV fluid, repeat vital signs are BP 94/56 mm Hg, pulse 135/min; then BP 80/50 mm Hg, pulse 150/min. With these vital signs, the patient is likely to require blood products after how many liters of IV fluid?
    a. 1
    b. 2
    c. 4
    d. 5

33. The nurse is caring for a patient with a head injury whose Glasgow coma scale score is 3. This score indicates the patient is most likely to do what?
    a. Withdraw from painful stimuli
    b. Open eyes spontaneously
    c. Moan with incoherent speech
    d. Present as totally unresponsive

34. The ED clinical nurse specialist (CNS) is designing ways to teach newly graduated nurses about priority setting in the triage area. Which strategy is the CNS most likely to recommend?
    a. Assign new nurses to triage during low-volume periods.
    b. Pair a new nurse with an experienced nurse in the triage area.
    c. Prepare handouts and tip sheets for the principles of triage.
    d. Have the new nurses observe the triage process for several days.

35. A patient comes to the ED with severe respiratory distress. He has a long history of chronic respiratory disease and now requires endotracheal intubation. How does the nurse assess this patient's lung compliance?
    a. Auscultate the lung fields, especially for coarse crackles.
    b. Sense the degree of difficulty in ventilating with a bag-valve-mask.
    c. Monitor the pulse oximeter for decreasing saturation levels.
    d. Count the respiratory rate and observe the respiratory effort.

36. Each patient listed below has entered the ED's waiting area. Place them in order of priority, with 1 being the highest priority and 4 being the lowest priority.
    _____ a. 3-year-old child with inconsolable high-pitched crying, high fever, headache, and nuchal rigidity
    _____ b. 65-year-old man having diaphoresis with left anterior crushing chest pain
    _____ c. 32-year-old woman reporting upper abdominal pain and vomiting green bile emesis
    _____ d. 16-year-old boy with a broken arm from skateboarding, pulse and sensation intact

37. Based on the nurse's knowledge of normal versus abnormal findings related to growth and development, which assessment finding concerns the nurse the most?
    a. Mottling of extremities in a newborn
    b. Dry skin with tenting in an elderly woman
    c. Anxiety and fearfulness in an 18-month-old child
    d. Rapid, shallow respirations in a 7-year-old child

38. A patient is brought to the ED by the paramedics. The patient is alert but disoriented, and the left lower leg has swelling and deformity. Which question is most essential to ask the paramedics?
    a. "Does the patient have insurance coverage?"
    b. "Are friends or family en route to the hospital?"
    c. "What was the mechanism of injury?"
    d. "Does the patient have a primary care provider?"

39. A patient has been admitted to the ED following a motor vehicle accident and has a history of substance abuse. What is a priority for the nurse to include in the assessment?
    a. Assess the time the patient last ate.
    b. Assess the patient's risk factors for suicide.
    c. Evaluate the patient's spiritual beliefs.
    d. Identify an individual who emotionally supports the patient.

40. A patient was involved in a high-speed motor vehicle accident. The health care provider instructs the nurse to prepare for several urgent procedures because of severe injury and physical compromise. Which procedure does the nurse prepare for first?
    a. Central line insertion
    b. Peritoneal lavage
    c. Chest tube insertion
    d. Endotracheal intubation

41. A patient in the ED has sustained a closed fracture after falling 50 feet while rock climbing. What are the assessments and interventions the nurse would perform for this patient in priority order? *(Select in order of priority, with 1 being the highest priority.)*

    _____ a. Evaluate the neuromuscular status of the left lower extremity.

    _____ b. Assess the head, chest, and abdomen for injuries.

    _____ c. Assess airway, breathing, and circulation.

    _____ d. Immobilize the injured extremity.

    _____ e. Monitor the degree of pain or discomfort.

42. Which factor is most likely to hinder the nurse's ability to objectively and accurately triage patients?
    a. Ambiguity about which triage model is the best for selected patients
    b. Several patients arrive simultaneously at the triage area
    c. Nurse is personally experiencing compassion fatigue and burnout
    d. Patient has a complex health history, and is a poor historian

43. A patient comes to the ED for gastric distress with vomiting large amounts of dark-brown emesis and passing small amounts of bright-red blood. Which preexisting health condition is most likely to be a factor in determining triage classification?
    a. History of diabetes mellitus
    b. History of anticoagulant use
    c. History of high blood pressure
    d. History of childhood appendectomy

44. An elderly man is brought to the ED by the patient's son. The patient is alert, but is disoriented to person, place, and time, and is unable to follow simple instructions. Which question is the most important to ask the son?
    a. "Does your father have any health conditions?"
    b. "Are you the primary caregiver for your father?"
    c. "Do you think your father would consent to emergency care?"
    d. "Who is your father's primary care provider?"

45. A patient with a sprained ankle says, "I have been here for 4 hours and other people who came after me have been taken back to see the doctor. My ankle hurts! Why am I being ignored?" What is the best response?
    a. "Sir, other patients have problems that are more serious than yours."
    b. "This is a system fault, if you would like to complain, I'll call a supervisor."
    c. "We have to attend to life-threatening or unstable conditions first."
    d. "Sir, I see that you are frustrated, but please sit down and wait your turn."

46. An experienced nurse is working in triage. For which circumstance is the nurse most likely to seek input from the emergency physician or advanced-practice nurse about acuity level of the patient?
    a. A 65-year-old man is having severe anterior chest pain and shortness of breath.
    b. A 35-year-old man with history of kidney stones has severe back pain and hematuria.
    c. A 1-year-old child with history of frequent ear infections is screaming and pulling at his ear.
    d. A 23-year-old female with previous good health has sudden, severe flulike symptoms.

47. Based on mechanism of injury, which patient is most likely to automatically require trauma team intervention?
    a. Stab wound to the leg
    b. Gunshot wound to the chest
    c. Possible drowning
    d. Unwitnessed cardiac arrest

48. The patient died in the ED despite resuscitation efforts. Homicide is suspected. Which nursing action would be incorrect, due to the likelihood of forensic investigation?
    a. Invites the family to spend time with the deceased patient
    b. Gives the patient's clothes and other belongings to the family
    c. Declines to give information to friends of the deceased
    d. Leaves intravenous lines and indwelling tubes in place

49. The nurse sees that the emergency provider has written an order to discharge an elderly patient to go home. The patient cannot walk independently and has no relatives. What should the nurse do first?
    a. Talk to the provider about the patient's self-care abilities.
    b. Ask the patient if a friend could come to the hospital.
    c. Obtain a taxicab voucher for the patient.
    d. Consult social services for nursing home placement.

50. A patient died in the ED after sustaining multiple injuries that occurred during an aggravated assault. The family arrives after the patient is pronounced dead and they ask to see the body. What does the nurse do?
    a. Explain that viewing the body would be too traumatic because all the tubes must remain in place for the forensic exam.
    b. Remove any tubes or debris that are near the patient's face and then cover the rest of the body with a blanket.
    c. Explain what they will see; dim the lights; leave the patient's face exposed, but cover the rest of the body with a blanket.
    d. Suggest that the family could spend time with their loved one at the mortuary after the medical examiner is finished.

51. The emergency physician and the nurse go together to tell the family that a patient died despite resuscitation efforts. What is the best way to inform the family?
    a. "We did everything that we could, but Mr. S. expired."
    b. "He never woke up, but we are sure that he passed on without discomfort."
    c. "We are sorry to inform you that Mr. S. died due to extensive injuries."
    d. "We want to extend our sympathies because Mr. S. is not with us anymore."

52. Which action would typically be performed by the ED bereavement committee?
    a. Assigns a staff nurse to sit with the family during resuscitation efforts of patient
    b. Advocates that one or two family members be allowed at bedside during resuscitation
    c. Provides grief counseling and group support for nurses who care for patients who code
    d. Attends funerals, sends sympathy cards, and makes follow-up calls to family

53. The nurse observes that a homeless woman frequently comes to the ED during the winter for symptoms of dizziness and generalized pain. The patient typically stays for several hours, undergoes diagnostic testing and is discharged with a referral to a primary care provider. What should the nurse do?
    a. Assess and treat the patient as if she were any other patient.
    b. Offer food and a blanket and encourage her to leave after she warms up.
    c. Develop an individual care plan using an interdisciplinary team approach.
    d. Talk to the patient and attempt to establish validity of symptoms.

54. The nurse is interviewing a homeless patient in the triage area. The patient says, "I'm a nurse too. Flying pictures say God is me. I'm a god, taking noise away." The patient then stands up and kicks over the garbage can. What should the nurse do first?
    a. Remain calm and slowly step away from the patient.
    b. Run towards the panic button and immediately push it.
    c. Gently take the patient's arm and lead her to a quiet space.
    d. Call for help and instruct bystanders to get out of the way.

55. The nurse is working at a level III trauma center. A patient involved in a chemical plant explosion arrives with burns, probable closed head injury, extremity fractures, and blunt trauma to the abdomen. What action is the nurse most likely to perform in the care of this patient?
    a. Preparing the patient for emergency surgery
    b. Débriding and cleansing the burned areas
    c. Initiating large-bore intravenous access for fluids
    d. Assisting with procedures to diagnose internal hemorrhage

56. The patient was repeatedly kicked and punched in the abdomen. The initial assessment and diagnostic testing reveals no life-threatening damage. The emergency provider tells the nurse that the patient should remain in the ED for observation. What is the most important action for the nurse to perform?
    a. Administer pain medication in a timely fashion.
    b. Initiate serial abdominal assessments.
    c. Instruct the UAP to take vital signs every 4 hours.
    d. Find a quiet space where the patient can rest.

9

CHAPTER

Care of Patients with Common Environmental Emergencies

1. Which predisposing factors are associated with heat-related illness? *(Select all that apply.)*
   a. High humidity
   b. Beta-adrenergic blockers
   c. Obesity
   d. Anemia
   e. Seizures
   f. Dehydration

2. The nurse is providing patient education about the prevention of heat-related illness. Which statements are correct? *(Select all that apply.)*
   a. "Wear lightweight, dark-colored clothing when working outside."
   b. "Plan to limit activities at the hottest time of day."
   c. "Avoid fluids with electrolytes before, during, and after exercise."
   d. "Wear loose-fitting clothing."
   e. "Rest frequently when working in a hot environment."

3. A patient reports being outside when temperatures reached 110° F and he forgot to drink water. Now he reports weakness, a headache, and nausea with dizziness. His body temperature is 98.9° F. What is this patient suffering from?
   a. Classic heat stroke
   b. Exertional heatstroke
   c. Heat exhaustion
   d. Fluid overload

4. Which prehospital interventions are appropriate for a patient with heat exhaustion? *(Select all that apply.)*
   a. Provide salted snacks for him to eat.
   b. Call for emergency medical services.
   c. Provide oral hydration such as a sports drink.
   d. Fan or spray water on his skin.
   e. Avoid giving him salt tablets.

5. During a summer marathon, the temperature is over 100° F and the humidity is high. Suddenly a runner collapses after running in the race for 1 hour. The runner's body temperature is 105.2° F, she is confused and sweating. What is this patient suffering from?
   a. Classic heat stroke
   b. Exertional heat stroke
   c. Heat exhaustion
   d. Dehydration

6. The nurse is participating in a local community sports day. The day is hot and humid and older adults are walking around. Prevention of heat-related injuries would include which intervention?
   a. Encouraging participants to eat high-energy snacks, such as sports bars
   b. Advising that people with disabilities should not participate
   c. Setting up a shade tent with areas for rest and relaxed activity
   d. Limiting direct sun exposure to 2 hours during the hottest time of the day

7. The nurse is volunteering at the first-aid station at a local community fair. The weather is predicted to be hot and humid. In planning care for people who may experience heat-related illness in this setting, what should the nurse obtain?
   a. Supply of salt tablets and bottles of water
   b. Bags of IV normal saline and IV insertion equipment
   c. Several water spray bottles and a portable fan
   d. Supply of educational pamphlets and sunscreen samples

8. It is the middle of summer and the weather has been hot and humid for several weeks. Which patient has the highest risk for severe heat-related illness?
   a. Older adult woman who lives alone in an apartment with no air conditioning
   b. Well-conditioned athlete who is participating in a marathon
   c. Experienced construction worker who is working on an outdoor structure
   d. Young child who is participating in an organized team sport

9. The nurse has received reports on several patients who were admitted for heat-related illnesses. The patient who has the most severe case of heat-related illness exhibits which signs/symptoms?
   a. Headache, heavy perspiration, temperature of 101° F
   b. Feeling of illness, nausea, and vomiting
   c. Significant sunburn to extremities, face, and neck; temperature of 102° F
   d. Hot and dry skin, alert and oriented to person, pulse of 120/min

10. A homeless man is found lying in a vacant lot in the middle of July. He is lethargic and confused and he has sustained severe sunburns on the exposed areas of his skin. His core temperature is 106° F. What do prehospital emergency cooling measures include for this patient? (Select all that apply.)
    a. Administering cold IV fluid
    b. Stripping off all clothing
    c. Packing the axilla and groin with ice
    d. Encouraging sips of cool water
    e. Sponging with cool water and fanning

11. A young migrant worker has been living in a garden shed for several months. He is brought to the emergency department (ED) and is alert and conversant, but appears fearful and confused. His skin is hot and dry and his lips are cracked and bleeding. His skin turgor is poor and he is malnourished. His blood pressure is 96/60 mm Hg, pulse is 120, respirations 30, temperature is 105° F. In addition to high-flow oxygen, what does the nurse anticipate the ED health care provider will initially order?
    a. IV normal saline and a Foley catheter
    b. IV Ringer's lactate and an NG tube
    c. IV 5% dextrose and acetaminophen (Tylenol)
    d. IV 45% saline and chlorpromazine (Thorazine)

12. An older adult man in the ED has sustained a snakebite. What key questions does the nurse ask to assess the risk for envenomation? (Select all that apply.)
    a. "What color was the snake?"
    b. "Did the snake have a triangle-shaped head?"
    c. "Was the swelling localized or did it extend beyond the bite site?"
    d. "Did the bite leave any secretions on the skin?"
    e. "Was the fang mark immediately evident on the skin?"

13. A patient sustained a bite from a pit viper and is admitted for observation. Which potential complications does the nurse observe for? *(Select all that apply.)*
    a. Local tissue necrosis
    b. Diarrhea
    c. Massive tissue swelling
    d. Renal failure
    e. Hypovolemic shock
    f. Increased intracranial pressure

14. The nurse is participating in a summer hike with a group of children. Suddenly the children start screaming, "Snake! Snake!" One little girl is sitting in a tall grassy area, clutching her ankle and crying. What is the first priority in the field care of this child?
    a. Remove any constricting clothing.
    b. Maintain the extremity below the level of the heart.
    c. Move the child to a safe area and encourage rest.
    d. Keep the child warm and provide calm reassurance.

15. The nurse is on a backpacking trip. One of the hikers sustains a pit viper bite to the lower leg. Which first-aid measure will the nurse perform while waiting for transportation to the hospital?
    a. Elevate the leg and apply cool packs.
    b. Incise the fang marks with a pocket knife.
    c. Immobilize the leg with a splint in a functional position.
    d. Apply a constricting band proximal to the fang marks.

16. A patient arrives in the ED after sustaining a cottonmouth snakebite. What is included in the immediate interventions for this patient?
    a. Assessing for cranial nerve deficits
    b. Applying a pressure bandage
    c. Monitoring blood pressure and cardiac function
    d. Administering antivenin

17. A patient is admitted for a poisonous snakebite. The nurse observes that the patient has hemorrhagic complications of hematuria, hemoptysis, petechiae, and extensive bruising. These clinical observations indicate to the nurse that the patient may be experiencing which complication associated with snakebite?
    a. Disseminated intravascular coagulation
    b. Agranulocytosis
    c. Thrombocytopenia
    d. Aplastic anemia

18. Antivenin polyvalent is given to patients with caution when they exhibit which preexisting factors? *(Select all that apply.)*
    a. Previous allergic reaction to antivenom therapy
    b. Older adults who were bitten several hours prior to arrival at the ED
    c. Sensitivity to mercury-containing products
    d. Pregnancy
    e. Hypersensitivity to bovine protein

19. Which symptoms indicate that the patient may have the beginning of serum sickness?
    a. Skin rash with pruritus
    b. Nausea and vomiting
    c. Dizziness and lightheadedness
    d. Malaise and excessive fatigue

20. A patient is transported to the ED by a family member after sustaining a snakebite on a hiking trip. The patient may be a potential candidate for Crotalidae Polyvalent Immune Fab (CroFab). In order to safely administer therapy, which question would the nurse ask?
    a. "What type of snake inflicted the bite?"
    b. "How much time has passed since the snakebite occurred?"
    c. "Do you have a history of deep vein thrombosis (DVT) or do you take Coumadin?"
    d. "Do you have allergies to papaya or pineapple?"

21. A patient sustained a snakebite 2 hours ago and the health care provider orders CroFab. What is the priority nursing intervention in administering this medication to the patient?
    a. Monitor for symptom control after the first dose.
    b. Monitor the patient closely for hives, rash, or difficulty breathing.
    c. Give the bolus dose slowly over 10 minutes.
    d. Give the medication within 3 hours of the snakebite.

22. A patient sustained a coral snakebite on the forearm approximately 12 hours ago and he has been admitted for observation. He reported a mild transient pain, but was otherwise asymptomatic on admission. Which clinical manifestations are early signs of envenomation?
    a. Nausea, vomiting, and pallor
    b. Difficulty speaking and swallowing
    c. Total flaccid paralysis
    d. Severe pain and swelling at the site

23. A patient sustained a coral snakebite and developed severe complications. Which diagnostic test results reveal the physiologic damage that occurs with envenomation?
    a. Complete blood count (CBC)
    b. Coagulation profile
    c. Creatine kinase
    d. Electrolytes

24. The nurse is assisting a neighbor with a gardening project. The neighbor sustains a snakebite when reaching to move a rock. What is the best action to perform in order to identify the snake?
    a. Crush the body of the snake with a rock but preserve the head.
    b. Note the markings of the snake and seek pictures on the Internet.
    c. Stand at a distance and take a digital picture of the snake.
    d. Trap the snake using a long garden tool and bucket.

25. A patient sustained a coral snakebite and calls the ED for instructions. Besides calling for an ambulance, what does the nurse instruct the patient to do?
    a. Apply ice to the wound.
    b. Incise the wound to allow the blood to flow freely.
    c. Use an elastic bandage to impede lymphatic flow and apply a splint.
    d. Place a tourniquet that is tight enough to reduce arterial flow of the venom.

26. When administering antivenom for pit viper bites, which signs/symptoms does the nurse observe for that would signal the most likely adverse reaction to the treatment?
    a. Elevated blood pressure
    b. Pain at the injection site
    c. Pruritus and hives
    d. Disorientation

27. A patient calls the health care provider's office after sustaining a spider bite on the arm 3 hours ago asking for advice about whether to come into the office or hospital for evaluation. She denies any allergic reactions or shortness of breath. Which question would be the most relevant in helping the patient to make the decision?
    a. "Do you have diphenhydramine (Benadryl) at the house?"
    b. "Is your arm painful or swollen?"
    c. "Were you able to identify the spider?"
    d. "Was the spider hiding in a dark secluded area?"

28. A patient calls the ED for advice on immediate first aid for a brown recluse spider bite on his hand. He denies allergic response or shortness of breath and states that he plans to see his health care provider, but is currently about 2 to 3 hours away. What does the nurse advise the patient to do?
    a. Apply a warm pack and elevate the extremity.
    b. Wash the bite area several times with soap and water.
    c. Apply cold compresses and rest as much as possible.
    d. Apply a snug constricting band at the wrist level.

29. A patient sustained a brown recluse bite and has been admitted for IV antibiotics and wound management. Which laboratory value indicates that the patient may be developing severe systemic complications from the bite?
    a. Increased red blood count
    b. Increased glucose level
    c. Decreased platelet count
    d. Decreased blood urea nitrogen

30. A patient was bitten by a brown recluse spider 4 days ago. The nurse observes prolonged bleeding after venipunctures and notes that the patient has a low platelet count. What do these findings indicate?
    a. Thrombocytopenia
    b. Hemolytic anemia
    c. Aplastic anemia
    d. Agranulocytosis

31. Which complications are related to a black widow spider bite? *(Select all that apply.)*
    a. Muscle rigidity and spasms of large muscles
    b. Severe dizziness and tinnitus
    c. Severe abdominal pain
    d. Latrodectism
    e. Hypertension

32. The nurse is assessing a patient who reports being bitten by a black widow spider. The patient may have clinical signs and symptoms that mimic which disorder?
    a. Myocardial infarction
    b. Acute abdomen
    c. Small bowel obstruction
    d. Deep vein thrombosis

33. A patient who has been bitten by a black widow spider requires the following interventions in which priority order? *(Select in order of priority.)*
    _____ a. Administration of antivenin for severe reaction (respiratory arrest and uncontrolled hypertension)
    _____ b. Application of an ice pack to the site
    _____ c. Monitoring of vital signs
    _____ d. Administration of diazepam (Valium) for seizures

34. Which patient is most likely to be treated with antivenin for a black widow spider bite?
    a. Patient in the second trimester of pregnancy
    b. Patient who relapsed 2 weeks after being bitten
    c. Patient who has severe pain and swelling at the site
    d. Patient who is asymptomatic with a cardiac history

35. A patient reports a scorpion sting to the back of the hand. There is no obvious redness or inflammation at the suspected sting site. Which assessment technique does the nurse use to confirm a bark scorpion sting?
    a. Raise the arm and observe for blanching.
    b. Observe for the stinger embedded in the skin.
    c. Look for puncture marks surrounded by fine hairs.
    d. Gently tap at the suspected area to elicit pain.

36. A patient is admitted for observation following a bark scorpion sting. The nurse monitors the patient for which type of systemic complications? *(Select all that apply.)*
    a. Gastrointestinal disorders
    b. Tachycardia
    c. Hypotension
    d. Temperature of 100.7° F (38.2° C)
    e. Pulmonary edema

37. A patient is being treated for a bark scorpion sting. He is currently alert, but somewhat confused. He complains of localized pain (5/10) at the site and requires frequent oral suction. Vital signs are temperature 102° F, pulse 95/min, respirations 12/min, and blood pressure 140/85 mm Hg. Which medication order does the nurse question?
    a. Acetaminophen 650 mg prn (as needed) for fever
    b. Tetanus toxoid 0.5 mL intramuscularly x 1 dose
    c. Morphine 20 mg intravenous push for severe pain
    d. Atropine 0.4 mg subcutaneously for hypersalivation

38. A person is stung by a wasp at a picnic. The person has no difficulty breathing and no history of allergic reaction to bee or wasp stings. What is the priority first-aid action for this person?
    a. Place a tourniquet proximal to the sting.
    b. Gently scrape the stinger off with the edge of a credit card.
    c. Apply an ice pack to the area and elevate.
    d. Observe the area for signs of inflammation prior to taking any action.

39. A teenager is brought to the ED with a reported bee sting. The nurse observes facial swelling, an audible wheeze, and labored rapid breathing. The teen's girlfriend reports he has been vomiting and having trouble speaking and breathing. What does the nurse anticipate the priority medication order will be?
    a. IV normal saline bolus of 400 mL
    b. 50 mg diphenhydramine (Benadryl) PO (by mouth)
    c. 0.5 mL of 1:1000 epinephrine IM
    d. 100 mg methylprednisolone sodium succinate (Solu-Medrol) IV infusion

40. The health care provider orders IV infusion of epinephrine for an older adult patient who is not responding to the IM epinephrine that was administered for an allergic reaction to a bee sting. In conjunction with the epinephrine administration, which action does the nurse take?
    a. Place the patient on a cardiac monitor.
    b. Place the patient on continuous pulse oximetry.
    c. Obtain an order for an electrocardiogram (ECG).
    d. Obtain an order for an arterial blood gas.

41. The school nurse is preparing for an outside field trip to a farm with middle school–aged children. What instructions does the nurse provide to the children for bee and wasp sting prevention? *(Select all that apply.)*
    a. Place all jackets or sweaters in a pile on the ground.
    b. Do not try to outrun bees if attacked by a swarm.
    c. Keep garbage or leftover food in covered containers.
    d. Inspect clothes and shoes for insects before putting on.
    e. Do not swat at bees or wasps close to you.

42. A patient calls the health care provider's office asking for advice about whether to seek immediate medical attention for a bee sting. She has no shortness of breath or swelling to the face, throat, or lips. Which question will elicit information to assist the patient in making the decision?
    a. "Were you stung by an African 'killer bee'?"
    b. "Is the affected area red, painful, or swollen?"
    c. "Did you receive multiple stings?"
    d. "Were you able to remove the stinger?"

43. At a park, the nurse observes a mother of a toddler attempting to remove the stinger of bee with tweezers. What should the nurse do?
    a. Instruct the mother to stop, because tweezing the stinger injects additional venom.
    b. Reinforce that the correct action is to immediately remove the stinger with tweezers or by scraping.
    c. Suggest applying an ice pack for local anesthesia before removing the stinger.
    d. Place a bandage over the stinger and suggest immediately going to the ED.

44. A 37-year-old woman was stung by a bee while gardening. What will cause her to develop a systemic effect?
    a. Multiple bee stings
    b. Immediate local reaction
    c. Desensitization to the venom
    d. No prior allergic reaction to bee stings

45. An anaphylactic reaction to a wasp or bee sting manifests as which conditions? *(Select all that apply.)*
    a. Hypertension
    b. Respiratory distress
    c. Hypoglycemia
    d. Laryngeal edema
    e. Deterioration in mental status

46. A patient with which situation would best benefit from always carrying an epinephrine autoinjector (EpiPen)?
    a. Frequently works outside in the yard
    b. Allergies to poison ivy, grass, and pollens
    c. Previous allergic reaction to a wasp sting
    d. History of severe pain with bee or wasp stings

47. The nurse is administering a first dose of epinephrine to a patient with laryngeal edema after a bee sting. Which route of administration is recommended?
    a. Subcutaneous
    b. Intramuscular
    c. Intravenous
    d. Mucosal

48. A man who was stung by a wasp is treated and observed for symptoms of urticaria, pruritus, and swelling of the lips and then discharged home with medication instructions. Which medication is most likely to be prescribed to prevent delayed allergic effects?
    a. EpiPen
    b. Acetaminophen (Tylenol) as needed
    c. Corticosteroids in tapered doses
    d. Albuterol (Proventil)

49. The nurse is instructing a patient who has a history of allergic reaction to bee stings on what to do if he or she experiences a bee sting in the future. What information does the nurse relay to the patient? *(Select all that apply.)*
    a. Wear a medical alert bracelet.
    b. Take an antihistamine before administering an EpiPen injection.
    c. Administer epinephrine immediately.
    d. Call 911 to be transported to a medical facility.
    e. Take an aspirin immediately.

50. A patient treated for a severe allergic reaction to a bee sting tells the nurse, "The doctor told me that I had to be careful about getting bee stings in the future, because I could have another allergic reaction." Based on the patient's statement, what is the nurse's first action?
    a. Repeat the information that the health care provider gave her.
    b. Assess the patient's understanding of allergic reactions and first aid.
    c. Advise the patient to obtain a medical alert bracelet.
    d. Ensure that the patient has a prescription for an EpiPen.

51. Which person has the greatest risk for injury from lightning strike?
    a. Jogger in the park at mid-morning in December
    b. Deer hunter walking through the woods in the evening in October
    c. Golfer out on the green in the late afternoon in June
    d. Camper walking on the beach during the early morning in April

52. Which lightning-strike victim should receive attention first?
    a. Teenager who is motionless except for shallow respirations; he has a weak pulse
    b. Middle-aged man, unconscious, with no palpable pulse
    c. Confused older adult woman with apparent paralysis in lower extremities
    d. Child crying, bleeding from ears, mottled skin, and decreased pulses in left leg

53. A construction worker who was struck by lightning is brought to the ED. He was reported to be unconscious, but cardiopulmonary resuscitation (CPR) was started immediately and he awoke just before the arrival of emergency medical services (EMS) personnel. In the ED, he is alert but confused, and reports pain to his right hand and foot with fernlike marks. Which assessment tool is the priority for this patient?
    a. Glasgow coma scale
    b. Pulse oximeter
    c. Cardiac monitor
    d. Rule of nines chart

54. The nurse receives a phone call from a child who says, "Mommy was hit by lightning! She's outside. I'm afraid to touch her! I'll get shocked too!" How does the nurse advise the child?
    a. "There is no danger in touching your mom. You won't get hurt."
    b. "It will be okay, just quickly run outside and see if she is breathing."
    c. "Is there anybody at home with you? Let me speak to an adult."
    d. "You stay in the house and someone will come to help very soon."

55. A patient was struck by lightning and sustained temporary paralysis of the lower limbs which resolved, with no physical effects, but the patient developed emotional problems. Which mental health disorder is the most likely complication?
    a. Generalized anxiety disorder
    b. Schizophrenia
    c. Posttraumatic stress disorder
    d. Acute-onset dementia

56. The nurse is caring for a patient who had cardiac and respiratory arrest after being struck by lightning. The patient was resuscitated, and he is now alert and appears to be progressing toward recovery. The nurse observes tea-colored urine in the Foley drainage bag. What does the nurse suspect?
    a. This is a normal finding associated with trauma and resuscitation
    b. Dehydration
    c. Urinary tract infection
    d. Excessive muscle damage affecting the kidneys

57. The nurse is advising parents who are organizing a winter cross-country skiing trip. In assisting the parents to develop an appropriate winter clothing list, which articles should be taken on the trip? *(Select all that apply.)*
    a. Synthetic socks
    b. Cotton underwear
    c. Polyester fleece shirt
    d. Windproof outer jacket
    e. Hat made from Gore-Tex
    f. Sunglasses

58. The day camp nurse is with a group of children who have been participating in hiking, swimming, and crafts. The nurse sees a child who is soaking wet, stumbling, and taking off all of her clothes. What does the nurse suspect is wrong with this child?
    a. Snakebite
    b. High-altitude sickness
    c. Hypothermia
    d. Nearly drowned

59. The nurse is conducting a community presentation on cold weather safety. Which point is the nurse sure to include in the presentation?
    a. Hydration and water intake are not an issue, so pack extra clothes, not extra water.
    b. Wear multiple layers of socks when participating in winter sports.
    c. When driving in cold winter weather, carry extra clothes, food, and fluids.
    d. Hypothermia occurs only in the winter months in the United States.

60. Which signs/symptoms indicate the most severe case of hypothermia? *(Select all that apply.)*
    a. Tachycardia
    b. Depressed respiratory rate
    c. Decreased pain response
    d. Acid-base imbalance
    e. Dysarthria

61. A patient involved in a boating accident has extensive injuries and comes to the ED in wet clothes. The nurse identifies a risk for hypothermia. Which interventions does the nurse implement? *(Select all that apply.)*
    a. Remove wet clothing.
    b. Infuse warm IV solutions.
    c. Set the room temperature at 90° F.
    d. Give sips of warm fluid.
    e. Use a heating blanket.

62. Several people on a cross-country ski trip return to the ski lodge with mild hypothermia. Which items does the nurse offer or obtain for the hypothermia victims? *(Select all that apply.)*
    a. Synthetic-fiber hats
    b. Cups of warm broth
    c. Caffeinated beverages
    d. Polyester fleece shirts
    e. Dry socks and gloves

63. A patient arrives at the ED after a prolonged cold exposure. The staff avoids rough and vigorous movements during the transfer from stretcher to bed to prevent which complication?
    a. Ventricular fibrillation related to rough handling
    b. Third-degree heart block related to cold autotransfusion
    c. After-drop due to cold blood moving to the central circulation
    d. Pulmonary emboli related to dislodgment of a clot

64. The health care provider orders core warming methods for a conscious patient with moderate hypothermia. What equipment would the nurse obtain in order to provide this therapy?
    a. Three-way Foley with warmed lavage fluid
    b. Axillary thermometer to monitor core temperature
    c. Bag-valve-mask with warmed humidified oxygen
    d. Several warm blankets and warming pads

65. A man is found lying in an alley in cold weather for an unknown length of time. His hands, toes, and face show evidence of frostbite; otherwise there are no obvious injuries. He is severely obtunded with a pulse of 43 beats/min, respirations of 9/min, and a core temperature of 27° C. What is this patient's most immediate physiologic risk?
    a. Acute respiratory distress syndrome
    b. Pulmonary edema
    c. Cardiac arrest
    d. Acute renal failure

66. The nurse has volunteered at a storm shelter to identify potential problems related to cold-related injuries. Which conditions predispose people to a greater risk for cold injury? *(Select all that apply.)*
    a. Hypothyroidism
    b. Advanced age
    c. Crohn's disease
    d. Osteoarthritis
    e. Malnutrition

67. The nurse is working in a mountain clinic where there is a high incidence of cold-related injuries. Which signs/symptoms indicate the most severe case of frostbite?
    a. Large fluid-filled blisters with partial-thickness skin necrosis
    b. Numbness, coldness, and bloodlessness of affected area
    c. Small blisters that contain dark fluid; skin is cool
    d. Pain, numbness, and pallor of the affected area

68. Which measures are correct when rewarming a victim of deep frostbite? *(Select all that apply.)*
    a. Rubbing the area helps speed the warming process.
    b. Rapid rewarming in a 40° C to 42° C water bath will be required.
    c. Rapid rewarming is avoided because of increased tissue damage.
    d. After rewarming, the extremity should be elevated above the heart level.
    e. An opioid analgesic may be given because of the pain associated with rewarming.
    f. Immunization for tetanus prophylaxis will be needed.

69. The nurse is conducting a class about cold-weather hiking. What are the early signs of frostbite, which hiking partners should frequently observe for?
    a. White, waxy, or pale gray appearance to ears, nose, and cheeks
    b. Edema and redness over the exposed skin
    c. Mottled coloring of the skin
    d. Small blisters that contain dark fluid and areas that do not blanch

70. The ED nurse receives a phone call from someone stating that he and his friend have been out in the cold weather and his friend's fingers 3 through 5 appear white and waxy. What does the nurse direct the caller to do?
    a. Seek shelter immediately and massage and briskly rub the fingers.
    b. Seek shelter immediately and place the hands under the armpits.
    c. Seek medical attention and place hands on car heating vents while en route.
    d. Seek medical attention and place fingers in cool water while en route.

71. A patient has sustained severe frostbite to the toes and lower legs. He received rewarming therapy in the ED and arrives to the medical-surgical unit with a splint on both legs. IV normal saline is infusing at 125 mL/hr. He reports severe pain in the lower extremities. Which health care provider order does the nurse question?
    a. Morphine 1-2 mg IV push prn for pain in extremities
    b. Elevate bilateral lower extremities above the level of the heart
    c. Neurologic and circulation checks every 1 hour to bilateral lower extremities
    d. Apply compression bandage to bilateral lower extremities

72. The nurse is reviewing the CBC results for a patient who lives in a high mountain town. The patient's red blood cell count (RBC) is 6.8 million/mm^3. What does this lab value combined with the patient's environment indicate?
    a. Anemia related to a decreased production of erythropoietin
    b. Polycythemia related to chronic hypoxia
    c. Pernicious anemia related to a regional dietary deficiency
    d. Hemolytic anemia related to cold temperature

73. A patient reports having a throbbing headache with nausea and vomiting "like the worst hangover of my life" after recently returning from a hiking trip to the mountains. The nurse suspects high-altitude sickness. Which question helps the nurse gather relevant information about this condition?
    a. "Did you experience any episodes of hypothermia during your trip?"
    b. "How quickly did you ascend to the top of the mountain range?"
    c. "Did you go skiing or hiking in a high-altitude area?"
    d. "Did you have trouble sleeping while you were in the mountains?"

74. A patient is admitted to the ED for high-altitude sickness. In the morning, he appears apathetic and declines to perform basic activities of daily living (ADLs). Later in the shift, the patient is unable to move himself in bed or to independently sit upright. What condition does the nurse suspect?
    a. High-altitude cerebral edema (HACE)
    b. Severe hypoxemia
    c. Acute mountain sickness (AMS)
    d. Severe hypothermia

75. What are the most common signs/symptoms of high-altitude pulmonary edema (HAPE)? *(Select all that apply.)*
    a. Dyspnea at rest
    b. Persistent dry cough
    c. Abdominal pain and cramping
    d. Pale lips and nail beds
    e. Cyanotic lips and nail beds

76. A Foreign Service employee normally lives in a coastal area, but he must take an emergency trip to a high-mountain area. He asks the nurse what he can do if AMS occurs when he is at a high altitude. What advice should the nurse give? *(Select all that apply.)*
    a. Stay at a higher altitude if a throbbing headache occurs.
    b. If available, administer oxygen.
    c. Take the oral form of furosemide (Lasix).
    d. Descend to a lower altitude.
    e. Get a prescription for sildenafil (Viagra).

77. Which occurrence in the patient treated for AMS indicates that treatment with acetazolamide (Diamox) was effective?
    a. Decreased pulse rate and decreased urine output
    b. Increased urine output and an increased respiratory rate
    c. Periodic respirations during sleep and decreased pulse
    d. Decreased sleep disturbance and decreased respiratory rate

78. A rescue team is attempting to take the patient to the hospital for symptoms of HAPE. The descent to the hospital is delayed due to severe weather conditions. What is the most important treatment for this patient during the delay?
    a. Dexamethasone (Decadron)
    b. Furosemide (Lasix)
    c. Oxygen administration
    d. Avoidance of cold stress

79. Two teenagers bring their friend to the ED because "he was drowning." The patient is unconscious but shows spontaneous breathing, and he is immediately taken to the resuscitation area. Which question is most important for the nurse to ask the patient's friends in determining the outcomes for the patient?
    a. "Was this a fresh water or salt water drowning?"
    b. "Does he have any medical conditions, such as seizures?"
    c. "Was the water contaminated with chemicals or algae?"
    d. "How long was he under the water and not breathing?"

80. What responses does the "diving reflex" cause in the body? *(Select all that apply.)*
    a. Tachycardia
    b. Metabolic alkalosis
    c. Bradycardia
    d. Increased cardiac output
    e. Vasoconstriction of vessels in the intestines and kidneys

81. Several people are looking out across a lake and pointing to a swimmer in the distance who appears to be struggling to stay afloat. What is the correct sequence of emergency steps to take? *(Select in order of priority.)*
    _____ a. Stabilize the spine with a board.
    _____ b. Safely rescue the victim.
    _____ c. Begin immediate CPR.
    _____ d. Assess neurologic status.
    _____ e. Assess airway patency.

82. The pathophysiology of drowning involves a washing out of surfactant, which leads to decreased surface tension, increased lung compliance, and increased airway resistance. What disorder is a result of the pathophysiology?
    a. Pulmonary emboli
    b. Pulmonary edema
    c. Chemical pneumonitis
    d. Aspiration pneumonia

83. A college student was drinking beer and dove from a 20-foot ledge into a lake. He was pulled from the lake by a friend and given mouth-to-mouth. The patient is currently in the ED, awake, and receiving supplemental oxygen. What serial assessments is the nurse most likely to initiate for this patient?
    a. Cardiac monitoring for possible myocardial infarction
    b. Level of consciousness and orientation to monitor for stroke
    c. Peripheral sensation and movement related to spinal cord injury
    d. Frequent blood glucose checks to monitor for hypoglycemia

84. The ED health care team is administering emergency treatment to a drowning victim. Which task can be delegated to a UAP?
    a. Insert the nasogastric tube.
    b. Advise the family about the patient's status.
    c. Take and report vital signs every 15 minutes.
    d. Assist with the bag-valve-mask during intubation.

85. Which combination of factors is likely to contribute to the highest survival rate for drowning victims?
    a. In very cold fresh water for 6 minutes; arrives in ED with pulse of 40
    b. In warm salt water for 6 minutes; arrives in ED with pulse of 70
    c. In very cold salt water for 10 minutes; arrives in ED with no pulse
    d. In warm contaminated water for 5 minutes; arrives in ED with no pulse

86. The nurse is teaching a class on water safety to a group of 5-year-old children. Which point is the nurse most likely to emphasize with this group?
    a. Take swimming lessons and learn how to use floatation devices.
    b. Never swim alone; a parent or other adult should always be with you.
    c. Always test the water depth before jumping in head-first.
    d. If your friends don't know how to swim, always watch out for them .

87. What might the nurse notice if the patient has impaired thermoregulation as a result of a cold-related injury? *(Select all that apply.)*
    a. Hyperemia and edema of fingers or toes
    b. Shivering
    c. Possible atrial fibrillation
    d. Numbness and pain of nose or ears
    e. Profuse diaphoresis

88. What should the nurse interpret for the patient with impaired thermoregulation as a result of a cold-related injury? *(Select all that apply.)*
    a. Temperature
    b. Cardiac assessment
    c. Neurologic assessment
    d. Gastrointestinal assessment
    e. Fluid status

89. How should the nurse respond to the patient with impaired thermoregulation as a result of a cold-related injury? *(Select all that apply.)*
    a. Thaw frozen body parts in a warm-water bath and handle gently.
    b. Provide pain control measures.
    c. Apply compression dressings.
    d. Administer tetanus prophylaxis and possible antibiotics for open wounds.
    e. Initiate passive external rewarming by covering with blankets.

90. On what should the nurse reflect in caring for the patient with impaired thermoregulation as a result of a cold-related injury? *(Select all that apply.)*
    a. Monitor the patient's response to pain medication and rewarming techniques.
    b. Monitor for further injury from rewarming techniques.
    c. Monitor for reccurrence of cardiac dysrhythmias.
    d. Evaluate the patient and family's knowledge about the injury and treatment plans.
    e. Educate the patient and family on ways to prevent future cold-related injury.

10 CHAPTER

Concepts of Emergency and Disaster Preparedness

1. For which event would a large urban hospital's emergency management plan typically be activated?
   a. Three-car collision on the freeway
   b. Fight between two local street gangs
   c. School bus involved in an accident
   d. Explosion at a chemical factory

2. Which event would be considered an internal disaster?
   a. A fire in a long-term care facility
   b. Gunfire in the hospital parking lot
   c. A tornado devastates the community
   d. Several people die from flulike symptoms

3. Which priority intervention would be more likely to occur during an internal disaster compared to an external disaster?
   a. Extra staff would be called in to assist.
   b. Emergency management plan would be activated.
   c. Patients and staff would be evacuated.
   d. Staff would don personal protective equipment.

4. A nurse working at a small rural hospital gets a frantic phone call about a rumor of a student attacking other students at a local high school. What is the most important data to verify in order to determine potential for a multicasualty event versus a mass casualty event?
   a. "How long ago did the event occur?"
   b. "What are the number and severity of the injuries?"
   c. "What are school officials saying about the incident?"
   d. "Have emergency medical services been notified?"

5. The hospital in a small mountain town is updating their emergency management plan to incorporate the "all hazards approach" and to address all credible threats to the area. Which disaster events are the likely priorities in this community's emergency management plan? *(Select all that apply.)*
   a. Avalanches
   b. Floods
   c. Burns
   d. Car accidents
   e. Tornados
   f. Bioterrorism

6. The hospital committee is reviewing the emergency management plan of their small community hospital in a suburban area of a large city. What is a priority to include in this hospital's emergency management plan?
   a. Plan for evacuation routes out of the city.
   b. Plan for transporting patients to other hospitals.
   c. Method to contact the National Disaster Medical System.
   d. Stockpiling postexposure prophylactic antibiotics.

7. The hospital staff is participating in a disaster drill and the nurse is assigned to organize personnel who are called in from home. Which task would be appropriate to delegate to a unlicensed assistive personnel (UAP) who usually works in the labor and delivery area?
   a. Stay with "black tag" patients in the holding area.
   b. Talk to the families of the "red tag" patients.
   c. Care for and support the "green tag" patients.
   d. Obtain vital signs of the "yellow tag" patients.

8. The nurse based in Iowa is a volunteer member of the Medical Reserve Corps (MRC) and has been called to serve in Ohio where he does not hold an active nursing license. What should the nurse do?
   a. Determine if Ohio has reciprocity with Iowa before accepting deployment.
   b. Decline deployment because his nursing license will not allow him to practice in Ohio.
   c. Prepare for deployment because he will be considered a federal employee with valid licensure.
   d. Delay deployment until he has reviewed the nurse practice act that is specific to Ohio.

9. The nursing director of a long-term care facility is designated as the "incident commander" for the facility's emergency management plan. What is the priority action for the incident commander?
   a. Call all the off-duty staff and ask them to come into work.
   b. Take inventory of supplies according to the emergency management plan.
   c. Activate the disaster management process according to the plan.
   d. Call the National Guard to move all patients to other facilities.

10. The nurse is assigned to assist the hospital incident commander during a disaster drill. Which responsibility is appropriate for the nurse in this capacity?
    a. Call all nursing units to determine the number of patients who could potentially be discharged.
    b. Call the physical therapy department and direct therapists to assist in the operating room or the intensive care unit (ICU).
    c. Go to the emergency department (ED) and assist with the triage of disaster victims to appropriate clinical areas.
    d. Contact the security department and instruct them to control the number of people who attempt to enter the hospital.

11. The nurse serves on a committee that is tasked to develop tools and aids that the medical command physician could use during a disaster event. What is an appropriate project for this purpose?
    a. Make a current list, including contact information, of trauma and orthopedic surgeons.
    b. Make a telephone tree for contacting the nursing and ancillary staff.
    c. Design a triage algorithm that addresses different types of disaster events.
    d. Design an algorithm for contacting the Federal Emergency Management Agency.

12. At 3:00 AM, the ED charge nurse of a large suburban hospital receives notification that a commercial plane has just crashed outside the city limits. What does the nurse do? *(Select all that apply.)*
    a. Collaborate with the medical command physician.
    b. Activate the hospital's emergency management plan.
    c. Initiate the staff telephone tree.
    d. Collaborate with the triage officer.
    e. Organize nursing and ancillary services.

13. A local news station calls the hospital seeking permission to verify the number of victims and details of a local disaster. What is the nurse's best response?
    a. "Please don't bother us now. We are swamped with victims."
    b. "We have a lot of stable victims and two people have died."
    c. "Please hold and I will connect you to the public information officer."
    d. "I will connect you with the emergency command center."

14. The emergency management plan is activated because a major earthquake has caused many serious and minor injuries. Which nurse reassignment is most likely to meet the needs of the patients, while best utilizing available personnel?
    a. Operating room nurse is reassigned to the ED to assist in triage.
    b. ED nurse is reassigned to care for patients on the medical-surgical unit.
    c. Critical care nurse is reassigned to the ED to care for "black tag" patients.
    d. Performance improvement nurse is reassigned to care for "green tag" patients..

15. A city committee reviews possible scenarios related to a disaster event. Which is an example of the "greatest good for the greatest number of people"?
    a. The city's supply of antibiotics is sent to one hospital that has 25 victims with exposure to a bioterrorism agent.
    b. Twenty victims infected by a bioterrorism agent are placed on life support and mechanical ventilation.
    c. Thirty people with possible exposure to a bioterrorism agent are quarantined including five children who are asymptomatic.
    d. Elderly community members are treated with prophylactic antibiotics for a bioterrorism agent.

16. The nurse is making a personal emergency preparedness plan. What is the nurse sure to include in the plan?
    a. Make a disaster supply kit with clothing and basic survival supplies.
    b. Resolve the ethical conflicts of family and professional obligations.
    c. Stockpile antibiotics, first-aid supplies, and resuscitation equipment.
    d. Teach family members about radiation and HAZMAT safety issues.

17. A patient comes to the ED worried that he has been exposed to an infectious bioterrorism agent that was sent to him through the mail. What is the priority action for the ED nurse take?
    a. Escort the patient to quarantined area.
    b. Take a history and assess for symptoms.
    c. Call local police and the Department of Public Health.
    d. Activate the emergency preparedness plan.

18. The nurse is assigned to assist the incident commander who is evaluating the feasibility of deactivating the emergency management plan. The commander directs the nurse to accomplish certain tasks. Which task is the priority?
    a. Contact all hospital departments and determine if needs have been met.
    b. Go to the ED and supervise the inventory and restocking of supplies.
    c. Arrange for temporary sleeping quarters for exhausted staff members.
    d. Assist in the preparations of the critical incident stress debriefing.

19. A multiple-car accident with mass casualties has occurred near an urban hospital. The hospital's emergency preparedness plan is activated. For what purposes is the postplan administrative review conducted? *(Select all that apply.)*
    a. To identify only the things that went wrong during the plan
    b. To identify employees who need financial assistance or reimbursement
    c. To establish a social networking system for the employees
    d. To provide all employees the opportunity to express positive and negative comments
    e. To solicit written critique forms for additional information

20. To prevent the development of posttraumatic stress disorder (PTSD) in hospital staff, what action is likely to be taken by the facility?
    a. Conducting administrative debriefings
    b. Providing employees with information on PTSD
    c. Offering employees psychological counseling
    d. Conducting critical incident stress debriefings

21. To protect hospital staff from experiencing posttraumatic stress disorder (PTSD), what are appropriate recommendations by the facility to its employees? *(Select all that apply.)*
    a. Drink plenty of water.
    b. Limit verbalizing feelings to family and friends.
    c. Use available counseling.
    d. Encourage and support coworkers.
    e. Do not work more than 14 hours per day.

22. To promote effective coping for survivors of a mass-casualty event, the nurse practices which principles while interacting with patients in crisis? *(Select all that apply.)*
    a. Listening to patients
    b. Encouraging patients to have solitude
    c. Promoting relaxation
    d. Allowing unstructured routines
    e. Offer choices whenever possible to increase feelings of control

23. A gang-related incident has occurred involving major casualties from gunshot wounds to 11 victims. Which type of debriefing is utilized by the hospital after handling this event?
    a. Critical stress incident
    b. Posttraumatic stress
    c. Administrative stress
    d. Restoring normalcy

24. A community hospital is reviewing the activation and implementation of its emergency preparedness plan after a recent mass-casualty event. What is the appropriate type of debriefing that will effectively evaluate these procedures?
    a. Hospital incident command
    b. Event resolution
    c. Administrative
    d. Critical incident

25. After a major city-wide environmental crisis, which type of debriefing is most appropriate for hospital staff?
    a. Administrative debriefing
    b. Critical incident stress debriefing
    c. Discussion within small groups that can be shared with close family and friends
    d. Referrals for mental health counseling

26. Which nurse activity would best help the hospital to meet the Joint Commission's mandate for emergency preparedness?
    a. Assist in planning drills that include patient simulations.
    b. Help other nurses make a personal emergency preparedness plan.
    c. Attend training classes to learn how to handle hazardous materials.
    d. Identify the credible threats to the safety of the community.

27. The ED nurse is instructing a group of ED UAPs on how to use personal protective equipment (PPE) when caring for patients who may have been exposed to bioterrorism agents. One of the group is clowning around and making jokes. What should the nurse do first?
    a. Threaten to report him to the supervisor, if he doesn't settle down and pay attention.
    b. Instruct him to demonstrate use of PPE in the care of a patient with Ebola.
    c. Advise him that PPE is for his safety, but ignoring safety protocols is a personal choice.
    d. Ignore him and continue instructing because clowning around is a coping method for him.

28. A long-term care facility formed a committee to review the facility's emergency preparedness plan. Which element needs to be resolved in order to meet the guidelines of the Life Safety Code, which is published by the National Fire Protection Association?
    a. Fire extinguishers are heavy and difficult to use.
    b. Fire safety training is difficult because of high staff turnover.
    c. Building has one main front door and side doors have sealed shut.
    d. Many residents are unwilling or incapable of participating in fire drills.

29. Using disaster triage principles, which patient has been correctly triaged and marked with the appropriate color tag?
    a. A toddler who has died of his injuries: green tag
    b. An older woman with a fractured ankle: yellow tag
    c. An older man with shortness of breath and a hemothorax: red tag
    d. A teenager with profuse bleeding from a severe arm laceration: black tag

30. A committee is reviewing the hospital's emergency management plan. In the event of a large-scale multi-casualty event, which group is likely to require the largest amount of physical space to accommodate the number of victims?
    a. Black-tagged patients
    b. Red-tagged patients
    c. Yellow-tagged patients
    d. Green-tagged patients

31. Which disaster situation is most likely to increase the complexity of managing the green-tagged patients who are more likely to self-transport from the scene of the incident to the health care facility?
    a. Collapse of a church roof during Sunday services
    b. Human stampede at a poorly controlled music festival
    c. Breach of containment at a nuclear plant
    d. Demonstration with rioting on a college campus

32. Which scenario is most likely to require activation of the emergency preparedness plan?
    a. A private six-passenger plane crashes at a large urban airport on Wednesday morning
    b. There is an outbreak of food-borne illness at a long-term care center on Tuesday afternoon.
    c. An ice storm strikes a city on Monday night and causes falls and vehicular accidents.
    d. A multi-car accident occurs in front of a small rural hospital after midnight on Sunday.

33. The triage method for multi-casualty or mass response utilizes what sorting methods? *(Select all that apply.)*
    a. Patients are alphabetized by name.
    b. Health care providers triage most critical patients.
    c. Patients are labeled by number.
    d. Patients are ranked by assessment scores.
    e. Patients are ranked using colored labels.

34. The nurse is working in the ED where several local gang members are being treated for gunshot and knife wounds. The nurse hears gunshots in the waiting room, followed by screaming and cries for help. What does the nurse do first?
    a. Grab the resuscitation box and run to the waiting room.
    b. Assist all the ambulatory patients to leave through a back entrance.
    c. Alert the ED health care provider that additional trauma victims need care.
    d. Assess the level of threat to self and others and call for help.

35. Following a tornado disaster, a charge nurse is assigned to be the group co-leader of a critical incident stress debriefing session. During the session, a nurse says, "We weren't prepared for this! The administration at this hospital is a joke." What is the best response?
    a. "This session is not about pointing fingers or fixing blame."
    b. "Tell us about what you experienced while you were caring for victims."
    c. "Improving the emergency plan will be discussed at the administrative review."
    d. "We are all pretty stressed out. Let's take a deep breath and calm down."

11 CHAPTER

Assessment and Care of Patients with Fluid and Electrolyte Imbalances

1. Which findings indicate that a patient may have hypervolemia? *(Select all that apply.)*
   a. Increased, bounding pulse
   b. Jugular venous distention
   c. Diminished peripheral pulses
   d. Presence of crackles
   e. Excessive thirst
   f. Elevated blood pressure
   g. Orthostatic hypotension
   h. Skin pale and cool to touch

2. What is the term for a difference in concentration of particles that is greater on one side of a permeable membrane than on the other side?
   a. Hydrostatic pressure
   b. Concentration gradient
   c. Passive transport
   d. Active transport

3. A patient's blood osmolarity is 302 mOsm/L. What manifestation does the nurse expect to see in the patient?
   a. Increased urine output
   b. Thirst
   c. Peripheral edema
   d. Nausea

4. An older adult patient at risk for fluid and electrolyte problems is vigilantly monitored by the nurse for the first indication of a fluid balance problem. What is this indication?
   a. Fever
   b. Elevated blood pressure
   c. Poor skin turgor
   d. Mental status changes

5. What are the consequences for a patient who does not meet the obligatory urine output? *(Select all that apply.)*
   a. Lethal electrolyte imbalances
   b. Alkalosis
   c. Urine becomes diluted
   d. Toxic buildup of nitrogen
   e. Acidosis

6. What is the minimum amount of urine output per day needed to excrete toxic waste products?
   a. 200 to 300 mL
   b. 400 to 600 mL
   c. 500 to 1000 mL
   d. 1000 to 1500 mL

7. Patients with which conditions are at greatest risk for deficient fluid volume? *(Select all that apply.)*
   a. Fever of 103° F
   b. Extensive burns
   c. Thyroid crisis
   d. Water intoxication
   e. Continuous fistula drainage
   f. Diabetes insipidus

8. The nurse is working in a long-term care facility where there are numerous patients who are immobile and at risk for dehydration. Which task is best to delegate to the unlicensed assistive personnel (UAP)?
   a. Offer patients a choice of fluids every 1 to 2 hours.
   b. Check patients at the beginning of the shift to see who is thirsty.
   c. Give patients extra fluids around medication times.
   d. Evaluate oral intake and urinary output.

9. The nurse is assisting a community group to plan a family sports day. In order to prevent dehydration, what beverage does the nurse suggest be supplied?
   a. Iced tea
   b. Light beer
   c. Diet soda
   d. Bottled water

10. Which factors affect the amount and distribution of body fluids? *(Select all that apply.)*
    a. Race
    b. Age
    c. Gender
    d. Height
    e. Body fat

11. The nurse is caring for a patient with hypovolemia secondary to severe diarrhea and vomiting. In evaluating the respiratory system for this patient, what does the nurse expect to find on assessment?
    a. No changes, because the respiratory system is not involved
    b. Hypoventilation, because the respiratory system is trying to compensate for low pH
    c. Increased respiratory rate, because the body perceives hypovolemia as hypoxia
    d. Normal respiratory rate, but a decreased oxygen saturation

12. The nurse is assessing skin turgor in a 65-year-old patient. What is the correct technique to use with this patient?
    a. Pinch the skin over the sternum and observe for tenting and resumption of skin to its normal position after release.
    b. Observe the skin for a dry, scaly appearance and compare it to a previous assessment.
    c. Pinch the skin over the back of the hand and observe for tenting; count the number of seconds for the skin to recover position.
    d. Observe the mucous membranes and tongue for cracks, fissures, or a pasty coating.

13. The emergency department (ED) nurse is caring for a patient who was brought in for significant alcohol intoxication and minor trauma to the wrist. What will serial hematocrits for this patient likely show?
    a. Hemoconcentration
    b. Normal and stable hematocrits
    c. Progressively lower hematocrits
    d. Decreasing osmolality

14. The nurse is caring for several older adult patients who are at risk for dehydration. Which task can be delegated to the UAP?
    a. Withhold fluids if patients are incontinent of bowels or bladder.
    b. Assess for and report any difficulties that patients are having in swallowing.
    c. Stay with patients while they drink and note the exact amount ingested.
    d. Divide the total amount of fluids needed over a 24-hour period and post a note.

15. The nurse assessing a patient notes a bounding pulse quality, neck vein distention when supine, presence of crackles in the lungs, and increasing peripheral edema. What fluid disorder do these findings reflect?
    a. Fluid volume deficit
    b. Fluid volume excess
    c. Fluid homeostasis
    d. Fluid dehydration

16. A patient is at risk for fluid volume excess and dependent edema. Which task does the nurse delegate to the UAP?
    a. Massage the legs and heels to stimulate circulation.
    b. Evaluate the effectiveness of a pressure-reducing mattress.
    c. Assess the coccyx, elbows, and hips daily for signs of redness.
    d. Assist the patient to change position every 2 hours.

17. The nurse is reviewing orders for several patients who have risk for fluid volume excess. For which patient condition does the nurse question an order for diuretics?
    a. Pulmonary edema
    b. Congestive heart failure
    c. End-stage renal disease
    d. Ascites

18. The UAP reports to the nurse that a patient being evaluated for kidney problems has produced a large amount of pale-yellow urine. What does the nurse do next?
    a. Instruct the UAP to measure the amount carefully and then discard the urine.
    b. Instruct the UAP to save the urine in a large bottle for a 24-hour urine specimen.
    c. Assess the patient for signs of fluid imbalance and check the specific gravity of the urine.
    d. Compare the amount of urine output to the fluid intake for the previous 8 hours.

19. On admission, a patient with pulmonary edema weighed 151 lbs.; now the patient's weight is 149 lbs. Assuming the patient was weighed both times with the same clothing, same scale, and same time of day, how many milliliters of fluid does the nurse estimate the patient has lost?
    a. 500
    b. 1000
    c. 2000
    d. 2500

20. The nurse is giving discharge instructions to the patient with advanced heart failure who is at continued risk for fluid volume excess. For which physical change does the nurse instruct the patient to call the health care provider?
    a. Greater than 3 lbs. gained in a week or greater than 1 to 2 lbs. gained in a 24-hour period
    b. Greater than 5 lbs. gained in a week or greater than 1 to 2 lbs. gained in a 24-hour period
    c. Greater than 15 lbs. gained in a month or greater than 5 lbs. gained in a week
    d. Greater than 20 lbs. gained in a month or greater than 5 lbs. gained in a week

21. The nurse is caring for several patients at risk for falls because of fluid and electrolyte imbalances. Which task related to patient safety and fall prevention does the nurse delegate to the UAP?
    a. Assess for orthostatic hypotension.
    b. Orient the patient to the environment.
    c. Help the incontinent patient to toilet every 1 to 2 hours.
    d. Encourage family members or significant other to stay with the patient.

22. The nurse is assessing a patient's urine specific gravity. The value is 1.035. How does the nurse interpret this result?
    a. Overhydration
    b. Dehydration
    c. Normal value for an adult
    d. Renal disease

23. What are the functions of potassium in the body? *(Select all that apply.)*
    a. Regulates hydration status
    b. Intracellular osmolarity and volume
    c. Stimulates the secretion of antidiuretic hormone (ADH)
    d. Regulates glucose use and storage
    e. Helps maintain normal cardiac rhythm

24. Which statements are true about the electrolyte chloride and its role in the cellular environment of the body? *(Select all that apply.)*
    a. It is a major cation in extracellular fluid (ECF).
    b. It maintains plasma acid-base balance.
    c. It provides electroneutrality in relation to sodium.
    d. Chloride imbalances occur with alterations in body water volume.
    e. Chloride concentration varies inversely with changes in bicarbonate concentration.

25. What impacts does sodium have on body function? *(Select all that apply.)*
    a. Maintains electroneutrality
    b. Maintains electrical membrane excitability
    c. Aids in carbohydrate and lipid metabolism
    d. Regulates water balance
    e. Regulates plasma osmolality

26. What impacts does phosphorus have in the body? *(Select all that apply.)*
    a. Adds strength/density to bones and teeth
    b. Activates vitamins and enzymes
    c. Aids in blood-clotting cascade
    d. Assists in the formation of adenosine triphosphate (ATP)
    e. Assists in cell growth and metabolism

27. The electrolyte magnesium is responsible for which functions? *(Select all that apply.)*
    a. Formation of hydrochloric acid
    b. Carbohydrate metabolism
    c. Contraction of skeletal muscle
    d. Regulation of intracellular osmolarity
    e. Formation of ATP

28. A patient is talking to the nurse about sodium intake. Which statement by the patient indicates an understanding of high-sodium food sources?
    a. "I have bacon and eggs every morning for breakfast."
    b. "We never eat seafood because of the salt water."
    c. "I love Chinese food, but I gave it up because of the soy sauce."
    d. "Pickled herring is a fish and my doctor told me to eat a lot of fish."

29. Which statement best explains how ADH affects urine output?
    a. It increases permeability to water in the tubules causing a decrease in urine output.
    b. It increases urine output as a result of water being absorbed by the tubules.
    c. Urine output is reduced as the posterior pituitary decreases ADH production.
    d. Increased urine output results from increased osmolarity and fluid in the extracellular space.

30. A patient with hyponatremia would have which gastrointestinal findings upon assessment? *(Select all that apply.)*
    a. Hyperactive bowel sounds on auscultation, mostly in the left lower quadrant
    b. Hard, dark-brown stools
    c. Hypoactive bowel sounds on auscultation
    d. Bowel movements that are frequent and watery
    e. Abdominal cramping

31. The nurse is caring for a patient with severe hypocalcemia. What safety measures does the nurse put in place for this patient? *(Select all that apply.)*
    a. Encourage the patient to use a cane when ambulating.
    b. Turn on a bed alarm when the patient is in bed.
    c. Obtain an order for zolpidem (Ambien) to ensure the patient sleeps at night.
    d. Place the patient on a low bed.
    e. Ensure the side rails are up when the patient is in bed.

32. Which patients are at risk for developing hyponatremia? *(Select all that apply.)*
    a. Postoperative patient who has been NPO (nothing by mouth) for 24 hours with no IV fluid infusing
    b. Patient with decreased fluid intake for several days
    c. Patient receiving excessive intravenous fluids with 5% dextrose
    d. Diabetic patient with blood glucose of 250 mg/dL
    e. Patient with overactive adrenal glands
    f. Tennis player in 100° F weather who has been drinking water

33. The nurse is evaluating the lab results of a patient with hyperaldosteronism. What abnormal electrolyte finding does the nurse expect to see?
    a. Hyponatremia
    b. Hyperkalemia
    c. Hypocalcemia
    d. Hypernatremia

34. The UAP informs the nurse that a patient with hypernatremia who was initially confused and disoriented on admission to the hospital is now trying to pull out the IV access and Foley catheter. What is the nurse's first action?
    a. Place bilateral soft wrist restraints.
    b. Inform the provider of the patient's change in behavior and obtain an order for restraints.
    c. Assess the patient.
    d. Offer the patient oral fluids.

35. Patients with which conditions are at risk for developing hypernatremia? *(Select all that apply.)*
    a. Chronic constipation
    b. Heart failure
    c. Severe diarrhea
    d. Poor kidney function
    e. Profound diaphoresis

36. The provider has ordered therapy for a patient with low sodium and signs of hypervolemia. Which diuretic is best for this patient?
    a. Conivaptan (Vaprisol)
    b. Furosemide (Lasix)
    c. Hydrochlorothiazide (HydroDIURIL)
    d. Bumetanide (Bumex)

37. The nurse is assessing a patient with a mild increase in sodium level. What early manifestation does the nurse observe in this patient?
    a. Muscle twitching and irregular muscle contractions
    b. Inability of muscles and nerves to respond to a stimulus
    c. Muscle weakness occurring bilaterally with no specific pattern
    d. Reduced or absent deep tendon reflexes

38. The nurse is caring for a patient with hypernatremia caused by fluid and sodium losses. What type of IV solution is best for treating this patient?
    a. Hypotonic 0.225% sodium chloride
    b. Small-volume infusions of hypertonic (2% to 3%) saline
    c. Isotonic sodium chloride (NaCl)
    d. 0.45% sodium chloride

39. Which serum value does the nurse expect to see for a patient with hyponatremia?
    a. Sodium less than 136 mEq/L
    b. Chloride less than 95 mEq/L
    c. Sodium less than 145 mEq/L
    d. Chloride less than 103 mEq/L

40. The nurse is caring for a psychiatric patient who is continuously drinking water. The nurse monitors for which complication related to potential hyponatremia?
    a. Proteinuria/prerenal failure
    b. Change in mental status/increased intracranial pressure
    c. Pitting edema/circulatory failure
    d. Possible stool for occult blood/gastrointestinal bleeding

41. What interventions are appropriate for a patient with mild hypernatremia caused by excessive fluid loss? *(Select all that apply.)*
    a. Hypotonic intravenous infusion
    b. 0.45% sodium chloride intravenous infusion
    c. D_5W intravenous infusion
    d. Administration of bumetanide (Bumex)
    e. Ensure adequate water intake

42. The nurse is caring for several patients at risk for fluid and electrolyte imbalances. Which patient problem or condition can result in a relative hypernatremia?
    a. Use of a salt substitute
    b. Presence of a feeding tube
    c. Drinking too much water
    d. NPO status

43. The nurse is caring for an older adult patient whose serum sodium level is 150 mEq/L. The nurse assesses the patient for which common manifestations associated with this sodium level? *(Select all that apply.)*
    a. Intact recall of recent events
    b. Increased pulse rate
    c. Rigidity of extremities
    d. Hyperactivity
    e. Muscle weakness

44. Which precaution or intervention does the nurse teach a patient at continued risk for hypernatremia?
    a. Avoid salt substitutes.
    b. Avoid aspirin and aspirin-containing products.
    c. Read labels on canned or packaged foods to determine sodium content.
    d. Increase daily intake of caffeine-containing foods and beverages.

45. The nurse identifies the priority problem of potential for injury for a patient with hyponatremia. What is the etiology of this priority patient problem?
    a. Altered mental capabilities
    b. Fragility of bones
    c. Immobility
    d. Altered senses

46. A patient with renal failure that results in hypernatremia will require which interventions? *(Select all that apply.)*
    a. Administration of furosemide (Lasix)
    b. Hemodialysis
    c. IV infusion of 0.9% sodium chloride
    d. Dietary sodium restriction
    e. Administration of bumetanide (Bumex)

47. The nurse is teaching a patient to recognize foods that are high in sodium. Which food items does the nurse use as examples? *(Select all that apply.)*
    a. Egg roll with soy sauce
    b. White rice
    c. Salad with oil and vinegar dressing
    d. Bacon and eggs
    e. Steak
    f. Soup with saltine crackers
    g. Steamed vegetables

48. A hospitalized patient who is known to be homeless has been diagnosed with severe malnutrition, end-stage renal disease, and anemia. He is transfused with 3 units of packed red blood cells. Which potential electrolyte imbalance does the nurse anticipate to occur in this patient?
    a. Hypernatremia
    b. Hyperkalemia
    c. Hypercalcemia
    d. Hypermagnesemia

49. A newly admitted patient with congestive heart failure has a potassium level of 5.7 mEq/L. How does the nurse identify contributing factors for the electrolyte imbalance? *(Select all that apply.)*
    a. Assess the patient for hypokalemia.
    b. Obtain a list of the patient's home medications.
    c. Assess the patient for hyperkalemia.
    d. Ask about the patient's method of taking medications at home.
    e. Evaluate the patient's appetite.

50. A young adult patient is in the early stages of being treated for severe burns. Which electrolyte imbalance does the nurse expect to assess in this patient?
    a. Hypernatremia
    b. Hypokalemia
    c. Hypercalcemia
    d. Hyperkalemia

51. A patient with hypokalemia is likely to have which conditions? *(Select all that apply.)*
    a. Liver failure
    b. Metabolic alkalosis
    c. Chronic obstructive pulmonary disease
    d. Hypothyroidism
    e. Paralytic ileus

52. The nurse is taking care of a trauma patient who was in a motor vehicle accident. The patient has a history of hypertension, which is managed with spironolactone (Aldactone). This patient is at risk for developing which electrolyte imbalance?
    a. Hyperkalemia
    b. Hypernatremia
    c. Hypokalemia
    d. Hypocalcemia

53. A patient with lung cancer is admitted to the hospital for respiratory distress. Which imbalances does the nurse expect this patient to have?
    a. Metabolic alkalosis
    b. Hypokalemia
    c. Hypermagnesemia
    d. Respiratory acidosis

54. Which serum laboratory value does the nurse expect to see in the patient with hypokalemia?
    a. Calcium less than 8.0 mg/dL
    b. Potassium less than 5.0 mEq/L
    c. Calcium less than 11.0 mg/dL
    d. Potassium less than 3.5 mEq/L

55. The patient's potassium level is 2.5 mEq/L. Which clinical findings does the nurse expect to see when assessing this patient? *(Select all that apply.)*
    a. General skeletal muscle weakness
    b. Moist crackles and tachypnea
    c. Lethargy
    d. Increased specific gravity and decreased urine output
    e. Weak hand grasps

56. The nurse administering potassium to a patient carefully monitors the infusion because of the risk for which condition?
    a. Pulmonary edema
    b. Cardiac dysrhythmia
    c. Postural hypotension
    d. Renal failure

57. Which changes on a patient's electrocardiogram (ECG) reflect hyperkalemia?
    a. Tall peaked T waves
    b. Narrow QRS complex
    c. Tall P waves
    d. Normal P-R interval

58. The nurse is teaching the patient about hypokalemia. Which statement by the patient indicates a correct understanding of the treatment of hypokalemia?
    a. "My wife does all the cooking. She shops for food high in calcium."
    b. "When I take the liquid potassium in the evening, I'll eat a snack beforehand."
    c. "I will avoid bananas, orange juice, and salt substitutes."
    d. "I hate being stuck with needles all the time to monitor how much sugar I can eat."

59. The nurse is caring for a patient who takes potassium and digoxin. For what reason does the nurse monitor both laboratory results?
    a. Digoxin increases potassium loss through the kidneys.
    b. Digoxin toxicity can result if hypokalemia is present.
    c. Digoxin may cause potassium levels to rise to toxic levels.
    d. Hypokalemia causes the cardiac muscle to be less sensitive to digoxin.

60. Which serum laboratory value does the nurse expect to see in a patient with hyperkalemia?
    a. Calcium greater than 8.0 mg/dL
    b. Potassium greater than 3.5 mEq/L
    c. Calcium greater than 11.0 mg/dL
    d. Potassium greater than 5.0 mEq/L

61. A patient has an elevated potassium level. Which assessment findings are associated with hyperkalemia? *(Select all that apply.)*
    a. Wheezing on exhalation
    b. Numbness in hands, feet, and around the mouth
    c. Frequent, explosive diarrhea stools
    d. Irregular heart rate and hypotension
    e. Circumoral cyanosis

62. The nurse is teaching a patient with hypokalemia about foods high in potassium. Which food items does the nurse recommend to this patient? *(Select all that apply.)*
    a. Soybeans
    b. Lettuce
    c. Cantaloupe
    d. Potatoes
    e. Peaches

63. A patient's serum potassium value is below 2.8 mEq/L. The patient is also on digoxin. The nurse quickly assesses the patient for which cardiac problem before notifying the provider?
    a. Cardiac murmur
    b. Cardiac dysrhythmia
    c. Congestive heart failure
    d. Cardiac tamponade

64. Which potassium levels are within normal limits? *(Select all that apply.)*
    a. 2.0 mmol/L
    b. 3.5 mmol/L
    c. 4.5 mmol/L
    d. 5.0 mmol/L
    e. 6.0 mmol/L

65. A patient has hyperkalemia resulting from dehydration. Which additional laboratory findings does the nurse anticipate for this patient?
    a. Increased hematocrit and hemoglobin levels
    b. Decreased serum electrolyte levels
    c. Increased urine potassium levels
    d. Decreased serum creatinine

66. A 65-year-old patient has a potassium laboratory value of 5.0 mEq/L. How does the nurse interpret this value?
    a. High for the patient's age
    b. Low for the patient's age
    c. Normal for the patient's age
    d. Dependent upon the medical diagnosis

67. A patient's potassium level is low. What change in the cardiovascular system does the nurse expect to see related to hypokalemia?
    a. Tall, peaked T waves
    b. Weak, thready pulse
    c. Malignant hypertension
    d. Distended neck vein

68. Plasma is part of which components? *(Select all that apply.)*
    a. The intracellular compartment
    b. The extracellular compartment
    c. All fluid within the cells
    d. Interstitial fluid
    e. Intravascular fluid

69. Which fluid has the highest corresponding electrolyte content?
    a. Intracellular fluid is highest in potassium.
    b. Extracellular fluid is highest in sodium.
    c. Extracellular fluid is highest in sodium and chloride.
    d. Intracellular fluid is highest in magnesium and sodium.

70. Which component has a high content of potassium and phosphorus?
    a. Extracellular fluid
    b. Intracellular fluid
    c. Extracellular fluid and the intravascular space
    d. Intracellular fluid and lymph fluid

71. A patient with low potassium must have an IV potassium infusion. The pharmacy sends a 250-mL IV bag of dextrose in water with 40 mEq of potassium. The label is marked "to infuse over 1 hour." What is the nurse's best action?
    a. Obtain a pump and administer the solution.
    b. Double-check the provider's order and call the pharmacy.
    c. Hold the infusion because there is an error in labeling.
    d. Recalculate the rate so that it is safe for the patient.

72. An older adult patient needs an oral potassium solution, but is refusing it because it has a strong and unpleasant taste. What is the best strategy the nurse uses to administer the drug?
    a. Tell the patient that failure to take the drug could result in serious heart problems.
    b. Ask the patient's preference of juice and mix the drug with a small amount.
    c. Mix the solution into food on the patient's meal tray and encourage the patient to eat everything.
    d. Offer the drug to the patient several times and then document the patient's refusal.

73. A patient has a low potassium level and the provider has ordered an IV infusion. Before starting an IV potassium infusion, what does the nurse assess?
    a. Intravenous line patency
    b. Oxygen saturation level
    c. Baseline mental status
    d. Apical pulse

74. Which foods will the nurse instruct a patient with kidney disease and hyperkalemia to avoid? *(Select all that apply.)*
    a. Canned apricots
    b. Dried beans
    c. Potatoes
    d. Cabbage
    e. Cantaloupe

75. Which assessment findings are related to prolonged hypercalcemia? *(Select all that apply.)*
    a. Prolonged bradycardia
    b. Paresthesia
    c. Leg cramping
    d. Hyperactive bowel sounds
    e. Shortened QT interval
    f. Impaired blood flow
    g. Profound muscle weakness

76. Which nursing interventions apply to patients with hypercalcemia? *(Select all that apply.)*
    a. Administer IV normal saline (0.9% sodium chloride).
    b. Assess the patient for a positive Homans' sign.
    c. Measure the abdominal girth.
    d. Massage calves to encourage blood return to the heart.
    e. Monitor for ECG changes.
    f. Provide adequate intake of vitamin D.
    g. During treatment, monitor for tetany.

77. The nurse is reviewing the laboratory calcium level results for a patient. Which value indicates mild hypocalcemia?
    a. 5.0 mg/dL
    b. 8.0 mg/dL
    c. 10.0 mg/dL
    d. 12.0 mg/dL

78. A patient with a recent history of anterior neck injury reports muscle twitching and spasms with tingling in the lips, nose, and ears. The nurse suspects these symptoms may be caused by which condition?
    a. Hypocalcemia
    b. Hypokalemia
    c. Hyponatremia
    d. Hypomagnesemia

79. Which conditions cause a patient to be at risk for hypocalcemia? *(Select all that apply.)*
    a. Crohn's disease
    b. Acute pancreatitis
    c. Removal or destruction of parathyroid glands
    d. Immobility
    e. Use of digitalis

80. The nurse is assessing the patient with a risk for hypocalcemia. What is the correct technique to test for Chvostek's sign?
    a. Patient flexes arms against the chest and examiner attempts to pull the arms away from the chest.
    b. Place a blood pressure cuff around the upper arm and inflate the cuff to greater than the patient's systolic pressure.
    c. Tap the patient's face just below and in front of the ear to trigger facial twitching of one side of the mouth, nose, and cheek.
    d. Lightly tap the patient's patellar and Achilles tendons with a reflex hammer and measure the movement.

81. The nurse is caring for several patients with electrolyte imbalances. Which intervention is included in the plan of care for a patient with hypocalcemia?
    a. Implementing an oral fluid restriction of 1500 mL/day
    b. Implementing a renal diet
    c. Providing moderate environmental stimulation with music
    d. Placing the patient on seizure precautions

82. Which clinical condition can result from hypocalcemia?
    a. Stimulated cardiac muscle contraction
    b. Increased intestinal and gastric motility
    c. Decreased peripheral nerve excitability
    d. Increased bone density

83. Which patient is at greatest risk of developing hypocalcemia?
    a. 30-year-old Asian woman with breast cancer
    b. 45-year-old Caucasian man with hypertension and diuretic therapy
    c. 60-year-old African-American woman with a recent ileostomy
    d. 70-year-old Caucasian man on long-term lithium therapy

84. Which is a preventive measure for patients at risk for developing hypocalcemia?
    a. Increase daily dietary calcium and vitamin D intake.
    b. Increase intake of phosphorus.
    c. Apply sunblock and wear protective clothing whenever outdoors.
    d. Administer calcium-containing IV fluids to patients receiving multiple blood transfusions.

85. The patient who has undergone which surgical procedure is most at risk for hypocalcemia?
    a. Thyroidectomy
    b. Adrenalectomy
    c. Pancreatectomy
    d. Gastrectomy

86. Which medication order does the nurse clarify before administering the drug to a patient with hypomagnesemia?
    a. Magnesium sulfate 1 g IM every 6 hours for four doses
    b. Aluminum hydroxide (AlternaGEL) 15 mL orally three times a day and at bedtime
    c. Calcium carbonate 1000 mg orally after meals and at bedtime
    d. Calcium gluconate 5 mEq IV prn for tetany

87. Which are typical nursing assessment findings for a patient with hypocalcemia? (Select all that apply.)
    a. Positive Chvostek's sign
    b. Hypertension
    c. Diarrhea
    d. Prolonged ST interval
    e. Elevated T wave

88. Which intervention does the nurse implement for a patient with hypocalcemia?
    a. Encourage activity by the patient as tolerated, including weight-lifting.
    b. Encourage socialization and active participation in stimulating activities.
    c. Include a tracheostomy tray at the bedside for emergency use.
    d. Provide adequate intake of vitamin D and calcium-rich foods.

89. A patient has chronic kidney disease (CKD). Which electrolyte imbalance often associated with hypocalcaemia and CKD does the nurse monitor for?
    a. Hypophosphatemia
    b. Hyperphosphatemia
    c. Hyperkalemia
    d. Hyponatremia

90. A patient with hypocalcemia is in need of supplemental diet therapy. Which foods does the nurse recommend to provide both calcium and vitamin D? *(Select all that apply.)*
    a. Tofu
    b. Cheese
    c. Eggs
    d. Broccoli
    e. Milk

91. A patient shows a positive Trousseau's or Chvostek's sign. The nurse prepares to give the patient which urgent treatment?
    a. IV calcium
    b. Calcitonin (Calcimar)
    c. IV potassium chloride
    d. Large doses of oral calcium

92. Which are preventive nursing interventions for a patient at risk for developing hypercalcemia? *(Select all that apply.)*
    a. Administer D$_5$W.
    b. Administer furosemide (Lasix).
    c. Ensure adequate hydration.
    d. Administer plicamycin (Mithracin).
    e. Discourage weight-bearing activity such as walking.

93. The nurse caring for a patient with hypercalcemia anticipates orders for which medications? *(Select all that apply.)*
    a. Magnesium sulfate
    b. Calcitonin (Calcimar)
    c. Furosemide (Lasix)
    d. Plicamycin (Mithracin)
    e. Calcium gluconate
    f. Aluminum hydroxide

94. The nurse instructs the UAP to use precautions with moving and using a lift sheet for which patient with an electrolyte imbalance?
    a. Young diabetic woman with hyperkalemia
    b. Psychiatric patient with hyponatremia
    c. Older woman with hypocalcemia
    d. Child with severe diarrhea and hypomagnesemia

95. A patient's laboratory results show a decrease in serum phosphorus level. The nurse expects to see a reciprocal increased change in which serum level?
    a. Calcium
    b. Potassium
    c. Sodium
    d. Magnesium

96. Which intervention does the nurse include for a patient with moderate hypophosphatemia?
    a. Aggressive treatment with parenteral phosphorous
    b. Administration of oral vitamin D and phosphorus supplements
    c. Concurrent administration of calcium supplements
    d. Elimination of beef, pork, and legumes from the diet

97. Which manifestations reflect severe hypophosphatemia? *(Select all that apply.)*
    a. Profound muscle weakness
    b. Decreased peristalsis
    c. Elevated T wave
    d. Irritability
    e. Cardiac muscle damage

98. Which factors can cause hyperphosphatemia? *(Select all that apply.)*
    a. Tumor lysis syndrome
    b. Decreased intake of phosphorus
    c. Hypoparathyroidism
    d. Decreased renal excretion
    e. Hyperthyroidism

99. What are common causes of hypophosphate-mia? *(Select all that apply.)*
    a. Increased intake of phosphorus
    b. Hypercalcemia
    c. Immobility
    d. Uncontrolled diabetes
    e. Use of magnesium-based antacids

100. A patient with which condition would need priority nursing assessment?
    a. Renal insufficiency
    b. Potassium level of 3.4 mEq/L
    c. Sodium level of 133 mEq/L
    d. Irritability

101. The health care provider orders magnesium sulfate (MgSO$_4$) for a patient with severe hypomagnesemia. What is the preferred route of administration for this drug?
    a. Oral
    b. Subcutaneous
    c. Intramuscular
    d. Intravenous

102. The nurse is assessing a patient with severe hypermagnesemia. Which assessment findings are associated with this electrolyte imbalance?
    a. Bradycardia and hypotension
    b. Tachycardia and weak palpable pulse
    c. Hypertension and irritability
    d. Irregular pulse and deep respirations

103. A patient in the hospital has a severely elevated magnesium level. Which intervention should the nurse complete first?
    a. Discontinue oral magnesium.
    b. Administer furosemide (Lasix).
    c. Discontinue parenteral magnesium.
    d. Administer calcium to treat bradycardia.

104. A patient has a magnesium level of 0.8 mg/dL. Which treatment does the nurse expect to be ordered for this patient?
    a. Intramuscular magnesium sulfate
    b. Increased intake of fruits and vegetables
    c. Oral preparations of magnesium sulfate
    d. IV magnesium sulfate and discontinuation of diuretic therapy

105. The nurse monitors the effectiveness of magnesium sulfate by assessing which factor every hour?
    a. Deep tendon reflexes
    b. Vital signs
    c. Serum laboratory values
    d. Urine output

106. Which condition places a patient at risk for hypocalcemia, hyperkalemia, and hypernatremia?
    a. Hypothyroidism
    b. Diabetes mellitus
    c. Chronic kidney disease
    d. Adrenal insufficiency

107. A patient with congestive heart failure is receiving a loop diuretic. The nurse monitors for which electrolyte imbalances? *(Select all that apply.)*
    a. Hypocalcemia
    b. Hypokalemia
    c. Hyponatremia
    d. Hypercalcemia
    e. Hyperkalemia
    f. Hypernatremia

12 CHAPTER

Assessment and Care of Patients with Acid-Base Imbalances

1. A patient with chronic obstructive pulmonary disease (COPD) has just developed respiratory distress. Vital signs are: pulse oximetry 88% on 2 L nasal cannula oxygen; dyspnea at rest; respirations 32 per minute. The patient reports shortness of breath. Which statements apply to this clinical situation? *(Select all that apply.)*
   a. Interference in alveolar-capillary diffusion results in carbon dioxide retention.
   b. The nurse should instruct the patient to use pursed-lip breathing.
   c. Position the patient with the head of the bed at less than 20 degrees.
   d. Interference in alveolar-capillary diffusion results in acidemia.
   e. The nurse should explain to the patient that the need for rapid breathing will relieve the shortness of breath.

2. The unlicensed assistive personnel (UAP) notifies the nurse that the patient with emphysema on oxygen at 2 L via nasal cannula is short of breath after morning care. What is the nurse's best first action?
   a. Page the provider immediately.
   b. Ask the UAP to check the patient's SaO_2 level.
   c. Instruct the UAP to check vital signs.
   d. Document the incident in the patient's chart.

3. A patient with bilateral lower lobe pneumonia is diagnosed with respiratory acidosis based on arterial blood gas (ABG) results. What is the likely cause of the patient's respiratory acidosis?
   a. Underelimination of carbon dioxide from the lungs
   b. Buffering of extracellular fluid by ammonium
   c. Overelimination of carbon dioxide from the lungs
   d. An increased bicarbonate level due to respiratory elimination of acid

4. A patient is admitted to the hospital for diabetic ketoacidosis. Which ABG results should the nurse expect? *(Select all that apply.)*
   a. pH 7.32
   b. $Paco_2$ 55 mm Hg
   c. Bicarbonate (Bicarb) 18 mEq/L
   d. pH 7.46
   e. Bicarb 29 mEq/L

5. A patient who recently emigrated to the U.S. from Germany, but speaks fluent English, has been admitted to the emergency department (ED) with diabetic ketoacidosis. On intake assessment, the patient cannot recall the medications she takes. What first action does the nurse take?
   a. Instruct the patient to compare a hospital list of medications to her home medications.
   b. Ask the patient's significant other to bring the patient's medications from home.
   c. Request that the patient complete a meal recall for the past 24 hours.
   d. Teach the patient about the importance of keeping a list of current medications in her purse.

6. A patient who has pancreatitis with nausea and vomiting will likely have which related alterations in acid-base balance? *(Select all that apply.)*
   a. Overproduction of hydrogen ions
   b. Metabolic acidosis
   c. Serum pH value that is directly related to the concentration of hydrogen ions
   d. Underproduction of bicarbonate
   e. Metabolic alkalosis

7. Which statements correctly apply to acid-base balance in the body? *(Select all that apply.)*
   a. Renal mechanisms are stronger in regulating acid-base balance, but slower to respond than respiratory mechanisms.
   b. The immediate binding of excess hydrogen ions occurs primarily in the red blood cells.
   c. Combined acidosis is less severe than either metabolic acidosis or respiratory acidosis alone.
   d. Respiratory acidosis is caused by a patent airway.
   e. Acid-base balance occurs through control of hydrogen ion production and elimination.

8. The nurse is interpreting the ABG results of a patient with acute respiratory insufficiency. As the $Paco_2$ level increases, which result would the nurse expect?
   a. Decreased pH
   b. Decreased Bicarb
   c. Increased Pao_2
   d. Increased pH

9. The nurse is admitting a patient with acute kidney injury to the medical unit. Which ABG results would she expect for this patient?
   a. Respiratory acidosis
   b. Metabolic acidosis
   c. Respiratory alkalosis
   d. Metabolic alkalosis

10. For which conditions will the plasma pH decrease? *(Select all that apply.)*
    a. Increase in $Paco_2$
    b. Decrease in HCO_3^-
    c. Increase in lactic acid
    d. Increase in HCO_3^-
    e. Decrease in CO_2

11. Which blood pH value does the nurse interpret as within normal limits?
    a. 7.27
    b. 7.37
    c. 7.47
    d. 7.5

12. The early stage of incomplete breakdown of glucose occurs whenever cells metabolize under anaerobic conditions to form lactic acid. Based on this knowledge of pathophysiology, which conditions could cause the patient to develop acidosis? *(Select all that apply.)*
    a. Sepsis
    b. Hypovolemic shock
    c. Use of a mechanical ventilator
    d. Prolonged nasogastric suctioning
    e. Hypoventilation

13. Which patient with the highest risk for acidosis must the nurse care for first?
    a. Patient in mild pain with a kidney stone
    b. Patient with chronic obstructive pulmonary disease, pulse oximetry 88% on 2 L oxygen
    c. Patient who just had a seizure with pulse oximetry of 91%
    d. Patient with a rectal tube in place for frequent diarrhea

14. A patient's ABG results show an increase in pH. Which condition is most likely to contribute to this laboratory value?
    a. Mechanical ventilation
    b. Ketoacidosis
    c. Nasogastric suction
    d. Diarrhea

15. Which patient is most likely to have a decrease in bicarbonate?
    a. Patient with pancreatitis
    b. Patient with hypoventilation
    c. Patient who is vomiting
    d. Patient with emphysema

16. A patient has a new onset of shallow and slow respirations. While the patient's body attempts to compensate, what happens to the patient's pH level?
    a. Increases
    b. Decreases
    c. Stabilizes
    d. Fluctuates

17. A patient is at risk for acid-base imbalance. Which laboratory value indicates that the patient is acidotic?
    a. $Paco_2$ = 55 mm Hg
    b. HCO_3^- = 25 mEq/L
    c. Lactate = 2.5 mmol/L
    d. pH = 7.30

18. Which type of medication increases an older adult patient's risk for acid-base imbalance?
    a. Antilipemics
    b. Hormonal therapy
    c. Diuretics
    d. Antidysrhythmics

19. Which medication usage could cause metabolic acidosis?
    a. Aspirin overdose
    b. Overuse of antacids
    c. Prolonged use of antihistamines
    d. Vitamin overdose

20. Which nursing assessment finding indicates a worsening of respiratory acidosis?
    a. Decreased respiratory rate
    b. Decreased blood pressure
    c. Use of accessory respiratory muscles
    d. Pale nail beds

21. Which patient is most likely to have respiratory acidosis?
    a. Patient who is anxious and breathing rapidly
    b. Patient with multiple rib fractures
    c. Patient with IV normal saline bolus
    d. Patient with increased urinary output

22. Which patient requires assessment related to inadequate chest expansion that would place the patient at risk for respiratory acidosis? *(Select all that apply.)*
    a. Patient with lordosis
    b. Patient with emphysema
    c. Severely obese patient on prolonged bedrest
    d. Patient in the first trimester of pregnancy
    e. Patient 2 days postoperative for cholecystectomy

23. The nurse reviews the electrocardiogram (ECG) and cardiovascular status of a patient. Which findings are early changes associated with mild acidosis?
    a. Decreased heart rate with hypertension
    b. Hypotension and faint peripheral pulses
    c. Increased heart rate and increased cardiac output
    d. Peaked T waves and wide QRS complexes

24. The nurse is assessing a patient with an acid-base imbalance by using Gordon's Functional Health Patterns. What primary areas are affected? *(Select all that apply.)*
    a. Values/Beliefs
    b. Activity-Exercise
    c. Health Perception–Health Management
    d. Elimination
    e. Sleep–Rest
    f. Coping–Stress Tolerance

25. The nurse is testing the muscle strength of a patient at risk for acid-base imbalance. Which technique does the nurse use to test arm strength?
    a. Asks the patient to hold the arms straight out in front and the nurse observes for drift.
    b. The patient flexes the arms against the chest; the nurse tries to pull the arms from the chest.
    c. Asks the patient to pick up an object that weighs at least 10 lbs.
    d. The patient clasps the hands together and pushes as hard as possible.

26. The nurse assesses an acidotic patient's lower extremities for strength as part of the nursing shift assessment. What finding does the nurse expect to see?
    a. Bilateral weakness
    b. Weakness on the dominant side
    c. No change from baseline
    d. Cramping, but no weakness

27. The nurse observes tall peaked T waves on the ECG of a patient with metabolic acidosis. Before notifying the health care provider, the nurse would assess the results of which laboratory test?
    a. Serum calcium
    b. Serum glucose
    c. Serum potassium
    d. Serum magnesium

28. Which signs and symptoms would the nurse expect to assess in a patient with metabolic acidosis? *(Select all that apply.)*
    a. Kussmaul's respirations
    b. Shallow, rapid respirations
    c. Warm, flushed skin
    d. Skin pale to cyanotic
    e. Elevated $Paco_2$
    f. Decreased bicarbonate

29. What interventions are included in the plan of care for a patient with metabolic ketoacidosis? *(Select all that apply.)*
    a. Monitor ABG levels for decreasing pH level, as appropriate.
    b. Maintain patent IV access.
    c. Administer fluids as prescribed.
    d. Monitor for irritability and muscle tetany.
    e. Monitor loss of bicarbonate through the gastrointestinal tract such as diarrhea.

30. What is the priority intervention for a patient with diabetic ketoacidosis?
    a. Administer bicarbonate.
    b. Administer oxygen.
    c. Administer insulin.
    d. Administer potassium.

31. Which statement made by the patient indicates that he or she may have an alkaline condition?
    a. "I am more and more tired and can't concentrate."
    b. "I have tingling in my fingers and toes."
    c. "My feet and ankles are swollen."
    d. "I am short of breath all of the time."

32. Which patient is most likely to have respiratory alkalosis?
    a. Hypoxic patient
    b. Patient with a body cast
    c. Patient having a panic attack
    d. Morbidly obese patient

33. Which type of electrolyte imbalance does the nurse expect to see in a patient with metabolic alkalosis?
    a. Hyperkalemia
    b. Hypophosphatemia
    c. Hyperchloremia
    d. Hypocalcemia

34. Which patient is most likely to develop metabolic alkalosis as a result of base excess?
    a. Patient taking thiazide diuretics
    b. Patient who is having nasogastric suction
    c. Patient with severe vomiting
    d. Patient who had a massive blood transfusion

35. The nurse is assessing a patient with metabolic alkalosis. Which neuromuscular finding is the most ominous and warrants immediate notification of the health care provider?
    a. Muscle cramps
    b. Muscle twitching
    c. Hyperactive deep tendon reflexes
    d. Tetany

36. The nurse is caring for a patient with metabolic alkalosis secondary to diuretic medication. Which equipment does the nurse obtain to administer the correct therapy to this patient?
    a. Oxygen tubing and cannula or mask
    b. IV catheter and IV start kit
    c. Foley catheter and drainage bag
    d. Antiemetic drug and emesis basin

37. Which occurrence can be a result of hyperventilation?
    a. Hypocalcemia
    b. Anxiety
    c. Respiratory alkalosis
    d. Respiratory acidosis

38. Which patient showing symptoms of an acid-base imbalance must the nurse see first?
    a. Patient who exhibits increased heart rate of 110/min and increased cardiac output
    b. Patient showing activity weakness and lethargy
    c. Patient who has a reduced attention span
    d. Patient who has asymptomatic bradycardia with a heart rate of 57/min

39. A patient has taken antacids for the past 3 days to relieve "heartburn." What alteration in acid-base balance would the nurse expect for this patient?
    a. Respiratory alkalosis
    b. Metabolic acidosis
    c. Metabolic alkalosis
    d. Respiratory acidosis

40. A patient with anemia has completed a blood transfusion of 2 units of packed red blood cells. Which imbalance should the nurse monitor for after the blood transfusion?
    a. Metabolic alkalosis
    b. Respiratory acidosis
    c. Metabolic acidosis
    d. Respiratory alkalosis

41. A patient is hospitalized with hyperglycemia and has a blood glucose of 476 mg/dL. Which signs and symptoms does the nurse expect to see in this patient? *(Select all that apply.)*
    a. Hyperventilation
    b. Kussmaul's respirations
    c. Respiratory acidosis
    d. Hypotension
    e. Metabolic acidosis

42. A patient has had diarrhea for the past 2 days. Which acid-base abnormalities would the nurse monitor for? *(Select all that apply.)*
    a. Overelimination of bicarbonate
    b. Respiratory alkalosis
    c. Metabolic acidosis
    d. Underelimination of hydrogen ions
    e. Overproduction of hydrogen ions

43. A patient who has advanced muscular dystrophy may develop which complications related to the disease? *(Select all that apply.)*
    a. Hyperventilation
    b. Hypoventilation
    c. Underproduction of bicarbonate
    d. Respiratory acidosis
    e. Underelimination of hydrogen ions

44. A patient who has a decreased amount of hydrogen ions and a decreased amount of carbon dioxide in the body will have what response?
    a. Decreased rate and depth of respirations
    b. Decreased renal absorption of hydrogen ions
    c. Increased rate and depth of respirations
    d. Decreased renal excretions of bicarbonate

45. A patient's ABG results reveal respiratory acidosis. How does the body compensate for this imbalance?
    a. Loss of bicarbonate
    b. Regular, unlabored respirations
    c. Hypoventilation
    d. Renal reabsorption of bicarbonate

46. The nurse is caring for a patient with excessive alcohol ingestion and salicylate intoxication. What is the most likely acid-base imbalance this patient will have?
    a. Bicarbonate underelimination
    b. Bicarbonate loss
    c. Metabolic acidosis
    d. Metabolic alkalosis

47. Which ABG results would the nurse interpret as metabolic alkalosis? *(Select all that apply.)*
    a. pH 7.30, $Paco_2$ 66, bicarbonate 38, Pao_2 70
    b. pH 7.52, $Paco_2$ 45, bicarbonate 36, Pao_2 95
    c. pH 7.55, $Paco_2$ 24, bicarbonate 20, Pao_2 95
    d. pH 7.28, $Paco_2$ 24, bicarbonate 15, Pao_2 95
    e. pH 7.45, $Paco_2$ 50, bicarbonate 42, Pao_2 80

48. Which arterial blood gas results would the nurse interpret as within normal limits?
    a. pH 7.28, $Paco_2$ 24, bicarbonate 15, Pao_2 95
    b. pH 7.45, $Paco_2$ 41, bicarbonate 25, Pao_2 97
    c. pH 7.35, $Paco_2$ 24, bicarbonate 15, Pao_2 95
    d. pH 7.30, $Paco_2$ 66, bicarbonate 38, Pao_2 70

49. A patient has a low pH level. Which other concurrent change does the nurse expect to see in this patient?
    a. Elevated serum sodium level
    b. Elevated serum potassium
    c. Decreased serum chloride level
    d. Decreased serum calcium level

50. What is the safest way to administer oxygen to a patient with chronic respiratory acidosis?
    a. High-volume intermittent positive pressure
    b. Low-flow oxygen (2 L/min) via nasal cannula
    c. High-flow 40% oxygen via facemask
    d. Positive end-expiratory pressure (PEEP)

51. Which assessment finding indicates that a patient with chronic respiratory acidosis is responding favorably to treatment?
    a. Nail beds pale, extremities cool
    b. Respiratory stridor with inspiration
    c. Expectorating clear, thin mucus
    d. Diffuse crackles auscultated bilaterally

52. In order to ensure the safety of a patient with metabolic alkalosis, which task is best to delegate to the UAP?
    a. Watch the patient when he or she eats or drinks anything.
    b. Sit with the patient to prevent wandering.
    c. Clean up spills immediately.
    d. Remove all sharp objects from the bedside table.

53. Which ABG values indicate an alkaline condition?
    a. $Paco_2 = 66$
    b. Bicarbonate = 16
    c. pH = 7.55
    d. pH = 7.32

54. Which conditions cause the underproduction of bicarbonate? *(Select all that apply.)*
    a. Heavy exercise
    b. Kidney failure
    c. Liver failure
    d. Seizure activity
    e. Dehydration
    f. Diarrhea

13 CHAPTER

Infusion Therapy

1. The nurse is preparing to start an infusion of 10% dextrose. Why would the nurse infuse the solution through a central line?
   a. Osmolarity of the solution could cause phlebitis or thrombosis.
   b. The patient could be at risk for fluid overload.
   c. Viscosity of the solution would slow the infusion.
   d. The solution should not be mixed with other drugs or solutions.

2. A patient is in the hospital for his first chemotherapy treatment for lung cancer. Which IV access methods are appropriate for this patient? *(Select all that apply.)*
   a. Peripheral IV access
   b. Peripherally inserted central catheter (PICC)
   c. Dialysis catheter
   d. Tunneled central venous catheter
   e. Implanted port

3. A patient has a peripherally inserted central catheter (PICC) placed and is ordered to receive IV cisplatin (Platinol). The drug has infiltrated into the tissue and redness is observed in the right lower side of the neck. What is the nurse's first action?
   a. Apply cold compresses to the site of swelling.
   b. Stop the infusion and disconnect the IV line from the administration set.
   c. Aspirate the drug from the IV access device.
   d. Monitor the patient and document.

4. The nurse is preparing to give a patient IV drug therapy. What information does the nurse need before administering the drug? *(Select all that apply.)*
   a. Indications, contraindications, and precautions for IV therapy
   b. Appropriate dilution, pH, and osmolarity of solution
   c. Rate of infusion and dosage of drugs
   d. Compatibility with other IV medications
   e. Percentage of adverse events for the drug
   f. Specifics of monitoring because of immediate effect

5. The charge nurse is reviewing IV therapy orders. What information must be included in each order? *(Select all that apply.)*
   a. Specific type of solution
   b. Rate of administration
   c. Specific drug dose to be added to the solution
   d. Method for diluting drugs for the solution
   e. Specific type of administration equipment

6. The nurse must insert a short peripheral IV catheter. In order to decrease the risk of deep vein thrombosis or phlebitis, which vein does the nurse choose for the infusion site?
   a. Wrist
   b. Foot
   c. Forearm
   d. Antecubital

7. A patient requires IV therapy via a peripheral line. What considerations does the nurse use when inserting the peripheral IV? *(Select all that apply.)*
   a. Use either an upper or lower extremity for the insertion site.
   b. Start with more distal sites, such as the hand veins.
   c. Start with more proximal sites, such as the forearm.
   d. Choose the patient's nondominant arm.
   e. Do not use the arm if the patient had a mastectomy on that side.
   f. If the vein is hard and cordlike, use an indirect approach.
   g. Avoid placing an IV over the palm side of the wrist.

8. The nurse is assessing a patient's IV site and identifies signs and symptoms of infiltration. What is the first action that the nurse implements for this patient?
   a. Elevates the extremity
   b. Applies a sterile dressing if weeping from the tissue has occurred
   c. Removes the IV access
   d. Stops the infusion

9. Which items does the nurse include in the documentation after completing the insertion of a PICC? *(Select all that apply.)*
   a. Type of dressing applied
   b. Response of the family to IV access
   c. Type of IV access device used
   d. How long it took to place the IV access
   e. Location and vein that was used for insertion

10. The nurse is selecting a site for peripheral IV insertion. Which patient condition influences the choice of left versus right upper extremity?
   a. Pneumothorax with a chest tube on the right side
   b. Myocardial infarction with pain radiating down the left arm
   c. Right hip fracture with immobilization and traction in place
   d. Regular renal dialysis with a shunt in the left upper forearm

11. The nurse is attempting to insert a peripheral IV when the patient reports tingling and a feeling like "pins and needles." What does the nurse do next?
   a. Change to a short-winged butterfly needle.
   b. Stop immediately, remove the catheter, and choose a new site.
   c. Ask the patient to wiggle the fingers to stimulate circulation.
   d. Pause the procedure and gently massage the fingers.

12. A patient has been on prolonged steroid therapy. In assessing the patient for IV insertion, what finding does the nurse expect to see?
   a. Ecchymosis and possibly a hematoma
   b. Skin that is thick, tough, dry, and difficult to puncture
   c. Edema or puffiness, making visualization of veins difficult
   d. Rash with excoriation from scratching, which limits site selection

13. Under what circumstances does the nurse elect to use only one secondary set rather than a secondary set for each medication?
   a. When multiple intermittent medications are required
   b. To eliminate the cost of using multiple secondary sets
   c. When the nurse is using the back-priming method
   d. When the medications are compatible

14. When using an intermittent administration set to deliver medications, how often does the Infusion Nurses Society recommend that the set be changed?
   a. Every 24 hours
   b. Every shift
   c. Every morning
   d. After every dose

15. The nurse is supervising a student nurse who is preparing an IV bag with IV administration tubing. For which action by the student nurse must the nurse intervene?
    a. The student touches the drip chamber.
    b. The sterile cap from the distal end of the set is removed.
    c. The distal end is attached to a needleless connector.
    d. The student touches the tubing spike.

16. The nurse is caring for a patient with a Groshong catheter. According to the manufacturer's recommendations, which technique does the nurse use in maintaining this type of catheter?
    a. Flush the catheter with heparin.
    b. Flush the catheter with saline.
    c. Avoid flushing the catheter.
    d. Aspirate the catheter to remove clots.

17. A patient has a PICC placed by an IV therapy nurse at the bedside. Before using the catheter, how is its placement verified?
    a. The provider who ordered the procedure verifies placement.
    b. The line is aspirated gently and the nurse watches for blood return.
    c. A chest x-ray is taken, which shows the catheter tip in the lower superior vena cava.
    d. The line is slowly flushed with 10 mL of saline while the nurse notes the ease of flow.

18. A patient requires a nontunneled percutaneous central catheter. What is the nurse's role in this procedure?
    a. Insert the catheter using sterile technique.
    b. Place the patient in Trendelenburg position.
    c. Read the chest x-ray to validate placement.
    d. Select and prepare the insertion site.

19. A patient requires an infusion of packed red blood cells (PRBCs). Which factor allows the nurse to infuse the PRBCs through the patient's PICC?
    a. Length of the PICC allows infusion within 6 hours.
    b. The nurse is unable to obtain an infusion pump.
    c. Lumen size of the PICC is 4 Fr or larger.
    d. PRBCs can be warmed before infusion.

20. Which patient is the most likely candidate for a tunneled central venous catheter?
    a. Patient with trauma from a motor vehicle accident
    b. Patient in need of IV antibiotics for several weeks
    c. Patient in need of permanent parental nutrition
    d. Patient in need of intermittent chemotherapy

21. Which nursing interventions are implemented when caring for a patient with an implanted port? *(Select all that apply.)*
    a. Before puncture, palpate the port to locate the septum.
    b. Use a large-bore needle to access the port.
    c. Flush the port before each use.
    d. Use a noncoring needle to access the port.
    e. Flush the port at least once a month.

22. A 65-year-old patient has been receiving IV fluids at 100 mL/hr of $D_5$1/2% normal saline (NS) for the past 3 days, along with IV antibiotic therapy. After receiving the new antibiotic, the patient reports chills and a headache. On assessment, the patient's temperature is elevated. What complication do these assessment findings indicate?
    a. Catheter-related infection in the blood
    b. Allergic reaction to the antibiotics
    c. Speed shock
    d. Circulatory overload

23. A patient has a central line inserted in the vena cava. The nurse assesses the patient for which potential complications related to the procedure? *(Select all that apply.)*
    a. Phlebitis
    b. Hemothorax
    c. Air embolism
    d. Cardiac tamponade
    e. Arterial puncture

24. The nurse is helping the provider insert a central line when the patient develops chest pain and shortness of breath with decreased breath sounds and restlessness. What does the nurse do next?
    a. Tell the patient "Relax, the procedure will soon be over" and administer pain medication.
    b. Administer pain medication to minimize the pain of insertion and order a stat chest x-ray.
    c. Administer oxygen, remove the catheter, place an occlusive dressing, and order a stat chest x-ray.
    d. Monitor ongoing pulse oximetry and respiratory changes after placing an occlusive dressing over the catheter site.

25. A triple-lumen catheter central line is inserted in a patient. What does the nurse do immediately after the procedure?
    a. Start IV fluids, but at a slower rate to prevent any fluid overload.
    b. Watch and wait for any complications before using the site.
    c. Get a portable chest x-ray and hold IV fluids until results are obtained.
    d. Assess vital signs and assess the patient; if patient is stable, start IV fluids.

26. After a tubing change to a patient's central line, the line is later found to be disconnected from the catheter. The patient develops chest pain and restlessness, heart rate of 120 beats/min, blood pressure drops to 90/40 mm Hg, and pulse oximetry is 89%. What does the nurse do next?
    a. Place the patient in Trendelenburg position on the left side, clamp the catheter, and notify the provider.
    b. Assess for patency of the catheter, change the tubing, and resume IV fluids.
    c. Notify the provider, remove the central line, apply pressure, and place the patient in a semi-Fowler's position.
    d. Notify the provider and administer urokinase to unclot the catheter.

27. Which nursing interventions are essential to prevent an infection in a patient with a central line? *(Select all that apply.)*
    a. Assess the dressing and insertion site of the central line.
    b. Use aseptic technique when administering medications and changing tubing.
    c. Change the catheter every 72 hours and tubing every 24 hours.
    d. Monitor the patient's temperature for any elevation and give acetaminophen as needed.
    e. Use sterile technique when inserting a central line.
    f. Use proper handwashing and nonsterile gloves before coming into contact with a central line.

28. A patient with an implanted port is discharged home and will receive long-term therapy on an outpatient basis. How frequently must the port be flushed between courses of therapy?
    a. Daily
    b. Weekly
    c. Monthly
    d. When therapy resumes

29. The nurse is preparing to deliver IV infusion therapy through an implanted port. What technique does the nurse use to access the port?
    a. Palpate the port to locate the septum, scrub, and access with a Huber needle.
    b. Scrub the port with alcohol and access with a needleless device.
    c. Scrub the port with Betadine and flush using a 10-mL syringe.
    d. Palpate the port, scrub, and access with a winged butterfly needle.

30. A patient is to be discharged home with an implanted port and needs discharge instructions on prescribed medication administration. Which instructions must the nurse give to the patient and family member who will be assisting the patient? *(Select all that apply.)*
    a. The device must be flushed every 24 hours.
    b. When the port is not accessed, an occlusive dressing should be applied.
    c. The skin will be punctured over the port when the port is accessed.
    d. When the port is not accessed, no dressing needs to be applied.
    e. The port must be flushed after each use.

31. The nurse is preparing to administer IV infusion therapy to a patient. When is the choice of using a glass container appropriate?
    a. When the patient needs a rapid infusion of fluids
    b. When the patient needs emergency transportation
    c. When the nurse must accurately read the container
    d. When the drug is incompatible with a plastic container

32. A patient requires a 2-month course of antibiotics to treat a resistant infection. Which device is chosen for this therapy?
    a. Short peripheral catheter
    b. Midline catheter
    c. Nontunneled percutaneous central catheter
    d. PICC

33. The nurse is attaching an administration set to a central venous catheter. Which type of equipment decreases the risk of accidental disconnection or leakage?
    a. Slip lock connector
    b. Luer-Lok connector
    c. Extension set
    d. Needleless connector

34. The nurse is adding a filter to an IV administration setup. Where is the best place to add the filter to the IV line?
    a. As close to the solution container as possible
    b. Immediately below the infusion pump
    c. At any convenient connection point
    d. As close as possible to the catheter hub

35. Which safety measures does the nurse apply to decrease the risk of catheter-related bloodstream infection (CR-BSI) related to needleless systems? *(Select all that apply.)*
    a. Clean needleless system connections vigorously every 24 hours.
    b. Do not tape connections between tubing sets.
    c. Use evidence-based hand hygiene guidelines from the Centers for Disease Control and Prevention (CDC) and the Occupational Safety and Health Administration (OSHA).
    d. Minimize traffic in and out of the patient's room during insertion of the device.
    e. Use needleless systems only when necessary.
    f. Discard needleless equipment in a biohazard container.

36. A patient is receiving IV therapy via an infusion pump. What is a nursing responsibility related to the therapy and equipment?
    a. Count the number of drops per minute.
    b. Monitor the patient's infusion site and rate.
    c. Check the equipment at the end of the infusion.
    d. Position the container for gravity flow.

37. Which characteristics apply to IV infusion pumps? *(Select all that apply.)*
    a. Delivers fluids under pressure
    b. Relies on gravity to create fluid flow
    c. Is pole-mounted or ambulatory and portable
    d. Is best for accurate infusion
    e. Counts drops to regulate flow

38. The nurse is assessing a patient's IV insertion site. What features must the nurse look for during the assessment? *(Select all that apply.)*
    a. Observe for redness and swelling.
    b. Check that the dressing is clean and dry.
    c. Ensure that the dressing is adherent to the skin.
    d. Observe for yellow discoloration.
    e. Observe for hardness or drainage.

39. A patient's central venous IV site is covered with a transparent membrane dressing. How often does the nurse change this dressing?
    a. Every 24 hours
    b. Every 48 hours
    c. At least every 7 days
    d. The dressing does not need changing

40. A patient is ordered to receive peripheral parenteral nutrition (PPN). What type of access device is appropriate for this patient?
    a. Peripheral 20-gauge IV needle
    b. Nontunneled percutaneous central catheter
    c. Peripheral 22-gauge IV needle
    d. PICC

41. An external long-term IV catheter is required for hemodialysis of a hospitalized patient. Which statements are true about this patient's venous access device? *(Select all that apply.)*
    a. It should not be used for administration of other fluids or medications except in an emergency.
    b. A nontunneled catheter with large lumen is required for hemodialysis.
    c. Venous thrombosis is a common problem with hemodialysis access.
    d. A device for hemodialysis has a port to access the catheter.
    e. A tunneled catheter with large lumen is required for hemodialysis.

42. The nurse has removed the dressing from a patient's central venous catheter site. In order to monitor the catheter position, what does the nurse do?
    a. Gently push the catheter into the insertion site.
    b. Slightly retract the catheter and observe the position.
    c. Mark the catheter with a pen to monitor the length.
    d. Note the length of the catheter external to the insertion site.

43. The nurse is caring for a patient with a central venous catheter. What measures does the nurse use to prevent air emboli when changing the administration set or connectors? *(Select all that apply.)*
    a. The patient lies flat so the catheter site is below the heart.
    b. Use the pinch clamp that can be closed during the procedure.
    c. Use sterile technique when handling the equipment.
    d. Have an assistant apply pressure at the insertion site.
    e. Ask the patient to perform the Valsalva maneuver by holding the breath and bearing down.

44. After assessing the patency of a patient's IV catheter, the nurse attempts to flush the catheter and meets resistance. What does the nurse do next?
    a. Get a larger-sized syringe and repeat the flush attempt.
    b. Use a heparinized solution and repeat the flush attempt.
    c. Gently force-flush the catheter using the push-pause method.
    d. Stop the flush attempt and discontinue the IV.

45. The nurse is flushing a patient's short peripheral IV catheter. What does the nurse typically use for this procedure?
    a. 3 mL of normal saline
    b. 5 mL of heparin
    c. 10 mL of normal saline
    d. 30 mL of bacteriostatic saline

46. The patient is ready for discharge. Which actions must the nurse follow to remove the patient's peripheral catheter? *(Select all that apply.)*
    a. Hold pressure on the site until hemostasis is achieved.
    b. Flush the peripheral catheter with normal saline before removing.
    c. Assess the catheter tip to make sure it is intact and completely removed.
    d. Slowly withdraw the catheter from the skin.
    e. Remove the peripheral catheter dressing.
    f. Document catheter removal and the appearance of the IV site.

47. The nurse is attempting to remove a PICC line and feels resistance. What technique does the nurse use first to attempt to resolve this problem?
    a. Gently pull on the catheter while the patient holds his or her breath.
    b. Place a cold pack on the extremity and give the patient a cold drink.
    c. Use simple distraction techniques and deep breathing.
    d. Place the patient in Trendelenburg position.

48. The nurse is assessing a short peripheral catheter after removal and it appears that the catheter tip is missing. What does the nurse do next?
    a. Notify the health care provider.
    b. Assess the patient for symptoms of emboli.
    c. Apply firm pressure to the insertion site.
    d. Assess the extremity for coldness, cyanosis, or numbness.

49. A patient has a local complication from a peripheral IV access with 0.9% normal saline infusing at 100 mL/hour. What does the nurse assess at the insertion site? *(Select all that apply.)*
    a. Blood returns in the catheter when nurse draws back on the IV access.
    b. A red streak is present proximal to the site.
    c. Edema is present proximal to the site.
    d. A scant amount of blood is noted beneath the clear dressing at the site.
    e. The IV fluids are not infusing.

50. The nurse is caring for the patient receiving arterial therapy via the carotid artery. What important nursing action is specific to this therapy?
    a. Assess the extremities for sensation and pulses.
    b. Monitor respirations for rate and regularity.
    c. Perform frequent neurologic assessments.
    d. Place antiembolic stockings on the patient's lower extremities.

51. Which statements are correct about intraperitoneal infusion (IP)? *(Select all that apply.)*
    a. Sterile technique is used with IP access and supplies.
    b. IP can be accessed by a catheter with an implanted port and large internal lumens.
    c. Strict aseptic technique is used with IP access and supplies.
    d. IP is used for patients who are receiving medications for diagnostic tests.
    e. IP can be accessed by a tunneled catheter with capped ports and large internal lumens.
    f. IP is used for patients who are receiving chemotherapy agents.

52. During intraperitoneal therapy, a patient reports nausea and vomiting. What does the nurse do next?
    a. Help the patient move from side to side.
    b. Flush the catheter with normal saline.
    c. Reduce the flow rate and give antiemetics.
    d. Obtain an order for an abdominal x-ray.

53. In what position does the nurse place a patient before starting intraperitoneal therapy?
    a. Semi-Fowler's
    b. Prone
    c. Supine
    d. Side-lying

54. Hypodermoclysis can be used for a patient under which types of circumstances? *(Select all that apply.)*
    a. If the patient requires palliative care
    b. For IV fluid replacement that is less than 2000 mL
    c. When a subcutaneous IV infusion is warranted
    d. If the patient requires acute care
    e. When short-term fluid volume replacement is warranted

55. The nurse is preparing to start a hypodermoclysis treatment on a patient. What is the preferred insertion site?
    a. Anterior forearm
    b. Anterior tibial area
    c. Lateral aspect of the upper arm
    d. Area under the clavicle

56. The home health nurse is adjusting the rate for a hypodermoclysis treatment. What is the usual maximum rate for this therapy?
    a. 2 mL/hr
    b. 30 mL/hr
    c. 80 mL/hr
    d. 125 mL/hr

57. The home health nurse is caring for a patient receiving hypodermoclysis therapy. How often are the subcutaneous sites rotated?
    a. Every 4 hours
    b. Every 24 hours
    c. At least every 3 days
    d. At least once a week

58. The nurse is caring for a patient receiving intrathecal pain medication. Which agent is preferred for cleaning the access site?
    a. Alcohol
    b. Soap and water
    c. Povidone iodine
    d. Chlorhexidine gluconate

59. A patient is receiving epidural medication therapy. The nurse assesses for which potential problem specific to this type of therapy?
    a. Meningitis
    b. Loss of bowel function
    c. Respiratory distress
    d. Cardiac dysrhythmias

60. A patient is brought to the emergency department (ED) after a serious motor vehicle accident. Which factor makes the patient a candidate for intraosseous (IO) therapy?
    a. Patient has a history of chronic renal failure.
    b. Endotracheal intubation is difficult to accomplish.
    c. Patient is an older adult and very thin.
    d. IV access cannot be achieved within a few minutes.

61. A patient has an IO needle in place. Why does the nurse advocate for removal of the device within 24 hours after insertion?
    a. There is an increased risk for osteomyelitis.
    b. There is an increased risk for arterial insufficiency.
    c. The device hinders patient mobility.
    d. The device is unstable and easily dislodged.

62. The patient has an order for a unit of PRBCs. Which priority action must the nurse complete before starting this infusion?
    a. Place a new IV line designated only for blood product infusion.
    b. Ensure that the IV line to be used for infusion is larger than a 22-gauge.
    c. Check patient identification with another RN using two identifiers.
    d. Ensure that the unit of PRBCs has been warmed to body temperature.

14 CHAPTER

Care of Preoperative Patients

1. Which is the top priority for nurses during the perioperative period?
   a. Patient teaching
   b. Patient diagnostic testing
   c. Patient safety
   d. Patient care documentation

2. Which statements best describe the preoperative period? *(Select all that apply.)*
   a. It begins when the patient makes the appointment with the surgeon to discuss the need for surgery.
   b. It ends at the time of transfer to the surgical suite.
   c. It is a time during which the patient's need for surgery is established.
   d. It begins when the patient is scheduled for surgery.
   e. It is a time during which the patient receives testing and education related to impending surgery.

3. Which are the focus areas for the Surgical Care Improvement Project (SCIP)? *(Select all that apply.)*
   a. Prevention of infection
   b. Prevention of respiratory complications
   c. Prevention of serious cardiac events
   d. Prevention of venous thromboembolism
   e. Prevention of acute kidney injury

4. A female patient is having a biopsy of a nodule found in the right breast. Which classification identifies this surgery?
   a. Urgent
   b. Minor
   c. Cosmetic
   d. Diagnostic

5. A patient who can barely ambulate with a walker at home is having a left total knee replacement. What is the most appropriate category for this surgery?
   a. Urgent
   b. Restorative
   c. Simple
   d. Palliative

6. A colostomy is scheduled to be done on a patient who has severe Crohn's disease. What is the correct classification for this surgery?
   a. Palliative
   b. Minor
   c. Restorative
   d. Curative

7. A male patient has a scar on his forehead from a third-degree burn. What is the correct classification for this surgery?
   a. Major
   b. Restorative
   c. Cosmetic
   d. Curative

8. An appendectomy is being performed on a patient with appendicitis. What is the correct classification for this surgery?
   a. Curative
   b. Diagnostic
   c. Urgent
   d. Radical

9. A patient with an abdominal aortic aneurysm is having surgical repair. What is the correct classification for this surgery?
   a. Restorative
   b. Emergent
   c. Urgent
   d. Minor

10. A 76-year-old patient is having a bilateral cataract removal. What is the correct classification for this surgery?
    a. Major
    b. Cosmetic
    c. Elective
    d. Emergent

11. A 47-year-old patient is having surgery to remove kidney stones. What is the correct classification for this surgery?
    a. Restorative
    b. Emergent
    c. Palliative
    d. Urgent

12. The nurse screens a preoperative patient for conditions that may increase the risk for complications during the perioperative period. Which conditions are possible risk factors? *(Select all that apply.)*
    a. Emotionally stable
    b. 67 years old
    c. Obesity
    d. Marathon runner
    e. Pulmonary disease

13. A 75-year-old patient is having an exploratory laparotomy tomorrow. The wife tells the nurse that at night the patient gets up and walks around his room. What priority action does the nurse take after hearing this information?
    a. Notifies the provider
    b. Develops a plan to keep the patient safe
    c. Obtains an order for sleep medication
    d. Tells the patient not to get out of bed at night

14. The nurse has received a patient in the holding area who is scheduled for a left femoral-popliteal bypass. What are the priority safety measures for this patient before surgery? *(Select all that apply.)*
    a. The operative limb is marked by the surgeon.
    b. The patient is positively identified by checking the name and date of birth.
    c. The patient is asked to confirm the marked operative limb.
    d. The patient is identified by checking the name and room number.
    e. The patient is instructed to verify any family members waiting.

15. The 79-year-old patient with type 2 diabetes is scheduled for surgery to remove his left great toe. Which risk factors for complications of surgery does the nurse assess for in this patient? *(Select all that apply.)*
    a. Presence of chronic illnesses
    b. Problems with healing
    c. Absence of smoking history
    d. Dehydration
    e. Electrolyte imbalances
    f. Daily exercise routine

16. During preoperative screening, the nurse discovers that the patient is allergic to shellfish. What is the nurse's best first action?
    a. Notifies the surgeon
    b. Develops a plan to keep the patient safe
    c. Obtains an order for a shellfish-free diet
    d. Asks the patient if any other family members have the same allergy

17. The preoperative patient tells the nurse that she is afraid that she may experience a reaction if she must receive blood during or after her surgery. What is the nurse's best response to the patient's concern?
    a. "The likelihood that you will need a blood transfusion for your surgery is minimal, so do not worry about this."
    b. "You could donate some of your own blood (autologous donation) a few weeks before your surgery."
    c. "With today's technology and procedures, it is very unlikely that you would have a reaction to donated blood."
    d. "The nursing staff follows strict procedures to prevent such an event from ever happening."

18. The nurse is preparing the patient for surgery. Which common laboratory tests does the nurse anticipate to be ordered? *(Select all that apply.)*
    a. Total cholesterol
    b. Urinalysis
    c. Electrolyte levels
    d. Uric acid
    e. Clotting studies
    f. Serum creatinine

19. Which statement is true regarding the patient who has given consent for a surgical procedure?
    a. Information necessary to understand the nature of and reason for the surgery has been provided.
    b. The length of stay in the hospital has been preapproved by the managed care provider.
    c. Information about the surgeon's experience has been provided.
    d. The nurse has provided detailed information about the surgical procedure.

20. Which statement best describes the collaborative roles of the nurse and surgeon when obtaining the informed consent?
    a. The nurse is responsible for having the informed consent form on the chart for the physician to witness.
    b. The nurse may serve as a witness that the patient has been informed by the physician before surgery is performed.
    c. The nurse may serve as witness to the patient's signature after the physician has the consent form signed before preoperative sedation is given and before surgery is performed.
    d. The nurse has no duties regarding the consent form if the patient has signed the informed consent form for the physician, even if the patient then asks additional questions about the surgery.

21. A patient with type 1 diabetes mellitus is scheduled for surgery at 0700. Which actions must the nurse perform for this patient before he goes to the operating room? *(Select based on priority order.)*
    a. Modify the dose of insulin given based on the patient's blood glucose.
    b. Complete the preoperative checklist before transfer to surgical suite.
    c. Teach the patient about foot care and properly fitted shoes.
    d. Delegate obtaining the patient's Accucheck and vital signs to the unlicensed assistive personnel (UAP).
    e. Check if the patient has any jewelry on and call security to secure valuables.

22. The nurse has given the ordered preoperative medications to the patient. What actions must the nurse take after administering these drugs? *(Select all that apply.)*
    a. Raise the side rails.
    b. Place the call light within the patient's reach.
    c. Ask the patient to sign the consent form.
    d. Instruct the patient not to get out of bed.
    e. Place the bed in its lowest position.

23. Which postoperative interventions will the nurse typically teach a patient to prevent complications following surgery? *(Select all that apply.)*
    a. Range-of-motion exercises
    b. Massaging of lower extremities
    c. Taking pain medication only when experiencing severe pain
    d. Incision splinting
    e. Deep-breathing exercises

15 CHAPTER

Care of Intraoperative Patients

1. Which nursing intervention is most appropriate for the patient in the operative setting?
   a. Provide a climate of privacy, comfort, and confidentiality when caring for the patient.
   b. Instruct the patient that after the preoperative medication has taken effect, he or she will be drowsy.
   c. Avoid discussing the activities taking place around the patient while in the holding area.
   d. Assist members of the surgical team readying the operating room suite.

2. Which interventions must the operating room (OR) nurses provide for patient physiological integrity during the intraoperative period? *(Select all that apply.)*
   a. Apply padding to the OR bed to protect skin integrity.
   b. Communicate patient's fears about anesthesia to the nurse anesthetist.
   c. Monitor patient's airway, vital signs, electrocardiogram (ECG), and oxygen saturation during and after sedation.
   d. Assess and document skin condition before transferring patient to the postanesthesia care unit (PACU).
   e. Ensure that patient's wishes with regard to advance directives are respected.

3. A patient with breast cancer is scheduled for a left mastectomy. The patient has informed the surgeon and nurse that she is a Jehovah's Witness and does not want any blood transfusions. In preparation for intraoperative care of this patient, what measures does the nurse take? *(Select all that apply.)*
   a. Obtain 2 units of packed red blood cells, typed and crossmatched.
   b. Make provider aware of patient's request for no blood transfusions.
   c. Ensure autotransfusion device is in place intraoperatively.
   d. Ensure patient has a medical necessity order for emergency blood transfusion.
   e. Inform the patient of potential risks if blood transfusion is not given.

4. To reduce the incidence of patients with a known history or risk of malignant hyperthermia (MH), what best practices are put in place in the operating room? *(Select all that apply.)*
   a. List of medications available for emergency treatment of MH
   b. Genetic counseling after each episode of MH
   c. Dedicated MH cart with treatment medications
   d. Treatment before, during, and after surgery if the patient has a known history or risk
   e. Additional nursing support on call if MH develops
   f. Available MH hotline number

5. A patient has an MH incident during surgery. To whom does the nurse report this incident?
   a. North American Malignant Hyperthermia Registry
   b. The Joint Commission
   c. Centers for Disease Control
   d. Occupational Safety and Health Administration

6. Which duties are within the scope of practice of the circulating nurse in the operative setting?
   a. Manages the patient's care while the patient is in this area and initiates documentation on a perioperative nursing record.
   b. Sets up the sterile field; assists with the draping of the patient; and hands sterile supplies, equipment, and instruments to the surgeon.
   c. Assumes responsibility for the surgical procedure and any surgical judgments about the patient.
   d. Coordinates, oversees, and participates in the patient's nursing care while the patient is in the operating room.

7. During surgery, what things do anesthesia personnel monitor, measure, and assess? *(Select all that apply.)*
   a. Intake and output
   b. Room temperature
   c. Cardiopulmonary function
   d. Level of anesthesia
   e. Family concerns
   f. Vital signs

8. Which nursing interventions are appropriate during stage 2 of anesthesia?
   a. Prepare for and assist in treatment of cardiovascular and/or pulmonary arrest. Document in record.
   b. Shield patient from extra noise and physical stimuli. Protect the patient's extremities. Assist anesthesia personnel as needed. Stay with patient.
   c. Close operating room doors and control traffic in and out of room. Position patient securely with safety belts. Maintain minimal discussion in operating room.
   d. Assist anesthesia personnel with intubation of patient. Place the patient in position for surgery. Prep the patient's skin in area of operative site.

9. The acute, life-threatening complication of MH results from the use of which agents?
   a. Hypnotics and neuromuscular blocking agents
   b. Succinylcholine and inhalation agents
   c. Nitrous oxide and pancuronium for muscle relaxation
   d. Fentanyl and regional anesthesia for spinal block

10. Which clinical features are found in an MH crisis? *(Select all that apply.)*
    a. Sinus tachycardia
    b. Tightness and rigidity of the patient's jaw area
    c. Lowering of the blood pressure
    d. A decrease in the end-tidal carbon dioxide level
    e. Skin mottling and cyanosis
    f. An extremely elevated temperature at onset
    g. Tachypnea

11. The surgical team understands that time is crucial in recognizing and treating an MH crisis. Once recognized, what is the treatment of choice?
    a. Danazol gluconate (Danocrine)
    b. Phenytoin sodium (Dilantin)
    c. Diazepam sulfate (Valium)
    d. Dantrolene sodium (Dantrium)

12. Which factors may lead to an anesthetic over-dose in a patient? *(Select all that apply.)*
    a. Amount of anesthesia retained by fat cells
    b. Patient who is older
    c. Slowed metabolism and drug elimination
    d. An uncooperative patient
    e. Liver or kidney disease

13. A patient experiences MH immediately after induction of anesthesia. What is the nurse anesthetist's first priority action?
    a. Administer IV dantrolene sodium (Dantrium) 2 to 3 mg/kg.
    b. Apply a cooling blanket over the torso.
    c. Assess arterial blood gases (ABGs) and serum chemistries.
    d. Stop all inhalation anesthetic agents and succinylcholine.
    e. Monitor cardiac rhythm by electrocardiography to assess for dysrhythmias.

14. What techniques are essential to performing a proper surgical scrub of the hands by the surgeon, assistants, and scrub nurse? *(Select all that apply.)*
    a. Use a broad-spectrum, surgical antimicrobial solution.
    b. Scrub for 2 minutes, followed by a rinse with water.
    c. Use an alcohol-based antimicrobial solution.
    d. Hold hands higher than the elbows during the scrub and rinse.
    e. Scrub for 3-5 minutes, followed by a rinse with water.
    f. Hold hands below the elbows during the scrub and rinse.

15. Which nursing interventions will prevent the potential intraoperative complication of radial joint stiffness, pain, and inflammation?
    a. Support the wrist with padding; do not overtighten wrist straps.
    b. Place pillow or foam padding under bony prominences; maintain good body alignment; slightly flex joints and support with pillows, trochanter rolls, and pads.
    c. Pad the elbow, avoid excessive abduction, secure the arm firmly on an arm board positioned at shoulder level.
    d. Place a safety strap above or below the area. Place a pillow or padding under the knees.

16. In which situations is regional anesthesia used instead of general anesthesia? *(Select all that apply.)*
    a. For an endoscopy or cardiac catheterization
    b. In patients who have had an adverse reaction to general anesthesia
    c. In some cases when pain management after surgery is enhanced by regional anesthesia
    d. In patients with serious medical problems
    e. When the patient has a preference and a choice is possible

17. Which characteristics are appropriate to the anesthetic agent ketamine HCl?
    a. Can depress respiratory and cardiac functions
    b. May increase heart rate and lower blood pressure (BP) during induction
    c. Short-acting; patient becomes responsive quickly postoperatively
    d. Dissociative emergence reactions; can induce nausea and vomiting

18. To avoid electrical safety problems during surgery, what does the nurse do?
    a. Observes for breaks in sterile technique
    b. Continuously assists the anesthesia provider
    c. Ensures proper placement of the grounding pads
    d. Monitors the operating room with available cameras

19. Which medical condition increases a patient's risk for surgical wound infection?
    a. Anxiety
    b. Hiatal hernia
    c. Diabetes mellitus
    d. Amnesia

20. Which definition is appropriate for local anesthesia?
    a. Injection of anesthetic agent into or around a nerve or group of nerves, resulting in blocked sensation and motor impulse transmission.
    b. Injection of the anesthetic agent into the epidural space; the spinal cord areas are never entered.
    c. Injection of an anesthetic agent directly into the tissue around an incision, wound, or lesion.
    d. Injection of anesthetic agent into or around a nerve or group of nerves, resulting in blocked sensation and motor impulse transmission.

21. Which patient would be a candidate for moderate sedation? *(Select all that apply.)*
    a. Endoscopy
    b. Cesarean section delivery
    c. Closed fracture reduction
    d. Cardiac catheterization
    e. Suturing a laceration
    f. Abdominal surgery
    g. Cardioversion

22. A patient is requesting moderate sedation for repair of a torn meniscus and has no medical contraindications. How does the nurse respond to this patient's request?
    a. "Your surgeon will decide if you will receive moderate sedation or general anesthesia."
    b. "You can discuss your request for moderate sedation with your surgeon and anesthesiologist."
    c. "Most patients prefer general anesthesia. Can you tell me why you want moderate sedation?"
    d. "It can be frightening to see surgery done on yourself. You need to think about that."

23. The patient is scheduled to have minimally invasive surgery (MIS) for a laparoscopic cholecystectomy. Part of this surgery is the injection of air (insufflation) into the abdomen to separate and better see the organs. What patient teaching must the nurse do about the insufflation?
    a. "Your surgeon will make several small incisions instead of a large one."
    b. "You will be able to go home once your surgery is completed and you are awake."
    c. "You may experience some abdominal discomfort from the air injected with the surgery."
    d. "You will have a tube for drainage for a few days after your surgery is completed."

24. The patient in the OR holding area tells the nurse that his surgery is for the right foot. The patient's chart states that the surgery is for his left foot. What is the nurse's best action?
    a. Do nothing because the patient is confused after receiving premedications.
    b. Make a note about this in the nursing notes of the patient's chart.
    c. Call the nurse anesthetist to check whether the chart or patient is correct.
    d. Notify the surgeon immediately before the patient goes into the OR about this discrepancy.

25. The patient received moderate sedation (conscious sedation) by IV prior to a bronchoscopy procedure. Before allowing the patient to have oral liquids, what must the nurse assess in this patient?
    a. The patient is arousable.
    b. The patient is able to speak.
    c. The patient's gag reflex is working.
    d. The patient is able to rotate his head.

16 CHAPTER

Care of Postoperative Patients

1. Which description illustrates the beginning of the postoperative period?
   a. Completion of the surgical procedure and arousal of the patient from anesthesia in the operating room (OR)
   b. Discharge planning initiated in the preoperative setting
   c. Closure of the patient's surgical incision with sutures
   d. Completion of the surgical procedure and transfer of the patient to the postanesthesia care unit (PACU)

2. What is the primary purpose of a PACU?
   a. Follow-through on the surgeon's postoperative orders
   b. Ongoing critical evaluation and stabilization of the patient
   c. Prevention of lengthened hospital stay
   d. Arousal of patient following the use of conscious sedation

3. A patient develops respiratory distress after having a left total hip replacement. The patient develops labored breathing and a pulse oximetry reading is 83% on 2 L oxygen via nasal cannula. Which intervention is appropriate for the nurse to delegate to unlicensed assistive personnel (UAP)?
   a. Assess change in patient's respiratory status.
   b. Order necessary medications to be administered.
   c. Intubate the patient for maintenance of airway and assisted breathing.
   d. Check the patient's vital signs.

4. Which signs/symptoms are considered postoperative complications? *(Select all that apply.)*
   a. Sedation
   b. Pain at the surgical site
   c. Pulmonary embolism
   d. Hypothermia
   e. Wound evisceration

5. If a patient experiences a wound dehiscence, which description illustrates what is happening with the wound?
   a. Purulent drainage is present at incision site because of infection.
   b. Extreme pain is present at incision site.
   c. A partial or complete separation of outer layers is present at incision site.
   d. The inner and outer layers of the incision are separated.

6. A patient who is 2 days postoperative for abdominal surgery states, "I coughed and heard something pop." The nurse's immediate assessment reveals an opened incision with a portion of large intestine protruding. Which statements apply to this clinical situation? *(Select all that apply.)*
   a. Incision dehiscence has occurred.
   b. This is an emergency situation.
   c. The wound must be kept moist with normal saline-soaked sterile dressings.
   d. This is an urgent situation.
   e. Incision evisceration has occurred.

7. In the PACU, the nurse assesses that a patient is bleeding profusely from an abdominal incision. What is the nurse's best first action?
   a. Notify the surgeon.
   b. Apply pressure to the wound dressing.
   c. Instruct the UAP to get additional dressing supplies.
   d. Request and draw a complete blood count.

8. The nurse transfers a patient to the PACU with an incision and drainage of an abscess in the right groin under general anesthesia. Blood pressure is 80/47 mm Hg, heart rate 117/min in sinus tachycardia, respiratory rate 28/min, pulse oximetry reading 93% on oxygen at 3 L nasal cannula, temp is 38.5° C. The Jackson-Pratt drain has 70 mL of a cream-colored output. Normal saline is infusing at 150 mL/hr. The surgeon orders a bolus of 500 mL IV over 1 hour of normal saline, two sets of blood cultures, and culture drainage from the Jackson-Pratt drain. The patient's history includes vulvar cancer with a needle biopsy of the right groin, hypertension treated with lisinopril (Zestril) 5 mg PO daily, and no known drug allergies. The patient is a full code. Using the SBAR (situation, background, assessment, recommendation) charting format, which information should be included in assessment?
   a. Nurse transfers patient to the PACU with an incision and drainage of an abscess in the right groin with general anesthesia.
   b. Surgeon sending orders to bolus the patient with 500 mL normal saline over an hour, draw two sets of blood cultures and send a culture of drainage from the Jackson-Pratt drain.
   c. Blood pressure 80/47 mm Hg, heart rate 117/min, sinus tachycardia, respirations 28/min, pulse oximetry 93% on O_2 at 3 L nasal cannula, temp 38.5° C, Jackson-Pratt drain with 70 mL cream-colored output.
   d. Patient had a right groin abscess. History of vulvar cancer. Needle biopsy of right groin completed 1 week ago. History of hypertension treated with lisinopril (Zestril) 5 mg. No known drug allergies. Full code.

9. A postoperative patient in the PACU has had an open reduction internal fixation of a left fractured femur. Vital signs are blood pressure 87/49 mm Hg, heart rate 100/min sinus rhythm, respirations 22/min, temperature 98.3° F. The Foley catheter has a total amount of 110 mL of clear, yellow urine in the last 4 hours. Which body systems have been assessed by the nurse? *(Select all that apply.)*
   a. Respiratory
   b. Cardiovascular
   c. Neurovascular
   d. Integumentary
   e. Renal/urinary

10. A patient cared for in the PACU has had a colostomy placed for treatment of Crohn's disease. The nurse assesses that an abdominal dressing is 25% saturated with serosanguineous drainage and notes that the incision is intact. An IV is infusing with D_5/lactated Ringer's at 100 mL/hr through a 20-g peripheral IV access. Auscultation of abdomen reveals hypoactive bowel sounds in all four quadrants, abdomen soft, and no distention. Foley catheter is in place and draining yellow urine with sediment, 375 mL output in Foley bag. Which body systems have been assessed by the nurse? *(Select all that apply.)*
   a. Renal/urinary
   b. Gastrointestinal
   c. Respiratory
   d. Musculoskeletal
   e. Integumentary

11. A 49-year-old patient is in the PACU following a frontal craniotomy for repair of a ruptured cerebral aneurysm. The nurse assesses that the patient's eyes open on verbal stimulation. Pupils are equal, reactive to light, and diameter is 3 mm. The patient's hand grasps are equal and strong. When the nurse asks the patient to state name, the patient states name correctly. The patient has had one episode of nausea and vomiting. Incision edges are dry and approximated with sutures. Lung sounds are slightly diminished per auscultation and the nurse observes the patient is using abdominal accessory muscles to breathe. Which body systems has the nurse assessed? *(Select all that apply.)*
    a. Cardiovascular
    b. Gastrointestinal
    c. Neurologic
    d. Integumentary
    e. Respiratory

12. The PACU nurse is assessing a patient transferred in from the OR. Which assessment findings apply to assessment of the cardiovascular system? *(Select all that apply.)*
    a. Opens eyes on command.
    b. Absent dorsalis pedis pulse left foot.
    c. Foley catheter in place with clear yellow drainage.
    d. Monitor shows normal sinus rhythm.
    e. States name correctly when asked.
    f. Apical pulse 85 beats/minute.

13. A patient arrives in the PACU. Which action does the nurse perform first?
    a. Assess for a patent airway and adequate gas exchange.
    b. Rate the patient's pain using the 0-10 pain assessment scale.
    c. Position the patient in a supine position to prevent aspiration.
    d. Calculate the patient-controlled analgesia (PCA) pump maximum dose per hour to avoid an overdose.

14. A patient arrives at the PACU and the nurse notes a respiratory rate of 10 with sternal retractions. The report from anesthesia personnel indicates that the patient had received fentanyl during surgery. What is the nurse's best priority first action?
    a. Monitor the patient for effects of anesthetic for at least 1 hour.
    b. Closely monitor vital signs and pulse oximetry readings until the patient is responsive.
    c. Administer oxygen as ordered, monitoring pulse oximetry.
    d. Maintain an open airway through positioning and suction if needed.

15. The nurse is teaching incisional care to a patient who has been discharged after abdominal surgery. Which priority instruction must the nurse include?
    a. Do not rub or touch the incision site.
    b. Practice proper handwashing.
    c. Clean the incision site two times a day with soap and water.
    d. Splint the incisional site as often as needed for comfort.

16. The health care team determines a patient's readiness for discharge from the PACU by noting a postanesthesia recovery score of at least 10. After determining that all criteria have been met, the patient is discharged to the hospital unit or home. Review the patient profiles after 1 hour in the PACU listed below. Which patient should the nurse expect to be discharged from the PACU first?
    a. 10-year-old girl, tonsillectomy, general anesthesia. Duration of surgery 30 minutes. Immediate response to voice. Alert to place and person. Able to move all extremities. Respirations even, deep, rate of 20. Vital signs (VS) are within normal limits. IV solution is D_5RL. Has voided on bedpan. Eating ice chips. Complaining of sore throat.
    b. 55-year-old man, repair of fractured lower left leg. General anesthesia. Duration of surgery 1 hour, 30 minutes. Drowsy, but responds to voice. Nausea and vomiting twice in PACU. No urge to void at this time. IV infusing D_5NS. Pedal pulses noted in both lower extremities. VS: temperature 98.6° F; pulse 130 beats/min; respiratory rate 24/min; blood pressure 124/76 mm Hg.
    c. 24-year-old man, reconstruction of facial scar. General anesthesia. Duration of surgery 2 hours. Sleeping, groans to voice command. VS are within normal limits. Respirations 10 breaths/min. No urge to void. IV of D_5RL infusing. Complains of pain in surgical area.
    d. 42-year-old woman, colonoscopy. IV conscious sedation. Awake and alert. Up to bathroom to void. IV discontinued. Resting quietly in chair. VS are within normal limits.

17. The nurse is caring for a patient who has had abdominal surgery. After a hard sneeze, the patient reports pain in the surgical area, and the nurse immediately sees that the patient has a wound evisceration. What priority action must the nurse do first?
    a. The nurse calls for help and stays with the patient.
    b. The nurse leaves the patient to immediately call the surgeon.
    c. The nurse covers the wound with a nonadherent dressing moistened with normal saline.
    d. The nurse takes the patient's vital signs.

18. Which intervention for postsurgical care of a patient is correct?
    a. When positioning the patient, use the knee gatch of the bed to bend the knees and relieve pressure.
    b. Gentle massage on the lower legs and calves helps promote venous blood return to the heart.
    c. Encourage bedrest for 3 days after surgery to prevent complications.
    d. The patient should splint the surgical wound for support and comfort when getting out of bed.

19. The morning after a patient's lower leg surgery, the nurse notes that the dressing is wet from drainage. The surgeon has not yet been in to see the patient on rounds. What does the nurse do about the dressing?
    a. Removes the dressing and puts on a dry, sterile dressing
    b. Reinforces the dressing by adding dry, sterile dressing material on top of the existing dressing
    c. Applies dry, sterile dressing material directly to the wound, then retapes the original dressing
    d. Does nothing to the dressing but calls the surgeon to evaluate the patient immediately

20. The PACU nurse is caring for a postoperative patient. The patient's oxygen saturation drops from 98% to 88%. What is the nurse's priority action?
    a. Call the anesthesia provider.
    b. Call the surgeon.
    c. Call the Rapid Response Team.
    d. Call the respiratory therapist.

21. What criteria guide the handoff report when a patient is transferred from the OR to the PACU? *(Select all that apply.)*
    a. It is a two-way verbal interaction.
    b. The language is clear.
    c. Reporting nurse asks questions about PACU procedures.
    d. Standardized reports help avoid omissions.
    e. Receiving nurse repeats information to verify what was said.

22. The nurse on the medical-surgical unit is caring for a postoperative patient. Which assessment criteria indicate to the nurse that the patient is experiencing respiratory difficulty? *(Select all that apply.)*
    a. The patient's oxygen saturation drops from 98% to 94%.
    b. The patient is using accessory muscles to breathe.
    c. The patient makes a high-pitched crowing sound when breathing.
    d. The patient's blood pressure drops from 120/80 to 110/78 mm Hg.
    e. The patient's respiratory rate is 26/min.

23. When assessing the older postoperative patient for hydration status, where must the nurse assess for tenting of the skin? *(Select all that apply.)*
    a. On the back of the hand
    b. On the forehead
    c. On the forearm
    d. On the sternum
    e. On the abdomen

24. Which patient is most at risk for postoperative nausea and vomiting (PONV)?
    a. The patient with a history of motion sickness
    b. The patient with a nasogastric tube
    c. The patient who recently experienced a weight loss of 50 pounds
    d. The patient who had minimally invasive surgery (MIS)

25. The nurse is assessing a postoperative patient's gastrointestinal system. What is the best indicator that peristaltic activity has resumed?
    a. Presence of bowel sounds
    b. Patient states he is hungry
    c. Passing of flatus or stool
    d. Presence of abdominal cramping

26. The PACU nurse is assessing an older adult postoperative patient for pain. Which nonverbal manifestations by the patient suggest pain to the nurse? *(Select all that apply.)*
    a. Restlessness
    b. Profuse sweating
    c. Difficult to arouse
    d. Confusion
    e. Increased blood pressure

27. The medical-surgical nurse is caring for a postoperative patient whose lab values reveal an increase in band cells (immature neutrophils). What is the nurse's best interpretation of this value?
    a. The patient may need a transfusion.
    b. The patient is using up clotting factors.
    c. The patient is developing an infection.
    d. The patient's result is expected postoperatively.

28. Which are interventions for the medical-surgical nurse to use in preventing hypoxemia for the postoperative patient? *(Select all that apply.)*
    a. Monitor the patient's oxygen saturation.
    b. Position the patient supine.
    c. Encourage the patient to cough and breathe deeply.
    d. Get the patient up ambulating as soon as possible.
    e. Instruct the patient to rest as much as possible.

29. The health care provider removed a patient's original surgical dressing 2 days after surgery and is discharging the patient home on daily dressing changes. Which actions does the nurse take for this patient's discharge teaching? *(Select all that apply.)*

    a. Ask the patient's family or significant other to observe the dressing change.

    b. Ask the UAP to get dressing supplies for the patient.

    c. Instruct that the drainage will appear sero-sanguineous.

    d. Instruct the patient to go to the emergency department (ED) for problems related to dressing changes.

    e. Have the case manager arrange for a home health nurse to ensure that dressing changes are done and there are no complications of infection.

17 CHAPTER
Inflammation and Immunity

1. Which statements about the purpose of the immune system are true? *(Select all that apply.)*
   a. The immune system provides protection from and eliminates or destroys microorganisms.
   b. The immune system is able to identify nonself-proteins and cells.
   c. The immune system removes foreign proteins and other substances.
   d. The immune system protects against allergic/anaphylactic reactions.
   e. The immune system is able to prevent healthy body cells from being destroyed.

2. Which factors may affect the function of the immune system? *(Select all that apply.)*
   a. Nutritional status
   b. Environmental conditions
   c. Drugs
   d. Family health history
   e. Age

3. The immune system is responsible for self-tolerance. Which functions related to self-tolerance are included the immune system's responsibilities? *(Select all that apply.)*
   a. Recognize self versus nonself.
   b. Be recognized by T-lymphocyte helper/inducer T cells.
   c. Recognize different proteins on cell membranes.
   d. Recognize self versus the inflammatory response.
   e. Identify nonself, which includes all invading cells and organisms.

4. From where do most immune cells originate?
   a. Thymus
   b. Spleen
   c. Liver
   d. Bone marrow

5. How does the body determine self from nonself cells?
   a. Red blood cells use T-lymphocyte helper cells.
   b. Leukocytes use human leukocyte antigens.
   c. Leukocytes use the macrophages.
   d. White blood cells use the stem cells.

6. A patient has sustained a severe right ankle sprain, and the nurse is explaining the process of inflammation to the patient and family. Which information does the nurse include in this teaching? *(Select all that apply.)*
   a. The presence of inflammation does not always indicate that an infection is present.
   b. It occurs in response to tissue injury.
   c. It provides long-term protection.
   d. It is a specific body defense to invasion or injury.
   e. How widespread the symptoms are depends on the intensity and severity of the initiating injury.

7. The nurse is instructing a patient with an immune system disease about what the major functions of immunity are. Which information must the nurse include? *(Select all that apply.)*
   a. Immunity requires three immunity processes.
   b. Inflammation process is natural immunity.
   c. The gastrointestinal system is part of natural immunity.
   d. Antibody-mediated immunity produces new white blood cells.
   e. Cell-mediated immunity circulates T-lymphocytes.

8. The actions of leukocytes provide the body protection against invading organisms. Which are actions of leukocytes? *(Select all that apply.)*
   a. Phagocytic destruction of foreign invaders and unhealthy or abnormal self cells
   b. Lytic destruction of foreign invaders and unhealthy self cells
   c. Stimulate maturational pathway of stem cells
   d. Production of antibodies directed against invaders
   e. Production of cytokines that decrease specific leukocyte growth and activity

9. Which statement about the inflammatory response is true?
   a. Response is different with each incident.
   b. Response is the same whether the insult to the body is a burn or otitis media.
   c. Response depends on the location in the body.
   d. Response is specific to the cell type invaded or injured.

10. In which conditions is the inflammatory response present? *(Select all that apply.)*
    a. Sprain injuries to joints
    b. Appendicitis
    c. Diabetes mellitus
    d. Myocardial infarction
    e. Contact dermatitis

11. Which cell types associated with the inflammatory response participate in phagocytosis?
    a. Neutrophils and eosinophils
    b. Macrophages and neutrophils
    c. Macrophages and eosinophils
    d. Eosinophils and basophils

12. Which type of white blood cell does the body produce most?
    a. Macrophages
    b. Eosinophils
    c. Neutrophils
    d. Band neutrophils

13. Which are characteristics of neutrophils? *(Select all that apply.)*
    a. Contain chemicals such as histamine
    b. 12- to 18-hour life span
    c. Clinical sign of left shift indicates not enough mature cells being produced
    d. Liver and spleen have greatest concentration
    e. When mature, capable of phagocytosis
    f. The number in circulation increases during an allergic response

14. Which statements about phagocytosis are true? *(Select all that apply.)*
    a. It is a process that engulfs invaders and destroys them by enzymatic degradation.
    b. It is a function of all leukocytes.
    c. It rids the body of debris and destroys foreign invaders.
    d. It is done in a predictable manner.
    e. Phagocytosis involves six very important steps.

15. When an injury or invasion occurs, which functions will the phagocytic cell perform? *(Select all that apply.)*
    a. Release chemotaxins or leukotaxins
    b. Initiate repair of damaged tissue
    c. Generate specific antibodies
    d. Interrupt the process of an allergic response
    e. Gain direct contact with the antigen or invader
    f. Recognize nonself

16. What are phagocytes capable of doing?
    a. Making antibodies
    b. Ingesting cells
    c. Secreting complement
    d. Producing insulin

17. A patient is seen in the emergency department for a scalding burn to the left dorsal surface of the hands and fingers that occurred one day ago. The nurse assesses the injury to have redness, swelling, warmth to touch, and the patient reports pain in the hand. The nurse observes that the patient has limited ability to hold a pen and limited range of motion. What do these findings indicate? *(Select all that apply.)*
    a. Stage II of inflammation
    b. The result of an antigen-antibody interaction
    c. Cardinal signs of inflammation
    d. A vascular response
    e. Stage I of inflammation

18. The nurse is caring for a patient prescribed a new oral antibiotic, who has elevation in level of eosinophils and basophils. What is the nurse's best interpretation of this result?
    a. The patient may be having an allergic reaction to the antibiotic.
    b. The patient's body is fighting off an infection.
    c. The patient's white blood cells are phagocytizing the invasive organisms.
    d. The patient is at high risk for pneumonia and other respiratory infections.

19. The patient's wound has increased blood flow (hyperemia) and swelling. Which stage of inflammation does the nurse recognize?
    a. Stage I
    b. Stage II
    c. Stage III
    d. Stage IV

20. At the time of inflammation, a colony-stimulating factor stimulates bone marrow to perform which action?
    a. Produce leukocytes in less time
    b. Produce immature leukocytes
    c. Release immature leukocytes
    d. Synthesize immunoglobulins

21. The nurse is providing care for a patient whose wound is producing the substance commonly called "pus" as exudate. Which stage of inflammation does the nurse recognize?
    a. Stage I
    b. Stage II
    c. Stage III
    d. Stage IV

22. Which statements correctly describe characteristics of the phagocytosis process? *(Select all that apply.)*
    a. Neutrophils are a functional part of phagocytosis.
    b. Platelets are a functional part of phagocytosis.
    c. During phagocytosis, invading microorganisms are attacked and destroyed.
    d. During phagocytosis, dead tissue is removed.
    e. Immunoglobulins are critical to the defense of the host against pathogenic bacteria and fungi.

23. When B-lymphocytes, part of the antibody-mediated immunity (AMI) response, become sensitized to an antigen, what do they do next?
    a. Release colony-stimulating factors.
    b. Cause leukocytes to aggregate.
    c. Generate specific antibodies.
    d. Suppress phagocytosis.

24. When a person is exposed to an antigen, seven special actions take place in sequence. In which step do antibodies bind to the antigen and form an immune complex?
    a. 2
    b. 4
    c. 5
    d. 7

25. Which cells interact in the presence of an antigen to start antibody production? *(Select all that apply.)*
    a. B-lymphocytes
    b. Macrophages
    c. Neutrophils
    d. T-helper/inducer cells
    e. T-suppressor cells

26. Which statement about B-lymphocytes sensitizing to one antigen is true?
    a. Once sensitized, B-lymphocytes are always sensitized to that antigen.
    b. Plasma cells produce the antigen.
    c. The plasma cell lies dormant until the next exposure.
    d. Memory cells prevent plasma cells from oversecreting antibodies.

27. In what way is AMI different from cell-mediated immunity (CMI)?
    a. AMI is more powerful than CMI.
    b. AMI can be transferred from one person to another; CMI cannot.
    c. CMI requires constant reexposure for "boosting;" AMI does not.
    d. CMI requires inflammatory actions for best function; AMI function is independent of inflammatory actions.

28. Which action occurs during the antibody-binding reaction, agglutination?
    a. Cell membrane destruction
    b. Clumping-like antibody action
    c. Activation of IgG and IgM
    d. Covering of antigen's active site

29. Which statement is true about innate-native immunity?
    a. It is genetically determined, nonspecific, and cannot be transferred.
    b. It adapts to individual exposure and invasion.
    c. It can be altered by environmental or physiologic changes.
    d. It requires a special interaction with antibody-mediated immunity for activation.

30. Which characteristic is correct for active immunity?
    a. Antigens enter the body and the body makes antibodies against the antigen.
    b. Protection is developed by vaccination or immunization.
    c. Immunity, which is a naturally occurring feature of a person.
    d. Immunity that occurs when antibodies are created in another person or animal.

31. Which cells are the T-lymphocyte subsets that are critically important to CMI? *(Select all that apply.)*
    a. Helper/inducer T-cell
    b. Suppressor T-cell
    c. Cytotoxic/cytolytic T-cell
    d. Natural killer cells
    e. Cytokines

32. Which statement best describes the function of CD4+ (cluster of differentiation 4, or T4+) cells?
    a. They participate in specialized episodes of phagocytosis directed against cancer cells.
    b. They provide a frame or lattice for tissue repair and regeneration after inflammatory events.
    c. They secrete lymphokines that can enhance the activity of other white blood cells (WBCs).
    d. They deliver a "lethal hit" of lytic substance to a target cell in response to antibody-dependent lysis.

33. Which statement best describe the function of natural killer cells?
    a. Prevent overreaction.
    b. Exert cytotoxic effect without first undergoing period of sensitization.
    c. Bind with infected cell's antigen that results in death of affected cell.
    d. Secrete lymphokines that stimulate activities of other cells of the immune system.

34. A patient who is in good health is naturally assisted in cancer prevention by which type of immunity?
    a. Cell-mediated
    b. Innate
    c. Lymphokine
    d. Humoral

35. The action of which cell types must be suppressed to prevent acute rejection of transplanted organs? *(Select all that apply.)*
    a. Eosinophils
    b. Suppressor T-cells
    c. Natural killer cells
    d. Cytotoxic/cytolytic T-cells
    e. Helper/inducer T-cells

36. During surgery, a patient who had a heart transplant is experiencing rejection of the organ. What type of rejection is this?
    a. Acute
    b. Chronic
    c. Hyperacute
    d. Transplant

37. Which type of organ transplant rejection does not always mean immediate loss of the organ?
    a. Rejection of suppressor T-cells
    b. Chronic
    c. Acute
    d. Hyperacute

38. A patient who had an organ transplant 2 months ago is experiencing rejection of the organ. What type of rejection is this?
    a. Acute
    b. Hyperacute
    c. Delayed
    d. Chronic

39. Which characteristics describe a hyperacute rejection? *(Select all that apply.)*
    a. Immediate
    b. Rejection cannot be stopped
    c. Leads to organ destruction
    d. Does not mean loss of transplant
    e. Is antibody-mediated
    f. Triggers blood clotting cascade

40. A patient was admitted to the hospital for acute rejection after a kidney transplant that occurred 2 months ago. What are the appropriate interventions for this patient? *(Select all that apply.)*
    a. Immunosuppressant therapy to limit damage and save the organ
    b. Counseling for the patient and family about the inability to save the organ
    c. Cardiac catheterization
    d. Organ biopsy to diagnose impaired function
    e. Immediate removal of the transplanted kidney

41. How does the immune system respond to a graft when a transplant rejection occurs? *(Select all that apply.)*
    a. Anticoagulation causes damage to the graft cells.
    b. Natural killer cells cause lysis of the organ cells.
    c. Interleukin-1 causes clotting and leads to necrosis.
    d. Cytotoxic/cytolytic T-cells destroy and eliminate nonself cells.
    e. The host's immune system starts inflammation and immunologic actions to destroy nonself cells.

42. What precaution or intervention has the highest priority for a patient going home on maintenance drugs after receiving a kidney transplant?
    a. Monitoring for bacterial and fungal infections
    b. Avoiding the use of table salt
    c. Measuring abdominal girth daily
    d. Avoiding blood donation

43. Which statement is characteristic of the antibody type IgE?
    a. Mediates many types of allergic reactions
    b. Mediates ABO incompatibility reactions in blood transfusions
    c. Present in body secretions such as tears, mucus, saliva
    d. Has the highest percentage in the blood

44. The nurse is instructing a patient who has undergone an organ transplant about immunosuppressant medications. What information does the nurse include? *(Select all that apply.)*
    a. All immunosuppressive medications increase the risk of infection and cancer.
    b. These medications are used for maintenance therapy of the graft.
    c. These medications will be gradually discontinued.
    d. These medications are essential to preventing transplant rejection.
    e. Some are intravenous drugs and must be given periodically by the health care provider.

45. In order to combat rejection of a transplanted kidney, what medication given before and after the transplant surgery and that uses monoclonal antibodies is administered to the patient?
    a. Daclizumab (Zenapax)
    b. Tacrolimus FK 506 (Prograf)
    c. Cyclosporin
    d. Muromonab-CD3 (OKT3)

46. Muromonab-CD3 (OKT3) is another essential drug given to patients who are having an organ transplant. Which characteristics apply to taking this medication? *(Select all that apply.)*
    a. There is a high incidence of flulike symptoms.
    b. Induction of capillary leak syndrome is common.
    c. An antibody is also used to prevent T-cell activities.
    d. It mediates many types of immunosuppression.

47. A patient is admitted with pneumonia and has developed sepsis. What can the findings from a differential WBC count reveal about this patient? *(Select all that apply.)*
    a. If an infection is present
    b. Whether an infection is bacterial or viral
    c. The tissue type from the human leukocyte antigen
    d. Whether the patient has active immunity
    e. The type of antibody response occurring

48. The patient has experienced a myocardial infarction 6 months ago during which 25% of his left ventricle was damaged and replaced by scar tissue. Which statement does the nurse recognize as accurate?
    a. The patient will have lost 25% of effectiveness of his left ventricular contraction.
    b. The patient will have lost 50% of his ejection fraction.
    c. The patient will have regained most of the effectiveness of his left ventricle due to healing.
    d. The patient will have regained all of his activity tolerance.

49. The health care provider writes an order for the patient to be immunized with the flu vaccine. Which type of immunity does the nurse provide the patient by injecting this vaccine?
    a. Natural active immunity
    b. Artificial active immunity
    c. Adaptive immunity
    d. Passive immunity

18 CHAPTER

Care of Patients with Arthritis and Other Connective Tissue Diseases

1. A rheumatic disease is any condition or disease of which body system?
   a. Cardiovascular
   b. Hematopoietic
   c. Integumentary
   d. Musculoskeletal

2. Connective tissue diseases are characterized by which features? *(Select all that apply.)*
   a. Chronic pain
   b. Dry skin
   c. Decreased function
   d. Joint deterioration
   e. Autoimmune disorder

3. What are the known causes of osteoarthritis (OA)? *(Select all that apply.)*
   a. Smoking
   b. Aging
   c. Decrease in the production of synovial fluid
   d. Decrease in proteoglycans
   e. Obesity

4. Which are features of OA? *(Select all that apply.)*
   a. Excessive formation of scar tissue
   b. Narrowing of the joint space and formation of bone spurs
   c. Nerve degeneration resulting in joint paresthesias
   d. Bone cyst formation and joint subluxation
   e. Progressive deterioration of the loss of cartilage in one or more joints
   f. Thinning cartilage

5. The nurse is caring for an obese patient with OA. The patient asks the nurse what caused the OA. Which statement about obesity's influence on the development of osteoarthritis is accurate?
   a. The obese person has a reduced inflammatory response with less joint swelling.
   b. The high body fat levels of the obese patient lubricate joints and improve mobility.
   c. The extra weight of obesity increases the degeneration rate of hip and knee joints.
   d. Obesity has no positive or negative influence on development of OA.

6. Which patients are at risk for developing OA? *(Select all that apply.)*
   a. Obese older woman living alone
   b. Slender, nonsmoking, middle-aged man
   c. Middle-aged man with 25 years working construction
   d. Young woman with family history of rheumatoid arthritis
   e. Middle-aged adult with multiple knee injuries from playing soccer in high school

7. Which phrase is a patient most likely to use when describing crepitus associated with OA to the nurse?
   a. Increasing joint pain and stiffness
   b. A grating sound
   c. Protruding bony lumps
   d. Limited movement

8. The nurse is preparing an educational session for a group of patients newly diagnosed with OA. What lifestyle changes that may slow joint degeneration does the nurse suggest? *(Select all that apply.)*
   a. Keep body weight within normal limits.
   b. Quit smoking.
   c. Do not participate in any strenuous activity.
   d. Avoid risk-taking behaviors that may result in trauma.
   e. Avoid high-intensity exercise.

9. The presence of fluid in the knees may be diagnosed as which condition?
   a. Subcutaneous swelling
   b. Joint nodules
   c. Joint effusions
   d. Joint deformities

10. OA affecting the spine presents as what type of symptoms?
    a. Localized pain at L3-4, bone spurs, stiffness, and muscle spasm
    b. Radiating pain at L3-4, C4-6, stiffness, muscle spasms, and bone spurs
    c. Localized pain at T6-12, stiffness, and muscle atrophy
    d. Radiating pain throughout the spine, stiffness, and muscle spasms

11. Which responses from a patient with advanced OA alerts the nurse to a problem coping with the image and role changes necessitated by disease progression? *(Select all that apply.)*
    a. "I used to be a playground assistant; now I work with children who need help with reading."
    b. "I must be getting younger. I used to tie my shoes; now I am using Velcro closures just like my kids."
    c. "I find it easier to do my ironing sitting down rather than standing up."
    d. "I try to avoid public places so no one will see my ugly hands."
    e. "My joints are so stiff all the time; I can't be bothered to go outside."

12. To determine an alteration in a patient's body image and self-esteem, what does the nurse assess as priorities? *(Select all that apply.)*
    a. Church affiliation
    b. Personal care of self
    c. Demeanor as happy or sad
    d. Expression of feeling of reacting to change
    e. Number of years the patient has been married

13. The nurse is evaluating laboratory results from a patient with OA. Which lab results could the nurse expect to find elevated?
    a. White blood cells including neutrophils, basophils, macrophages, and eosinophils
    b. Erythrocyte sedimentation rate (ESR) and high-sensitivity C-reactive protein (hsCRP)
    c. Electrolytes such as potassium and calcium
    d. Clotting studies such as partial thromboplastin time (PTT) and International Normalized Ratio (INR)

14. The nurse is teaching a patient with OA about taking prescribed ibuprofen (Motrin). Which statement by the patient indicate a correct understanding of the medication?
    a. "I'll take the medication between meals."
    b. "The medication will affect my appetite."
    c. "The medication will help my pain and swelling."
    d. "I should stop the medication if my joints swell."

15. Which treatment modalities might the nurse expect for a patient who is undergoing nonsurgical management of chronic joint pain? *(Select all that apply.)*
    a. Immobilization to promote rest
    b. Weight control
    c. Anesthetics
    d. Exercise balanced with rest
    e. Thermal modalities

16. When educating a patient about total joint arthroplasty (TJA), what does the nurse do first?
    a. Asks whether the patient has insurance
    b. Reviews instructions and asks the patient to repeat them back
    c. Assesses the patient's knowledge about TJA
    d. Asks if the provider has explained the procedure

17. For preoperative care of a patient scheduled for TJA, what does the nurse plan to do? *(Select all that apply.)*
    a. Provide written or videotaped information about the procedure.
    b. Assess the patient's understanding of the procedure.
    c. Assess and include the patient's support people or family.
    d. Include interdisciplinary providers, if possible.
    e. Assist in scheduling needed dental procedures after the surgery.

18. Which are contraindications for TJA? *(Select all that apply.)*
    a. Infection
    b. Severe pain
    c. Advanced osteoporosis
    d. Severe inflammation
    e. Open wound

19. The nurse is preparing an educational session for a patient who is scheduled to undergo hip replacement. Which potential complications does the nurse make the patient aware of? *(Select all that apply.)*
    a. Venous thromboembolism
    b. Hip dislocation
    c. Overgrowth of bone
    d. Neurovascular compromise
    e. Infection

20. The nurse is preparing an educational program for student nurses on the orthopedic unit. Which three signs of hip dislocation would be included in this offering? *(Select all that apply.)*
    a. Increased pain
    b. Hip flexing of 45 degrees
    c. Shortening of affected leg
    d. Leg rotation
    e. Skin breakdown near the incision

21. Which interventions can the nurse use to prevent or manage infections in patients who have undergone total joint replacement (TJR)? *(Select all that apply.)*
    a. Use aseptic technique for wound care and emptying of drains.
    b. Wash hands thoroughly when caring for patients.
    c. Culture drainage fluid if a change is observed.
    d. Encourage early ambulation along with leg exercises.
    e. Report excessive inflammation or drainage to the provider.

22. The patient has returned from the postanesthesia care unit (PACU) after TJR. Which interventions will the nurse use to prevent venous thromboembolism? *(Select all that apply.)*
    a. Apply sequential compression devices (SCDs).
    b. Administer subcutaneous enoxaparin (Lovenox) as ordered.
    c. Keep the patient on bedrest for the first and second days postoperatively.
    d. Teach the patient to perform leg exercises such flexion and dorsiflexion.
    e. Instruct the patient to have blood drawn for INR every month.

23. Which preoperative tests are performed for a patient scheduled to undergo a total hip arthroplasty (THA)? *(Select all that apply.)*
    a. X-ray of nonoperative hip
    b. X-ray of operative hip
    c. Computed tomography (CT) of operative hip
    d. Biopsy of operative hip
    e. Magnetic resonance imaging (MRI) of operative hip

24. A patient is reluctant to consider hip surgery because of a fear of blood transfusion reaction. What is the nurse's best response?
    a. "No one will force you to receive blood if you don't want it."
    b. "You could donate your own blood for several weeks before the surgery."
    c. "Why do you think you are going to have a blood transfusion reaction?"
    d. "Blood products are very safe these days and there are numerous safety protocols."

25. A patient is receiving low–molecular-weight heparin (LMWH) therapy to prevent postoperative deep vein thrombosis (DVT). Which routine assessments are most important for this patient during anticoagulation therapy? *(Select all that apply.)*
    a. Ensure that antiembolic stockings or sequential compression devices are in use.
    b. Monitor complete blood count (CBC) and platelet counts.
    c. Monitor activated partial thromboplastin time (aPTT) levels.
    d. Check stools for occult blood.
    e. Monitor the surgical site for bleeding.

26. The nurse is providing care for a patient scheduled for a THA. Which medications should the patient receive before surgery?
    a. Enoxaparin by subcutaneous injection
    b. Bisacodyl (Dulcolax) tablet orally
    c. Antihypertensive tablet orally
    d. Aspirin 2 tablets for headache orally

27. How does a continuous peripheral nerve blockade (CPNB) device work?
    a. Infuses intravenous opioids.
    b. Infuses a local anesthetic into the surgical site.
    c. Circulates cold liquids within a wrap around the incision site.
    d. Stimulates vibration-sensitive receptors in the incision area to "close the gate" on pain.

28. Adlea is a refined capsaicin product. What is the advantage of infusing this drug directly into the surgical joint during knee surgery?
    a. Patients experience less acute postoperative pain.
    b. Capsaicin shuts down C fiber receptors.
    c. It depletes calcium stores in nerve cells and blocks pain transmission.
    d. It works as a local anesthetic, numbing nerves in the operative region.

29. Postoperative total hip replacement (THR) patients can develop numerous complications. Which interventions are most important in preventing complications? *(Select all that apply.)*
    a. Bedrest with pillow between the legs
    b. Adequate diet and fluid intake
    c. Getting out of bed on the first postoperative day
    d. Sitting on the side of the bed
    e. Frequent assessment of the patient's pain

30. For patients who have TJAs, the risk of DVT is high. Which statements are true? *(Select all that apply.)*
    a. Older adults are at high risk for DVT and compromised circulation.
    b. Thinner patients are more at risk than obese patients.
    c. Patients with a history of DVT are at high risk for recurrence.
    d. Leg exercises must be started in the immediate postoperative period.
    e. Use of an abduction splint will decrease the risk of DVT.

31. To prevent a DVT, several types of anticoagulant medications can be ordered. Which is the most commonly used drug during hospitalization?
    a. Oral or parenteral aspirin
    b. Warfarin
    c. Intravenous tPA
    d. Subcutaneous LMWH

32. It is important to monitor which laboratory test for patients on anticoagulant therapy with LMWH after TJA? *(Select all that apply.)*
    a. Prothrombin time and INR
    b. Oxygen saturation
    c. CBC
    d. Activated partial thromboplastin time
    e. Platelet count

33. Postoperative care for total knee replacement (TKR) may include which techniques? *(Select all that apply.)*
    a. Hot compresses to the incisional area
    b. Continuous passive motion (CPM) used immediately or several days postoperatively
    c. Ice packs or cold packs to the incisional area
    d. The use of a CPM machine in the daytime and an immobilizer at night
    e. Maintaining abduction

34. Postoperative care following finger and wrist replacements includes which techniques? *(Select all that apply.)*
    a. Traction
    b. Joint wrapped in a bulky dressing
    c. Splint, brace, or cast
    d. Abduction pillow
    e. Elevation of the arm to prevent edema
    f. CPM machine

35. Which interventions does the nurse implement to improve mobility for a patient who has undergone a THR? *(Select all that apply.)*
    a. Encourage use of assistive devices such as a walker when ambulating.
    b. Recommend to quickly decrease rest periods between activities.
    c. Instruct to flex the hips 90 degrees or greater.
    d. Instruct to sit on a soft chair with a raised back.
    e. Instruct in the use of a raised toilet seat.

36. What is an important health teaching point for a patient with TJA?
    a. "Do as much as you can as often as you can."
    b. "Reach beyond the physical therapist's instructions."
    c. "Protect the joint."
    d. "No pain, no gain."

37. Although arthritis is not curable, many "cures" are marketed to patients with the disease. What does the nurse encourage the patient to do?
    a. Take advantage of clinical trials or experimental therapy.
    b. Check with the Arthritis Foundation for appropriate modalities.
    c. Buy special liniments and creams.
    d. Take herbals and vitamins.

38. The nurse assesses a postoperative TKR patient for neurovascular compromise. Which assessments must the nurse document? *(Select all that apply.)*
    a. Skin color and temperature
    b. Presence or absence of distal peripheral pulses
    c. Flexion of the hips 180 degrees or greater
    d. Capillary refill of operative leg
    e. Comparison of operative leg to nonoperative leg

39. Which statements regarding rheumatoid arthritis (RA) are true? *(Select all that apply.)*
    a. It is a chronic, progressive, systemic, inflammatory process.
    b. It primarily affects the synovial joints.
    c. It is known to have periods of remission.
    d. It occurs most often in older men and women.
    e. It often involves an inflamed, red rash.

40. Because of the inflammatory process in RA, a pannus forms in the joint. What is a pannus?
    a. Scar tissue restricting the joint
    b. Vascular granulation tissue in the joint
    c. Necrotic tissue sloughing into the joint
    d. Fluid encapsulated in the joint

41. What common musculoskeletal health problem is often associated with RA?
    a. Paget's disease
    b. Fibromyalgia
    c. Marfan syndrome
    d. Osteoporosis

42. Although the etiology of RA is unknown, it is considered to be what type of disorder?
    a. An autoimmune disease
    b. Associated with aging
    c. Genetic
    d. The result of joint misuse

43. The nurse is assessing a patient admitted with RA. Which manifestations indicate to the nurse that the patient is experiencing late RA? *(Select all that apply.)*
    a. Joint deformities
    b. Joint inflammation
    c. Vasculitis
    d. Subcutaneous nodules
    e. Paresthesias
    f. Low-grade fever
    g. Anemia

44. Which patient-reported symptoms are typical of RA? *(Select all that apply.)*
    a. "My hands are stiff, swollen, and tender."
    b. "My right hand is weak."
    c. "My pain and stiffness is worse in the morning."
    d. "My knees are swollen and stiff."
    e. "I am weak and fatigued."

45. When a patient has RA of the temporomandibular joint, what is the major complaint?
    a. Pain on chewing and opening the mouth
    b. Headache at the temple
    c. Toothache
    d. Earache

46. What is the most common area of involvement of RA in the spine?
    a. Lumbar spine
    b. Sacral spine
    c. Cervical spine
    d. Thoracic spine

47. Complications of spinal involvement in RA may be seen as which signs/symptoms? *(Select all that apply.)*
    a. Compression of the phrenic nerve that controls the diaphragm
    b. Resulting subluxation of the first and second vertebrae
    c. Becoming quadriplegic or quadriparetic
    d. Bilateral sciatic pain in the legs
    e. Numbness of the hands and feet

48. In patients with RA, where might Baker's cysts be located?
    a. Ankles
    b. Wrists
    c. Popliteal bursae
    d. Achilles tendon

49. In late RA, the patient may have systemic involvement called "flareups." How are these characterized? *(Select all that apply.)*
    a. Moderate to severe weight loss
    b. Fever and fatigue
    c. Muscle atrophy
    d. Joint contractures
    e. Complete loss of mobility

50. What might a psychosocial examination of a patient with advanced RA reveal? *(Select all that apply.)*
    a. Role changes
    b. Poor self-esteem and body image
    c. Grieving and depression
    d. Loss of control and independence
    e. Inability to perform relaxation techniques

51. In RA, autoantibodies (rheumatoid factors [RFs]) are formed that attack healthy tissue, especially synovium, causing which condition?
    a. Nerve pain
    b. Bone porosity
    c. Ischemia
    d. Inflammation

52. The nurse is providing teaching for a patient with RA who is receiving methotrexate (Rheumatrex). Which teaching points must the nurse include? *(Select all that apply.)*
    a. The medication is given in a low dose once a week.
    b. Methotrexate is an immunosuppressant medication.
    c. Expect some increase in swelling while taking this medication.
    d. Avoid crowds of people and people who are ill.
    e. Report any mouth sores to the health care provider immediately.

53. What CBC laboratory values does the nurse expect to be low for a patient with RA? *(Select all that apply.)*
    a. Hemoglobin
    b. Hematocrit
    c. Red blood cell count (RBC)
    d. White blood cell count (WBC)
    e. Platelets

54. Arthrocentesis done on the patient with RA may reveal which elements in the synovial fluid of the joint? *(Select all that apply.)*
    a. Glucose and glycogen
    b. Inflammatory cells and immune complexes
    c. Protein, such as albumin
    d. Platelet aggregation
    e. Increased WBCs

55. The nurse is teaching a patient about the common side effects of chronic salicylate and nonsteroidal antiinflammatory (NSAID) therapy. Which body system side effects does the nurse focus on in the teaching plan?
    a. Central nervous system
    b. Skin
    c. Gastrointestinal
    d. Cardiovascular

56. The nurse is performing an assessment of a patient with RA. Which findings does the nurse expect?
    a. Head and neck pain
    b. Early morning joint pain
    c. Increased range of motion (ROM) in the hands
    d. Absence of joint swelling

57. The nurse's plan of care for a patient with RA includes which interventions? *(Select all that apply.)*
    a. Ensure optimal pain relief.
    b. Utilize the prone position.
    c. Encourage frequent rest periods.
    d. Decrease exercise to every other day.
    e. Recommend liberal use of arthritic creams.

58. Which statement best describes discoid lupus?
    a. It is the most frequently diagnosed type of lupus.
    b. It results in an increase in immune complexes within the joint cavity.
    c. It is not a systemic condition and is limited to involvement of the skin.
    d. It is a lupus-like syndrome that occurs in patients taking certain medications.

59. What can be expected for a patient with recently diagnosed systemic lupus erythematosus (SLE)?
    a. An acute inflammatory disorder
    b. Spontaneous remission and exacerbations
    c. Symptoms limited to arthritis
    d. Symptoms limited to skin lesions

60. What is the most common cause of death in patients with SLE?
    a. Cardiac failure
    b. Skin involvement
    c. Central nervous system involvement
    d. Renal failure

61. Which laboratory test is the only significant test for diagnosing a patient with discoid lupus?
    a. Antinuclear antibody
    b. Serum complement
    c. CBC
    d. Skin biopsy

62. A patient with scleroderma may have which problems? *(Select all that apply.)*
    a. Dysphagia
    b. Smooth tongue
    c. Malabsorption problems causing malodorous diarrhea stools
    d. Butterfly lesions on the face and nose
    e. Spiderlike hemangiomas

63. Raynaud's phenomenon in a patient with scleroderma may present as which signs/symptoms? *(Select all that apply.)*
    a. Digit necrosis
    b. Excruciating pain
    c. Autoamputations of digits
    d. Periungual lesions
    e. Peripheral neuropathy

64. What are characteristics of primary gout? *(Select all that apply.)*
    a. Results from medications such as diuretics
    b. Sodium urate deposited in the synovium
    c. Affects large joints most commonly
    d. Affects middle-aged and older men
    e. Peak time of onset after age 50

65. The patient with SLE is taking hydroxychloroquine (Plaquenil). What essential teaching point must the nurse include when teaching the patient about this drug?
    a. Watch for signs of malaria as this is an antimalarial drug.
    b. You are at risk for an increase in skin lesions while taking this drug.
    c. Have eye examinations before and every 6 months after starting this drug.
    d. Be sure to get lots of the sunlight while taking this drug.

66. A patient was prescribed the combination drug of probenicid (Lannett's Probalan) and colchicine (Colcrys) for the treatment of gout. How does the health care team evaluate the effectiveness of the therapy?
    a. Monitor the serum uric acid level.
    b. Check the results of urinalysis.
    c. Review the patient's compliance with a low-purine diet.
    d. Assess the mobility of affected joints.

67. Polymyalgia rheumatica and temporal arteritis present with which symptoms? *(Select all that apply.)*
    a. Stiffness
    b. Low-grade fever
    c. Arthralgias
    d. Decreased ESR
    e. Polycythemia

68. Patients with ankylosing spondylitis have the risk of which condition?
    a. Compromised respiratory function
    b. Cardiac involvement
    c. Hip pain
    d. Dysphagia

69. Which are common findings in a patient with Reiter's syndrome? *(Select all that apply.)*
    a. Conjunctivitis
    b. Erythema and psoriasis
    c. Arthritis
    d. Paresthesias and fatigue
    e. Urethritis

70. Which manifestations are expected in a patient with Marfan syndrome? *(Select all that apply.)*
    a. Obesity
    b. Shortened hands and feet
    c. Short, swollen fingers
    d. Excessive height
    e. Elongated hands and feet

71. Lyme disease is identified early by which signs/symptoms? *(Select all that apply.)*
    a. Known bite from deer tick
    b. Bull's-eye rash at onset
    c. Facial paralysis
    d. Dysphagia
    e. Generalized erythema

72. The nurse assessing a patient with fibromyalgia identifies the trigger points by palpation. In which specific areas does the nurse expect to elicit pain and tenderness? *(Select all that apply.)*
    a. Neck
    b. Lips
    c. Trunk
    d. Lower back
    e. Upper back

73. A patient is prescribed amitriptyline (Elavil) for the diagnosis of fibromyalgia. What kind of drug is this medication?
    a. Antiinflammatory
    b. Antirheumatic
    c. Antidepressant
    d. Antipsychotic

19 CHAPTER

Care of Patients with HIV Disease and Other Immune Deficiencies

1. Which statements about immunodeficiency are true? *(Select all that apply.)*
   a. It causes a decrease in the patient's risk for infection.
   b. It may be acquired or congenital.
   c. It occurs when a person's body cannot recognize antigens.
   d. It is the same as autoimmunity.
   e. It may cause varied reactions from mild, localized health problems to total immune system failure.

2. Which definition of immunodeficiency is accurate?
   a. Disease/deficiency acquired as a result of viral infection, contact with a toxin, or medical therapy
   b. Deficient immune response as a result of impaired or missing immune components
   c. Chronic infection with immunodeficiency virus
   d. Disease/deficiency present since birth

3. Which statements about the human immunodeficiency virus (HIV) are accurate? *(Select all that apply.)*
   a. It may be acquired or congenital.
   b. It is a retrovirus.
   c. It always progresses to acquired immunodeficiency syndrome (AIDS).
   d. It is a virus that attacks the immune system.
   e. It is a parasite that forces cells to make copies of itself.

4. Which immune function abnormalities are a result of HIV infection? *(Select all that apply.)*
   a. Lymphocytosis
   b. CD4+ cell depletion
   c. Increased CD8+ cell activity
   d. Long macrophage life span
   e. Lymphocytopenia

5. The health care provider prescribed an integrase inhibitor drug for the patient with HIV. The patient asks the nurse how this drug works. What is the nurse's best response?
   a. "It reduces how well HIV genetic material can be converted into human genetic material."
   b. "It reinforces the immune system's ability to fight off an HIV infection."
   c. "It prevents viral deoxyribonucleic acid (DNA) from integrating into the host's (your) DNA.
   d. "It will prevent your HIV infection from progressing to AIDS."

6. Which groups are experiencing increased numbers of HIV infections? *(Select all that apply.)*
   a. Men having sex with other men
   b. Intravenous drug users
   c. Women having sex with men
   d. African Americans
   e. Hispanics

7. Which descriptions are characteristic of a nonprogressor? *(Select all that apply.)*
   a. Has been infected for 10 years
   b. Is asymptomatic
   c. Has no CD4+ or T-lymphocytes
   d. Is immunocompetent
   e. Are functional antibodies

8. Which statements about the transmission of HIV are true? *(Select all that apply.)*
   a. HIV may only be transmitted during the end stages of the disease.
   b. Those with recent HIV infection and high viral load are very infectious.
   c. Those with end-stage HIV and no drug therapy are very infectious.
   d. HIV is only transmitted with sexual contact with an infected person.
   e. All people infected with HIV will quickly progress to AIDS.

9. Which conditions may be the first signs of HIV in women? *(Select all that apply.)*
   a. Vaginal candidiasis
   b. Bladder infections
   c. Cervical cancer
   d. Pelvic inflammatory disease (PID)
   e. Mononucleosis

10. Which statement regarding HIV/AIDS among older adults are true?
    a. The risk for HIV infection after exposure is minimal for older adults.
    b. Older men are more susceptible to HIV infection than are older women.
    c. It is not necessary to assess an older adult for a history of drug abuse.
    d. Older adults who participate in high-risk behaviors are susceptible to HIV infection.

11. What is the most important means of preventing HIV spread or transmission?
    a. Engineering
    b. Education
    c. Isolation
    d. Counseling

12. HIV is most commonly transmitted by which routes? *(Select all that apply.)*
    a. Oral
    b. Sexual
    c. Parenteral
    d. Airborne
    e. Perinatal

13. Highly activated antiretroviral therapy (HAART) causes what effect?
    a. Reversal of a patient's antibody status
    b. Decrease of the viral load
    c. Increase of the viral load
    d. More detectable HIV

14. The HIV-positive patient tells the nurse that that his HIV-negative partner will be using the preexposure drug emtricitabine (Truvada). Which statement indicates to the nurse the need for additional teaching about this drug?
    a. "My partner will need to be tested for HIV every 3 months."
    b. "This drug will decrease the chances of my partner becoming HIV positive."
    c. "Once we start using Truvada I will no longer need to use a condom."
    d. "My partner will need to be monitored for any side effects of this drug."

15. A patient is an IV drug user who regularly shares needles and syringes with friends. What information does the nurse provide to decrease the patient's risk of HIV through shared needles and syringes after each use?
    a. Fill and flush the syringe with clear water, then fill the syringe with bleach, shake approximately 30-60 seconds, and rinse with clear water.
    b. Fill and flush the syringe with water, then fill the syringe with soap and hot water, shake 2 minutes, and rinse with cold water.
    c. Rinse needles after each use with a bleach and water solution, then allow to air dry.
    d. Rinse needles after each use with rubbing alcohol and water solution, then rinse with water.

16. Which practices are recommended to prevent sexual transmission of HIV? *(Select all that apply.)*
    a. Use of latex or polyurethane condoms for genital and anal intercourse
    b. Use of natural-membrane condoms for genital and anal intercourse
    c. Use of topical contraceptives
    d. Use of antiviral medications
    e. Use of a latex barrier for genital and anal intercourse

17. An HIV-positive woman who is pregnant asks if her baby is at risk for HIV. Which points must the nurse be sure to include when teaching this patient? *(Select all that apply.)*
    a. "The HIV virus can cross the placenta during pregnancy."
    b. "The infant can contract HIV with exposure to blood and vaginal secretions during birth."
    c. "Once your baby is born, you should be able to breastfeed.
    d. "There is a risk of perinatal transmission of HIV from you to your child. Because you are using HIV drug therapy, that risk is about 8%."
    e. "You should consider the use of oral contraceptives to protect yourself from other sexually transmitted infections."

18. Which is the most common route for health care providers to contract the HIV virus? Exposure to HIV-positive:
    a. blood.
    b. body fluids.
    c. mucous membranes.
    d. needlesticks.

19. You are orienting a new graduate RN to the medical unit. Which point would you be sure to include when teaching this nurse to prevent HIV transmission from patients?
    a. Wear gloves when in contact with patients' mucous membranes or nonintact skin.
    b. Be sure to wear protective gear when providing any care to HIV-positive patients.
    c. Always wear a mask when entering an HIV-positive patient's room.
    d. Use postexposure prophylaxis (PEP), whether the patient is HIV-positive or not.

20. Which opportunistic infections can be observed in AIDS? *(Select all that apply.)*
    a. Toxoplasmosis
    b. Gastroenteritis
    c. Tuberculosis
    d. Candidiasis
    e. Cytomegalovirus

21. A patient with *Pneumocystis jiroveci* pneumonia (PJP) usually presents with which symptoms?
    a. Dyspnea, tachypnea, persistent dry cough, and fever
    b. Cough with copious thick sputum, fever, and dyspnea
    c. Chest pain and difficulty swallowing
    d. Fever, persistent cough, and vomiting

22. A patient presenting with toxoplasmosis may have which signs and symptoms? *(Select all that apply.)*
    a. Speech difficulty
    b. Shortness of breath
    c. Visual changes
    d. Impaired gait
    e. Mental status changes

23. Cryptosporidiosis is a form of intestinal infection in which diarrhea can amount to a loss of how many liters of fluid per day?
    a. 1 to 2
    b. 3 to 5
    c. 5 to 8
    d. 15 to 20

24. The patient with HIV/AIDS tells the nurse that food tastes funny and is difficult to swallow. What is the nurse's priority action at this time?
    a. Check the patient's gag reflex.
    b. Ask the health care provider to order blood cultures.
    c. Examine the patient's mouth and throat.
    d. Collaborate with the dietitian to provide a soft diet.

25. Where can candidiasis occur in the body? *(Select all that apply.)*
    a. Nose
    b. Esophagus
    c. Vagina
    d. Mouth
    e. Ears

26. Where in the body can cytomegalovirus (CMV) present with symptoms? *(Select all that apply.)*
    a. Eyes, causing visual impairment
    b. The kidneys as glomerulonephritis
    c. Respiratory tract, causing pneumonitis
    d. Gastrointestinal tract, causing diarrhea
    e. The heart as cardiomyopathy

27. The patient with HIV/AIDS develops manifestations of tuberculosis. What type of precautions does the nurse institute at this time?
    a. Universal precautions
    b. Airborne precautions
    c. Enteric precautions
    d. Protective isolation

28. How does the herpes simplex virus (HSV) manifest itself in patients with HIV and AIDS? *(Select all that apply.)*
    a. Maculopapular lesions that can spread
    b. A chronic ulceration after vesicles rupture
    c. Vesicles located in the perirectal, oral, and genital areas
    d. Numbness and tingling occurring before the vesicle forms
    e. Itching localized in the perianal area

29. Shingles results from varicella zoster virus (VZV) leaving the nerve ganglia and entering the body by which route?
    a. Mucous membranes
    b. Pulmonary spaces
    c. Body fluids and other tissue areas
    d. Bone marrow

30. Which malignancy is most common in patients with HIV/AIDS?
    a. Non-Hodgkin's B cell lymphoma
    b. Anal cancer
    c. Primary brain cancer
    d. Kaposi's sarcoma

31. Which treatments are intended to boost the immune system?
    a. Protease inhibitors
    b. Hematopoietic growth factors
    c. Lymphocyte transfusion
    d. Interleukin-2 infusion

32. The patient with HIV/AIDS appears emaciated and has diarrhea, anorexia, mouth lesions, and persistent weight loss. What condition does the nurse suspect this patient is developing?
    a. AIDS dementia complex
    b. AIDS wasting syndrome
    c. AIDS gastrointestinal opportunistic infection
    d. AIDS candidiasis opportunistic infection

33. Which conditions cause severe pain in HIV disease and AIDS? *(Select all that apply.)*
    a. Enlarged organs
    b. Peripheral neuropathy
    c. Tumors
    d. High fevers
    e. Dry skin

34. What methods or agents are used to treat Kaposi's sarcoma? *(Select all that apply.)*
    a. Radiotherapy
    b. Chemotherapy
    c. Antibiotics
    d. Cryotherapy
    e. Surgery

35. Which actions are useful in helping orient a patient? *(Select all that apply.)*
    a. Repeating person, place, and time
    b. Using clocks and calendars
    c. Using the Mini-Mental State Examination (MMSE) screening test
    d. Having familiar items present
    e. Providing uninterrupted time

36. The nurse assesses a patient diagnosed with advanced AIDS for malnutrition. Which findings does the nurse most likely assess? *(Select all that apply.)*
    a. Pain
    b. Anorexia
    c. Urinary incontinence
    d. Diarrhea
    e. Vomiting

37. Which nursing actions can the nurse delegate to the unlicensed assistive personnel (UAP) who will be giving mouth care to a patient with HIV/AIDS? *(Select all that apply.)*
    a. Offer the patient mouth rinses with sodium bicarbonate and sterile water several times a day.
    b. Assess the patient's mouth for increased presence of candidiasis lesions.
    c. Encourage the patient to drink plenty of fluids.
    d. Provide the patient with a soft toothbrush.
    e. Administer an oral analgesic gel as needed.

38. The HIV-positive patient is receiving HAART drugs and asks the nurse why it is essential that the drugs be taken every day at the same time. What is the nurse's best response?
    a. "Missing or delaying doses of these drugs decreases the blood concentrations needed to inhibit viral replication."
    b. "Missing or delaying doses of these drugs decreases the risk of developing opportunistic infections."
    c. "Missing or delaying doses of these drugs decreases the effectiveness of the therapy."
    d. "Missing or delaying doses of these drugs decreases the risk of developing HIV resistant mutations."

39. Corticosteroids perform which actions? *(Select all that apply.)*
    a. Block the movement of neutrophils and monocytes through cell membranes.
    b. Increase cell production in the bone marrow.
    c. Reduce the number of circulating T cells, resulting in suppressed cell-mediated immunity.
    d. Decrease intracranial pressure.
    e. Constrict blood vessels.

40. Which methods or items are means of transmitting HIV? *(Select all that apply.)*
    a. Sexual intercourse
    b. Household utensils
    c. Breast milk
    d. Toilet facilities
    e. Mosquitoes

41. The nurse is teaching a patient about preventing HIV infection through sexual contact. Which statement made by the patient indicates effective teaching?
    a. "A latex condom with spermicide provides the best protection against getting infected with HIV."
    b. "Mutually monogamous sex with a noninfected partner will best prevent HIV infection."
    c. "Contraceptive methods like implants and injections are recommended to prevent HIV transmission."
    d. "If my partner and I are both HIV-positive, unprotected sex is permitted."

42. Which laboratory results will the nurse expect to decrease in a patient who has HIV/AIDS? *(Select all that apply.)*
    a. CD4+
    b. CD8+
    c. WBC
    d. Lymphocytes
    e. HIV antibodies

43. A patient diagnosed with HIV is receiving medications to reduce the viral load and improve CD4+ lymphocyte counts. Which term accurately describes this HIV/AIDS drug regimen?
    a. Interferon treatment
    b. Antiviremia
    c. ELISA administration
    d. HAART therapy

20
CHAPTER

Care of Patients with Immune Function Excess: Hypersensitivity (Allergy) and Autoimmunity

1. Which type I hypersensitivity reaction requires immediate intervention by the nurse?
   a. Purified protein derivative (PPD) test result of 10 mm
   b. Anaphylaxis
   c. Vasculitis
   d. Fever

2. "Overreactions" to invaders or foreign antigens can be the result of which of the following? *(Select all that apply.)*
   a. Hypersensitivity
   b. Allergic response
   c. Autoimmune response
   d. Phagocytosis
   e. Increased cardiac output

3. Which statement best describes allergy or hypersensitivity?
   a. Excessive response to the presence of an antigen
   b. Excessive response against self cells and cell products
   c. Failure of the immune system to recognize self cells as normal
   d. Failure of the immune system to recognize foreign cells and microbial invaders

4. Which clinical examples are type I immediate hypersensitivities? *(Select all that apply.)*
   a. Graft rejection
   b. Hay fever
   c. Serum sickness
   d. Anaphylaxis
   e. Autoimmune hemolytic anemia
   f. Allergic asthma

5. Which clinical example is an example of type V stimulated hypersensitivity?
   a. Poison ivy
   b. Graves' disease
   c. Myasthenia gravis
   d. Vasculitis

6. Which type of therapy for allergy management administers small increasing amounts of identified allergens subcutaneously?
   a. Alternative
   b. Progressive
   c. Symptomatic
   d. Desensitization

7. During assessment of a newly admitted patient, the nurse notes a runny nose with clear drainage; pink, swollen mucosa; itchy, watery eyes; and a nasal-sounding voice. What does the nurse expect is the patient's diagnosis?
   a. Hypersensitivity
   b. Allergic response
   c. Allergic rhinitis
   d. Autoimmune response

8. Which techniques are used for allergy management? *(Select all that apply.)*
   a. Avoidance
   b. Desensitization
   c. Conization
   d. Antibiotics
   e. Injections

9. Which methods are used for testing for allergies? *(Select all that apply.)*
   a. Topical serums
   b. Scratch test
   c. Intravenous
   d. Intradermal
   e. Skin biopsy

10. The nurse is teaching a patient who is to have allergy scratch testing. Which key points would the nurse be sure to include? *(Select all that apply.)*
    a. The results will be available within 15-20 minutes.
    b. Be sure to take your antihistamine medication immediately before the test.
    c. Stop taking systemic glucocorticoids 2 weeks before the test.
    d. You may use a nasal spray to reduce mucous membrane swelling.
    e. The testing will be done on the inside of your forearm or your back.

11. The nurse is preparing to discharge a patient prescribed a decongestant drug. What must the nurse be sure to include when teaching about this drug?
    a. "This drug will prevent vasodilation and decrease secretions."
    b. "This drug works by causing vasoconstriction reducing the swelling."
    c. "This drug will decrease inflammation."
    d. "This drug will desensitize your allergic reactions."

12. The nurse is reviewing the health history of a patient who reports allergic rhinitis, and who has been taking over-the-counter (OTC) decongestants for these symptoms. Which chronic health problems cause the nurse to recommend that the patient stop taking the OTC medication immediately? *(Select all that apply.)*
    a. Osteoarthritis
    b. Hypertension
    c. Diabetes mellitus
    d. Glaucoma
    e. Pancreatitis

13. For a patient who is having an anaphylactic reaction, which common symptoms will manifest almost immediately after being exposed to an allergen? *(Select all that apply.)*
    a. Angioedema
    b. Apprehension
    c. Chills
    d. Fever
    e. Urticaria

14. A patient in anaphylaxis who is going into respiratory failure will demonstrate which symptoms? *(Select all that apply.)*
    a. Laryngeal edema
    b. Hypoxemia
    c. Hypocapnia
    d. Dehydration
    e. Crackles
    f. Wheezing

15. The patient has a documented allergy to bananas and avocadoes. What specific priority precaution must the nurse take when providing care for this patient? Ask the patient about:
    a. other food allergies.
    b. antibiotic drug allergies.
    c. allergies to pets.
    d. latex allergies.

16. The nurse is caring for a patient and suspects anaphylaxis. What first priority action does the nurse take at this time?
    a. Place the patient on a cardiac monitor.
    b. Insert a large-bore intravenous (IV) line.
    c. Call the Rapid Response Team.
    d. Apply oxygen by nasal cannula.

17. For the patient with anaphylaxis described above, which priority treatment does the nurse expect to administer?
    a. Education regarding the use of the EpiPen
    b. Epinephrine injection
    c. Intravenous 0.9% normal saline
    d. Intravenous corticosteroids

18. The nurse is assessing a patient experiencing a cytotoxic reaction to IV drugs. What is the nurse's first action?
    a. Discontinue drug administration.
    b. Decrease the infusion rate.
    c. Call the health care provider.
    d. Call the Rapid Response Team.

19. What are the clinical manifestations of systemic lupus erythematosus that are caused by immune complex reaction? *(Select all that apply.)*
    a. Vasculitis, glomerulonephritis nephritis
    b. Hypertension, anemia
    c. Destruction of mucus-producing glands
    d. Increased urinary output
    e. Arthritis

20. Which therapies are appropriate for the treatment of serum sickness? *(Select all that apply.)*
    a. Antihistamines for itching
    b. Aspirin for arthralgias
    c. Penicillin for infection
    d. Prednisone if manifestations are severe
    e. Plasmapheresis to remove antibodies

21. Which responses are characterized as type IV delayed hypersensitivity reactions? *(Select all that apply.)*
    a. Positive PPD test for tuberculosis
    b. Anaphylaxis after insect sting
    c. Thrombocytopenic purpura
    d. Contact dermatitis
    e. Graft rejection

22. What is the most important aspect of treating type V stimulating reactions?
    a. Medication management and observation for adverse effects
    b. Removing stimulated tissue to return the organ to normal functioning
    c. Monitoring for other organ involvement
    d. Surgical removal of secondary immune tissue

23. Which descriptions best characterize autoimmunity? *(Select all that apply.)*
    a. Cell-mediated immune response that does not cause an antibody-mediated response
    b. The synthetic substances used to stimulate or suppress the response of the immune system
    c. Inappropriate immune response to one's own healthy cells and tissues
    d. An altered immune response that results in an immediate hypersensitivity reaction
    e. Immune system failing to recognize certain body cells or tissues as self, triggering immune reactions

24. Which disorders are types of autoimmune diseases? *(Select all that apply.)*
    a. Polyarteritis nodosa
    b. Systemic lupus erythematosus
    c. Hypothyroidism
    d. Rheumatic fever
    e. Hashimoto's thyroiditis

25. Which management strategy does the nurse expect when caring for a patient with an autoimmune disease?
    a. Antibiotic drugs
    b. Antihistamine drugs
    c. Antiinflammatory drugs
    d. Bronchodilator drugs

26. What is the most common cause of Sjögren's syndrome thought to be?
    a. A bacterial infection
    b. A viral infection
    c. Inflammation
    d. An allergic reaction

27. The nurse suspects Sjögren's syndrome because the patient reports which common symptoms? *(Select all that apply.)*
    a. Increased tooth decay
    b. Burning and itching of the eyes
    c. Painful intercourse
    d. Nosebleeds
    e. Shortness of breath

28. The nurse expects the lab values on a patient with Sjögren's syndrome to include which results? *(Select all that apply.)*
    a. Increased presence of general antinuclear antibodies
    b. Elevated levels of IgM rheumatoid factor
    c. Decreased presence of anti-SS-A or anti-SS-B antibodies
    d. Decreased erythrocyte sedimentation rate
    e. Increased circulating platelets

29. Which symptomatic treatments does the nurse expect to implement for a patient with Sjögren's syndrome? *(Select all that apply.)*
    a. Water-soluble lubricants
    b. Artificial tears
    c. Beta-blockers
    d. Room humidifiers
    e. Nonsteroidal antiinflammatory drugs (NSAIDs)

30. Goodpasture's syndrome is an autoimmune disorder in which autoantibodies attack which two body components?
    a. Myocardial muscle and conduction system cells
    b. Mucous membranes of the mouth and nose
    c. Glomerular basement membrane and neutrophils
    d. Blood vessel walls in the skin and joints

31. The nurse is assessing a patient with suspected Goodpasture's syndrome. What symptoms would the nurse expect? *(Select all that apply.)*
    a. Hemoptysis
    b. Increased urine output
    c. Bradycardia
    d. Shortness of breath
    e. Weight loss
    f. Generalized edema

32. Which organs are often damaged in Goodpasture's syndrome, which can cause death?
    a. Heart and lungs
    b. Liver and kidneys
    c. Lungs and kidneys
    d. Heart and Liver

33. A patient has been diagnosed with Goodpasture's syndrome. Which drug therapies does the nurse expect to administer? *(Select all that apply.)*
    a. Vasopressors
    b. Low-dose chemotherapy
    c. Antibiotics
    d. Corticosteroids
    e. Muscle relaxants

34. The patient with Goodpasture's syndrome is to receive plasmapheresis. The nurse is preparing to teach about this treatment. Which statement best describes plasmapheresis?
    a. Blood is circulated through a machine that removes excess fluids.
    b. 300 to 500 mL of blood is intermittently removed to decrease immune complexes.
    c. Autoantibodies are removed from blood plasma.
    d. IV immunoglobulins (IVIGs) are infused.

35. Which nursing intervention is most important for the nurse to perform before administering any drug or therapeutic agent to a patient?
    a. Ask the patient about allergies to drugs or other substances.
    b. Compare the wristband name with the drug administration record.
    c. Verify the order with the prescriber.
    d. Calculate the prescribed drug dosage twice.

36. A patient who had a PPD test has redness and a 9-mm induration at the injection site. The nurse suspects which type of hypersensitivity reaction?
    a. Type I, immediate
    b. Type II, cytotoxic
    c. Type III, immune complex-mediated
    d. Type IV, delayed

37. A patient reports a runny nose with clear drainage, watery eyes, and a scratchy throat. The nurse determines the patient has been in close contact with several cats. Which hypersensitivity reaction does the nurse suspect the patient is experiencing?
    a. Type I, immediate
    b. Type II, cytotoxic
    c. Type III, immune complex-mediated
    d. Type IV, delayed

38. The nurse is preparing a teaching plan for the patient and family on how to care for an automatic epinephrine injector. Which essential points must the nurse include? *(Select all that apply.)*
    a. "Keep the device with you at all times."
    b. "You can inject the drug right through your pants."
    c. "Whenever you use the device, call your doctor and rest in bed for the next 24 to 48 hours."
    d. "Protect the device from light and avoid temperature extremes."
    e. "Keep safety cap in place until you are ready to use the device."

21 CHAPTER

Cancer Development

1. Which task is the nurse most likely to perform related to cancer disorders or the care of a patient with cancer?
   a. Informs a 36-year-old woman about the initial diagnosis of breast cancer
   b. Explains recommendations for yearly mammograms to a 50-year-old woman
   c. Suggests treatments based on staging of breast tumor to a 65-year-old woman
   d. Advises a 23-year-old woman to have surgery for breast cancer

2. In affluent countries such as the United States, which factor has contributed to the increase of certain types of cancer?
   a. Life expectancy has increased.
   b. Screening for cancer is more common.
   c. Obesity is common at an early age.
   d. Use of tobacco has increased.

3. Which body tissue will undergo normal growth through the process of hypertrophy?
   a. Skin
   b. Heart muscle
   c. Stomach lining
   d. Brain

4. In which circumstance would mitosis be considered a normal physiologic process?
   a. A 25-year-old woman is diagnosed with endometriosis.
   b. A 45-year-old woman notices several skin tags on her neck.
   c. A 35-year-old male has ulcer disease that is slowly resolving.
   d. A 65-year-old man has a benign tumor that seems to be enlarging.

5. The nurse reads a laboratory report that indicates that the tissue sample of a patient is essentially neoplastic. How does the nurse interpret this report?
   a. Cell growth is abnormal and not needed for tissue replacement.
   b. The tissue specimen shows malignant cell growth.
   c. The parent cell was abnormal, but new growth is benign.
   d. Early cell death is inevitable, because the morphology is abnormal.

6. Which cells would normally not produce fibronectin?
   a. Cells with a large nuclear-cytoplasmic ratio
   b. Normal cardiac muscle cells
   c. Normal red blood cells
   d. Cells that are undergoing normal mitosis

7. Which areas of the body contain cells that grow throughout the life span? *(Select all that apply.)*
   a. Heart
   b. Hair
   c. Brain
   d. Bone marrow
   e. Skin

8. Which biologic process demonstrates the differentiated function of red blood cells (RBCs)?
   a. RBCs float freely through the circulatory system.
   b. RBCs die according to programmed cell death.
   c. RBCs make hemoglobin, which carries oxygen.
   d. RBCs are formed with 23 pairs of chromosomes.

9. Which biologic process demonstrates that there is a problem with cellular regulation?
   a. Living cells spend most of their time in G_0 state.
   b. Mitosis occurs to replace damaged tissue.
   c. Cyclin activity is balanced by suppressor genes.
   d. Cells continue to divide despite contact inhibition.

10. Place the activities of the phases of the cell cycle in the correct order.

    _____ a. The single cell splits into two during the M phase.

    _____ b. In the G_1 phase, the cell takes on nutrients, makes energy, and grows extra membrane.

    _____ c. The cell makes proteins for division and normal function in the G_2 phase.

    _____ d. During the S phase, the cell doubles its deoxyribonucleic acid (DNA) content.

11. If apoptosis is occurring within a patient's body, what is the expected outcome of this physiologic process?
    a. Rapid growth of malignant tumors metastasizing through the body.
    b. Organs have an adequate number of cells at their functional peak.
    c. Normal tissue continues to function in an abnormal place.
    d. Cells will initially resemble parent cells, but will rapidly mutate.

12. Benign cells have which characteristics? (Select all that apply.)
    a. Tissue unnecessary for normal function
    b. Resemble the parent tissue
    c. Orderly growth with normal growth patterns
    d. Perform their differentiated function
    e. Invade other tissues

13. Which features are specific to cancer cells?
    a. They grow very slowly, but eventually harm the body.
    b. They have a small, fragile nucleus that is easily damaged.
    c. They produce fibronectin that strengthens the cell wall.
    d. They have an unlimited life span and can metastasize.

14. What is an action of carcinogens?
    a. Damages the DNA
    b. Increases migration of cells
    c. Turn offs oncogenes
    d. Stimulates viral activity

15. Why do cancer cells spread throughout the body? (Select all that apply.)
    a. They deplete available nutrients at the original site.
    b. They are able to metastasize.
    c. They are persistent in their growth.
    d. Cell division does not respond to contact inhibition.
    e. They have only one enzyme on their surface.

16. Ideally, the health care team should encourage primary prevention measures to target which step of carcinogenesis?
    a. Initiation
    b. Promotion
    c. Progression
    d. Metastasis

17. What role do normal hormones and proteins such as insulin and estrogen play in the development of cancer?
    a. They prolong or delay the latency period.
    b. They can promote frequent division of cells.
    c. They act like carcinogens under certain conditions.
    d. They turn off the suppressor genes.

18. What is the minimum size for a detectable tumor?
    a. 1 millimeter
    b. 1 centimeter
    c. Depends on type of tumor
    d. Depends on site of tumor

19. If a primary tumor is located in a vital organ, what happens?
    a. The organ's rate of cell division is increased.
    b. The organ's response to injury is decreased.
    c. There is interference with the organ's functioning.
    d. Function of the organ is initially increased.

20. Which statement correctly describes metastatic tumors?
    a. They are caused by cells breaking off from the primary tumor.
    b. They become less malignant over time.
    c. They are usually less harmful than a primary tumor.
    d. They become the tissue of the organ where they spread.

21. What role does vascular endothelial growth factor (VEGF) have in the metastasis of cancer?
    a. VEGF triggers capillary growth to ensure blood supply to the tumor.
    b. Use of VEGF helps to stop the growth and spread of the primary tumor.
    c. VEGF is a carcinogen that activates when cancer cells reach the vascular system.
    d. For cancers with a genetic link, VEGF must be present before metastasis occurs.

22. Which information can be obtained from grading a tumor?
    a. Cause of the cancer
    b. Location of metastasis
    c. Evaluating prognosis and appropriate therapy
    d. How long the cancer has been present

23. What information can be obtained by surgical staging? *(Select all that apply.)*
    a. Assessment of tumor size
    b. Number of tumors
    c. Sites of tumors
    d. Pattern of spread of tumors
    e. Pain related to tumors

24. On the figure below, identify the step where "tumor vascularization" is occurring during the process of metastasis. _____

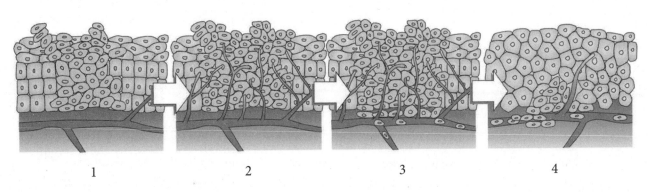

1   2   3   4

25. From a primary prevention perspective, what is the most important information that the nurse should emphasize when teaching patients about tobacco and cancer risk?
    a. Tobacco is the single most preventable source of carcinogenesis.
    b. Tobacco use is linked to many different types of cancer.
    c. A person's risk for cancer depends on the amount of tobacco use.
    d. A person's risk for cancer increases when tobacco and alcohol are used.

26. The nurse is talking to a young woman who "is using a tanning salon, because it is a safer way to get a tan than lying in the sun." What is the best response?
    a. "Even if you use a tanning salon, you should still use a sunscreen."
    b. "Tanning salons are safer because exposure to radiation is very controlled."
    c. "Ultraviolet (UV) radiation from sun exposure or tanning salons can cause skin cancer."
    d. "Ionizing radiation is dangerous, but tanning salons use UV radiation."

27. Which person has the greatest risk for developing cancer?
    a. 10-year-old African American with asthma
    b. 32-year-old Asian immigrant with low income
    c. 23-year-old white American who is diabetic
    d. 62-year-old African American with AIDS

28. African Americans have the highest rate of and highest death rate from cancer. Which intervention targets the most likely explanation for this disparity?
    a. Increase local efforts to dispense cancer information to this vulnerable group.
    b. Develop educational materials that are culturally sensitive towards African Americans.
    c. Provide referral information to health care facilities that are affordable and accessible.
    d. Continue research which further clarifies the genetic or racial risk for cancer.

29. The nurse hears in report that the patient is diagnosed with glioblastoma. Which question is the most important to ask the off-going nurse?
    a. "What is the patient's current mental status?"
    b. "Does the patient have leg pain during ambulation?"
    c. "Is the patient able to eat a normal diet?"
    d. "Does the patient have trouble passing urine?"

30. Which patient would have the best prognosis for survival based on the TNM staging classification listed?
    a. $T_{IS}N_0M_0$
    b. $T_xN_xM_x$
    c. $T_2N_1M_0$
    d. $T_2N_3M_1$

31. Which patient report should be investigated as one of the seven warning signs of cancer?
    a. Soreness and stiffness to joints in the morning
    b. Abdominal pain associated with menstrual cycle
    c. Redness to skin with pain after sun exposure
    d. Sore on nipple present for several months

32. Which are cancers that have genetic predisposition? (Select all that apply.)
    a. Breast
    b. Colorectal
    c. Melanoma
    d. Bladder
    e. Lung

33. The American Cancer Society reports that the cancer incidence and survival rate are related to which factor?
    a. Gender of patient and gender of family care giver
    b. Availability of health care services
    c. Belief in effectiveness of cancer treatment
    d. Age at initiation of lifestyle modification

34. Which lunch tray represents a diet that would decrease the risk of cancer?
    a. Plain chicken breast on white bread
    b. Vegetable plate with a bran muffin
    c. Grilled cheese sandwich with fruit salad
    d. Bacon cheeseburger with French fries

35. The nurse is preparing a brochure to inform patients about secondary prevention of cancer. Which information would be included?
    a. Yearly mammography for women over age 40
    b. Chemoprevention with vitamin therapy
    c. Removing colon polyps
    d. Using sunscreen when outdoors

36. Which woman would be the most likely candidate to consider removal of "at risk" breast tissue?
    a. Has a family history of breast and colon cancer
    b. Has a family history of breast cancer and smokes cigarettes
    c. Has mutations in the BRCA1 and BRCA2 genes
    d. Has mammogram results that suggest a biopsy is needed

22 CHAPTER

Care of Patients with Cancer

1. Which patient with cancer has the greatest risk for infection?
   a. Recently diagnosed with breast cancer
   b. Has leukemia with neutropenia
   c. Has lung cancer with a persistent cough
   d. Diagnosed with prostate cancer 3 years ago

2. The health care provider informs the nurse that it is likely that the patient's cancer has invaded the bone marrow. Based on this information, the nurse will be vigilant for which signs and symptoms? *(Select all that apply.)*
   a. Nausea and vomiting
   b. Fatigue and weakness
   c. Decreasing white blood cell counts
   d. Confusion with memory loss
   e. Bruises or other bleeding signs

3. A patient asks the nurse why untreated cancers cause gastrointestinal problems. Which responses are appropriate? *(Select all that apply.)*
   a. "A tumor in the bowel can decrease your ability to absorb necessary nutrients."
   b. "The spread or metastasis of the cancer to the stomach occurs very frequently."
   c. "Changes in taste can decrease appetite or cause food aversions."
   d. "Cancer is treated with radiation therapy that usually alters bowel function."
   e. "Tumors may increase metabolic needs which you are unable to meet."

4. The nurse hears in report that the patient has cachexia. Which assessment will the nurse plan to perform?
   a. Ability to ambulate independently
   b. Appetite and nutritional intake
   c. Mental status and cognition
   d. Sensation and pulses in extremities

5. The patient has breast cancer with bone metastasis. Based on this information, which laboratory result would the nurse expect to see?
   a. Increase in serum calcium level
   b. Decrease in blood glucose
   c. Increase in platelet count
   d. Decrease in serum sodium level

6. Which factors determine the type of therapy for cancer? *(Select all that apply.)*
   a. Type and location of cancer
   b. Overall health of the patient
   c. Whether the cancer has metastasized
   d. Family history and genetics
   e. Previous lymph node biopsy

7. Which example best illustrates appropriate prophylactic cancer surgery?
   a. Removal of breast tissue for strong family history of breast cancer
   b. Biopsy of lymph node at a site distal to the primary tumor
   c. Breast reconstruction after a mastectomy
   d. Partial removal of a tumor to provide pain relief

8. Which therapy is an example of the cornerstone for cancer treatment?
   a. Use of ionizing radiation to destroy cancer cells
   b. Physical rehabilitation exercises to restore function
   c. Surgical removal of the visible and microscopic tumor
   d. Chemotherapy to cure or increase survival time

9. Which word best describes the purpose of cytoreductive surgery for cancer?
   a. Prevention
   b. Control
   c. Cure
   d. Restore

10. Which cancer patient is the most likely candidate for palliative surgery?
    a. Needs extensive cosmetic repair after treatment of neck cancer
    b. Has continuous vomiting because tumor is obstructing the gastrointestinal (GI) tract
    c. Has a suspicious skin lesion that requires further investigation
    d. Has been treated for cancer and is currently asymptomatic

11. Which cancer patient is the most likely candidate for reconstructive surgery?
    a. Has severe back pain and decreased sensation in the lower extremities
    b. Has significant scarring of the face and neck after completing treatments
    c. Requires lymph node removal for possible metastasis of primary tumor
    d. Has leukemia that is not responding to transfusion therapy

12. The nurse is talking to a young athlete who needs lung removal for treatment of lung cancer. Which statement best indicates that the patient is coping with the uncertainty of cancer and long-term impact on his physical activities?
    a. "If I delay the surgery, I could still compete for a couple of months."
    b. "My coach says I might be able to compete even with one lung."
    c. "Competing in sports is important to me and I eventually I will recover."
    d. "I love to compete in sports, but I like to do a lot of other things too."

13. The nurse is caring for a 56-year-old woman who had a modified mastectomy for breast cancer. The woman jokes, "That breast was too saggy anyway. Good riddance to it." Later, the nurse sees the woman crying. What should the nurse do first?
    a. Encourage the woman to accept body changes by looking at the surgical site.
    b. Suggest participation in a support group sponsored by the American Cancer Society.
    c. Invite a breast cancer survivor who successfully coped with mastectomy.
    d. Sit with the woman and encourage her to express her feelings and concerns.

14. Which factors are used to determine a cancer patient's absorbed radiation dose? (Select all that apply.)
    a. Intensity of radiation exposure
    b. Proximity of radiation source to the cells
    c. Duration of exposure
    d. Age of the patient
    e. Previous radiation therapy

15. Based on the "inverse square law" for radiation exposure, which patient received the smallest radiation dose?
    a. Received radiation dose at a distance of 0.5 meter
    b. Received radiation dose at a distance of 1 meter
    c. Received radiation dose at a distance of 2.5 meters
    d. Received radiation dose at a distance of 3 meters

16. What is the most typical schedule for radiation therapy?
    a. Small doses of radiation given on a daily basis for a set time period
    b. Large one-time dose of radiation given after completing chemotherapy
    c. Small doses of radiation given several days apart to minimize side effects
    d. Large doses administered monthly for a set period of months

17. How does the nurse apply the "inverse square law" in caring for a patient with cancer who is treated with a radiation implant?
    a. Assists the health care provider to calculate the radiation dose
    b. Reminds unlicensed assistive personnel (UAP) to wear a dosimeter film badge for protection
    c. Stands at a distance from the patient as much as possible
    d. Monitors condition of skin after therapy with gamma rays

18. The nurse is caring for a patient who will receive stereotactic body radiotherapy. Which intervention is the nurse most likely to use in the care of this patient?
    a. Post a sign to remind pregnant visitors to avoid entering the patient's room.
    b. Assess the UAP's understanding of how to handle radioactive urine and stool.
    c. Teach the patient about the need for exact positioning during the treatment.
    d. Assess the patient for history of allergies to iodine or contrast media.

19. At what point is a patient radioactive when receiving radiation treatment by teletherapy and is therefore a potential danger to other people?
    a. The patient is never radioactive
    b. During the mechanical delivery of gamma rays
    c. For the first 24 to 48 hours after treatment
    d. Until the radiation source has decayed by one half-life

20. What are the side effects of radiation? *(Select all that apply.)*
    a. Altered taste sensation
    b. Skin changes and permanent local hair loss
    c. Diarrhea and tooth loss
    d. Weight gain and fluid retention
    e. Fatigue

21. For a patient undergoing external radiation therapy, what do the nurse's instructions include? *(Select all that apply.)*
    a. Do not remove the markings.
    b. Do not use lotions or ointments.
    c. Avoid direct skin exposure to sunlight for up to a year.
    d. Use mild soap and water on the affected skin.
    e. Gently rub treated areas to stimulate circulation

22. Why does the nurse wear a dosimeter when providing care to a patient receiving brachytherapy?
    a. Indicates special expertise in radiation therapy.
    b. Protects the nurse from absorbing radiation.
    c. Measures the nurse's exposure to radiation.
    d. Ensures that the radiation dosage is accurate.

23. The patient has thyroid cancer and will be treated with injection of the radionuclide iodine-131 (brachytherapy). Which guideline is the most relevant to correctly instructing the UAP about assisting the patient with hygiene and activities of daily living (ADLs)?
    a. Oncology Nursing Society practice guidelines
    b. American Cancer Society treatment guidelines
    c. Institutional evidence-based policies for infection control
    d. Institutional policies for handling body fluids and wastes

24. The nurse is supervising a nursing student who is giving care to a patient with a sealed implant. The nurse would intervene if the student performed which action?
    a. Places a "Caution: Radioactive Material" sign on the door of the patient's room
    b. Wears a dosimeter film badge at all times while caring for patient
    c. Wears a lead apron while providing care, but turns away from the patient
    d. Saves all dressings and bed linens in the patient's room

25. The nurse hears in report that the patient has xerostomia. Which teaching point does the nurse plan to review with the patient?
    a. Regular dental visits are essential because of increased risk for dental caries.
    b. Use mild soap and apply unscented moisturizers to reduce itching sensation.
    c. Avoid rigorous sports because bones are more prone to pathologic fractures.
    d. Avoid direct sun exposure for at least 1 year because skin will be sensitive.

26. What are the rationales for chemotherapy as a cancer treatment? *(Select all that apply.)*
    a. Increases survival time for the patient
    b. Decreases the patient's risk for life-threatening complications
    c. Systemic treatment for cancer cells that may have escaped from the primary tumor
    d. Concentrates in secondary lymphoid tissues and prevents widespread metastasis
    e. Less expensive and safer than radiation therapy

27. The nurse works at an institution where pharmacogenomics is incorporated into the care of cancer patients. How does this newer approach impact nursing care?
    a. Nurse is likely to see fewer cancers that are linked to a genetic etiology.
    b. Targeted chemotherapy selection will eliminate side effects.
    c. Prophylactic treatment of first-degree family members is likely to increase.
    d. Patients' risk for the more dangerous side effects is decreased.

28. Which laboratory result is the most important in relation to the nadir?
    a. Red blood cell count
    b. White blood cell count
    c. Platelet count
    d. Serum calcium level

29. Each chemotherapeutic agent has a specific nadir. What is important to do when giving combination therapy?
    a. Give two agents with similar nadirs.
    b. Avoid giving agents with similar nadirs at the same time.
    c. Allow for one agent's nadir to recover before giving another agent.
    d. Give two agents from the same drug class.

30. Chemotherapy drug dosage is based on total body surface area (TBSA); therefore, what assessment will the nurse perform?
    a. Measure the patient's height and weight.
    b. Compare the patient's weight to a nomogram.
    c. Calculate body mass index.
    d. Measure abdominal girth.

31. What does a course of chemotherapy normally include? *(Select all that apply.)*
    a. Rounds every week for a total of 6 weeks
    b. Variance with patient's responses to therapy
    c. Timed dosing of the therapy to minimize normal cell damage
    d. A concurrent dose of radiation
    e. The administration of one specific anticancer drug

32. A patient is on a newer protocol, dose-dense chemotherapy. Which factor is most likely to contribute to patient noncompliance if the nurse fails to educate the patient and the family?
    a. Treatment is expensive and less likely to be covered by insurance.
    b. Length of therapy is prolonged and progress is slow to manifest.
    c. Side effects are likely to be more intense and unpleasant.
    d. Administration is painful and pain does not respond to medications.

33. The charge nurse sees an order for intravenous (IV) chemotherapy. According to the Oncology Nursing Society, who should the charge nurse assign to administer the medication?
    a. Any nurse who studied pharmacology and has IV therapy training
    b. Advanced-practice nurse who specializes in oncology education
    c. Registered nurse who completed an approved chemotherapy course
    d. Licensed practical nurse with years of experience in giving medications

34. The nurse is caring for a patient who must receive an IV chemotherapy infusion. What is the most important intervention related to extravasation?
    a. Identify the specific antidote and make sure it is readily available.
    b. Frequently monitor the access site to prevent leakage of large volumes.
    c. Advocate that an implanted port be established prior to administration.
    d. Check institutional policy to see if warm or cold compresses are prescribed.

35. What is the major side effect that limits the dose of chemotherapy?
    a. Nausea and vomiting
    b. Peripheral neuropathy
    c. Bone marrow suppression
    d. "Chemo brain"

36. A patient is being discharged with a prescription for an oral cancer agent. Based on recent research studies, which teaching point will the nurse emphasize?
    a. Oral anticancer medications are less toxic and can be handled like regular medications.
    b. Oral forms are more convenient for home use and cost less than IV medications.
    c. Crushing the medication and mixing it with pudding or juice will mask the unpleasant taste.
    d. Adherence to therapy schedule is more of a problem, but do not skip or reduce doses.

37. The nurse hears in report that the patient is distressed by the prospect of developing alopecia. Which question is the nurse most likely to ask to assess the patient's concerns?
    a. "Would you like additional information about side effects of chemotherapy?"
    b. "What questions do you have about hair and skin care products?"
    c. "How would losing your hair affect your life and activities?"
    d. "How would you feel about talking to someone who experienced hair loss?"

38. The nurse reads in the patient's chart that the health care provider is concerned about myelosuppression. Which laboratory results will the nurse closely monitor and report to the provider? *(Select all that apply.)*
    a. White blood cell count
    b. Serum potassium level
    c. Red blood cell count
    d. Platelet count
    e. Blood glucose level

39. The nurse is reviewing the medication list of an older patient who is getting chemotherapy and filgrastim (Neupogen). Which intervention is the nurse most likely to use to facilitate the purpose of the filgrastim (Neupogen)?
    a. Teach patient, family, and all visitors about scrupulous hand hygiene.
    b. Administer the filgrastim (Neupogen) prior to chemotherapy to prevent nausea.
    c. Teach and assess for bleeding signs such as bruising or bleeding gums.
    d. Assess the patient for fatigue and plan for periods of uninterrupted rest.

40. What instructions will the nurse give to the UAP regarding the hygienic care of a patient with neutropenia?
    a. Do not enter the room unless absolutely necessary and then minimize time spent in the room.
    b. Mouth care and washing of the axillary and perianal regions must be done during the shift.
    c. If the patient seems very tired, assist with toileting, but defer all other aspects of hygienic care.
    d. Assist the patient to perform hygienic care according to the standard routine for all patients.

41. A patient is taking oprelvekin (Neumega). Which assessment data finding indicates that the therapy is working?
    a. Weight has increased by 2 pounds.
    b. Nausea and vomiting are relieved.
    c. Platelet count is increasing.
    d. Hemoglobin level is normalizing.

42. The patient is having nausea and vomiting, so the nurse checks the medication orders for an antiemetic. The orders indicate to give Avandemet (rosiglitazone maleate and metformin hydrochloride) as needed (prn) for nausea and vomiting. What should the nurse do?
    a. Give the Avandemet as ordered and observe for symptom relief.
    b. Contact the provider for clarification, because Avandemet is not an antiemetic.
    c. Check the medication administration record for time of last Avandemet.
    d. Assess the patient for delayed nausea before giving the Avandemet.

43. An older adult is having frequent and severe chemotherapy-induced nausea and vomiting (CINV) which seems to be anticipatory and acute. Which assessment is the most important to make?
    a. Fears and feelings associated with chemotherapy
    b. Patient's self-management of distressing symptoms
    c. Signs of dehydration or electrolyte imbalance
    d. Willingness to try complementary or alternative therapies

44. What technique is used in oral care for a patient with stomatitis?
    a. Apply petrolatum jelly to lips after each mouth care.
    b. Brush teeth and tongue with a hard-bristled toothbrush every 8 hours.
    c. "Swish and spit" room-temperature tap water at least four times a day.
    d. Use commercial mouthwashes and glycerin swabs to refresh mouth.

45. The nurse is responsible for teaching the immunosuppressed patient and the family about health-promoting activities. Which information is correct?
    a. Wash hands thoroughly with an antimicrobial soap.
    b. Do not drink water, milk, juice, or other cold liquids.
    c. Boil dishes or use disposables whenever possible.
    d. Don a mask before entering the patient's personal space.

46. Biologic response modifiers have which positive effects on patients receiving chemotherapy? *(Select all that apply.)*
    a. Less risk of life-threatening infections
    b. Reduced incidence of alopecia
    c. Reduced severity of nausea
    d. Able to tolerate higher doses of chemotherapy
    e. Euphoria and increased libido

47. The nurse is caring for several patients who are receiving chemotherapy. Which patient is the most likely to need transfer to the intensive care unit?
    a. Patient receiving interleukin therapy for renal cell carcinoma develops edema
    b. Patient receiving estrogen therapy develops calf pain with redness and swelling
    c. Patient receiving vascular endothelial growth factor/receptor inhibitor has high blood pressure
    d. Patient receiving an antiandrogen receptor develops gynecomastia

48. A patient with cancer tells the nurse she has numbness and weakness in her legs. What is the nurse's best response?
    a. "Are you having any back pain?"
    b. "Have you been exercising vigorously?"
    c. "When was your last dose of pain medication?"
    d. "This is a normal response to chemotherapy."

49. Which interventions does the nurse implement for a patient receiving chemotherapy to prevent the serious side effects of sepsis and disseminated intravascular coagulation? *(Select all that apply.)*
    a. Strict handwashing
    b. Monitor WBCs and clotting factors
    c. Educate patient and family
    d. Administer prophylactic IV heparin
    e. Frequently assess for signs of infection

50. A patient with lymphoma reports severe facial swelling, tightness of the gown collar, and epistaxis. Which complication does the nurse suspect?
    a. Tumor lysis syndrome
    b. Cancer-induced hypercalcemia
    c. Superior vena cava syndrome
    d. Congestive heart failure

51. A patient has a diagnosis of cancer with a gram-negative infection. The nurse assesses bleeding from many sites throughout the body. For which condition does the nurse expect to perform nursing interventions?
    a. Sepsis
    b. Anemia
    c. Disseminated intravascular coagulation
    d. Syndrome of inappropriate antidiuretic hormone

52. A patient diagnosed with bone cancer reports fatigue, loss of appetite, and constipation. Which laboratory result does the nurse report immediately?
    a. Potassium level of 4.2 mEq/L
    b. Magnesium level of 2.0 mg/dL
    c. Sodium level of 140 mEq/L
    d. Calcium level of 10.5 mEq/dL

53. A patient with advanced breast cancer reports severe back pain and leg weakness. Based on these symptoms, what does the nurse suspect?
    a. Tumor lysis syndrome
    b. Lower back cancer
    c. Spinal cord compression
    d. Bladder tumor

23 CHAPTER

Care of Patients with Infection

1. Which term describes a patient who has pathogenic microbes within the body but remains asymptomatic?
   a. Communicable
   b. Virulence
   c. Colonization
   d. Susceptibility

2. Which term best describes an organism's ability to cause disease?
   a. Pathogenicity
   b. Colonization
   c. Virulence
   d. Communicable

3. Transmissions of infection require a reservoir. Which is an example of an animate reservoir?
   a. People
   b. Water
   c. Soil
   d. Intravenous (IV) solution

4. Which factors are essential for transmission of organisms to occur? *(Select all that apply.)*
   a. Normal flora
   b. Reservoir source
   c. Susceptible host
   d. Bacterial organism
   e. Transmission mode

5. Which type of pathogen is a substance produced in cell walls of certain bacteria and released by cell lysis?
   a. Enterotoxin
   b. Toxin
   c. Exotoxin
   d. Endotoxin

6. Which factors increase a patient's susceptibility to infection? *(Select all that apply.)*
   a. Alcohol consumption
   b. Diabetes mellitus
   c. Nicotine use
   d. Oral contraceptives
   e. High-protein diet
   f. Advanced age

7. Which nursing intervention best decreases a patient's susceptibility to infection?
   a. Using standard precautions
   b. Removing soiled linens
   c. Restricting all visitors
   d. Avoiding direct contact

8. Which methods of transmission can result in organisms directly entering a patient's bloodstream? *(Select all that apply.)*
   a. Ingestion
   b. Insect bite
   c. Laceration
   d. Intravascular device
   e. Catheterization

9. The nurse is caring for a patient with a cold who is sneezing. Which modes of organism transmission does the nurse need to protect the patient's roommate against? *(Select all that apply.)*
   a. Direct
   b. Indirect
   c. Airborne
   d. Droplet
   e. Vector

10. A patient admitted with a postoperative abdominal wound infection is diagnosed with methicillin-resistant *Staphylococcus aureus* (MRSA). While performing a physical examination on this patient, which personal protective equipment must the nurse wear? *(Select all that apply.)*
    a. Gown
    b. Mask
    c. Gloves
    d. Shoe covers
    e. Goggles

11. The nurse is preparing to hang an IV of 1 g vancomycin in 250 mL of normal saline for a patient diagnosed with MRSA infection. The medication is to infuse over 1.5 hours. At what rate in mL per hour does the nurse set the IV pump?
    a. 109 mL/hr
    b. 127 mL/hr
    c. 153 mL/hr
    d. 167 mL/hr

12. Which is the most important physiologic barrier to infection?
    a. Immune system
    b. Lysozymes
    c. Intact skin
    d. Phagocytosis

13. The new graduate nurse is discussing planned interventions to reduce the risk of a patient feeling isolated while on airborne precautions. Which statement by the new nurse requires that the preceptor intervene?
    a. "I have arranged to have the newspaper delivered to the room daily."
    b. "I will leave the door propped open to increase auditory and visual stimuli."
    c. "I have demonstrated the use of television and radio controls for the patient."
    d. "I will bundle my activities in order to have more time to talk to the patient while in the room."

14. Handwashing, rather than using alcohol-based hand rub, must be performed during which situation?
    a. After setting up a basin and towels for a patient's AM care
    b. Before having direct contact with patients
    c. Before donning and after removing sterile gloves
    d. After contact with a patient who has had diarrhea for 3 days

15. Appropriate methods of infection control include which precautions? *(Select all that apply.)*
    a. Utilizing effective hand hygiene
    b. Using appropriate personal protective equipment
    c. Limiting time spent with patients
    d. Using standard precautions
    e. Administering prophylactic antibiotics

16. During the shift-to-shift handoff, the nurse is informed that a patient is experiencing urticaria. What question does the nurse ask to clarify the condition of urticaria?
    a. "Were isolation precautions initiated?"
    b. "Did the patient receive an antibiotic before the onset?"
    c. "Was a culture specimen obtained from the site?"
    d. "Does the patient have a history of MRSA?"

17. The nurse is observing a new graduate nurse perform hand hygiene. Which observation indicates a need for further instruction?
    a. Wetting hands before applying soap
    b. Holding hands higher than the elbows
    c. Using friction under running water
    d. Washing for at least 15 seconds

18. Which situation requires that the nurse use soap and water for handwashing?
    a. Before a sterile dressing change
    b. After removing sterile gloves
    c. Dry skin
    d. Hands feeling sticky

19. Which type of transmission-based precautions must the nurse use to prevent transmission by touch from a patient or environment with vancomycin-resistant enterococcus (VRE)?
    a. Contact precautions
    b. Droplet precautions
    c. Standard precautions
    d. Airborne precautions

20. Which type of transmission-based precautions must the nurse use to prevent transmission from a patient with tuberculosis?
    a. Contact precautions
    b. Droplet precautions
    c. Standard precautions
    d. Airborne precautions

21. Which patient is at most risk for developing hospital-acquired methicillin-resistant *Staphylococcus aureus* (HA-MRSA)?
    a. 78-year-old ICU patient receiving IV antibiotics with pneumonia
    b. 45-year-old orthopedic patient with a total knee replacement
    c. 53-year-old medical patient with a venous thromboembolism (VTE)
    d. 67-year-old gynecologic patient who had a hysterectomy

22. The unlicensed assistive personnel (UAP) tells the nurse that an 88-year-old patient has a temperature of 100.2° F. What is the nurse's best action?
    a. Document the temperature.
    b. Administer 2 tablets of acetaminophen (Tylenol).
    c. Instruct the UAP to recheck the temperature in 4 hours.
    d. Report the elevated temperature to the health care provider.

23. A localized infection may include which symptoms? *(Select all that apply.)*
    a. Cool and clammy skin
    b. Pain
    c. Fever
    d. Redness
    e. Swelling

24. A patient has had a bacterial infection for 3 days and laboratory results show the percentage of immature neutrophils has increased at a greater rate than mature neutrophils. How does the nurse interpret these findings?
    a. The patient is very sick and immunocompromised.
    b. There is a unilateral shift to the right in the differential.
    c. The infection was caused by antimicrobial agents.
    d. There is a shift to the left in the differential.

25. The health care provider orders a serum trough level of vancomycin. When must the nurse assure that blood for this level is drawn?
    a. 30 minutes after the next ordered dose of vancomycin
    b. 30 minutes prior to the next ordered dose of vancomycin
    c. 60 minutes after the next ordered dose of vancomycin
    d. 60 minutes prior to the next ordered dose of vancomycin

26. In a patient with an infection, which common interventions may be used to reduce fever? *(Select all that apply.)*
    a. Antipyretic drugs such as aspirin or acetaminophen
    b. External cooling, cooling blankets, cool compresses
    c. Use of electric fans
    d. Oral and IV fluid administration
    e. Antimicrobial therapy with antibiotic, antiviral, or antifungal agents
    f. Opening the windows and door to the patient's room

27. A patient has been prescribed gentamicin drug therapy. Which nursing intervention ensures effective antimicrobial therapy?
    a. Avoid the use of acetaminophen while on this medication.
    b. Deliver a sufficient dosage and duration of therapy.
    c. Take the medication with food.
    d. Closely monitor the patient's temperature.

28. A patient is diagnosed with *Mycobacterium tuberculosis*. Which nursing intervention does the nurse implement for this patient?
    a. Wash hands before and after entering the room.
    b. Ensure the patient has a private room with negative airflow.
    c. Use contact and droplet precautions.
    d. Place contaminated gloves outside the room.

29. Which individual is at greatest risk for exposure to a blood-borne pathogen?
    a. Nursing assistant who is helping a patient ambulate
    b. Nurse who is changing the tubing on a patient's IV infusion
    c. Provider who is injecting a patient with a local anesthetic
    d. Janitorial worker who is mopping an area where a patient vomited

30. A patient reports fever, chills, headache, and swollen glands in the groin and axillary areas. When the nurse assesses multiple reddened areas on both lower extremities, the patient states, "Those are flea bites from the refugee camp mission that I went to." What does the nurse suspect?
    a. Plague (*Yersinia pestis*)
    b. Erythema multiforme (Stevens-Johnson syndrome)
    c. Smallpox (variola virus)
    d. Measles (rubeola)

31. A patient who had previously reported flu-like symptoms which seemed to be improving woke up today with severe dyspnea, tachycardia, fever, and diaphoresis. What does the nurse suspect?
    a. Meningitis
    b. Influenza
    c. Inhalation anthrax (*Bacillus anthracis*)
    d. Respiratory syncytial virus

32. A patient who has returned from a camping trip reports severe vomiting and diarrhea and is experiencing symmetrical flaccid paralysis. The patient reports eating mostly canned foods during the trip. What does the nurse suspect?
    a. Meningitis
    b. Botulism
    c. Variola virus
    d. Inhalation anthrax

33. The nurse is caring for multiple patients in a temporary hospital after severe flooding in the area. Several patients have high fever, headache, and a papular rash over the face and extremities, including the palms of the hands. Some of the skin lesions are vesicular and pustular. What does the nurse suspect?
    a. Pandemic infection
    b. Superinfection
    c. Plague (*Yersinia pestis*)
    d. Smallpox (variola virus)

34. Which interventions should be included when a patient is placed on droplet precautions? (*Select all that apply.*)
    a. Place patient in a private room.
    b. Wear a disposable gown whenever entering the patient's room.
    c. Use a mask when within 3 feet of the patient.
    d. Put a mask on the patient whenever transport is necessary.
    e. Wear gloves when entering the patient's room.

35. Which factors increase the risk of infection in the older adult? (*Select all that apply.*)
    a. Increased antibody production
    b. Thin, delicate skin
    c. Decreased gag reflex
    d. Increased gastrointestinal motility
    e. Increased immobility

24

CHAPTER

Assessment of the Skin, Hair, and Nails

1. A dark-skinned patient is admitted for pneumonia. What is the most accurate method to assess for cyanosis in this patient?
    a. Observe for shallow and rapid respirations.
    b. Check the tongue and lips for a gray color.
    c. Auscultate for decreased breath sounds in lung fields.
    d. Inspect the palms and soles for a yellow-tinged color.

2. A patient is at risk for hypovolemia. The nurse assesses this patient's skin using which assessment technique?
    a. Brush the skin surface and observe for flaking.
    b. Push on the skin and observe for blanching.
    c. Gently pinch the skin on the chest and observe for tenting.
    d. Push on the skin over the tibia and observe for depth of indentation.

3. A patient with a history of heart failure goes to the outpatient clinic for a follow-up appointment. How does the nurse assess for dependent edema in this patient?
    a. Palpate the dorsum of the foot or the medial ankle.
    b. Weigh the patient and compare to the baseline weight.
    c. Check the patient's buttocks or lower back.
    d. Ask the patient about intake and output.

4. The nurse is assessing the skin of an older adult patient who is at risk for dehydration due to excessive vomiting. The skin appears dry and loose. Where is the best site for the nurse to check skin turgor on this patient?
    a. Lower abdomen
    b. Forearm
    c. Forehead
    d. Mid-thigh

5. The nurse is preparing patient education material about healthy skin. What is the single most important preventive health behavior the nurse promotes?
    a. Limit continuous sun exposure.
    b. Drink plenty of water.
    c. Practice good skin hygiene.
    d. Eat a well-balanced diet.

6. The nursing student must perform a skin assessment on an older adult patient and observe for signs of skin breakdown. What does the student do to meet the clinical objective and demonstrate good time-management skills?
    a. Examine the skin while bathing or assisting the patient with hygiene.
    b. Complete the assessment before the end of the clinical experience.
    c. Check to see if the primary nurse has already completed the assessment.
    d. Perform the examination when the patient willingly consents and agrees.

7. A patient is being referred to a dermatologist for evaluation of a rash of unknown origin. The patient has trouble articulating specific information because of "nervousness." Which questions does the nurse use to help the patient practice for the specialist appointment? *(Select all that apply.)*
   a. "Why do you have the rash?"
   b. "When did you first notice the rash?"
   c. "Where on the body did the rash first start?"
   d. "How do you feel about the skin rash?"
   e. "Are you having an itching or burning sensation?"
   f. "Have you been having fever or sore throat?"

8. In regulating body temperature, how much evaporative water loss can occur during hot weather or exercise?
   a. 600 mL/day
   b. 900 mL/day
   c. 2 L/day
   d. 10 to 12 L/day

9. The nurse is caring for a very dark-skinned patient who has high risk for thrombocytopenia. Which area of the patient's body is the best place to check for petechiae?
   a. Anterior chest
   b. Oral mucosa
   c. Palmar surface
   d. Periorbital area

10. The nurse is performing a skin assessment on a patient and notes an area on the forearm that feels hard or "woody." How does the nurse interpret this physical finding?
    a. Inflammation
    b. Subcutaneous fat
    c. Psoriasis
    d. Skin cancer

11. Age-related changes in the integumentary system include a decrease in which factors? *(Select all that apply.)*
    a. Vitamin D production
    b. Thickness of epidermis
    c. Thickness of dermis
    d. Epidermal permeability
    e. Dermal blood flow

12. During handoff report, the nurse is informed that the patient has lichenified areas on the bilateral lower extremities. Based on this information, the nurse expects to observe which clinical finding on the lower extremities?
    a. Loss of hair
    b. Liver spots
    c. Thickened skin
    d. Yellow discoloration

13. A decreased number of active melanocytes in an older adult leads to which result?
    a. Decreased wound healing
    b. Decreased skin tone and elasticity
    c. Increased skin transparency
    d. Increased sensitivity to sun exposure

14. It is important for the nurse to avoid taping the skin of an older adult patient due to a decrease in which integumentary factor?
    a. Vitamin D production
    b. Thickness of epidermis
    c. Dermal blood flow
    d. Epidermal permeability

15. In an older adult, decreased vitamin D production increases the patient's susceptibility to which condition?
    a. Osteomalacia
    b. Osteodystrophy
    c. Hypothermia
    d. Dry skin

16. In caring for an older adult patient, the room may need to be kept warmer because of a decrease in which integumentary factor?
    a. Sebum production
    b. Subcutaneous fat layer
    c. Thickness of epidermis
    d. Number of active melanocytes

17. While obtaining a health history on a patient with a chronic skin condition, the nurse observes that the patient does not make eye contact and keeps the affected area covered with a scarf. What is the most appropriate nursing action?
    a. Explain all actions and procedures to the patient.
    b. Explain to the patient that it is normal to be embarrassed.
    c. Discuss the patient's behavior with another nurse for validation.
    d. Explore the patient's feelings about the condition.

18. The nurse is assessing the skin of an older patient. Which assessment finding needs follow-up?
    a. Multiple liver spots on the arms
    b. Dry, flaking skin on the lower extremities
    c. Presence of cherry hemangiomas
    d. Light-brown macule (6.5 cm) on the right scapula

19. A patient reports a rash that itches, but denies fever, shortness of breath, or other symptoms. Which questions does the nurse ask to help determine if the patient is having an allergic reaction? *(Select all that apply.)*
    a. "Are you taking any new medications?"
    b. "Have you been using any different soaps, cosmetics, or lotions?"
    c. "Is your skin unusually dry or flaky?"
    d. "Have you been exposed to any new cleaning solutions?"
    e. "Have you noticed any new bruises or brownish discolorations?"
    f. "Have you had any recent changes in your diet?"

20. The nurse is performing a physical exam on a patient and observes a dark asymmetrical lesion on the patient's back. The patient states, "I can't see back there and I don't know how long it has been there." What is the most important intervention for this patient?
    a. Encourage the patient to make an appointment with a dermatologist.
    b. Teach the patient how to do a total skin self-evaluation.
    c. Instruct the patient on self-care measures, such as use of sunscreen.
    d. Obtain an order for a fungal culture and take a fungal specimen.

21. To differentiate between color changes in the nailbed related to vascular supply and those from pigment disposition, what does the nurse do?
    a. Examine the nail plate under a Wood's light.
    b. Assess for thickness.
    c. Blanch the nailbed.
    d. Evaluate for lesions.

22. The nurse is taking a medication history of a patient and performing a physical assessment of the skin. During the assessment, the nurse notes that the skin is thin, fragile, and papery. The nurse specifically asks if the patient takes which type of medication?
    a. Anticoagulants
    b. Oral hypoglycemics
    c. Long-term steroids
    d. Herbal preparations

23. A young female patient reports an unusual increase in facial hair. Which question helps the nurse identify the need for a genital examination?
    a. "Have you noticed any bruising or unusual bleeding?"
    b. "Have you noticed any deepening of your voice quality?"
    c. "Are you having any trouble urinating?"
    d. "Does your skin seem unusually dry and flaky?"

24. What is the best rationale for encouraging the patient to follow through and seek treatment for dandruff?
    a. Dandruff flakes are caused by a dry scalp and suggest possible dehydration.
    b. Dandruff is merely a cosmetic problem, but appearance is important to self-esteem.
    c. Severe dandruff is caused by excessive oiliness and could cause hair loss.
    d. Brushing the hair every day prevents dandruff, but it weakens the hair follicle.

25. The nurse is caring for several older adult patients in a long-term care facility. Which patient has the greatest risk to develop a staphylococcal infection secondary to an ingrown toenail?
    a. A patient with chronic obstructive pulmonary disease who requires oxygen therapy
    b. A patient with hypertension, which is well controlled by medication
    c. A patient with osteoarthritis with some loss of mobility and strength
    d. A patient with diabetes mellitus who frequently eats sweets and carbohydrates

26. The nurse is assessing a patient who is African American with very dark skin. Which technique does the nurse use to assess the health of the nail?
    a. Gently squeeze the end of the finger, exert downward pressure, then release the pressure.
    b. Obtain a color chart to identify the normal color of nails for the dark-skinned patient.
    c. Observe the nailbed for a pale pink color and a shiny, smooth surface.
    d. Soak the fingertips in warm water, then gently push back the cuticle.

27. A patient reports a subjective sensation of pain and tenderness "because my arthritis is flaring up." In order to assess for inflammation, what does the nurse do?
    a. Place the hand just above the area and feel for radiant warmth.
    b. Use fingertips to depress tissue area and then release and observe.
    c. Use the back of the hand to palpate the area for warmth.
    d. Use the palm and make a circular motion over the area.

28. A patient has a history of heart failure and demonstrates some mild shortness of breath, with crackles on auscultation. The skin is tight and shiny over the patient's lower extremities, with pitting edema. How does the nurse interpret these findings?
    a. Fluid retention and edema
    b. Early signs of poor circulation
    c. Early stage of infection
    d. Normal for this patient

29. The nurse is caring for a patient who is several days postoperative. The unlicensed assistive personnel (UAP) reports that the patient's linens were changed, but are wet again. The nurse notes that the patient's skin is excessively warm and moist. What is the nurse's priority action?
    a. Initiate intake and output
    b. Take the patient's temperature
    c. Direct the UAP to change the linens
    d. Help the patient with hygiene

30. The nurse is assessing a patient's skin and notes a slightly darkened area over the left ankle. The patient denies pain, but reports a recent problem with the area. Based on the skin appearance and the patient's report, what does the nurse do next?
    a. Ask the patient if there was a serious and deep burn to the area.
    b. Observe the area for scar tissue.
    c. Ask the patient if there was an inflammation to the area.
    d. Take a scraping of the skin for culture.

31. The nurse is caring for an older adult patient with very dark skin. The patient has a low hemoglobin and hematocrit. How does the nurse assess for pallor in this patient?
    a. Observe the mucous membranes for an ash-gray color.
    b. Use indirect, low fluorescent lighting.
    c. Gently push on the skin and watch for blanching.
    d. Inspect the conjunctivae for a yellowish color.

32. The nurse is interviewing a patient who has come to the walk-in clinic and observes the patient has matted hair, body odor, and soiled clothes. Which conditions does the nurse assess for that could be contributing to the patient's overall hygiene? *(Select all that apply.)*
    a. Range of motion and strength to perform self-care
    b. Access to shower facilities and a laundry
    c. Patient's knowledge (or memory) of how to perform hygiene care
    d. Patient's perception of how he or she appears to others
    e. Diabetes mellitus or hypertension
    f. Intactness of sensory functions (i.e., sight, smell)

33. The health care provider has ordered diagnostic testing to determine whether a patient has a fungal infection of the skin. Which test does the nurse prepare the patient for?
    a. Shave biopsy
    b. Punch biopsy
    c. Wood's light examination
    d. KOH test

34. A fair-skinned patient has a history of chronic liver problems; liver enzyme tests and bilirubin results are pending. In order to assess for jaundice, where is the best place for the nurse to look for a yellowish discoloration?
    a. Hard palate
    b. Sclera
    c. Palms
    d. Conjunctivae

35. The nurse is collecting a superficial specimen for a suspected fungal infection from a patient's groin area. What is the correct technique to obtain this specimen?
    a. Obtain a small sample of tissue by using a biopsy needle.
    b. Express exudate from a lesion and use a sterile swab to collect the fluid.
    c. Gently scrape scales with a tongue blade into a clean container.
    d. Aspirate fluid from the lesion using sterile technique.

36. The nurse has collected several specimens from patients who have skin conditions. Which specimen must be immediately placed on ice?
    a. Punch biopsy performed with sterile technique for collection of a tissue piece.
    b. Exudate taken by sterile technique and swabbed on a bacterial culture medium.
    c. Aspirate taken by sterile technique, placed in a bacterial culture tube.
    d. Vesicle fluid taken by sterile technique and placed in a viral culture tube.

37. A patient is scheduled to have a punch biopsy for a lesion on the mid-back. What does the nurse tell the patient about the procedure?
    a. There will be a small scar similar to any surgical procedure.
    b. The surgeon uses a scalpel to punch through the lesion.
    c. A local anesthetic is used and it causes a temporary burning sensation.
    d. The health care provider uses a lens that punches the skin to reveal the shape of the lesion.

38. The nurse is caring for a patient who had an excisional biopsy of a skin lesion. What does the postprocedural care for this patient include?
    a. Monitor the biopsy site for bleeding and infection.
    b. Keep the site clean and dry for at least 24 hours.
    c. Remove dried blood or crusts with diluted hydrogen peroxide.
    d. Return for suture removal in 2 to 3 days.

39. The health care provider instructs the nurse to prepare a light-skinned patient for examination, which includes evaluation of skin pigment changes. Which piece of equipment does the nurse obtain to assist the provider with this examination?
    a. Wood's light
    b. Glass slide
    c. Biopsy tray
    d. Nonfluorescent light

40. The nurse is interviewing a patient who wants evaluation of a skin problem. When the nurse attempts to collect demographic data the patient states, "My age, race, occupation, and hobbies should not affect my access to health care." What is the best response?
    a. "The information obtained has nothing to do with access to care."
    b. "I understand your concerns, but we will see you regardless of your answers."
    c. "Age, race, occupation, and hobbies can be contributing factors to skin problems."
    d. "We are happy to see you, but you have to answer these questions."

41. Which skin disorder is most associated with a familial disposition?
    a. Psoriasis
    b. Ringworm
    c. Cellulitis
    d. Paronychia

42. The nurse is caring for a patient who sustained trauma and blood loss. The patient is alert and anxious, blood pressure is low, and the heart rate is high. Which skin characteristics are most likely to manifest during impending shock?
    a. Dry, flushed appearance
    b. White or pale, cool skin
    c. Bluish color that blanches
    d. Poor turgor with a rough texture

43. The nurse is interviewing a patient with a red rash that itches and burns. Which question would the nurse ask to help identify a transmittable disorder?
    a. "When did you first notice the redness and itching?"
    b. "Is there a family history of chronic skin problems?"
    c. "Have you recently traveled outside of the United States?"
    d. "Have any of your family members had recent skin problems?"

44. An obese elderly patient who has been living alone presents with overall poor hygiene. Her clothes are dirty, and she has a strong body odor. The nurse systematically assesses the patient's skin surface and will give special attention to which area?
    a. Scalp
    b. Skinfolds
    c. Nails
    d. Mucous membranes

45. The health care provider tells the nurse that the patient is likely to have polycythemia vera. Based on this information, what skin discoloration does the nurse expect to observe?
    a. Localized café au lait spots
    b. Nonblanching pallor to nailbeds
    c. Generalized reddish-blue tinge
    d. Yellowish tinge to sclera

46. The nurse is teaching the patient about total skin self-examination (TSSE). According to the American Cancer Society, when should the patient perform TSSE?
    a. After every bath or shower
    b. When a change of a lesion occurs
    c. On a monthly basis
    d. Depends on personal or family history

47. A home health nurse is visiting an older patient in January who lives alone in a small mobile home in the southwestern United States. The patient is recovering from a hip fracture. What is an expected finding for this patient?
    a. Wound healing is delayed.
    b. Skin is generally very dry.
    c. Affected leg has edema.
    d. Surgical site has petechiae.

48. The nurse observes that the patient has large areas of ecchymoses. Which laboratory result is the nurse most likely to check?
    a. Total serum bilirubin
    b. Platelet count
    c. Hemoglobin level
    d. White cell count

49. For which nursing action is the nurse most likely to don clean gloves?
    a. Inspecting for purpura, petechiae, or ecchymosis
    b. Comparing temperature between affected and nonaffected extremity
    c. Obtaining a bacterial culture from a primary lesion (vesicle)
    d. Gently pinching up the skin on the forehead to check for "tenting"

50. Which assessment finding is the best indicator of a healthy nail?
    a. Nailbed color is normal for the patient.
    b. Nailbed blanches with gentle pressure.
    c. Nails are well-groomed and nicely shaped.
    d. Nail surface is smooth and transparent.

51. Which condition is most likely to result in clubbing of the fingernails?
    a. Chronic hypoxia
    b. Prolonged vitamin D deficiency
    c. Uncontrolled blood glucose
    d. Prolonged febrile state

52. Which individual has the highest risk for chronic paronychia?
    a. Construction worker
    b. Nurse
    c. Homeless veteran
    d. Immigrant from southeast Asia

53. The nurse is assisting the health care provider to obtain specimens for diagnostic testing. For which test should the nurse obtain a vial of sterile nonbacteriostatic saline?
    a. Culture for a fungal infection
    b. Vesicle fluid to culture for viral infection
    c. Punch biopsy of a superficial skin lesion
    d. Biopsy for suspected deep cellulitis

54. The nurse and the UAP are assisting patients to move in bed. For which patient are they most likely to use a lift sheet?
    a. Elderly patient on steroids with thin, fragile skin
    b. Obese patient at risk for sacral pressure ulcer
    c. Child with a total body rash with vesicular oozing
    d. Patient with diabetes and delayed wound healing

55. Which teaching point will the nurse emphasize with the older patient to address changes of the subcutaneous layer of the skin related to aging?
    a. Teach to wear sunscreen and hat and avoid direct sun exposure during midday.
    b. Urge use of a multivitamin or a calcium supplement with vitamin D.
    c. Encourage application of moisturizers while skin is still moist.
    d. Teach to dress warmly in cold weather and change position every 2 hours.

56. Extensive destruction of the epidermis will result in the loss of the body's ability to perform which function?
    a. Cellular regeneration for wound healing and skin repair
    b. Photoconversion of 7-dehydrocholesterol to active vitamin D
    c. Cutaneous vascular promotion or inhibition of heat loss
    d. Storage of extra energy reserve for periods of decreased intake

57. The nurse is caring for a patient with a liver disorder. In addition to observing for a yellow-orange discoloration of the skin, which laboratory test is the nurse most likely to monitor?
    a. Hemoglobin level
    b. Vitamin D level
    c. Total serum bilirubin
    d. Serum calcium level

58. The nurse is caring for a postsurgical patient and observes that the patient's skin is red, moist, and hot to the touch. Which vital sign is of primary interest?
    a. Temperature
    b. Pulse
    c. Respirations
    d. Blood pressure

59. The nurse is caring for a patient with liver failure who has been unable to get out of bed for several days. In which area is the nurse most likely to find evidence of dependent edema?
    a. Dorsum of foot
    b. Medial ankle
    c. Buttocks and sacrum
    d. Lower abdomen

60. In which chronic health condition is the nurse most likely to observe increased moisture of the patient's skin?
    a. Kidney disease
    b. Diabetes mellitus
    c. Polycythemia vera
    d. Hyperthyroidism

61. The patient reports a red, raised, itchy rash over most of his body. What terms would the nurse use to document the patient's skin problem?
    a. Red, macular, lichenified
    b. Erythematous, diffuse, pruritic
    c. Cyanotic, annular, papular
    d. Red, universal, circinate

62. The home health nurse reads in the documentation that the patient has chronic venous stasis. Which assessment finding does the nurse expect to observe?
    a. Reddish-blue color to the hands
    b. Grayish-tan color in the lower legs
    c. Warmth and redness in lower legs
    d. Yellowish tinge to soles of the feet

63. The nurse is caring for a patient with myxedema. Which area of the body is the nurse most likely to assess for evidence of nonpitting edema?
    a. Tibia
    b. Forehead
    c. Ankle
    d. Sacrum

64. What should the nurse notice in a patient with adequate tissue integrity and body protection related to skin function?
    a. Body temperature is normal after dose of antipyretic.
    b. Oral mucous membranes are moist and pink.
    c. Areas of uneven pigmentations are covered with clothing.
    d. Hair is patchy and brittle, but clean and well-groomed.

65. The nurse is examining a patient's skin and sees large, sore-looking, raised bumps with pustular heads. Which method does the nurse use to obtain a specimen to test for a bacterial infection?
    a. Take a culture swab of the purulent material.
    b. Take cells from the base of a lesion for a Tzanck's smear.
    c. Scrape scales from the lesions and prepare a slide with KOH.
    d. Assist the health care provider with a skin biopsy.

25 CHAPTER

Care of Patients with Skin Problems

1. The nurse sees in the patient's record that the patient has a Braden score of 20. Which nursing action is the nurse most likely to perform in the care of this patient?
   a. Continue routine assessments.
   b. Turn patient every 2 hours.
   c. Consult with the nutritionist.
   d. Assist to keep skin clean and dry.

2. A patient weighs 110 pounds. The nurse knows that the patient must have an intake of 30 to 35 calories per kilogram of body weight in order to maintain a positive nitrogen balance. The patient needs _____ total calories per day.

3. A thin, malnourished patient requires emergency abdominal surgery. After the operation, in order to promote wound healing, what does the nurse encourage?
   a. High-calorie diet
   b. Low-sodium and low-carbohydrate diet
   c. High-quality protein diet
   d. Low-fat diet with vitamin supplements

4. The nurse is directing the home health unlicensed assistive personnel (UAP) in the care of an older adult patient. The patient reports dry skin and wants help in applying an emollient cream. What does the nurse direct the UAP to do?
   a. Assist the patient to soak for 10 minutes in a warm bath and then apply the cream to slightly damp skin within 2 to 3 minutes after bathing.
   b. Generously apply the cream and leave it on for 20 minutes, then bathe the patient, especially the genital and axillary areas.
   c. Use an antimicrobial skin soap and wash the patient carefully, then apply the emollient cream, especially to the leg area.
   d. Use hot water with added bath oil, then gently pat the patient dry and apply more oil and cream to the skin.

5. Which patients are at risk for pressure ulcers? *(Select all that apply.)*
   a. A confused patient who likes to wander through the halls
   b. A middle-aged quadriplegic patient who is alert and conversant
   c. A bedridden patient who is in the late stage of Alzheimer's
   d. A very overweight patient who must be assisted to move in the bed
   e. An ambulatory patient who has occasional urinary incontinence
   f. A thin patient who sits for long periods and refuses meals

6. The nurse is caring for an obese patient who has been on bedrest for several days. The nurse observes that the patient is beginning to develop redness on the sacral area. What intervention is used to decrease the shearing force?
   a. Place the patient in a high Fowler's position.
   b. Instruct the patient to use arms and legs to push when moving self in bed.
   c. Obtain an order for the patient to be up 3 to 4 times per day in a recliner chair.
   d. Place the patient in a side-lying position.

7. The nurse is reviewing the results of a pressure mapping on a patient at high risk for pressure ulcers. The map shows a red area over the hips. How does the nurse interpret this evidence?
   a. Normal finding because there is always pressure on the hip area
   b. Greater heat production associated with greater pressure
   c. Validation of observable skin redness and breakdown
   d. Cool and well-hydrated skin associated with lower pressure

8. The nurse is assessing the nutritional status of a patient at risk for skin breakdown who has been refusing to eat the hospital food. Which indicator is the most sensitive in identifying inadequate nutrition for this patient?
   a. Serum albumin level of 3.5 mg/dL
   b. Prealbumin level of 17.5 mg/dL
   c. Lymphocyte count of 1900/mm^3
   d. Weight loss of 10% of total body weight

9. Seeing a reddened area on a patient's skin, the nurse presses firmly with fingers at the center of the area and sees that the area blanches with pressure. The nurse interprets this finding as changes related to which factor?
   a. Inflammation
   b. Infection
   c. Blood vessel dilation
   d. Tissue damage

10. The nurse is assessing a wound on a patient's abdomen. What is the correct technique?
    a. Stand on the right side of the bed and lay a sterile cotton swab across the width and the length of the wound.
    b. Read the previous nursing documentation and follow the same pattern that other nurses are using for standardization.
    c. Assess the wound as a clock face with 12 o'clock toward the patient's head and 6 o'clock toward the patient's feet.
    d. Observe the wound after the dressing is removed and estimate the shape and record the appearance.

11. The nurse is assessing a patient's wound every day for signs of healing or infection. Which finding is a positive indication that healing is progressing as expected?
    a. Eschar starts to lift and separate from the tissue beneath which appears dry and pale.
    b. Area appears pale pink, progressing to a spongy texture with a beefy red color.
    c. Tissue is softer and more yellow and wound exudate increases substantially.
    d. Ulcer surface is excessively moist with a deep reddish-purple color.

12. The nurse is irrigating a large pressure ulcer on a patient's hip, and notes a small opening in the skin with purulent drainage. Which technique does the nurse use to check for tunneling?
    a. Ask the health care provider to order an ultrasound.
    b. Palpate the surface of the wound to identify spongy areas.
    c. Continue to flush the wound and watch the flow of the fluid.
    d. Use a sterile cotton-tipped applicator to probe gently for a tunnel.

13. The nurse is assessing a patient's skin and notes a 2" × 2" purplish-colored area on the coccyx with skin intact. These findings suggest which stage of a pressure ulcer?
    a. Suspected deep tissue injury
    b. Stage I pressure ulcer
    c. Stage II pressure ulcer
    d. Unstageable

14. When developing a plan of care for a patient who is at high risk for skin breakdown, what does the nurse include in the plan of care? *(Select all that apply.)*
    a. Applying a pressure reduction overlay to the mattress
    b. Frequent repositioning of the patient
    c. Instructing UAP to assess the patient's skin daily
    d. Instructing UAP to massage reddened areas
    e. Using positioning devices to keep heels pressure-free

15. Which expected outcome is most appropriate for a patient with a 1" × 1" stage II sacral decubitus ulcer?
    a. Wound will show healing and no infection
    b. Patient will verbalize that wound is smaller.
    c. Wound will show granulation and decrease in size.
    d. Patient will rate pain at an acceptable level.

16. A patient receiving negative pressure wound therapy (NPWT) should be monitored closely for which potential complication?
    a. Bleeding
    b. Infection
    c. Pain
    d. Nausea

17. Which class of medication would exclude a patient from participating in NPWT?
    a. Antihypertensives
    b. Anticoagulants
    c. Nonsteroidal antiinflammatory drugs
    d. Antidepressants

18. A patient on the unit has herpes zoster. Which staff members would be best to assign to the care of this patient?
    a. Any staff member, as long as personal protective equipment (PPE) is utilized
    b. Staff members who have had chickenpox
    c. Staff members who have completed training on herpes zoster
    d. Staff members with no small children at home

19. The emergency department (ED) nurse is giving discharge instructions to the parents of a child who has been diagnosed with bedbug bites. What instructions does the nurse give to the parents?
    a. Washing linens in hot soapy water will eliminate the problem.
    b. Using a topical insecticide kills bedbugs on the body surface.
    c. Repeatedly vacuuming surfaces of furniture or mattresses will help.
    d. Hiring a pest control company with bedbug experience is an option.

20. A patient diagnosed with bedbug bites says to the nurse "I am so embarrassed. I shower daily and do not live in an unclean environment." Which response by the nurse is most appropriate?
    a. "No need to be embarrassed. These things happen."
    b. "Showering will not kill bedbugs."
    c. "Have you been traveling or staying in a hotel?"
    d. "Have you seen bedbugs or their eggs on your clothing?"

21. The nurse reads in the chart that the patient has palmoplantar pustulosis (PPP). Which area of the patient's body will the nurse assess for this condition?
    a. Skinfold areas, such as axillae or beneath breasts
    b. Mouth area and oral mucous membranes
    c. Bony prominences such as heels, sacrum, or trochanters
    d. Palms of the hands and the soles of the feet

22. A mother reports that her child has dry skin with itching that seems to worsen at night. What nonpharmacologic interventions does the nurse teach to the mother? *(Select all that apply.)*
    a. Keep the child's fingernails trimmed short and filed to reduce skin damage.
    b. Place mittens or splints on the child's hands at night if the scratching is causing skin tears.
    c. Ensure a warm and moderately humid sleeping environment.
    d. Read the child a relaxing and familiar story to reduce stress.
    e. Use antibacterial soap during bathing to decrease risk of infection.

23. The health care provider recommended over-the-counter diphenhydramine (Benadryl) to treat the patient's hives. What does the nurse suggest to the patient for self-care?
    a. Avoid alcohol consumption, which can potentiate the sedative effect of Benadryl.
    b. Warm environments and warm showers will accelerate metabolism and recovery.
    c. Use an emollient cream or lotion after bathing to reduce the itching.
    d. Apply a topical antibiotic cream after bathing in the evening.

24. In order to assist the health care provider in determining if avoidance therapy is appropriate for a patient, which question would the nurse ask?
    a. Do you have a history of surgery for removal of skin growths?
    b. Have you noticed a change in appearance of a mole?
    c. Does anyone residing in your household have a similar skin problem?
    d. Have you used any new soaps, detergents, or personal care products?

25. The nurse is teaching a patient about self-care for a minor bacterial skin infection. What is the most important aspect the nurse emphasizes?
    a. Apply cool compresses twice a day.
    b. Do not squeeze any pustules or crusts.
    c. Apply astringent compresses.
    d. Bathe daily with an antibacterial soap.

26. A patient is diagnosed with psoriasis vulgaris. Which description of the characteristic lesions of psoriasis would the nurse expect to see in the patient's documentation?
    a. Plaques surmounted by silvery-white scales
    b. Circular areas of redness
    c. Multiple blisters with a yellowish crust
    d. Patches of tender, raised areas limited to extremities

27. What does the treatment for psoriasis include? *(Select all that apply.)*
    a. Ultraviolet light therapy
    b. Calcipotriene (Dovonex) topical cream
    c. Topical methotrexate (Folex)
    d. Oral ciprofloxacin (Cipro)
    e. Corticosteroids

28. The health care provider informs the nurse that the patient is having severe pruritus. Based on this information, the nurse is most likely to observe which assessment finding?
    a. Fluid-filled, weeping blisters
    b. Excoriations from scratching
    c. Dry, flaking skin with peeling
    d. Signs or symptoms of infection

29. The nurse is teaching an older adult about how to deal with and prevent dry skin. What information does the nurse include? *(Select all that apply.)*
    a. Use a room humidifier during the winter months or whenever the furnace is in use.
    b. Take a complete bath or shower every day.
    c. Maintain a daily fluid intake of 1000 mL unless contraindicated.
    d. Avoid clothing that continuously rubs the skin, such as tight belts or pantyhose.
    e. Thoroughly rinse soap from the skin.
    f. Vigorously rub the skin until it is free of moisture.

30. The nurse is teaching a patient about treatment of pediculosis pubis. What information does the nurse include? *(Select all that apply.)*
    a. Proper use of topical sprays or creams, such as permethrin (Elimite)
    b. Abstinence from sexual intercourse with the infected person
    c. Treatment of the patient's social contacts
    d. Side effects of ciprofloxacin (Cipro) or doxycycline (Doryx, Vibramycin)
    e. Washing clothing and bedding in hot water with detergent

31. The school nurse is examining a child and observes linear ridges on the inner aspect of wrists. The child reports intense itching, especially at night. The nurse scrapes the lesion and examines it under a microscope. Which condition does the nurse suspect?
    a. Head lice
    b. Scabies
    c. Body lice
    d. Dermatitis

32. The school nurse discovers a child has tinea capitis. What does the nurse instruct the parents to do?
    a. Treat the family pet and temporarily isolate the pet.
    b. Refrain from sharing items like combs or hats.
    c. Scrub the shower area and keep the feet dry.
    d. Ensure all family members carefully wash their hands.

33. The nurse is giving discharge instructions to a patient and family who must continue dressing changes and wound care at home. Which point does the nurse emphasize to help the family prevent infection and minimize cost?
    a. Scrupulous handwashing before and after wound care
    b. Use of sterile water for flushing and sterile dressing materials
    c. Use of clean gloves for performing dressing changes
    d. Careful disposal of contaminated dressings in a biohazard bag

34. The nurse is caring for a 25-year-old patient who recently had a rhinoplasty as part of reconstruction after cancer treatment. Which complication is cause for the greatest concern?
    a. Postnasal bleeding
    b. Difficulty swallowing
    c. Edema and swelling
    d. Preoccupation with appearance

35. A patient has been prescribed acetretin (Soriatane) for psoriasis. What information does the nurse tell the patient about this drug?
    a. Wear dark glasses after taking a dose.
    b. It is the first choice for psoriasis.
    c. Strict birth control measures are necessary.
    d. Apply it to superficial lesions.

36. A patient is diagnosed with Stevens-Johnson syndrome. What is the priority action for the health care team?
    a. Treat the subjective symptoms of pain and itching.
    b. Closely observe for signs of renal failure.
    c. Protect against localized skin infection.
    d. Identify the offending drug and discontinue it.

37. A patient is prescribed a topical steroid for treatment of contact dermatitis. Which instruction does the nurse provide to the patient about this drug?
    a. Moisten dressings with warm tap water; place over topical steroids for short periods.
    b. Apply topical steroids then cover with an occlusive dressing.
    c. Apply a topical corticosteroid sparingly on the face.
    d. Discontinue the use of topical steroids when symptoms subside.

38. Which statement is true about the application and use of topical preparations?
    a. Topical applications are generally much safer than oral medications.
    b. Using a water-soluble cream in the groin area could cause maceration.
    c. Using an oil-based ointment in the axillary area could cause folliculitis.
    d. An oil-based gel should be massaged into hairy areas.

39. A patient has a partial-thickness wound. How long does the nurse anticipate the healing by epithelialization will take?
    a. 24 hours
    b. 2 to 3 days
    c. 5 to 7 days
    d. 12 to 14 days

40. A toddler is miserable with itching from chickenpox. Which type of bath is the best to help relieve the toddler's discomfort?
    a. Sitz bath
    b. Bath with oil
    c. Sponge bath
    d. Colloidal oatmeal

41. The nurse is performing daily wound care and dressing changes on a patient with a full-thickness wound. The patient protests when the nurse attempts to débride the wound. What is the nurse's best response?
    a. "Reepithelialization, granulation, and contraction are natural body processes that will occur if this tissue is removed."
    b. "I know this is uncomfortable, but don't you want your wound to heal as fast as possible? This treatment allows the body to heal itself."
    c. "Harmful bacteria can grow in the dead tissue and it also interferes with the body's attempt to fill in the wound with new cells and collagen."
    d. "I would never force a patient to do anything, but this really is the best treatment for the wound that you have."

42. A patient has a stage III pressure ulcer over the left trochanter area that has a thick exudate. The wound bed is visible and beefy red, and the edges are surrounded with swollen pink tissue. The exudate has an odor. How does the nurse determine which dressing is best for this wound?
    a. Selects a hydrophilic dressing for heavy exudate
    b. Obtains an order to consult certified wound care specialist
    c. Obtains an order for the type of dressing from health care provider
    d. Applies a dry dressing and observes for "strike through"

43. The nurse is caring for a patient with arterial insufficiency in the lower right leg. In order to prevent leg ulcers, what does the nurse do?
    a. Elevates the leg frequently.
    b. Places the leg in a dependent position.
    c. Places a heel protector on the right foot.
    d. Encourages the patient to walk briskly.

44. Place the physiologic steps of healing of partial-thickness wounds in the correct order using the numbers 1 through 5.

    _____ a. Skin injury results in local inflammation and formation of a fibrin clot.

    _____ b. Stratification and keratin form to resemble normal skin.

    _____ c. Fibrin clot acts as a frame or scaffold to guide cell movement.

    _____ d. Regrowth is only one cell layer thick at first, then the cell layer thickens.

    _____ e. Growth factors stimulate epidermal cell division and new skin cells move into open spaces.

45. The nurse is caring for several patients who are incontinent of stool and urine. Which task is delegated to the UAP?
    a. Inspect the skin daily for any areas of redness.
    b. Massage the reddened areas after cleaning.
    c. Wash the skin with a pH-balanced soap to maintain normal acidity.
    d. Change the absorbent pads or garments every 4 hours.

46. The nurse is caring for a patient in a prolonged coma after a serious head injury. The nurse uses which interventions to prevent the development of pressure ulcers for this patient? *(Select all that apply.)*
    a. Use pillows or padding devices to keep heels pressure-free.
    b. Assess heel positioning every 8 hours.
    c. Delegate turning and positioning every 2 hours.
    d. Obtain an order for pressure-relief devices.
    e. Give special attention to fleshy or muscular areas.

47. The nurse is assessing a patient's skin and observes a superficial infection with a raised, red rash with small pustules. How does the nurse interpret this finding?
    a. Minor skin trauma
    b. Folliculitis
    c. Furuncles
    d. Cellulitis

48. An adolescent has a painful and unsightly herpes simplex blister on her lip, and would like to have her school photo delayed until after the lesion has resolved. What does the nurse tell the patient about the duration of the outbreak?
    a. Should resolve completely in 2 to 3 days.
    b. Within 3 to 5 days the blister is gone.
    c. Symptoms can last from 3 to 10 days.
    d. Begins to improve in 2 weeks.

49. The nurse is caring for a patient who needs frequent oral hygiene and endotracheal suctioning. In this particular circumstance, the nurse wears gloves to prevent contracting and spreading which organism?
    a. Herpetic whitlow
    b. Herpes zoster
    c. Methicillin-resistant *Staphylococcus aureus*
    d. Streptococcus

50. The nurse hears in report that a patient admitted for an elective surgery also has herpes zoster. The nurse initiates contact isolation for which factor?
    a. Fever and malaise are present as accompanying symptoms.
    b. Other patients or staff members have never had chickenpox.
    c. Lesions are present as fluid-filled blisters.
    d. Lesions are present and crusted over.

51. A patient is diagnosed with a primary herpetic infection. The nurse would question an order for which drug?
    a. Acyclovir (Zovirax)
    b. Valacyclovir (Valtrex)
    c. Ketoconazole (Nizoral)
    d. Famciclovir (Famvir)

52. The public health nurse is reviewing case files of people who were exposed to and treated for cutaneous anthrax. Which patient who develops the disease warrants further investigation as a possible bioterrorism exposure?
    a. Farmer
    b. Veterinarian
    c. Tannery worker
    d. Construction worker

53. A patient reported painless, raised vesicles that itched. Within a few days, there was bleeding in the center and then it sank inwards. Now it looks black and leathery. Which question does the nurse ask in order to elicit more information about this patient's condition?
    a. "Do you remember being bitten by an insect?"
    b. "Do you work with or around animals?"
    c. "Have you noticed any mite or lice infestations?"
    d. "Have you had exposure to new soaps, lotions, or foods?"

54. A patient is diagnosed with chronic psoriasis and is prescribed a topical therapy of anthralin (Lasan). What does the nurse teach the patient about proper use of this drug?
    a. Apply the paste every night before going to bed.
    b. Check for local tissue reaction.
    c. Apply the drug generously to the lesion and surrounding skin.
    d. Use two forms of contraception.

55. What does the nurse teach a patient about ultraviolet (UV) therapy for psoriasis?
    a. Use a commercial tanning bed service but limit exposure to 2 to 3 times per week.
    b. Use the sun as an inexpensive source of UV; inspect skin daily for overexposure.
    c. Wear dark glasses during and after treatment if psoralen is prescribed.
    d. Expect generalized redness with edema and tenderness after the treatment.

56. A patient is diagnosed with actinic keratoses. Which teaching point would the nurse emphasize?
    a. A follow-up appointment is needed for premalignant condition.
    b. Clean the skin with a mild soap and lukewarm water.
    c. Keep fingernails short to prevent infection from scratching.
    d. Apply the topical ointment while skin is moist.

57. The nurse is examining the nevi on a patient's back and neck. Because most malignant melanomas arise from moles, which finding is a concern to warrant further investigation?
    a. Regular, well-defined borders
    b. Uniform dark-brown color
    c. Rough surface
    d. Sudden report of itching

58. Which occurrence is an example of conditions associated with Koebner's phenomenon?
    a. Chronic overexposure to sunlight
    b. Exposure to a dermatophyte infection
    c. Dormant herpes simplex virus infection
    d. Itching that worsens during the night

59. Which patient is the most likely candidate to be referred for Mohs' surgery?
    a. Has joint contractures from burn wounds
    b. Has squamous cell carcinoma
    c. Has pressure ulcer with infection in deep tissue layers
    d. Has excessive breast tissue

60. The nurse is talking to a patient who is planning to have cosmetic plastic surgery. Which patient statement prompts the nurse to report concerns to the surgeon?
    a. "Having this surgery is going to help increase my self-confidence."
    b. "I know this surgery is going to solve my marital problems."
    c. "I have been thinking about having this surgery for a long time."
    d. "I am nervous about having the surgery, but I can't wait to see the outcome."

61. An older patient who is receiving chemotherapy is diagnosed with toxic epidermal necrolysis. In addition to identifying the causative agent, what does the nurse monitor for?
    a. Fluid and electrolyte imbalance, caloric intake, and hypothermia
    b. Shortness of breath, hypertension, and cardiac dysrhythmias
    c. Nausea, vomiting, diarrhea, and severe abdominal pain
    d. Severe itching with tenderness and edema of the skin

62. A patient with burns over a large amount of the body surface requires 2g/kg/day of protein for wound healing. The patient weighs 130 pounds. How many grams of protein does the patient need each day? _____

63. The nurse is instructing the UAP in how to perform skin care for a patient who is at risk for pressure ulcers because of immobility and incontinence. What instructions would the nurse give?
    a. After cleaning, apply a commercial skin barrier to areas exposed to urine or feces.
    b. After cleaning, apply a light layer of powder or talc directly on the perineum.
    c. Scrub and vigorously rub the skin to completely remove soil or dried feces.
    d. Use an antibiotic soap and rinse with hot water to remove soap residue.

64. Which chronic health condition is most likely to contribute to delayed wound healing or recurrence of a pressure ulcer after healing has occurred?
    a. Osteoporosis
    b. Hypertension
    c. Psoriasis
    d. Diabetes mellitus

65. A patient had surgery 5 days ago. What is the best way for the nurse to determine the current state of healing or deterioration of the patient's surgical wound?
    a. Consult the wound specialist to examine the wound.
    b. Compare existing wound features to those previously documented.
    c. Ask the patient for subjective sensations of pain or discomfort.
    d. Review the objective criteria for the desired outcomes of healing.

66. Which data set is most likely to prompt the nurse to call the health care provider to obtain an order for a wound culture?
    a. Patient reports pain along the incision site.
    b. Wound is accidentally contaminated during a dressing change.
    c. Tissue surrounding surgical site is pink and swollen.
    d. Wound has moderate exudate that has a foul odor.

67. The nurse is on a hiking trip and one of the hikers falls and sustains a laceration to the lower leg. It takes the group more than 36 hours to get to a health care facility. Which description of the drainage would be considered normal and expected within the first 48 hours?
    a. Greenish-blue pus
    b. Blood-tinged amber fluid
    c. Brownish drainage with a fecal odor
    d. Beige exudate with a fishy odor

68. At the hospital, the patient was receiving whirlpool treatments to débride dead tissue. What could the home health nurse suggest as a substitute?
    a. Soaking in a hot tub until tissue softens
    b. Sitting in a warm sitz bath for 20 minutes
    c. Forceful irrigation of the wound with a 35-mL syringe
    d. Gently scrubbing the wound with a moist sponge

69. The nurse hears in report that an older patient has postherpetic neuralgia. Which sign/symptom is the patient most likely to report?
    a. Pain
    b. Itching
    c. Unsightly rash
    d. Dry skin

70. A 60-year-old patient requests a Zostavax vaccination. Which health history needs further investigation before Zostavax is administered?
    a. Is being treated for an autoimmune disease
    b. Takes iron supplements for anemia
    c. Has history of deep vein thrombosis
    d. Is allergic to iodine and shellfish

26 CHAPTER

Care of Patients with Burns

1. A patient was burned on the forearm after tripping and falling against a wood-burning stove. There are currently several small blisters over the burn area. What does the nurse advise the patient to do about the blisters?
   a. Leave the blisters intact because they protect the wound from infection.
   b. Use a sterile needle to open a tiny hole in each blister to drain the fluid.
   c. Allow blisters to increase in size; then open them to prevent immunosuppression.
   d. Leave the blisters intact unless the pain and pressure increase.

2. The nurse is caring for a patient who has 30% total body surface area (TBSA) burn. During the first 12 to 36 hours, the nurse carefully monitors the patient for which status changes related to capillary leak syndrome?
   a. Bradycardia and pitting edema
   b. Hypertension and decreased urine output
   c. Tachycardia and hypotension
   d. Respiratory depression and lung crackles

3. The home health nurse is visiting an older couple for the initial visit. In observing the household, the nurse identifies several behaviors and environmental factors to address. Which identified factors increase the risk for burns and/or household fires? *(Select all that apply.)*
   a. Several potholders hanging within easy reach of the stove
   b. Ashtray with old cigarette butts on the bedside table
   c. Space heater very close to the bed
   d. Single smoke detector in the kitchen
   e. Back exit hall of the house used as a storage space

4. The nurse is caring for several patients on the burn unit who have sustained extensive tissue damage. The nurse should monitor for which electrolyte imbalance that is typically associated with the initial third-spacing fluid shift?
   a. Hypercalcemia
   b. Hypernatremia
   c. Hypokalemia
   d. Hyperkalemia

5. The nurse is reviewing the hemoglobin and hematocrit results for a patient recently admitted for a severe burn. Which result is most likely related to vascular dehydration?
   a. Hematocrit of 58%
   b. Hemoglobin of 14 g/dL
   c. Hematocrit of 42%
   d. Hemoglobin of 10 g/dL

6. The nurse is performing a morning assessment on a patient admitted for serious burns to the extremities. For what reason does the nurse assess the patient's abdomen?
   a. To perform a daily full head-to-toe assessment
   b. To assess for nausea and vomiting related to pain medication
   c. To assess for a paralytic ileus secondary to reduced blood flow
   d. To monitor increased motility that may result in cramps and diarrhea

7. The nurse is interviewing and assessing an electrician who was brought to the emergency department (ED) after being "electrocuted." Bystanders report that he was holding onto the electrical source "for a long time." The patient is currently alert with no respiratory distress. During the interview, what does the nurse assess for?
   a. Knowledge of electrical safety
   b. Burn marks on the dominant hand
   c. Injuries based on reports of pain
   d. Entrance and exit wounds

8. A patient was involved in a house fire and suffered extensive full-thickness burns. In the long-term, what issue may this patient have trouble with?
   a. Intolerance for vitamin C
   b. Metabolism of vitamin K
   c. Activation of vitamin D
   d. Absorption of vitamin A

9. During shift report, the nurse learns that a new patient was admitted for an inhalation injury. Auscultation of the lungs has revealed wheezing over the mainstem bronchi since admission. During the nurse's assessment of the patient, the wheezing sounds are absent. What does the nurse do next?
   a. Document these findings because they indicate that the patient is improving.
   b. Assess for respiratory distress because of potential airway obstruction.
   c. Obtain an order to discontinue oxygen therapy because it is no longer needed.
   d. Encourage use of incentive spirometry to prevent atelectasis.

10. The nurse is caring for several patients who have sustained burns. The patient with which initial injury is the least likely to experience severe pain when a sharp stimulus is applied?
    a. Severe sunburn after lying in the sun for several hours
    b. Deep full-thickness burn from an electrical accident
    c. Partial-thickness burn from picking up a hot pan
    d. Deep partial-thickness burn after a motorcycle accident

11. The nurse is reviewing arterial blood gas (ABG) results for a patient with 35% TBSA burn in the resuscitation phase: pH is 7.26; Pco_2 is 36 mm Hg; and HCO_3^- is 19 mEq/L. What condition does the nurse suspect the patient has?
    a. Metabolic alkalosis
    b. Metabolic acidosis
    c. Respiratory acidosis
    d. Respiratory alkalosis

12. A patient comes to the clinic to be treated for burns from a barbeque fire. Although the patient does not appear to be in any respiratory distress, the nurse suspects an inhalation injury after observing which findings? *(Select all that apply.)*
    a. Burns to the face
    b. Bright cherry-red color to lips
    c. Singed nose hairs
    d. Edema of the nasal septum
    e. Black carbon particles around the mouth
    f. Sweet, sugary smell to the breath

13. The nurse is caring for a burn patient who received rigorous fluid resuscitation in the ED for hypotension and hypovolemic shock. In assessing renal function for the first 24 hours, what finding does the nurse anticipate?
    a. Output will be approximately equal to fluid intake.
    b. Output will be decreased compared to fluid intake.
    c. Urine will have a very low specific gravity and a pale-yellow color.
    d. Output will be managed with diuretics.

14. A patient sustained a superficial-thickness burn over a large area of the body. The patient is crying with discomfort and is very concerned about the long-term effects. What does the nurse tell the patient to expect?
    a. "Healing should occur in 3 to 6 days with no scarring or complications."
    b. "The pain should be less because more of the nerve endings were destroyed."
    c. "The wound will appear red and dry with some white areas."
    d. "The leathery eschar will have to be removed before healing can occur."

15. The nurse is caring for a patient brought to the ED after bending over the engine of his car when it exploded in his face. What is the priority for this patient?
    a. Initiate fluid resuscitation
    b. Secure the airway
    c. Manage pain and discomfort
    d. Prevent infection

16. The nurse is caring for a patient who sustained carbon monoxide poisoning while working on his car engine in an enclosed space. What assessment finding does the nurse anticipate?
    a. Patient will be cyanotic because of hypoxia.
    b. Blood gas value of Pao_2 will be very low.
    c. Patient will report a headache.
    d. Patient will report a dry and irritated throat.

17. For which patient would the rule of nines method of calculating burn size be most appropriate?
    a. Child who weighs at least 50 pounds
    b. Adult whose weight is proportionate to height
    c. Adult who weighs under 300 pounds
    d. Child whose weight is proportionate to height

18. Which criterion describes a full-thickness burn wound? *(Select all that apply.)*
    a. The wound is red and moist and blanches easily.
    b. There is destruction to the epidermis and dermis.
    c. There are no skin cells for regrowth.
    d. The burned tissue is avascular.
    e. The burn wound will not be painful.

19. The nurse is assessing a patient with a burn wound to the back and chest area. Which assessment findings are consistent with a superficial-thickness burn wound? *(Select all that apply.)*
    a. Redness
    b. Pain
    c. Mild edema
    d. Moisture
    e. Eschar

20. The nurse observes peeling of dead skin on the legs of a patient with a superficial-thickness burn wound. What is the most accurate description of this assessment finding?
    a. Blanching
    b. Desquamation
    c. Slough
    d. Fluid shift

21. Which type of burn wound damages the epidermis, dermis, fascia, and tissues?
    a. Superficial
    b. Partial thickness
    c. Full thickness
    d. Deep full thickness

22. Which type of burn destroys the sweat glands, resulting in decreased excretory ability?
    a. Superficial
    b. Partial thickness
    c. Full thickness
    d. Deep full thickness

23. During the early phase of a burn injury, there is a drastic increase in capillary permeability. What does this physiologic change place the patient at risk for?
    a. Acute kidney injury
    b. Fluid overload
    c. Increased cardiac output
    d. Hypovolemic shock

24. An adult patient is admitted to the burn unit after being burned in a house fire. Assessment reveals burns to the entire face, back of the head, anterior torso, and circumferential burns to both arms. Using the rule of nines, what is the extent of the burn injury?
    a. 18%
    b. 24%
    c. 45%
    d. 54%

25. What is the most effective intervention for preventing transmission of infection to a burn patient?
    a. Use of personal protective equipment (PPE) for anyone entering the patient's room
    b. Maintaining reverse isolation during the resuscitation phase
    c. Equipment designated for patient use
    d. Performing hand hygiene correctly and when appropriate

26. Which vaccine is routinely administered when a burn patient is admitted to the hospital?
    a. Hepatitis B
    b. Tetanus
    c. Influenza
    d. Pneumonia

27. A patient has severe burns to the anterior surface of the body from a short exposure to high temperatures at a worksite furnace. Which area of the body is most vulnerable to a deep burn injury?
    a. Anterior chest
    b. Upper arms
    c. Palmar surface of hands
    d. Eyelids

28. A patient has sustained a burn which appears red and moist. The nurse gently applies pressure to the area to assess for what sign/symptom?
    a. Intensity of pain
    b. Blanching
    c. Pitting edema
    d. Fluid-filled blisters

29. What is the primary reason to prevent infection with burn injuries?
    a. Prevent extensive scar formation
    b. Avoid sepsis
    c. Avert worsening of pain
    d. Avoid fever and inflammation

30. The nurse is caring for several patients on the burn unit. Which patients have the greatest risk for developing respiratory problems? (Select all that apply.)
    a. Patient who was in a storage room where chemicals caught fire
    b. Patient who was working in an area where steam escaped from a pipe
    c. Patient who sustained a circumferential burn to the chest area
    d. Patient who was burned when a firecracker exploded prematurely
    e. Patient who was found unconscious in a slow-burning house fire

31. The nurse is caring for a firefighter who was trapped for a prolonged period of time by burning debris. During the shift, the nurse notes a progressive hoarseness, a brassy cough, and the patient reports increased difficulty with swallowing. How does the nurse interpret these changes?
    a. Temporary discomfort that can be treated with sips of cool fluids
    b. Signs and symptoms of probable carbon monoxide poisoning
    c. Signs indicating a pulmonary injury and possible airway obstruction
    d. Expected findings considering the mechanism of injury

32. The nurse has just received report on a patient admitted for steam inhalation burns. The patient is alert and conversant, but reports that his throat feels raw. His wife says that he sounds hoarse compared to usual. Considering these findings, which order should the nurse question?
    a. Continuous pulse oximetry
    b. Vital signs and airway assessment every shift
    c. Intubation equipment at the bedside
    d. Oxygen 2 L via nasal cannula to maintain saturation of greater than 90%

33. The nurse is caring for a burn patient who was stabilized by and transferred from a small rural hospital. The patient develops a new complaint of shortness of breath. On auscultation, the nurse hears crackles throughout the lung fields. What does the nurse suspect is causing this patient's symptoms?
    a. Pulmonary fluid overload due to fluid resuscitation
    b. Exposure to carbon monoxide that was undiagnosed
    c. Fat emboli secondary to extensive injury
    d. Excessive oxygen therapy at the first facility

34. The nurse is caring for several patients on the burn unit. Which of these patients has the most acute need for cardiac monitoring?
    a. Older adult woman who spilled hot water over her legs while boiling noodles
    b. Teenager with facial burns that occurred when he threw gasoline on a campfire
    c. Young woman who was struck by lightning while jogging on the beach
    d. Middle-aged man who fell asleep while smoking and sustained burns to the chest

35. A patient is transported to the ED for severe and extensive burns that occurred while he was trapped in a burning building. The patient is severely injured with respiratory distress and the resuscitation team must immediately begin multiple interventions. Which task is delegated to unlicensed assistive personnel (UAP)?
    a. Position the patient's head to open the airway and assist with intubation.
    b. Assist the respiratory therapist to maintain a seal during bag-valve-mask ventilation.
    c. Prepare the intubation equipment and set up the oxygen flowmeter.
    d. Elevate the head of the bed to achieve a high-Fowler's position.

36. The nursing student notes on the care plan that the burn patient she is caring for is at risk for organ ischemia. Based on the student's knowledge of the pathophysiology of burns, which etiology does the nursing student select?
    a. Related to hypovolemia and hypotension
    b. Related to fluid overload and peripheral edema
    c. Related to prolonged resuscitation and hypoxia
    d. Related to direct blunt trauma to the kidneys

37. The student nurse is caring for a patient who has been in the burn unit for several weeks. The patient needs assistance with the bedpan to have a bowel movement, and the student nurse notes that the stool is black with a tarry appearance. What is the most important priority action at this time?
    a. Report this finding to the primary nurse or the instructor.
    b. Ask if the patient is currently taking an iron supplement.
    c. Test for the presence of occult blood with a hemoccult card and reagent.
    d. Perform a dietary assessment to determine if the stool color is related to food.

38. A patient who lives in a rural community sustained severe burns during a house fire at 10 AM. The rural emergency medical services (EMS) started a peripheral IV at 11:00 AM at a keep-vein-open (KVO) rate. The patient was admitted to the hospital at 1:00 PM. In calculating the fluid replacement, at what time is the fluid for the first 8-hour period completed?
    a. 6:00 PM
    b. 7:00 PM
    c. 8:00 PM
    d. 9:00 PM

39. A patient in the burn intensive care unit weighed 80 kg (preburn weight). The provider orders titration of IV fluid to achieve 0.5 mL/kg/hr urine output. What is the minimal hourly urine output for this patient?
    a. 30 mL/hr
    b. 35 mL/hr
    c. 40 mL/hr
    d. 45 mL/hr

40. A burn patient with which condition is most likely to have mannitol (Osmitrol) ordered as part of the drug therapy?
    a. Peripheral edema associated with burns on the lower extremities
    b. Inhalation burns around the mouth causing mucosal swelling
    c. Electrical burn and myoglobin in the urine
    d. Smoke inhalation and superficial burns to the forearms

41. A patient was admitted to the burn unit approximately 6 hours ago after being rescued from a burning building. In the ED, he reported a dry, irritated throat "from breathing in the fumes," but otherwise had no airway complaints. During the shift, the nurse notes that the patient has suddenly developed marked stridor. The nurse anticipates preparing the patient for which emergency procedure?
    a. Bronchoscopy
    b. Intubation
    c. Needle thoracotomy
    d. Escharotomy

42. A patient was admitted for burns to the upper extremities after being trapped in a burning structure. The patient is also at risk for inadequate oxygenation related to inhalation of smoke and superheated fumes. Which diagnostic test best monitors this patient's gas exchange?
    a. Complete blood count
    b. Myoglobin level
    c. Carboxyhemoglobin level
    d. Chest x-ray

43. A patient in the burn intensive care unit is receiving vecuronium (Norcuron). What is the priority nursing intervention for this patient?
    a. Have emergency intubation equipment at the bedside.
    b. Ensure that all the equipment alarms are on and functional.
    c. Closely monitor the patient's urinary output every hour.
    d. Ensure that daily drug levels and electrolyte values are obtained.

44. The priority expected outcome during the resuscitation phase of a burn injury is to maintain which factor?
    a. The airway
    b. Cardiac output
    c. Fluid replacement
    d. Patient comfort

45. Which statement about the resuscitation phase of a burn injury is accurate?
    a. It occurs in the prehospital timeframe.
    b. It continues for about 4 hours after the burn.
    c. It continues for about 48 hours after the burn.
    d. It continues until the patient is stable.

46. The release of myoglobin from damaged muscle in patients with major burns can result in which potential complication?
    a. Paralytic ileus
    b. Acute kidney injury
    c. Limited mobility
    d. Hypovolemia

47. A burn patient in the fluid resuscitation phase is experiencing dyspnea. What are the priority interventions for this patient? *(Select all that apply.)*
    a. Elevate the head of bed to 45 degrees.
    b. Maintain patient in the supine position.
    c. Notify the Rapid Response Team.
    d. Administer an analgesic to calm the patient.
    e. Apply humidified oxygen.

48. The vasodilating effects of carbon monoxide in patients with carbon monoxide poisoning cause what clinical manifestation?
    a. Cyanosis around the lips
    b. Generalized pallor
    c. Cherry-red skin color
    d. Mottled skin color

49. The nurse is caring for a burn patient about to undergo hydrotherapy. Which complementary therapies are appropriate for pain management in this patient? *(Select all that apply.)*
    a. Administration of IV opioid analgesics
    b. Allowing the patient to make decisions regarding pain control
    c. Playing music in the background
    d. Use of meditative breathing
    e. Use of guided imagery

50. A burn patient refuses to eat. The potential problem of weight loss related to increased metabolic rate and reduced calorie intake is identified for this patient. What method does the nurse use to correctly weigh this patient?
    a. Weigh once a week after morning hygiene and compare to previous weight.
    b. Weigh daily at the same time of day and compare to preburn weight.
    c. Use a bed scale and subtract the estimated weight of linens.
    d. Weigh daily without dressings or splints and compare to preburn weight.

51. The student nurse is preparing to assist with hydrotherapy for a burn patient. The supervising nurse instructs the student to obtain the necessary equipment before beginning the procedure. What equipment does the student nurse obtain? *(Select all that apply.)*
    a. Scissors and forceps
    b. Hydrogen peroxide
    c. Mild soap or detergent
    d. Pressure dressings
    e. Washcloths and gauze sponges
    f. Chlorhexidine sponges

52. The nurse is applying a dressing to cover a burn on a patient's left leg. What technique does the nurse use?
    a. Consider the depth of the injury and amount of drainage, and work distal to proximal.
    b. Change the dressing every 4 hours or when the drainage leaks through the dressing.
    c. Consider the patient's mobility and the area of injury, and work proximal to distal.
    d. Use multiple gauze layers and roller gauze to pad and protect the joint areas.

53. The nurse has just received a phone report on a burn patient being transferred from the burn intensive care unit to the step-down burn unit. Which of these tasks are appropriate to delegate to UAP in order to prepare the room?
    a. Place sterile sheets and a sterile pillowcase on the bed.
    b. Place a new disposable stethoscope in the room.
    c. Clear a space in the corner for the patient's flowers.
    d. Hang a sign on the door to prohibit entry of visitors.

54. The nurse is monitoring the nutritional status of a burn patient. Which indicators will the nurse use? *(Select all that apply.)*
    a. Amount of food the patient eats
    b. Weight to height ratio
    c. Serum albumin
    d. Amount of water the patient drinks
    e. Blood glucose
    f. Serum potassium

55. The nurse is educating a patient who has sustained burns to the dominant hand. What kind of active range-of-motion exercises does the nurse instruct the patient to perform?
    a. Exercise the hand, thumb, and fingers every hour while awake.
    b. Exercise the fingers and thumb at least three times a day.
    c. Use the hands to perform activities of daily living.
    d. Squeeze a soft rubber ball several times a day.

56. A burn patient must have pressure dressings applied to prevent contractures and reduce scarring. For maximum effectiveness, what procedure pertaining to the pressure garments is implemented?
    a. Changed every 24 to 48 hours to prevent infection
    b. Worn at least 23 hours a day until the scar tissue matures
    c. Removed for hygiene and during sleeping
    d. Applied with aseptic technique

57. The family reports that the burn patient is unable to perform self-care measures, so someone has been "doing everything for her." The nurse finds that the patient has the knowledge and the physical capacity to independently perform self-care. What is the nurse's best response?
    a. "What can your family do to help you feel better and stronger?"
    b. "You should be doing these things for yourself to increase your self-esteem."
    c. "What has been happening since you were discharged from the hospital?"
    d. "Let's review the principles of self-care that you learned in the hospital."

58. A patient who sustained severe burns to the face with significant scarring and disfigurement will soon be discharged from the hospital. Which intervention is best to help the patient make the transition into the community?
    a. Discuss cosmetic surgery that could occur over the next several years.
    b. Focus on the positive aspects of going home and being with family.
    c. Teach the family to perform all aspects of care for the patient.
    d. Encourage visits from friends and short public appearances before discharge.

59. What does the process of full-thickness wound healing include? *(Select all that apply.)*
    a. Healing occurs by wound contraction.
    b. Eschar must be removed.
    c. Large blisters are protective and left undisturbed.
    d. Skin grafting may be necessary.
    e. Fasciotomy may be needed to relieve pressure and allow normal blood flow.

60. Which statement about the third-spacing or capillary leak syndrome in a patient with severe burns is accurate?
    a. It usually happens in the first 36 to 48 hours.
    b. It is a leak of plasma fluids into the interstitial space.
    c. It is present only in the burned tissues.
    d. It can usually be prevented with diuretics.

61. As a result of third-spacing, during the acute phase, which electrolyte imbalances may occur? *(Select all that apply.)*
    a. Hyperkalemia
    b. Hypokalemia
    c. Hypernatremia
    d. Hyponatremia
    e. Hypercalcemia

62. Because of the fluid shifts in burn patients, what effects on cardiac output does the nurse expect to see?
    a. An initial increase, then normalized in 24 to 48 hours
    b. Depressed up to 36 hours after the burn
    c. Improved with fluid restriction
    d. Responsive to diuretics as evidenced by urinary output

63. A patient with burn injuries is being discharged from the hospital. What important points does the nurse include in the discharge teaching? *(Select all that apply.)*
    a. Signs and symptoms of infection
    b. Drug regimens and potential medication side effects
    c. Definition of full-thickness burns
    d. Correct application and care of pressure garments
    e. Comfort measures to reduce scarring
    f. Dates for follow-up appointments

64. A patient has sustained significant burns which have created a hypermetabolic state. In planning care for this patient, what does the nurse consider?
    a. Increased retention of sodium
    b. Decreased secretion of catecholamines
    c. Increased caloric needs
    d. The decrease in core temperature

65. The nurse is reviewing the laboratory results for several burn patients who are approximately 24 to 36 hours postinjury. What laboratory results related to the fluid remobilization in these patients does the nurse expect to see?
    a. Anemia
    b. Metabolic alkalosis
    c. Hypernatremia
    d. Hyperkalemia

66. Local tissue resistance to electricity varies in different parts of the body. Which tissue has the most resistance?
    a. Skin epidermis
    b. Tendons and muscle
    c. Fatty tissue
    d. Nerve tissue and blood vessels

67. A patient was rescued from a burning house and treated with oxygen. Initially, the patient had audible wheezing and wheezing on auscultation, but after approximately 30 minutes the wheezing stopped. The patient now demonstrates substernal retractions and anxiety. What action does the nurse take at this time?
    a. Recognize an impending airway obstruction and prepare for immediate intubation.
    b. Continue to monitor the patient's respiratory status and initiate pulse oximetry.
    c. Document this finding as evidence of improvement and continue to observe.
    d. Stay with and encourage the patient to remain calm and breathe deeply.

68. The nurse is caring for a young woman who sustained burns on the upper extremities and anterior chest while attempting to put out a kitchen grease fire. Which laboratory results does the nurse expect to see during the resuscitation phase? *(Select all that apply.)*
    a. Potassium level of 3.2 mEq/L
    b. Glucose level of 180 mg/dL
    c. Hematocrit of 49%
    d. pH of 7.20
    e. Sodium level of 139 mEq/L

69. A patient has sustained a burn to the right ankle. The provider has applied the initial dressing to the ankle, and the nurse assists the patient into bed and positions the ankle to prevent contracture. What is the correct position the nurse uses?
    a. Dorsiflexion
    b. Adduction
    c. External rotation
    d. Hyperextension

70. A patient has sustained a severe burn greater than 30% TBSA. What is the best way to assess renal function in this patient?
    a. Measure urine output and compare this value with fluid intake.
    b. Weigh the patient every day and compare that to the dry weight.
    c. Note the amount of edema and measure abdominal girth.
    d. Assist the patient with a urinal or bedpan every 2 hours.

71. The nurse is caring for an African-American patient with a burn injury. The patient appears to be having severe pain and discomfort that are unrelated to the burned areas. The nurse advocates that the provider order which additional test?
    a. Sickle cell for trait
    b. Drug screen for opiate abuse
    c. X-rays to identify bone injuries
    d. ECG to identify cardiac dysrhythmias

72. The provider has ordered an escharotomy for a patient because of constriction around the patient's chest. The nurse is teaching the patient and family about the procedure. Which statement by the family indicates a need for additional teaching?
    a. "He doesn't do well under general anesthesia."
    b. "He'll be awake for the procedure."
    c. "He will receive medication for sedation and pain."
    d. "We could stay with him at the bedside during the procedure."

73. The nurse is caring for a firefighter who was brought in for burns around the face and upper chest. Airway maintenance for this patient with respiratory involvement includes what action?
    a. Monitoring for signs and symptoms of upper airway edema during fluid resuscitation
    b. Inserting a nasopharyngeal or oropharyngeal airway when the patient's airway is completely obstructed
    c. Obtaining an order for as-needed (prn) oxygen per nasal cannula
    d. Frequently suctioning the mouth with Yankauer suction

74. At what point does fluid mobilization occur in patients with burns?
    a. After the scar tissue is formed and fluids are no longer being lost.
    b. Within the first 4 hours after the burns were sustained.
    c. After 36 hours when the fluid is reabsorbed from the interstitial tissue.
    d. Immediately after the burns occur.

75. The nurse is caring for a patient with chronic pain associated with an old burn injury. Which nonpharmacologic intervention does the nurse use to help relieve the patient's pain?
    a. Nitrous oxide
    b. Cool room temperature to reduce discomfort
    c. Massaging nonburned areas
    d. Intravenous narcotics due to delayed tissue absorption

76. A patient with a burn injury had an autograft. The nurse learns in report that the donor site is on the upper thigh. What type of wound does the nurse expect to find at donor site?
    a. Stage 1
    b. Partial thickness
    c. Full thickness
    d. Stage 4

77. To prevent the complication of Curling's ulcer, what does the nurse anticipate the provider will order?
    a. Nasogastric tube insertion
    b. H2 histamine blockers
    c. Abdominal assessment every 4 hours
    d. Systemic antibiotic

78. Several patients are transported from an industrial fire to a local ED. Which factors increase the risk of death for these patients? *(Select all that apply.)*
    a. Male gender
    b. Age greater than 60 years
    c. Burn greater than 40% TBSA
    d. Presence of an inhalation injury
    e. Presence of contact burns

79. What is the most essential patient data needed for calculating the fluid rates, energy requirements, and drug doses for the burn patient?
    a. Age
    b. Health history
    c. Preburn weight
    d. Current weight

80. Which drug therapy reduces the risk of wound infection for burn patients?
    a. Large doses of oral antifungal medications every 4 hours
    b. Silver nitrate solution covered by dry dressings applied every 4 hours
    c. Silver sulfadiazine (Silvadene) on full-thickness injuries every 4 hours
    d. Broad-spectrum antibiotics given intravenously

81. A patient has sustained a relatively large burn. The nurse anticipates that the patient's nutritional requirements may exceed how many kcal/day?
    a. 1500
    b. 2000
    c. 3000
    d. 5000

82. Which feelings are most typically expressed by the burn patient? *(Select all that apply.)*
    a. Suspicion
    b. Regression
    c. Apathy
    d. Denial
    e. Suicidal ideations
    f. Anger

83. A patient has been depressed and withdrawn since her injury and has expressed that "life will never be the same." Which nursing intervention best promotes a positive image for this burn patient?
    a. Discussing the possibility of reconstructive surgery with the patient
    b. Allowing the patient to choose a colorful scarf to cover the burned area
    c. Playing cards or board games with the patient
    d. Encouraging the patient to consider how fortunate she is to be alive

84. A 28-year-old male patient sustained second- and third-degree burns on his legs (30%) when his clothing caught fire while he was burning leaves. He was hosed down by his neighbor and has arrived at the ED in severe discomfort. What is the priority problem for this patient at this time?
    a. Acute pain related to damaged or exposed nerve endings
    b. Decreased fluid volume related to electrolyte imbalance
    c. Potential for inadequate oxygenation
    d. Diminished self-image related to the appearance of legs

85. Which patient has the highest risk for a fatal burn injury?
    a. 4-year-old child
    b. 32-year-old man
    c. 45-year-old woman
    d. 77-year-old man

27 CHAPTER

Assessment of the Respiratory System

1. A patient comes to the health care provider's office for an annual physical. The patient reports having a persistent, nagging cough. Which question does the nurse ask first about this symptom?
   a. "When did the cough start?"
   b. "Do you have a family history of lung cancer?"
   c. "Have you been running a fever"
   d. "Do you have sneezing and congestion?"

2. When blood passes through the lungs, what happens to oxygen?
   a. It diffuses from the alveoli into the red blood cells.
   b. It diffuses from the red blood cells into the alveoli.
   c. It decreases concentration in the blood.
   d. It increases concentration in the alveoli.

3. Which substances from cigarette smoke have been implicated in the development of serious lung diseases? *(Select all that apply.)*
   a. Carbon dioxide
   b. Nicotine
   c. Tar
   d. Carbon monoxide
   e. Dust particles

4. A patient reports smoking a pack of cigarettes a day for 9 years. He then quit for 2 years, and then smoked 2 packs a day for the last 30 years. What are the pack-years for this patient?
   a. 39 years
   b. 69 years
   c. 19.5 years
   d. 41 years

5. Which is an example of third-hand passive smoking?
   a. Sitting in a car with a person who is smoking
   b. Exposure to smoke on the clothes of a smoker
   c. Walking through a group of people smoking outside
   d. Entering a room where several people have been smoking

6. Pulmonary function tests are scheduled for a patient with a history of smoking who reports dyspnea and chronic cough. What will patient teaching information about this procedure include?
   a. Do not smoke for at least 2 weeks before the test.
   b. Bronchodilator drugs may be withheld 2 days before the test.
   c. The patient will breathe through the mouth and wear a nose clip during the test.
   d. The patient will be expected to walk on a treadmill during the test.

7. The nurse is providing care for a patient who would like to quit smoking. Which important teaching points must be included when teaching this patient? *(Select all that apply.)*
   a. Talk with your health care provider about nicotine replacement therapies.
   b. Ask for help from family and friends who have quit smoking.
   c. Smoking while using a nicotine patch is acceptable as long as you are gradually decreasing how much you smoke.
   d. Remove all ashtrays, cigarettes, pipes, cigars, and lighters from your home to decrease the temptation to smoke.
   e. If you are used to having a cigarette after eating, get up from the table as soon as you are finished eating.
   f. Avoid starting an exercise program at the same time you quit smoking because making two big changes at the same time is setting yourself up for failure.

8. The health care provider has prescribed varenicline (Chantix) for the patient who wishes to quit smoking. What specific priority teaching must the nurse provide for the patient and his family?
   a. Avoid spending time in enclosed spaces with active smokers.
   b. Make a list of all the reasons that you wish to quit smoking cigarettes.
   c. Plan to reward yourself with the money you save from not smoking cigarettes.
   d. Be sure to report any changes in behavior or thought processes to your health care provider.

9. In which situation would the oxygen dissociation curve shift to the left?
   a. Decreased pH (acidosis)
   b. Increased pH (alkalosis)
   c. Increased body temperature
   d. Increased body carbon dioxide concentration

10. Which respiratory changes occur as a result of aging? *(Select all that apply.)*
    a. Increased elastic recoil
    b. Dilation of alveolar ducts
    c. Decreased ability to cough
    d. Alveolar surface tension increases
    e. Diffusion capacity decreases

11. A patient is scheduled to have a pulmonary function test (PFT). Which type of information does the nurse include in the nursing history so that PFT results can be appropriately determined?
    a. Age, gender, race, height, weight, and smoking status
    b. Occupational status, activity tolerance for activities of daily living
    c. Medication history and history of allergies to contrast media
    d. History of chronic medical conditions and surgical procedures

12. Which description best explains residual volume (RV)?
    a. Amount of air in the lungs at the end of maximal inhalation
    b. Amount of air remaining in lungs at the end of full forced exhalation
    c. Amount of air remaining in the lungs after normal exhalation
    d. Maximal amount of forced air that can be exhaled after maximal inspiration

13. The nurse is caring for an older adult who uses a wheelchair and spends over half of each day in bed. Which intervention is important in promoting pulmonary hygiene related to age and decreased mobility?
    a. Obtain an order for prn (as-needed) oxygen via nasal cannula.
    b. Encourage the patient to turn, cough, and deep-breathe.
    c. Reassure the patient that immobility is temporary.
    d. Monitor the respiratory rate and check pulse oximetry readings.

14. The nurse is assessing a middle-aged patient who reports a decreased tolerance for exercise and that she must work harder to breathe. Which questions assist the nurse in determining what these changes are related to? *(Select all that apply.)*
    a. "Do you have anemia?"
    b. "When did you first notice these symptoms?"
    c. "Do you or have you ever smoked cigarettes?"
    d. "How often do you exercise?"
    e. "Are you coughing up any colored sputum?"

15. A patient who received a bronchoscopy was NPO (nothing by mouth) for several hours before the test. Now a few hours after the test, the patient is hungry and would like to eat a meal. What does the nurse do before allowing the patient to eat?
    a. Order a meal because the patient is now alert and oriented.
    b. Check pulse oximetry to be sure oxygen saturation has returned to normal.
    c. Check for a gag reflex before allowing the patient to eat.
    d. Assess for nausea from the medications given for the test.

16. After a bronchoscopy procedure, the patient coughs up sputum which contains blood. What is the best nursing action at this time?
    a. Assess vital signs and respiratory status and notify the provider of the findings.
    b. Monitor the patient for 24 hours to see if blood continues in the sputum.
    c. Send the sputum to the lab for cytology for possible lung cancer.
    d. Reassure the patient this is a normal response after a bronchoscopy.

17. Before a bronchoscopy procedure, the patient received benzocaine spray as a topical anesthetic to numb the oropharynx. The nurse is assessing the patient after the procedure. Which finding suggests that the patient is developing methemoglobinemia?
    a. The patient has a decreased hematocrit level.
    b. The patient does not respond to supplemental oxygen.
    c. The blood sample is a bright cherry-red color.
    d. The patient experiences sedation and amnesia.

18. The nurse is caring for several patients who had diagnostic testing for respiratory disorders. Which diagnostic test has the highest risk for the postprocedure complication of pneumothorax?
    a. Bronchoscopy
    b. Laryngoscopy
    c. Computed tomography of lungs
    d. Percutaneous lung biopsy

19. A patient's pulse oximetry reading is 89%. What is the nurse's first priority action?
    a. Recheck the reading with a different oximeter.
    b. Apply supplemental oxygen and recheck the oximeter reading in 15 minutes.
    c. Assess the patient for respiratory distress and recheck the oximeter reading.
    d. Place the patient in the recovery position and monitor frequently.

20. A patient demonstrates labored, shallow respirations and a respiratory rate of 32/min with a pulse oximetry reading of 85%. What is the priority nursing intervention?
    a. Notify respiratory therapy to give the patient a breathing treatment.
    b. Start oxygen via nasal cannula at 2 L/min.
    c. Obtain an order for a stat arterial blood gas (ABG).
    d. Encourage coughing and deep-breathing exercises.

21. Which factors or conditions cause a decreased (below normal) PETCO$_2$ level due to abnormal ventilation? *(Select all that apply.)*
    a. Hyperthermia
    b. Hypotension
    c. Apnea
    d. Hyperventilation
    e. Hypothermia

22. The nurse is reviewing ABG results from an 86-year-old patient. Which results would be considered normal findings for a patient of this age?
    a. Normal pH, normal Pao$_2$, normal Paco$_2$
    b. Normal pH, decreased Pao$_2$, normal Paco$_2$
    c. Decreased pH, decreased Pao$_2$, normal Paco$_2$
    d. Decreased pH, decreased Pao$_2$, decreased Paco$_2$

23. Upon performing a lung sound assessment of the anterior chest, the nurse hears moderately loud sounds on inspiration that are equal in length with expiration. In what area is this lung sound considered normal?
    a. Trachea
    b. Primary bronchi
    c. Lung fields
    d. Larynx

24. Which sounds in the smaller bronchioles and the alveoli indicate normal lung sounds?
    a. Harsh, hollow, and tubular blowing
    b. Nothing; normally no sounds are heard
    c. Soft, low rustling; like wind in the trees
    d. Flat, dull tones with a moderate pitch

25. What is the characteristic of normal lung sounds that should be heard throughout the lung fields?
    a. Short inspiration, long expiration, loud, harsh
    b. Soft sound, long inspiration, short quiet expiration
    c. Mixed sounds of harsh and soft, long inspiration and long expiration
    d. Loud, long inspiration and short, loud expiration

26. Upon assessing the lungs, the nurse hears short, discrete popping sounds "like hair being rolled between fingers near the ear" in the bilateral lower lobes. How is this assessment documented?
    a. Rhonchi
    b. Wheezes
    c. Fine crackles
    d. Coarse crackles

27. The nurse is taking a history on a patient who reports sleeping in a recliner chair at night because lying on the bed causes shortness of breath. How is this documented?
    a. Orthopnea
    b. Paroxysmal nocturnal dyspnea
    c. Orthostatic nocturnal dyspnea
    d. Tachypnea

28. What conditions shift the curve to the right, meaning hemoglobin will dissociate oxygen? *(Select all that apply.)*
    a. Increased carbon dioxide concentration
    b. Decreased tissue concentration of glucose breakdown products
    c. Increased tissue pH (alkalosis)
    d. Decreased tissue temperature
    e. Decreased tissue pH (acidosis)

29. What observations does the nurse make when performing a general assessment of a patient's lungs and thorax? *(Select all that apply.)*
    a. Symmetry of chest movement
    b. Rate, rhythm, and depth of respirations
    c. Use of accessory muscles for breathing
    d. Comparison of the anteroposterior diameter with the lateral diameter
    e. Measurement of the length of the chest cavity
    f. Assessment of chest expansion and respiratory excursion

30. Which assessment finding is an objective sign of chronic oxygen deprivation?
    a. Continuous cough productive of clear sputum
    b. Audible inspiratory and expiratory wheeze
    c. Chest pain that increases with deep inspiration
    d. Clubbing of fingernails and a barrel-shaped chest

31. The nurse is palpating a patient's chest and identifies an increased tactile fremitus or vibration of the chest wall produced when the patient speaks. What does the nurse do next?
    a. Observe for other findings associated with subcutaneous emphysema.
    b. Document the observation as an expected normal finding.
    c. Observe the patient for other findings associated with a pneumothorax.
    d. Document the observation as a pleural friction rub.

32. The nurse reviews the complete blood count results for the patient who has chronic obstructive pulmonary disease (COPD) and lives in a high mountain area. What lab results does the nurse expect to see for this patient?
    a. Increased red blood cells
    b. Decreased neutrophils
    c. Decreased eosinophils
    d. Increased lymphocytes

33. The nurse is inspecting a patient's chest and observes an increase in anteroposterior diameter of the chest. When is this an expected finding?
    a. With a pulmonary mass
    b. Upon deep inhalation
    c. In older adult patients
    d. With chest trauma

34. While percussing a patient's chest and lung fields, the nurse notes a high, loud, musical, drumlike sound similar to tapping a cheek that is puffed out with air. What is the nurse's priority action?
    a. Document this expected finding using words like, "high," "loud," and "hollow."
    b. Immediately notify the provider because the patient has an airway obstruction.
    c. Assess the patient for air hunger or pain at the end of inhalation and exhalation.
    d. Palpate for crackling sensation underneath the skin or for localized tenderness.

35. What is the best position for a patient to assume for a thoracentesis?
    a. Side-lying, affected side exposed, head slightly raised
    b. Lying flat with arm on affected side across the chest
    c. Sitting up, leaning forward on the overbed table
    d. Prone position with arms above the head

36. Which procedure has a risk for the complication of pneumothorax?
    a. Thoracentesis
    b. Bronchoscopy
    c. PFT
    d. Ventilation-perfusion scan

37. A patient has undergone a percutaneous lung biopsy. After the procedure, what tests may be ordered to confirm that there is no pneumothorax? *(Select all that apply.)*
    a. Computed tomography
    b. Pulmonary function test
    c. Magnetic resonance imaging
    d. Digital chest radiography
    e. Chest x-ray

38. The respiratory therapist consults with and reports to the nurse that a patient is producing frothy pink sputum. What does the nurse suspect is occurring with this patient?
    a. Pneumothorax
    b. Pulmonary edema
    c. Pulmonary infection
    d. Pulmonary infarction

39. A patient who had a thoracentesis is now experiencing the following clinical manifestations: rapid shallow respirations, rapid heart rate, and pain on the affected side that is worse at the end of inhalation. What complication does the nurse suspect this patient has developed?
    a. Hemoptysis
    b. Lung abscess
    c. Pneumothorax
    d. Lung cancer

40. For what reasons would a patient have a bronchoscopy? *(Select all that apply.)*
    a. Obtain samples for cultures
    b. Diagnose pulmonary disease
    c. View upper airway structures
    d. Administer medications
    e. Obtain samples for biopsy

41. The nurse has just received a patient from the recovery room who is somewhat drowsy, but is capable of following instructions. Pulse oximetry has dropped from 95% to 90%. What is the priority nursing intervention?
    a. Administer oxygen at 2 L/min by nasal cannula, then reassess.
    b. Have the patient perform coughing and deep-breathing exercises, then reassess.
    c. Administer naloxone (Narcan) to reverse narcotic sedation effect.
    d. Withhold narcotic pain medication to reduce sedation effect.

42. What is a pulse oximeter used to measure?
    a. Oxygen perfusion in the extremities
    b. Pulse and perfusion in the extremities
    c. Generalized tissue perfusion
    d. Hemoglobin saturation

43. Which aspect of PFTs would be considered a normal result in the older adult?
    a. Increased forced vital capacity
    b. Decline in forced expiratory volume in 1 second
    c. Decrease in diffusion capacity of carbon monoxide
    d. Increased functional residual capacity

44. In the older adult with chronic pulmonary disease, there is a loss of elastic recoiling of the lung and decreased chest wall compliance. What is the result of this occurrence?
    a. The thoracic area becomes shorter.
    b. The patient has an increased activity tolerance.
    c. There is an increase in anteroposterior ratio.
    d. The patient has severe shortness of breath.

45. In the older adult, there are a decreased number of functional alveoli. To assist the patient to compensate for this change related to aging, what does the nurse do?
    a. Encourage the patient to ambulate and change positions.
    b. Allow the patient to rest and sleep frequently.
    c. Have face-to-face conversations when possible.
    d. Obtain an order for supplemental oxygen.

46. The nurse teaches a patient about the impact of cigarette smoking on the lower respiratory tract. Which statement by the patient indicates an understanding of the information?
    a. "Using nicotine replacement therapy will increase my chances of success."
    b. "If I stop smoking, the damage to my lungs will be reversed."
    c. "Cigarette smoke affects my ability to cough out secretions from the lungs."
    d. "Smoking makes the large and small airways get bigger."

47. A patient reports fatigue and shortness of breath when getting up to walk to the bathroom; however, the pulse oximetry reading is 99%. The nurse identifies a diagnosis of Activity intolerance. Which laboratory value is consistent with the patient's subjective symptoms?
    a. BUN of 15 mg/dL
    b. White blood cell count (WBC) of 8000/ mm^3
    c. Hemoglobin of 9 g/dL
    d. Glucose 160 mg/dL

48. The nurse is performing a respiratory assessment including pulse oximetry on several patients. Which conditions or situations may cause an artificially low reading? *(Select all that apply.)*
    a. Fever
    b. Anemia
    c. Receiving narcotic pain medications
    d. Peripheral artery disease
    e. History of respiratory disease such as cystic fibrosis or tuberculosis

49. A patient who had neck surgery for removal of a tumor reports "not being able to breathe very well." The nurse observes that the patient has decreased chest movement and an elevated pulse. A bronchoscopy is ordered. For what reason did the provider order a bronchoscopy for this patient?
    a. Reverse and relieve any obstruction caused during the neck surgery
    b. Assess the function of vocal cords or remove foreign bodies from the larynx
    c. Aspirate pleural fluid or air from the pleural space
    d. Visualize the larynx (airway structures) to use as a guide for intubation

50. A patient returns to the unit after bronchoscopy. In addition to respiratory status assessment, which assessment does the nurse make in order to prevent aspiration?
    a. Presence of pain or soreness in throat
    b. Time and amount of last oral fluid intake
    c. Type and location of chest pain
    d. Presence or absence of gag reflex

51. The nurse hears fine crackles during a lung assessment of the patient who is in the initial postoperative period. Which nursing intervention helps relieve this respiratory problem?
    a. Monitor the patient with a pulse oximeter.
    b. Encourage coughing and deep-breathing.
    c. Obtain an order for a chest x-ray.
    d. Obtain an order for high-flow oxygen.

52. A patient having respiratory difficulty has a pH of 7.48. What is the nurse's best interpretation of this value?
    a. Acidosis
    b. Alkalosis
    c. Chronic respiratory illness
    d. Shortness of breath

53. The nurse is performing a respiratory assessment on an older adult patient. Which questions are appropriate to ask when using Gordon's Functional Health Pattern Assessment approach? *(Select all that apply.)*
    a. "How has your general health been?"
    b. "Do you now or have you ever smoked?"
    c. "Have you had any colds this past year?"
    d. "Do you have sufficient energy to do what you like to do?"
    e. "When was the last time you were hospitalized?"

54. Tissue oxygen delivery through dissociation from hemoglobin is based on which factor?
    a. Saturation
    b. Oxygen tension
    c. Unloading from hemoglobin
    d. Tissues' need for oxygen

55. The nurse makes observations about several respiratory patients' abilities to perform activities of daily living in order to quantify the level of dyspnea. Which patient is considered to have class V dyspnea?
    a. Experiences subjective shortness of breath when walking up a flight of stairs
    b. Limited to bed or chair and experiences shortness of breath at rest
    c. Can independently shower and dress, but cannot keep pace with similarly aged people
    d. Experiences shortness of breath during aerobic exercise such as jogging

56. The nurse is reviewing the arterial blood gas results for a 25-year-old trauma patient who has new onset of shortness of breath and demonstrates shallow and irregular respirations. The arterial blood gas results are: pH, 7.26; Pco_2, 47%; Po_2, 89%; HCO_3^-, 24. What imbalance does the nurse suspect this patient has?
    a. Respiratory acidosis
    b. Respiratory alkalosis
    c. Metabolic acidosis
    d. Metabolic alkalosis

28 CHAPTER

Care of Patients Requiring Oxygen Therapy or Tracheostomy

1. At what times is oxygen therapy needed for a patient? *(Select all that apply.)*
   a. To treat hypoxia
   b. To treat hypothermia
   c. To treat hypoxemia
   d. When the normal 35% oxygen level in the air is inadequate
   e. When the normal 21% oxygen level in the air is inadequate

2. Which conditions will increase the body's need for more oxygen? *(Select all that apply.)*
   a. Hypothyroid
   b. Infection in the blood
   c. Diabetes mellitus
   d. Body temperature of 101° F
   e. Hemoglobin level of 8.7 g/dL

3. To improve a patient's oxygenation to a normal level, the amount of oxygen administered is based on which factors? *(Select all that apply.)*
   a. Symptom management only
   b. Pulse oximetry reading
   c. Respiratory assessment
   d. The patient's subjective complaints
   e. Arterial blood gas results

4. What are the hazards of administering oxygen therapy? *(Select all that apply.)*
   a. Oxygen supports and enhances combustion.
   b. Oxygen itself can burn.
   c. Each electrical outlet in the room must be covered if not in use.
   d. All electrical equipment in the room must be grounded to prevent fires.
   e. Solutions with high concentrations of alcohol or oil cannot be used in the room.

5. Which parameters does the nurse monitor to ensure that a patient's response to oxygen therapy gas exchange is adequate? *(Select all that apply.)*
   a. Level of consciousness
   b. Respiratory pattern
   c. Oxygen flow rate
   d. Pulse oximetry
   e. Respiratory rate

6. The patient has been on oxygen therapy at 70% for over 2 days. For which complication must the nurse monitor?
   a. Oxygen-induced hypoventilation
   b. Hypercarbia
   c. Oxygen toxicity
   d. Absorptive atelectasis

7. A patient requires home oxygen therapy. When the home health nurse enters the patient's home for the initial visit, he observes several issues that are safety hazards related to the patient's oxygen therapy. What hazards do these include? *(Select all that apply.)*
   a. Bottle of wine in the kitchen area
   b. Package of cigarettes on the coffee table
   c. Several decorative candles on the mantelpiece
   d. Grounded outlet with a green dot on the plate
   e. Electric fan with a frayed cord in the bathroom
   f. Computer with a three-pronged plug

8. The patient is receiving oxygen at 5 L/min by nasal cannula. What priority intervention must the nurse use at this time?
   a. Switch to a mask delivery system.
   b. Humidify the oxygen with sterile water.
   c. Monitor for manifestations of oxygen toxicity.
   d. Add extension tubing for patient mobility.

9. The home health nurse has been caring for a patient with a chronic respiratory disorder. Today the patient seems confused when she is normally alert and oriented x 3. What is the priority nursing action?
   a. Notify the provider about the mental status change.
   b. Check the pulse oximeter reading.
   c. Ask the patient's family when this behavior started.
   d. Perform a mental status examination.

10. The nurse is caring for several patients on a general medical-surgical unit. The nurse would question the need for oxygen therapy for a patient with which condition?
   a. Pulmonary edema with decreased arterial Po_2 levels
   b. Valve replacement with increased cardiac output
   c. Anemia with a decreased hemoglobin and hematocrit
   d. Sustained fever with an increased metabolic demand

11. When a patient is requiring oxygen therapy, what is important for the nurse to know?
   a. Patients require 1 to 10 L/min by nasal cannula in order for oxygen to be effective.
   b. Oxygen-induced hypoventilation is the priority when the $Paco_2$ levels are unknown.
   c. Why the patient is receiving oxygen, expected outcomes, and complications.
   d. The goal is the highest Fio_2 possible for the particular device being used.

12. The nurse is caring for a patient receiving humidified oxygen. Which precaution does the nurse take to prevent bacterial contamination and infection?
   a. Never drain fluid from the water trap back into the nebulizer.
   b. Always wear gloves when cleaning the patient's nasal cannula.
   c. Do not allow live or cut flowers into the patient's room.
   d. Administer routinely ordered antibiotic therapy.

13. The nurse is administering oxygen to a patient who is hypoxic and has chronic high levels of carbon dioxide. Which oxygen therapy prevents a respiratory complication for this patient?
   a. Fio_2 higher than the usual 2 to 4 L/min per nasal cannula
   b. Venturi mask of 40% for the delivery of oxygen
   c. Lower concentration of oxygen (1 to 2 L/min) per nasal cannula
   d. Variable Fio_2 via partial rebreather mask

14. A patient is receiving a high concentration of oxygen as a temporary emergency measure. Which nursing action is the most appropriate to prevent complications associated with high-flow oxygen?
   a. Auscultate the lungs every 4 hours for oxygen toxicity.
   b. Increase the oxygen if the Pao_2 level is less than 93 mm Hg.
   c. Monitor the prescribed oxygen level and length of therapy.
   d. Decrease the oxygen if the patient's condition does not respond.

15. Increased risk for oxygen toxicity is related to which factors? *(Select all that apply.)*
    a. Continuous delivery of oxygen at greater than 50% concentration
    b. Delivery of a high concentration of oxygen over 24 to 48 hours
    c. The severity and extent of lung disease
    d. Neglecting to monitor the patient's status and reducing oxygen concentration as soon as possible
    e. Adding continuous positive airway pressure (CPAP) or positive end-expiratory pressure (PEEP)

16. A patient is receiving warmed and humidified oxygen. The respiratory therapist informs the nurse that several other patients on other units have developed hospital-acquired infections and *Pseudomonas aeruginosa* has been identified as the organism. What does the nurse do?
    a. Place the patient in respiratory isolation.
    b. Obtain an order for a sputum culture.
    c. Change the humidifier every 24 hours.
    d. Obtain an order to discontinue the humidifier.

17. Which factors are considered hazards associated with oxygen therapy? *(Select all that apply.)*
    a. Increased combustion
    b. Oxygen narcosis
    c. Oxygen toxicity
    d. Absorption atelectasis
    e. Oxygen-induced hypoventilation

18. A patient is receiving warmed and humidified oxygen. In discarding the moisture formed by condensation, why does the nurse minimize the time that the tubing is disconnected?
    a. To prevent the patient from desaturating
    b. To reduce the patient's risk of infection
    c. To minimize the disturbance to the patient
    d. To facilitate overall time management

19. What is the best description of the nurse's role in the delivery of oxygen therapy?
    a. Receiving the therapy report from the respiratory therapist
    b. Evaluating the response to oxygen therapy
    c. Contacting respiratory therapy for the devices
    d. Being familiar with the devices and techniques used in order to provide proper care

20. Which complication is the result of constant pressure exerted by a tracheostomy cuff causing tracheal dilation and erosion of cartilage?
    a. Tracheomalacia
    b. Tracheal stenosis
    c. Tracheoesophageal fistula
    d. Trachea–innominate artery fistula

21. A patient requires oxygen therapy with a nasal cannula. Which interventions will the nurse teach the student nurse providing care for this patient? *(Select all that apply.)*
    a. "Make sure that the prongs on the nasal cannula are properly positioned in the nares."
    b. "Apply a water-soluble gel to the nares as needed."
    c. "Adjust the flow rate between 1 and 8 L/minute based on how the patient is feeling."
    d. "Be sure to assess that both nares are patent."
    e. "Assess the patient for any changes in respiratory rate and pattern."

22. A patient is receiving oxygen therapy through a nonrebreather mask. What is the correct nursing intervention?
    a. Maintain liter flow so that the reservoir bag is up to one-half full.
    b. Maintain 60% to 75% Fio_2 at 6 to 11 L/min.
    c. Ensure that valves and rubber flaps are patent, functional, and not stuck.
    d. Assess for effectiveness and switch to partial rebreather mask for more precise Fio_2.

23. A patient with a facemask at 5 L/min is able to eat. Which nursing intervention is performed at mealtimes?
    a. Change the mask to a nasal cannula of 6 L/min or more.
    b. Have the patient work around the facemask as best as possible.
    c. Obtain a provider order for a nasal cannula at 5 L/min.
    d. Obtain a provider order to remove the mask at meals.

24. The provider orders transtracheal oxygen therapy for a patient with respiratory difficulty. What does the nurse tell the patient's family is the purpose of this type of oxygen delivery system?
    a. Delivers oxygen directly into the lungs.
    b. Keeps the small air sacs open to improve gas exchange.
    c. Prevents the need for an endotracheal tube.
    d. Provides high humidity with oxygen delivery.

25. A patient is at risk for aspiration. Which instructions must the nurse provide to the unlicensed assistive personnel (UAP) prior to feeding the patient? *(Select all that apply.)*
    a. Position the patient in the most upright position possible.
    b. Provide adequate time; do not "hurry" the patient.
    c. Provide sips of water or milk between bites of food to help with swallowing.
    d. Encourage the patient to "tuck" his or her chin down and move the forehead forward while swallowing.
    e. If the patient coughs, stop the feeding until he or she indicates that the airway has been cleared.

26. A patient requires long-term airway maintenance following surgery for cancer of the neck. The nurse is using a piece of equipment to explain the procedure and mechanism that are associated with this long-term therapy. Which piece of equipment does the nurse most likely use for this patient teaching session?
    a. Tracheostomy tube
    b. Nasal trumpet
    c. Endotracheal tube
    d. Nasal cannula

27. A patient is receiving preoperative teaching for a partial laryngectomy and will have a tracheostomy postoperatively. How does the nurse define a tracheostomy to the patient?
    a. Opening in the trachea that enables breathing
    b. Temporary procedure that will be reversed at a later date
    c. Technique using positive pressure to improve gas exchange
    d. Procedure that holds open the upper airways

28. A patient returns from the operating room and the nurse assesses for subcutaneous emphysema, which is a potential complication associated with tracheostomy. How does the nurse assess for this complication?
    a. Checking the volume of the pilot balloon
    b. Listening for airflow through the tube
    c. Inspecting and palpating for air under the skin
    d. Assessing the tube for patency

29. A patient with a tracheostomy without a tube in place develops increased coughing, inability to expectorate secretions, and difficulty breathing. What are these assessment findings related to?
    a. Overinflation of the pilot balloon
    b. Tracheoesophageal fistula
    c. Cuff leak and rupture
    d. Tracheal stenosis

30. A patient returns from the operating room after having a tracheostomy. While assessing the patient, which observations made by the nurse warrant immediate notification of the provider?
    a. Patient is alert but unable to speak and has difficulty communicating his needs.
    b. Small amount of bleeding present at the incision.
    c. Skin is puffy at the neck area with a crackling sensation.
    d. Respirations are audible and noisy with an increased respiratory rate.

31. A patient was intubated for acute respiratory failure, and there is an endotracheal tube in place. Which nursing interventions are appropriate for this patient? *(Select all that apply.)*
    a. Ensure that the oxygen is warmed and humidified.
    b. Suction the airway, then the mouth, and give oral care.
    c. Suction the airway with the oral suction equipment.
    d. Position the tubing so it does not pull on the airway.
    e. Apply suction only when withdrawing the suction catheter.

32. To prevent accidental decannulation of a tracheostomy tube, what does the nurse do?
    a. Obtain an order for continuous upper extremity restraints.
    b. Secure the tube in place using ties or fabric fasteners.
    c. Allow some flexibility in motion of the tube while coughing.
    d. Instruct the patient to hold the tube with a tissue while coughing.

33. A patient has a recent tracheostomy. What necessary equipment does the nurse ensure is kept at the bedside? *(Select all that apply.)*
    a. Ambu bag
    b. Pair of wire cutters
    c. Oxygen tubing
    d. Suction equipment
    e. Tracheostomy tube with obturator

34. Which statement by the nursing student indicates an understanding of the purpose of administering oxygen by nasal cannula?
    a. "With a nasal cannula, a wide range of oxygen flow rates and concentrations can be delivered."
    b. "A minimum flow rate of 5 L/min is needed to prevent the rebreathing of exhaled air."
    c. "It works by pulling in a proportional amount of room air for each liter flow of oxygen."
    d. "It is often used for chronic lung disease and for any patient needing long-term oxygen therapy."

35. A patient has a temporary tracheostomy following surgery to the neck area to remove a benign tumor. Which nursing intervention is performed to prevent obstruction of the tracheostomy tube?
    a. Provide tracheal suctioning when there are noisy respirations.
    b. Provide oxygenation to maintain pulse oximeter readings.
    c. Inflate the cuff to maximum pressure and check it once per shift.
    d. Suction regularly and as needed (prn) with an oral suction device.

36. A patient sustained a serious crush injury to the neck and had a tracheostomy tube placed 3 days ago. As the nurse is performing tracheostomy care, the patient suddenly sneezes very forcefully and the tracheostomy tube falls out onto the bed linens. What does the nurse do?
    a. Ventilate the patient with 100% oxygen and notify the provider.
    b. Quickly and gently replace the tube with a clean cannula kept at the bedside.
    c. Quickly rinse the tube with sterile solution and gently replace it.
    d. Give the patient oxygen; call for assistance and a new tracheostomy kit.

37. Patients with a tracheostomy or endotracheal tube need suctioning. Which nursing interventions apply to proper suctioning technique? *(Select all that apply.)*
    a. Preoxygenate the patient for at least 30 seconds before suctioning.
    b. Instruct the patient that he or she is going to be suctioned.
    c. Quickly insert the suction catheter until resistance is met.
    d. Suction the patient for at least 30 seconds to remove secretions.
    e. Repeat suctioning as needed for four to five total suction passes.

38. What are possible complications that can occur with suctioning from an artificial airway? *(Select all that apply.)*
    a. Infection
    b. Coughing
    c. Hypoxia
    d. Tissue (mucosa) trauma
    e. Vagal stimulation
    f. Bronchospasm

39. A patient required emergency intubation and currently has an artificial airway in place. Oxygen is being administered directly from the wall source. Why would warmed and humidified oxygen be a more appropriate choice for this patient?
    a. Helps prevent drying damage to mucous membranes
    b. Promotes thick secretions which are easier to suction
    c. Is more comfortable for the patient
    d. Is less likely to cause oxygen toxicity

40. A patient has an endotracheal tube and requires frequent suctioning for copious secretions. What is a complication of tracheal suctioning?·
    a. Atelectasis
    b. Hypoxia
    c. Hypercarbia
    d. Bronchodilation

41. While the nursing student changes a patient's tracheostomy dressing, the nurse observes the student using a pair of scissors to cut a 4 × 4 gauze pad to make a split dressing that will fit around the tracheostomy tube. What is the nurse's best action?
    a. Give the student positive reinforcement for use of materials and technique.
    b. Report the student to the instructor for remediation of the skill.
    c. Change the dressing immediately after the student has left the room.
    d. Direct the student in the correct use of materials and explain the rationale.

42. The nurse is caring for a patient with a tracheostomy who has recently been transferred from the intensive care unit (ICU), but he has had no unusual occurrences related to the tracheostomy or his oxygenation status. What does the routine care for this patient include?
    a. Thorough respiratory assessment at least every 2 hours
    b. Maintaining the cuff pressure between 50 and 100 mm Hg
    c. Suctioning as needed; maximum suction time of 20 seconds
    d. Changing the tracheostomy dressing once a day

43. A patient with a tracheostomy is being discharged to home. In patient teaching, what does the nurse instruct the patient to do?
    a. Use sterile technique when suctioning.
    b. Instill tap water into the artificial airway.
    c. Clean the tracheostomy tube with soap and water.
    d. Increase the humidity in the home.

44. A patient with a permanent tracheostomy is interested in developing an exercise regimen. Which activity does the nurse advise the patient to avoid?
    a. Aerobics
    b. Tennis
    c. Golf
    d. Swimming

45. A patient with an endotracheal tube in place has dry mucous membranes and lips related to the tube and the partial open mouth position. What techniques does the nurse use to provide this patient with frequent oral care?
    a. Cleanses the mouth with glycerin swabs.
    b. Provides alcohol-based mouth rinse and oral suction.
    c. Cleanses with a mixture of hydrogen peroxide and water.
    d. Uses oral swabs or a soft-bristled brush moistened in water.

46. A patient with a tracheostomy who receives unnecessary suctioning can experience which complications? *(Select all that apply.)*
    a. Bronchospasm
    b. Mucosal damage
    c. Impaired gag reflex
    d. Bronchodilation
    e. Bleeding

47. A patient who is breathing on his own has a fenestrated tracheostomy tube with a cuff. Which precaution must the nurse instruct the student about when caring for this patient?
    a. Always keep the cuff inflated to prevent secretions from entering the lungs.
    b. Suction the patient every 30 to 60 minutes.
    c. Always deflate the cuff before capping the tube with the decannulation cap.
    d. To reduce the risk for tracheal damage, keep the cuff pressure between 22 and 30 mm Hg.

48. A patient has a cuffed tracheostomy tube without a pressure relief valve. To prevent tissue damage of the tracheal mucosa, what does the nurse do?
    a. Deflate the cuff every 2 to 4 hours and maintain as needed.
    b. Change the tracheostomy tube every 3 days or per hospital policy.
    c. Assess and record cuff pressures each shift using the occlusive technique.
    d. Assess and record cuff pressures each shift using minimal leak technique.

49. An older adult patient is at risk for aspirating food or fluids. Which are the most appropriate nursing actions to prevent this problem? *(Select all that apply.)*
    a. Provide close supervision when the patient is self-feeding.
    b. Instruct the patient to tilt the head back when swallowing.
    c. Obtain an order for a clear liquid diet and offer small, frequent amounts.
    d. Instruct the patient to tuck the chin down when swallowing.
    e. Place the patient in an upright position.

50. An older adult patient sustained a stroke several weeks ago and is having difficulty swallowing. To prevent aspiration during mealtimes, what does the nurse do?
    a. Hyperextend the head to allow food to enter the stomach and not the lungs.
    b. Give thin liquids after each bite of food to help "wash the food down."
    c. Encourage "dry swallowing" after each bite to clear residue from the throat.
    d. Maintain a low-Fowler's position during eating and for 2 hours afterwards.

51. A patient with a tracheostomy tube is currently alert and cooperative but seems to be coughing more frequently and producing more secretions than usual. The nurse determines that there is a need for suctioning. Which nursing intervention does the nurse use to prevent hypoxia for this patient?
    a. Allow the patient to breathe room air prior to suctioning.
    b. Avoid prolonged suctioning time.
    c. Suction frequently when the patient is coughing.
    d. Use the largest available catheter.

52. The nurse is suctioning the secretions from a patient's endotracheal tube. The patient demonstrates a vagal response by a drop in heart rate to 54/min and a drop in blood pressure to 90/50 mm Hg. After stopping suctioning, what is the nurse's priority action?
    a. Allow the patient to rest for at least 10 minutes.
    b. Monitor the patient and call the Rapid Response Team.
    c. Oxygenate with 100% oxygen and monitor the patient.
    d. Administer atropine according to standing orders.

53. A patient with a tracheostomy is unable to speak. He is not in acute distress, but is gesturing and trying to communicate with the nurse. Which nursing intervention is the best approach in this situation?
    a. Rely on the family to interpret for the patient.
    b. Ask questions that can be answered with a "yes" or "no" response.
    c. Obtain an immediate consult with the speech therapist.
    d. Encourage the patient to rest rather than struggle with communication.

54. Which clinical finding in a patient with a recent tracheostomy is the most serious and requires immediate intervention?
    a. Increased cough and difficulty expectorating secretions
    b. Food particles in the tracheal secretions
    c. Pulsating tracheostomy tube in synchrony with the heartbeat
    d. Set tidal volume on the ventilator not being received by the patient

29 CHAPTER

Care of Patients with Noninfectious Upper Respiratory Problems

1. The nurse is caring for a patient with a nasal fracture. The patient has clear secretions that react positively when tested for glucose. Which complication does the nurse suspect?
   a. Jaw fracture
   b. Facial fracture
   c. Vertebral fracture
   d. Skull fracture

2. The patient with a nasal fracture has clear fluid draining from the nose which dries on a piece of filter paper and leaves a yellow "halo" ring at the dried edge of the fluid. What is the nurse's best first action?
   a. Document the finding.
   b. Notify the health care provider.
   c. Send a sample to the lab.
   d. Place the patient in a supine position.

3. The nurse is caring for several patients who are at risk because of problems related to the upper airway. Which are the priority assessments and actions for these patients?
   a. Thickness of oral secretions; encourage ingestion of oral fluids
   b. Anxiety and pain; provide reassurance and nonsteroidal antiinflammatory drugs (NSAIDs)
   c. Adequacy of oxygenation; ensure an unobstructed air passageway
   d. Evidence of spinal cord injuries; obtain order for x-rays

4. On postoperative assessment, the nurse notes that the patient with a rhinoplasty repeatedly swallows. What is the nurse's best first action?
   a. Examine the throat for bleeding
   b. Provide ice chips to ease swallowing
   c. Notify the health care provider
   d. Ask if the patient is hungry

5. Which factors contribute to sleep apnea? (Select all that apply.)
   a. Smoking
   b. A short neck
   c. Athletic lifestyle
   d. Small uvula
   e. Enlarged tonsils or adenoids
   f. Underweight for height and gender

6. The patient with laryngeal trauma develops stridor. What is the nurse's highest priority intervention?
   a. Apply oxygen by nasal cannula
   b. Obtain an arterial blood gas sample
   c. Call the Rapid Response Team (RRT).
   d. Perform a maneuver to open the airway

7. A patient has been diagnosed with sleep apnea. Which assessment findings indicate that the patient is having complications associated with sleep apnea?
   a. Side effects of hypoxemia, hypercapnia, and sleep deprivation
   b. Decrease in arterial carbon dioxide levels and sleep deprivation
   c. Respiratory alkalosis with retention of carbon dioxide
   d. Irritability, obesity, and enlarged tonsils or adenoids

8. A patient has been diagnosed with airway obstruction during sleep. The nurse will likely include patient education about which device for home use?
   a. Continuous positive airway pressure (CPAP) to deliver a positive airway pressure
   b. Oxygen via facemask to prevent hypoxia
   c. Neck brace to support the head and facilitate breathing
   d. Nebulizer treatments with bronchodilators

9. The patient has a diagnosis of mild sleep apnea. Which interventions will the nurse teach the patient that may correct this condition? *(Select all that apply.)*
   a. Change sleeping positions
   b. Use CPAP every night
   c. Look into a weight loss program
   d. A position fixing device can prevent tongue subluxation
   e. You may need surgery to remodel your posterior oropharynx

10. A patient is at risk for aspiration related to open vocal cord paralysis. What does the nurse teach the patient to do? *(Select all that apply.)*
    a. Raise the chin while swallowing
    b. Breathe slowly through an open mouth immediately after swallowing
    c. Hold the breath during swallowing
    d. Tilt the head backward during and immediately after swallowing
    e. Tuck the chin down and tilt the head forward during swallowing

11. The nurse is assessing a patient who reports being struck in the face and head several times. During the assessment, a pink-tinged drainage from the nares is observed. Which nursing action provides relevant assessment data?
    a. Have the patient gently blow the nose and observe for bloody mucus.
    b. Test the drainage with a reagent to check the pH.
    c. Ask the patient to describe the appearance of the face before the incident.
    d. Place a drop of the drainage on a filter paper and look for a yellow ring.

12. While playing football at school, a patient injured his nose resulting in a possible simple fracture. The patient's parents call the nurse seeking advice. What does the nurse tell the parents to do?
    a. Ask the school nurse to insert a nasal airway to ensure patency.
    b. Apply an ice pack and allow the patient to rest in a supine position.
    c. Seek medical attention within 24 hours to minimize further complications.
    d. Monitor the symptoms for 24 hours and contact the provider if there is bleeding.

13. A patient had a rhinoplasty and is preparing for discharge home. A family member is instructed by the nurse to monitor the patient for postnasal drip by using a flashlight to look in the back of the throat. If bleeding is noted, what does the nurse tell the family member to do?
    a. Place ice packs on the back of the neck and apply pressure to the nose.
    b. Hyperextend the neck and apply pressure and ice packs as needed.
    c. Seek immediate medical attention for the bleeding.
    d. Monitor for 24 hours if the bleeding appears to be a small amount.

14. The nurse is teaching a patient about post-rhinoplasty care. Which patient statement indicates an understanding of the instruction?
    a. "I will have a very large dressing on my nose."
    b. "I will have bruising around my eyes, nose, and face."
    c. "There will be swelling that will cause a loss of sense of smell."
    d. "My nose will be three times its normal size for 3 weeks."

15. A patient with an active nosebleed is admitted to the emergency department. Which intervention does the nurse use first to attempt to stop the nosebleed?
    a. Have the patient sit upright with the head forward.
    b. Insert nasal packing.
    c. Apply direct lateral pressure to the nose.
    d. Place a nasal catheter.

16. After being treated in the emergency department for posterior nosebleed, the patient is admitted to the hospital. The nasal packing is in place and vital signs are stable. The patient has an IV of normal saline at 125 mL/hr. What is the priority for nursing care?
    a. Airway management
    b. Managing potential dehydration
    c. Managing potential decreased cardiac output
    d. Monitoring for potential infection

17. A patient is admitted for a posterior nosebleed. Posterior packing is in place and the patient is on oxygen therapy, antibiotics, and opioid analgesics. What is the priority assessment?
    a. Tolerance of packing or tubes
    b. Gag and cough reflexes
    c. Mouth breathing
    d. Skin breakdown around the nares

18. A patient returns from surgery following a rhinoplasty. The unlicensed assistive personnel (UAP) places the patient in a supine position to encourage rest and sleep. Which action should the nurse take first?
    a. Teach the patient how to use the bed controls to position herself.
    b. Explain the purpose of the semi-Fowler's position to the UAP.
    c. Place the patient in a semi-Fowler's position and assess for aspiration.
    d. Post a notice at the head of the bed to remind personnel about positioning.

19. The nurse is caring for a patient who had a nasoseptoplasty. Which action is the best to delegate to the licensed practical nurse?
    a. Administer a stool softener to ease bowel movements.
    b. Assess the patient's airway and breathing after general anesthesia.
    c. Evaluate the patient's emotional reaction to the facial edema and bruising.
    d. Take vital signs every 4 hours as ordered by the provider.

20. The nurse is providing postoperative nursing care for a patient with surgical correction of a deviated septum. Which intervention is part of the standard care for this patient?
    a. Apply ice to the nasal area and eyes to decrease swelling and pain.
    b. Encourage deep coughing to prevent atelectasis and clear secretions.
    c. Administer NSAIDs or Tylenol every 4 to 6 hours for pain relief.
    d. Apply moist heat and humidity to the nasal area for comfort and circulation.

21. A patient arrives in the emergency department with a severe crush injury to the face with blood gurgling from the mouth and nose and obvious respiratory distress. The nurse prepares to assist the provider with which procedure to manage the airway?
    a. Performing a needle thoracotomy
    b. Inserting an endotracheal tube
    c. Performing a tracheotomy
    d. Inserting a nasal airway and giving oxygen

22. A patient with facial trauma has undergone surgical intervention to wire the jaw shut. In performing discharge teaching with this patient, which topics does the nurse cover? *(Select all that apply.)*
    a. Oral care
    b. Activity
    c. Use of wire cutters
    d. Communication
    e. Aspiration prevention

23. The nurse is assessing a patient with significant and obvious facial trauma after being struck repeatedly in the face. Which finding is the priority and requires immediate intervention?
    a. Asymmetry of the mandible
    b. Restlessness with high pitched respirations
    c. Nonparallel extraocular movements
    d. Pain upon palpation over the nasal bridge

24. A patient has an inner maxillary fixation. The nurse encourages the patient to eat which kind of food?
    a. Milkshakes
    b. Cottage cheese
    c. Tea and toast
    d. Tuna and noodle casserole

25. A patient enters the emergency department after being punched in the throat. What does the nurse monitor for?
    a. Aphonia
    b. Dry cough
    c. Crepitus
    d. Loss of gag reflex

26. A patient has sustained a mandible fracture and the surgeon has explained that the repair will be made using a resorbable plate. The patient discloses to the nurse that he has not told the surgeon about his substance abuse and illicit drug dependence. What is the nurse's best response?
    a. "Why didn't you talk to your surgeon about this issue?"
    b. "You should tell the surgeon, but it is your choice."
    c. "It is important for your surgeon to know about this information."
    d. "You shouldn't be ashamed; your surgeon will still repair your fracture."

27. A patient has had an inner maxillary fixation for a mandibular fracture. Which piece of equipment should be kept at the bedside at all times?
    a. Water Pik
    b. Wire cutters
    c. Pair of hemostats
    d. Emesis basin

28. A patient who was in a motor vehicle accident and sustained laryngeal trauma is being treated in the emergency department with humidified oxygen and is being monitored every 15 to 30 minutes for respiratory distress. Which assessment finding indicates the urgent need for further intervention?
    a. Respiratory rate 24, PaO_2 80 to 100, no difficulty with communication
    b. Pulse oximetry 96%, anxious, fatigued, blood in sputum, abdominal breathing
    c. Confused and disoriented, difficulty producing sounds, pulse oximetry 80%
    d. Anxious, respiratory rate 30, talking rapidly about the accident, warm to touch

29. A patient in the emergency department with laryngeal trauma has developed shortness of breath with stridor and decreased oxygen saturation. What is the priority action?
    a. Insert an oral or nasal airway.
    b. Assess for tachypnea, anxiety, and nasal flaring.
    c. Obtain the equipment for a tracheostomy.
    d. Apply oxygen and stay with the patient.

30. An older adult patient who is talking and laughing while eating begins to choke on a piece of meat. What is the initial emergency management for this patient?
    a. Several sharp blows between the scapulae
    b. Call the Rapid Response Team
    c. Nasotracheal suctioning
    d. Abdominal thrusts (Heimlich maneuver)

31. Following radiation therapy for head and neck cancer, the nurse instructs the patient about which potential side effects? *(Select all that apply.)*
    a. Skin redness and tenderness
    b. Numbness of the mouth, lips, or face
    c. Dysphagia
    d. Hoarseness
    e. Dry mouth

32. What type of treatment has the highest cure rate for small cancers of the head and neck?
    a. Surgery
    b. Chemotherapy
    c. Laser surgery
    d. Radiation therapy

33. The nursing student is preparing patient teaching materials about head and neck cancer. Which statement is accurate and included in the patient teaching information?
    a. It metastasizes often to the brain.
    b. It usually develops over a short time.
    c. It is often seen as red edematous areas.
    d. It is often seen as white patchy mucosal lesions.

34. The nurse is interviewing a patient to assess for risk factors related to head and neck cancer. Which questions are appropriate to include? *(Select all that apply.)*
    a. "How many servings per day of alcohol would you typically drink?"
    b. "Have you had frequent episodes of acute or chronic visual problems?"
    c. "Have you had a problem with sores in your mouth?"
    d. "When was the last time you saw your dentist?"
    e. "Do you have recurrent laryngitis or frequent episodes of sore throat?"
    f. "How many packs per day do you smoke and for how many years?"

35. Which patient has the highest risk for developing cancer of the larynx and should be alerted about relevant lifestyle modifications to decrease this risk?
    a. 57-year-old male with alcoholism
    b. 18-year-old marijuana smoker
    c. 28-year-old female with diabetes
    d. 34-year-old male who snorts cocaine

36. The nurse is caring for a patient with a laryngeal tumor. In order to facilitate comfort and breathing for the patient, which type of position does the nurse use?
    a. Sims'
    b. Supine
    c. Fowler's
    d. Prone

37. A patient suffers from chronic xerostomia related to past radiation therapy treatments. Which intervention does the nurse use to assist the patient with this symptom?
    a. Offer small frequent meals.
    b. Suggest a moisturizing spray.
    c. Explain fluid restrictions.
    d. Teach to wash with mild soap and water.

38. The patient with laryngeal cancer that is being treated with radiation therapy is experiencing hoarseness. What teaching points must the nurse stress with this patient? *(Select all that apply.)*
    a. "Your voice should improve within 4 to 6 weeks after the radiation therapy is completed."
    b. "Typically the hoarseness becomes worse during the radiation therapy."
    c. "Gargle 4 to 6 times a day with an alcohol-based mouthwash."
    d. "Rest your voice and use alternative communication methods during radiation therapy."
    e. "Wash your neck 3 times daily with a strong antiseptic soap."

39. The nurse is assessing a patient's skin at the site of radiation therapy to the neck. Which skin condition is expected in relation to the radiation treatments?
    a. Red, tender, and peeling
    b. Shiny, pale, and tight
    c. Puffy and edematous
    d. Pale, dry, and cool

40. Which surgical procedure of the neck area poses no risk postoperatively for aspiration?
    a. Total laryngectomy
    b. Transoral cordectomy
    c. Hemilaryngectomy
    d. Partial laryngectomy

41. The patient with a total laryngectomy has a laryngectomy button in place. What important teaching points must the nurse include when teaching the patient about this device? *(Select all that apply.)*
    a. A laryngectomy button is shorter and softer than a laryngectomy tube.
    b. A laryngectomy button comes in only one size.
    c. A laryngectomy button is more comfortable than a laryngectomy tube.
    d. A laryngectomy button's requires use of an alternative form of communication.
    e. A laryngectomy button requires use of sterile procedure when it is changed.

42. The nurse is caring for a postoperative patient who had a neck dissection. Which assessment finding is expected?
    a. Bulky gauze dressing is present that is dry and intact over the site.
    b. The patient can speak normally, but reports a sore throat.
    c. Permanent gastrostomy tube is present with continuous tube feedings.
    d. The patient has shoulder muscle weakness and limited range of motion.

43. The nursing student is caring for an older adult patient who sustained a stroke and is confused and having trouble swallowing. Which statement by the nursing student indicates an understanding of aspiration precautions for this patient?
    a. "I will administer pills as whole tablets; they are easier to swallow."
    b. "If the patient coughs, I will discontinue feeding and contact the provider."
    c. "I will keep the head of bed elevated during and after feeding."
    d. "I will encourage small amounts of fluids such as water, tea, or juices."

44. The nurse observes that a patient is having difficulty swallowing and has initiated aspiration precautions. Which procedure does the nurse expect the provider to order for this patient?
    a. Chest x-ray of the neck and chest
    b. Computed tomography (CT) scan of the head and neck
    c. Dynamic study under fluoroscopy
    d. Direct and indirect laryngoscopy

45. A patient has had neck dissection surgery with a reconstructive flap over the carotid artery. Which intervention is appropriate for the flap care?
    a. Evaluate the flap every hour for the first 72 hours.
    b. Monitor the flap by gently placing a Doppler on the flap.
    c. Position the patient so that the flap is in the dependent position.
    d. Apply a wet-to-dry dressing to the flap.

46. The nurse is caring for several patients who require treatment for laryngeal cancer. Which treatment/procedure requires patient education about aspiration precautions?
    a. Total laryngectomy
    b. Laser surgery
    c. Radiation therapy
    d. Supraglottic laryngectomy

47. Which statement by the patient indicates understanding about radiation therapy for neck cancer?
    a. "My voice will initially be hoarse but should improve over time."
    b. "There are no side effects other than a hoarse voice."
    c. "Dry mouth after radiation therapy is temporary and short-term."
    d. "My throat is not directly affected by radiation."

48. What does the nurse include in the teaching session for a patient who is scheduled to have a partial laryngectomy?
    a. Supraglottic method of swallowing
    b. Presence of a tracheostomy tube and nasogastric tube for feeding due to postoperative swelling
    c. Not being able to eat solid foods
    d. Permanence of the tracheostomy, referred to as a laryngectomy stoma

49. A patient has been transferred from the intensive care unit to the medical-surgical unit after a laryngectomy. What does the nurse suggest to encourage the patient to participate in self-care?
    a. Changing the tracheostomy collar
    b. Suctioning the mouth with an oral suction device
    c. Checking the stoma with a flashlight
    d. Observing the color of the reconstructive flap

50. The nurse is caring for a patient who had reconstructive neck surgery and observes bright red blood spurting from the tissue flap that is covering the carotid artery. Which action must the nurse take first?
    a. Call the surgeon and alert the operating room.
    b. Call the Rapid Response Team.
    c. Apply immediate, direct pressure to the site.
    d. Apply a bulky sterile dressing and secure the airway.

51. A patient is experiencing acute anxiety related to hospitalization stress and an inability to accept changes related to laryngeal cancer. The patient wants to leave the hospital, but agrees to try a medication to "help me calm down." For which medication does the nurse obtain a PRN (as needed) order?
    a. Amitriptyline (Elavil)
    b. Modafinil (Provigil)
    c. Morphine sulfate (Statex)
    d. Lorazepam (Ativan)

52. A patient with a recent diagnosis of sinus cancer states that he wants another course of antibiotics because he believes he simply has another sinus infection. What is the nurse's best response?
    a. "I'll call the provider for the antibiotic prescription."
    b. "Why are you doubting your provider's diagnosis?"
    c. "Let me bring you some information about sinus cancer."
    d. "What did the provider say to you about your condition?"

53. A patient is unable to speak following a cordectomy. Which action is delegated to the UAP to help the patient deal with communication issues?
    a. Politely tell the patient not to communicate.
    b. Teach the patient how to use hand signals.
    c. Allow extra time to accomplish activities of daily living (ADLs) because of communication limitations.
    d. Give step-by-step instructions during the ADLs and discourage two-way communication.

54. The nurse is assessing a patient who has had a neck dissection with removal of muscle tissue, lymph nodes, and the eleventh cranial nerve. Which assessment finding is anticipated because of the surgical procedure?
    a. Shoulder drop with an increased limitation of movement
    b. Asymmetrical eye movements and a change in visual acuity
    c. Blood and serous fluid under the reconstructive flap
    d. Facial swelling with discoloration and bruising around the eyes

55. A patient is having radiation therapy to the neck and reports a sore throat and difficulty swallowing. Which statement by the nursing student indicates a correct understanding of symptom relief for this patient?
    a. "The patient should not swallow anything too cold or too hot."
    b. "I will give the patient a mouthwash with an alcohol base."
    c. "I will help the patient with a saline gargle."
    d. "The patient should be reassured that the sore throat is temporary."

56. The health care provider orders the discontinuation of the nasogastric tube for a patient with a total laryngectomy. Before discontinuing the tube, which action must be performed?
    a. The health care provider and the nurse will assess the patient's ability to swallow.
    b. Reassure the patient that eating and swallowing will be painless and natural.
    c. The nutritionist will evaluate the patient's nutritional status.
    d. The patient will be offered a prn analgesic or an anxiolytic medication.

57. A patient is learning esophageal speech and reports that he feels bloated after a practice session. To assist the patient with this issue, what does the nurse do?
    a. Refer the patient to the American Cancer Society Visitor Program.
    b. Obtain an order for prn antacids.
    c. Reassure the patient that the discomfort is worth the long-term benefit.
    d. Notify the speech therapist about the symptom.

58. A patient has had surgery for cancer of the neck. Which behavior indicates that the patient understands how to perform self-care to prevent aspiration?
    a. Chooses thin liquids that cause coughing, but knows to take small sips.
    b. Eats small, frequent meals that include a variety of textures and nutrients.
    c. Asks for small, frequent sips of nutrition supplement as a bedtime snack.
    d. Positions self upright before eating or drinking anything.

59. A patient is receiving enteral feedings and a nasogastric tube is in place. In order to prevent aspiration, which precautions are used? *(Select all that apply.)*
    a. No bolus feedings are given at night.
    b. Hold the feeding if the residual volume exceeds 20 mL.
    c. Vary the time of feedings according to the patient's preference.
    d. Elevate the head of bed during and after feedings.
    e. Evaluate the patient's tolerance of the feedings.

60. A patient has demonstrated anxiety since a diagnosis of neck cancer. The surgery and radiation therapy are completed. Which behavior indicates that the patient's fears are decreasing?
    a. Repeatedly asks the same questions and seeks to revalidate all information.
    b. States that he is less anxious, but is irritable and tense whenever questioned.
    c. Makes a plan to contact the American Cancer Society Visitor Program.
    d. Makes a plan to share personal belongings with friends and family.

61. Which side effects would a patient with obstructive sleep apnea report? *(Select all that apply.)*
    a. Excessive daytime sleepiness
    b. Excessive daytime hyperactivity
    c. Inability to concentrate
    d. Excessive production of sputum
    e. Irritability

30 CHAPTER

Care of Patients with Noninfectious Lower Respiratory Problems

1. Which of the following are characteristics of pulmonary emphysema? *(Select all that apply.)*
   a. Decreased surface area of alveoli
   b. Chronic thickening of bronchial walls
   c. Decreased respiratory rate
   d. Hypercapnia
   e. Arterial blood gases (ABGs) show chronic respiratory acidosis
   f. Increased eosinophils

2. Which are characteristics of asthma? *(Select all that apply.)*
   a. Narrowed airway lumen due to inflammation
   b. Increased eosinophils
   c. Decreased breathing cycle
   d. Intermittent bronchospasm
   e. Loss of elastic recoil
   f. Stimulation of disease process by allergies

3. The nurse is caring for an older adult patient with a chronic respiratory disorder. Which interventions are best to use in caring for this patient? *(Select all that apply.)*
   a. Provide rest periods between activities such as bathing, meals, and ambulation.
   b. Place the patient in a supine position after meals to allow for rest.
   c. Schedule drug administration around routine activities to increase adherence to drug therapy.
   d. Arrange chairs in strategic locations to allow the patient to walk and rest.
   e. Teach the patient to avoid getting the pneumococcal vaccine.
   f. Encourage the patient to have an annual flu vaccination.

4. The nurse is caring for an older adult patient with a history of chronic asthma. Which problem related to aging can influence the care and treatment of this patient?
   a. Asthma usually resolves with age, so the condition is less severe in older adult patients.
   b. It is more difficult to teach older adult patients about asthma than to teach younger patients.
   c. With aging, the beta-adrenergic drugs do not work as quickly or strongly.
   d. Older adult patients have difficulty manipulating handheld inhalers.

5. The nurse is presenting a community education lecture about respiratory disorders. Which statement by a participant indicates a correct understanding of the information?
   a. "Bronchitis is a genetic disease that affects many organs."
   b. "In bronchial asthma, an airway obstruction can be caused by inflammation."
   c. "In chronic bronchitis, the tissue damage is only temporary and is reversible."
   d. "Smoking cessation reverses the tissue damage caused by emphysema."

6. A patient with chronic obstructive pulmonary disease (COPD) is likely to have which findings on assessment? *(Select all that apply.)*
   a. Increased anteroposterior (AP) diameter of the chest
   b. Sitting in a chair leaning forward with elbows on knees
   c. Unintentional weight gain
   d. Decreased appetite
   e. Unexplained weight loss

7. The nurse is helping a patient learn about managing her asthma. What does the nurse instruct the patient to do?
   a. Keep a symptom diary to identify what triggers the asthma attacks.
   b. Make an appointment with an allergist for allergy therapy.
   c. Take a low dose of aspirin every day for the antiinflammatory action.
   d. Drink large amounts of clear fluid to keep mucus thin and watery.

8. The nurse is taking a medical history on a new patient who has come to the office for a check-up. The patient states that he was supposed to take a medication called montelukast (Singulair), but that he never got the prescription filled. What is the best response by the nurse?
   a. "When did you first get diagnosed with a respiratory disorder?"
   b. "Why didn't you get the prescription filled?"
   c. "Tell me how you feel about your decision to not fill the prescription."
   d. "Tell me about how your asthma has been recently?"

9. The nurse teaches a patient with asthma to monitor for which problem while exercising?
   a. Increased peak expiratory flow rates
   b. Wheezing from bronchospasm
   c. Swelling in the feet and ankles
   d. Respiratory muscle fatigue

10. A patient with asthma is repeatedly not compliant with the medication regimen, which has resulted in the patient being hospitalized for a severe asthma attack. Which interventions does the nurse suggest to help the patient manage asthma on a daily basis? (Select all that apply.)
    a. Encourage active participation in the plan of care.
    b. Help the patient develop a flexible plan of care.
    c. Have the pharmacist establish a plan of care.
    d. Teach the patient about asthma and its treatment plan.
    e. Assess symptom severity using a peak flowmeter 1 to 2 times per week.

11. An older adult patient experiences an asthma attack that is severe enough to warrant the use of a rescue drug. Which medication is best to use for the acute symptoms?
    a. Omalizumab (Xolair)
    b. Fluticasone (Flovent)
    c. Salmeterol (Serevent)
    d. Albuterol (Proventil)

12. Which are main purposes of asthma treatment? (Select all that apply.)
    a. Avoid secondhand smoke
    b. Improve airflow
    c. Relieve symptoms
    d. Improve exercise tolerance
    e. Prevent asthma episodes

13. For a patient who is a nonsmoker, which classic assessment finding of chronic airflow limitation is particularly important in diagnosing asthma?
    a. Cyanosis
    b. Dyspnea
    c. Audible wheezing
    d. Tachypnea

14. A patient who is allergic to dogs experiences a sudden "asthma attack." Which assessment findings does the nurse expect for this patient?
    a. Slow, deep, pursed-lip respirations
    b. Breathlessness and difficulty completing sentences
    c. Clubbing of the fingers and cyanosis of the nailbeds
    d. Bradycardia and irregular pulse

15. A patient is experiencing an asthma attack and shows an increased respiratory effort. Which arterial blood gas value is more associated with the early phase of the attack?
    a. $Paco_2$ of 60 mm Hg
    b. $Paco_2$ of 30 mm Hg
    c. pH of 7.40
    d. Pao_2 of 98 mm Hg

16. A patient who has well-controlled asthma has what kind of airway changes?
    a. Chronic, leading to hyperplasia
    b. Temporary and reversible
    c. Open alveoli
    d. Permanent and irreversible

17. What are the goals of drug therapy in the treatment of asthma? *(Select all that apply.)*
    a. Drugs are used to stop an attack once it has started.
    b. Weekly drugs are used to reduce the asthma response.
    c. Combination drugs are avoided in the treatment of asthma.
    d. Some patients only require drug therapy during an asthma episode.
    e. Drugs are used to change airway responsiveness.

18. The nurse is teaching a patient how to interpret peak expiratory flow readings and to use this information to manage drug therapy at home. Which statement by the patient indicates a need for additional teaching?
    a. "If the reading is in the green zone, there is no need to increase the drug therapy."
    b. "Red is 50% below my 'personal best'; I should try a rescue drug and seek help."
    c. "If the reading is in the yellow zone, I should increase my use of my inhalers."
    d. "If frequent yellow readings occur, I should see my provider for a change in medications."

19. A patient with chronic bronchitis often shows signs of hypoxia. Which clinical manifestation is the priority to look out for in this patient?
    a. Chronic, nonproductive, dry cough
    b. Clubbing of fingers
    c. Large amounts of thick mucus
    d. Barrel chest

20. The nurse is taking a history of a patient with chronic pulmonary disease. The patient reports often sleeping in a chair that allows his head to be elevated rather than sleeping in a bed. The patient's behavior is a strategy to deal with which condition?
    a. Paroxysmal nocturnal dyspnea
    b. Orthopnea
    c. Tachypnea
    d. Cheyne-Stokes respirations

21. A patient has chronic bronchitis. The nurse plans interventions for inadequate oxygenation based on which set of clinical manifestations?
    a. Chronic cough, thin secretions, and chronic infection
    b. Respiratory alkalosis, decreased $Paco_2$, and increased Pao_2
    c. Areas of chest tenderness and sputum production (often with hemoptysis)
    d. Large amounts of thick secretions and repeated infections

22. A patient has COPD with chronic difficult breathing. In planning this patient's care, what condition must the nurse acknowledge is present in this patient?
    a. Decreased need for calories and protein requirements since dyspnea causes activity intolerance
    b. COPD has no effect on calorie and protein needs, meal tolerance, satiety, appetite, and weight
    c. Increased metabolism and the need for additional calories and protein supplements
    d. Anabolic state, which creates conditions for building body strength and muscle mass

23. In obtaining a history for a patient with chronic airflow limitation, which risk factors are related to potentially causing or triggering the disease process? *(Select all that apply.)*
    a. Cigarette smoking
    b. Occupational and air pollution
    c. Genetic tendencies
    d. Smokeless tobacco
    e. Occupation

24. Which statement is true about the relationship of smoking cessation to the pathophysiology of COPD?
    a. Smoking cessation completely reverses the damage to the lungs.
    b. Smoking cessation slows the rate of disease progression.
    c. Smoking cessation is an important therapy for asthma but not for COPD.
    d. Smoking cessation reverses the effects on the airways but not the lungs.

25. A patient has a history of COPD but is admitted for a surgical procedure that is unrelated to the respiratory system. To prevent any complications related to the patient's COPD, what action does the nurse take?
    a. Assess the patient's respiratory system every 8 hours.
    b. Monitor for signs and symptoms of pneumonia.
    c. Give high-flow oxygen to maintain pulse oximetry readings.
    d. Instruct the patient to use a tissue if coughing or sneezing.

26. The nurse is instructing a patient regarding complications of COPD. Which statement by the patient indicates the need for additional teaching?
    a. "I have to be careful because I am susceptible to respiratory infections."
    b. "I could develop heart failure, which could be fatal if untreated."
    c. "My COPD is serious, but it can be reversed if I follow my doctor's orders."
    d. "The lack of oxygen could cause my heart to beat in an irregular pattern."

27. What is the purpose of pulmonary function testing?
    a. Determines the oxygen liter flow rates required by the patient
    b. Measures blood gas levels before bronchodilators are administered
    c. Evaluates the movement of oxygenated blood from the lung to the heart
    d. Distinguishes airway disease from restrictive lung disease

28. A patient with respiratory difficulty has completed a pulmonary function test before starting any treatment. The peak expiratory flow (PEF) is 15% to 20% below what is expected for this adult patient's age, gender, and size. The nurse anticipates this patient will need additional information about which topic?
    a. Further diagnostic tests to confirm pulmonary hypertension
    b. How to manage asthma medications and identify triggers
    c. Smoking cessation and its relationship to COPD
    d. How to manage the acute episode of respiratory infection

29. Patients with asthma are taught self-care activities and treatment modalities according to the "step method." Which symptoms and medication routines relate to step 3?
    a. Symptoms occur daily; daily use of inhaled corticosteroid, add a long-acting beta agonist.
    b. Symptoms occur more than once per week; daily use of antiinflammatory inhaler.
    c. Symptoms occur less than once per week; use of rescue inhalers once per week.
    d. Frequent exacerbations occur with limited physical activity; increased use of rescue inhalers.

30. What principle guides the nurse when providing oxygen therapy for a patient with COPD?
    a. The patient depends on a high serum carbon dioxide level to stimulate the drive to breathe.
    b. The patient requires a low serum oxygen level for the stimulus to breathe to work.
    c. The patient who receives oxygen therapy at a high flow rate is at risk for a respiratory arrest.
    d. The patient should receive oxygen therapy at rates to reduce hypoxia and bring Spo_2 levels up between 88% and 92%.

31. In assisting a patient with chronic airflow limitation to relieve dyspnea, which sitting positions are beneficial to the patient for breathing? *(Select all that apply.)*
    a. On edge of chair, leaning forward with arms folded and resting on a small table
    b. In a low semi-reclining position with the shoulders back and knees apart
    c. Forward in a chair with feet spread apart and elbows placed on the knees
    d. Head slightly flexed, with feet spread apart and shoulders relaxed
    e. Low semi-Fowler's position with knees elevated

32. The nurse is developing a teaching plan for a patient with chronic airflow limitation using the priority patient problem of insufficient knowledge related to energy conservation. What does the nurse advise the patient to avoid?
    a. Performing activities at a relaxed pace throughout the day with rest periods
    b. Working on activities that require using arms at chest level or lower
    c. Eating three large meals per day
    d. Talking and performing activities separately

33. A patient with COPD has meal-related dyspnea. To address this issue, which drug does the nurse offer the patient 30 minutes before the meal?
    a. Albuterol (Ventolin)
    b. Guaifenesin (Organidin)
    c. Fluticasone (Flovent)
    d. Pantoprazole sodium (Protonix)

34. The patient with COPD is taking systemic theophylline. What specific precautions must the nurse use when caring for this patient? *(Select all that apply.)*
    a. Monitor serum theophylline levels.
    b. Alert the health care provider for any abnormal values.
    c. Administer the drug using a metered-dose inhaler (MDI).
    d. Assess the patient for adverse reactions related to a toxic level.
    e. Monitor the patient's heart rate.

35. A patient is receiving ipratropium (Atrovent) and reports nausea, blurred vision, headache, and inability to sleep. What action does the nurse take?
    a. Administer a prn (as-needed) medication for nausea and a mild prn sedative.
    b. Report these symptoms to the provider as signs of overdose.
    c. Obtain a provider's request for an ipratropium level.
    d. Tell the patient that these side effects are normal and not to worry.

36. A patient with asthma has been prescribed a fluticasone (Flovent) inhaler. What is the purpose of this drug for the patient?
    a. Relaxes the smooth muscles of the airway
    b. Acts as a bronchodilator in severe episodes
    c. Reduces obstruction of airways by decreasing inflammation
    d. Reduces the histamine effect of the triggering agent

37. What is the advantage of using the aerosol route for administering short-acting beta$_2$ agonists?
    a. Achieves a rapid and effective antiinflammatory action
    b. Reduces the risk for fungal infections
    c. Increases patient compliance because it is easy to use
    d. Provides rapid therapy with fewer systemic side effects

38. The nurse is teaching a patient with chronic airflow limitation about his medications. What is the correct sequence for administering aerosol treatments?
    a. Bronchodilator should be taken 5 to 10 minutes after the steroid.
    b. Bronchodilator should be taken at least 5 minutes before other inhaled drugs.
    c. Bronchodilator should be taken immediately after the steroid.
    d. Bronchodilator and steroid are two different classes of drugs, so sequence is irrelevant.

39. A patient has been prescribed cromolyn sodium (Intal) for the treatment of asthma. Which statement by the patient indicates a correct understanding of this drug?
    a. "It opens my airways and provides short-term relief."
    b. "It is the medication that should be used 30 minutes before exercise."
    c. "It is not intended for use during acute episodes of asthma attacks."
    d. "It is a steroid medication, so there are severe side effects."

40. After the nurse has instructed a patient with COPD in the proper coughing technique, which action the next day by the patient indicates the need for additional teaching or intervention?
    a. Coughing upon rising in the morning
    b. Coughing before meals
    c. Coughing after meals
    d. Coughing at bedtime

41. A family member of a patient with COPD asks the nurse, "What is the purpose of making him cough on a routine basis?" What is the nurse's best response?
    a. "We have to check the color and consistency of his sputum."
    b. "We don't want him to feel embarrassed when coughing in public, so we actively encourage it."
    c. "It improves air exchange by increasing airflow in the larger airways."
    d. "If he cannot cough, the provider may elect to do a tracheostomy."

42. A patient with a history of bronchitis for more than 20 years is hospitalized. With this patient's history, what is a potential complication?
    a. Right-sided heart failure
    b. Left-sided heart failure
    c. Renal disease
    d. Stroke

43. The nurse is caring for a patient with chronic bronchitis, and notes the following clinical findings: fatigue, dependent edema, distended neck veins, and cyanotic lips. What condition is the patient exhibiting?
    a. COPD
    b. Cor pulmonale
    c. Asthma
    d. Lung cancer

44. A patient is admitted with asthma. Which assessment findings are most likely to indicate that the patient's asthma condition is deteriorating and progressing toward respiratory failure?
    a. Crackles, rhonchi, and productive cough with yellow sputum
    b. Tachypnea; thick, tenacious sputum; and hemoptysis
    c. Audible breath sounds, wheezing, and use of accessory muscles
    d. Respiratory alkalosis; slow, shallow respiratory rate

45. A patient has returned several times to the clinic for treatment of respiratory problems. Which action does the nurse perform first?
    a. Obtain a history of the patient's previous respiratory problems and response to therapy.
    b. Ask the patient to describe his compliance with the prescribed therapies.
    c. Obtain a request for diagnostic testing, including a tuberculosis and human immunodeficiency virus (HIV) evaluation.
    d. Listen to the patient's lungs, obtain a pulse oximetry reading, and count the respiratory rate.

46. The nurse assesses a patient and finds a dusky appearance with bluish mucous membranes and production of lots of mucus. What illness does the nurse suspect?
    a. Asthma
    b. Emphysema
    c. Chronic bronchitis
    d. Acute bronchitis

47. The patient with COPD is undergoing pulmonary rehabilitation by walking. What does the nurse teach this patient about when to increase his or her walking time?
    a. "You should increase your walking time when your rest periods decrease."
    b. "You should increase your walking time when your heart rate remains less than 80/minute."
    c. "You should increase your walking time when you are no longer short of breath."
    d. "You should increase your walking time when you do not need to use an inhaler."

48. A patient is undergoing diagnostic testing for possible cystic fibrosis (CF). Which nonpulmonary assessment findings does the nurse expect to observe in a patient with CF? (Select all that apply.)
    a. Peripheral edema
    b. Abdominal distention
    c. Steatorrhea
    d. Constipation
    e. Gastroesophageal reflux

49. The nurse is caring for a patient who has CF. Which assessment findings indicate the need for exacerbation therapy? (Select all that apply.)
    a. New-onset crackles
    b. Increased activity tolerance
    c. Increased frequency of coughing
    d. Increased chest congestion
    e. Increased Sao_2
    f. At least a 10% decrease in FEV_1

50. A patient with CF is admitted to the medical-surgical unit for an elective surgery. Which infection control measure is best for this patient?
    a. It is best to put two patients with CF in the same room.
    b. Standard precautions including handwashing are sufficient.
    c. The patient is to be placed on contact isolation.
    d. Measures that limit close contact between people with CF are needed.

51. The nurse is working for a manufacturing company and is responsible for routine employee health issues. Which primary prevention is most important for those employees at high risk for occupational pulmonary disease?
    a. Screen all employees by use of chest x-ray films twice a year.
    b. Advise employees not to smoke, and to use masks and ventilation equipment.
    c. Perform pulmonary function tests once a year on all employees.
    d. Refer at-risk employees to a social worker for information about pensions.

52. The nurse is caring for a patient with bronchiolitis obliterans organizing pneumonia (BOOP) that has been confirmed by biopsy. What treatment does the nurse expect for this patient?
    a. A course of 10 to 14 days of antibiotics
    b. Use of chest physiotherapy to mobilize secretions
    c. A short course of corticosteroid drug therapy
    d. Bronchodilation by MDI

53. A patient had prolonged occupational exposure to petroleum distillates and subsequently developed a chronic lung disease. This patient is advised to seek frequent health examinations because there is a high risk for developing which respiratory disease condition?
    a. Tuberculosis
    b. Cystic fibrosis
    c. Lung cancer
    d. Pulmonary hypertension

54. The nurse has completed a community presentation about lung cancer. Which statement from a participant demonstrates an understanding of the information presented?
    a. "The primary prevention for reducing the risk of lung cancer is to stop smoking and avoid secondhand smoke."
    b. "The overall 5-year survival rate for all patients with lung cancer is 85%."
    c. "The death rate for lung cancer is less than prostate, breast, and colon cancer combined."
    d. "Cures are most likely for patients who undergo treatment for stage III disease."

55. Which sites are commonly affected by lung cancer metastasis? *(Select all that apply.)*
    a. Heart
    b. Bone
    c. Liver
    d. Colon
    e. Brain

56. Which of the following may be warning signs of lung cancer? *(Select all that apply.)*
    a. Dyspnea
    b. Dark yellow-colored sputum
    c. Persistent cough or change in cough
    d. Abdominal pain and frequent stools
    e. Recurring episodes of pleural effusion

57. Which statement is true about radiation therapy for lung cancer patients?
    a. It is given daily in "cycles" over the course of several months.
    b. It causes hair loss, nausea, and vomiting for the duration of treatment.
    c. It causes dry skin at the radiation site, fatigue, and changes in appetite with nausea.
    d. It is the best method of treatment for systemic metastatic disease.

58. The nurse is taking a report on a patient who had a pneumonectomy 4 days ago. Which question is the best to ask during the shift report?
    a. "Does the provider want us to continue encouraging use of the spirometer?"
    b. "How much drainage did you see in the Pleur-Evac during your shift?"
    c. "Do we have a request to 'milk' the patient's chest tube?"
    d. "Does the surgeon want the patient placed on the nonoperative side?"

59. The nurse is caring for a patient with a chest tube. What is the correct nursing intervention for this patient?
    a. The patient is encouraged to cough and do deep-breathing exercises frequently.
    b. "Stripping" of the chest tubes is done routinely to prevent obstruction by blood clots.
    c. Water level in the suction chamber need not be monitored, just the collection chamber.
    d. Drainage containers are positioned upright or on the bed next to the patient.

60. Upon observation of a chest tube setup, the nurse reports to the provider that there is a leak in the chest tube and system. How has the nurse identified this problem?
    a. Drainage in the collection chamber has decreased.
    b. The bubbling in the suction chamber has suddenly increased.
    c. Fluctuation in the water seal chamber has stopped.
    d. There was onset of continuous vigorous bubbling in the water seal chamber.

61. The provider's prescriptions indicate an increase in the suction to –20 cm for a patient with a chest tube. To implement this, the nurse performs which intervention?
    a. Increases the wall suction to the medium setting, and observes gentle bubbling in the suction chamber
    b. Adds water to the suction and drainage chambers to the level of –20 cm
    c. Stops the suction, adds sterile water to level of –20 cm to the water seal chamber, and resumes the wall suction
    d. Has the patient cough and deep-breathe, and monitors level of fluctuation to achieve –20 cm

62. A patient is fearful that she might develop lung cancer because her father and grandfather died of cancer. She seeks advice about how to modify lifestyle factors that contribute to cancer. How does the nurse advise this patient?
    a. Not to worry about air pollution unless there is hydrocarbon exposure
    b. Quit her job if she has continuous exposure to lead or other heavy metals
    c. Avoid situations where she would be exposed to "secondhand" smoke
    d. Not to be concerned because there are no genetic factors associated with lung cancer

63. The nurse has determined that a patient with COPD has the priority problem of impaired oxygenation related to reduced airway size, ventilatory muscle fatigue, and excessive mucus production. Which action is best to delegate to the unlicensed assistive personnel (UAP)?
    a. Observe the patient for fatigue, shortness of breath, or change of breathing pattern during activities of daily living (ADLs).
    b. Report a respiratory rate of greater than 24/min at rest or 30/min after ambulating to the nurses' station.
    c. Encourage the patient to cough up sputum, and examine the color, consistency, and amount.
    d. Record and monitor the patient's intake and output, and give fluids to keep the secretions thin.

64. A patient is receiving a chemotherapy agent for lung cancer. The nurse anticipates that the patient is likely to have which common side effect?
    a. Diarrhea
    b. Nausea
    c. Flatulence
    d. Constipation

65. A patient is having pain resulting from bone metastases caused by lung cancer. What is the most effective intervention for relieving the patient's pain?
    a. Support the patient through chemotherapy.
    b. Handle and move the patient very gently.
    c. Administer analgesics around the clock.
    d. Reposition the patient, and use distraction.

66. A patient has a chest tube in place. What does the water in the water seal chamber do when the system is functioning correctly?
    a. Bubbles vigorously and continuously
    b. Bubbles gently and continuously
    c. Fluctuates with the patient's respirations
    d. Stops fluctuation, and bubbling is not observed

67. Which intervention promotes comfort in dyspnea management for a patient with lung cancer?
    a. Administer morphine only when the patient requests it.
    b. Place the patient in a supine position with a pillow under the knees and legs.
    c. Encourage coughing and deep-breathing and independent ambulation.
    d. Provide supplemental oxygen via cannula or mask.

68. A patient is diagnosed with cor pulmonale secondary to pulmonary hypertension and is receiving an infusion of epoprostenol (Flolan) through a small portable IV pump. What is the critical priority for this patient?
    a. Strict aseptic technique must be used to prevent sepsis.
    b. Infusion must not be interrupted, even for a few minutes.
    c. The patient must have a daily dose of warfarin (Coumadin).
    d. The patient must be assessed for anginalike chest pain and fatigue.

69. A patient has developed pulmonary hypertension. What is the goal of drug therapy for this patient?
    a. Dilate pulmonary vessels and prevent clot formation.
    b. Decrease pain and make the patient comfortable.
    c. Improve or maintain gas exchange.
    d. Maintain and manage pulmonary exacerbation.

70. A patient is newly diagnosed with sarcoidosis. Which statement by the patient indicates an understanding of the disease?
    a. "Corticosteroids are the main type of therapy for sarcoidosis."
    b. "Sarcoidosis is a type of lung cancer that is treatable if diagnosed early."
    c. "My condition can be treated with antibiotics."
    d. "Sarcoidosis is a type of pneumonia that is highly contagious."

71. The nurse is providing discharge instructions to a patient with pulmonary fibrosis and the family. What instructions are appropriate for this patient's diagnosis? *(Select all that apply.)*
    a. Using home oxygen
    b. Maintaining activity level as before
    c. Preventing respiratory infections
    d. Limiting fluid intake
    e. Energy conservation measures

72. A patient with a history of asthma enters the emergency department with severe dyspnea, accessory muscle involvement, neck vein distention, and severe inspiratory/expiratory wheezing. The nurse is prepared to assist the provider with which emergency procedure if the patient does not respond to initial interventions?
    a. Intubation
    b. Needle thoracentesis
    c. Chest tube insertion
    d. Pleurodesis

73. A patient presents to the walk-in clinic with extremely labored breathing and a history of asthma that is unresponsive to prescribed inhalers or medications. What is the priority nursing action?
    a. Establish IV access to give emergency medications.
    b. Obtain the equipment and prepare the patient for intubation.
    c. Place the patient in a high Fowler's position, and start oxygen.
    d. Call 911 and report that the patient has probable status asthmaticus.

74. The nurse is instructing a patient to use a flutter-valve mucus clearance device. What should the patient be taught to do?
    a. Inhale deeply and exhale forcefully through the device.
    b. Use an inhalation technique that is similar to the handheld inhaler.
    c. Use pursed-lip breathing before and after usage.
    d. Exhale slowly through the nose, and then inhale by sniffing.

31 CHAPTER

Care of Patients with Infectious Respiratory Problems

1. An adult patient diagnosed with rhinitis medicamentosa reports chronic nasal congestion. What does the nurse instruct the patient to do?
   a. Avoid exposure to older adults or immunosuppressed persons when symptoms flare.
   b. Damp-dust the house and clean the carpets to remove animal dander or mold.
   c. Discontinue the use of the current nose drops or sprays.
   d. Identify what triggers the hypersensitivity reaction by keeping a symptom diary.

2. The nurse notes that an older patient has a disorder that indicates drug therapy that the health care provider just prescribed for symptomatic relief of allergic rhinitis must be used with caution. Which disorder does the nurse report to the health care provider as a possible precaution for drug therapy?
   a. Sleep apnea
   b. Valvular heart disease
   c. Ménière's disease
   d. Urinary retention

3. Drug therapy with first-generation antihistamines to treat sinusitis is used with caution in the older adult because of which possible side effects? *(Select all that apply.)*
   a. Reduced clearance
   b. Hypotension
   c. Confusion
   d. Dry mouth
   e. Constipation

4. A patient comes to the walk-in clinic reporting seasonal nasal congestion; sneezing; rhinorrhea; and itchy, watery eyes. The nurse identifies that the patient most likely has rhinitis and should also be assessed for sinusitis. Which manifestations does the nurse assess in a patient with rhinosinusitis? *(Select all that apply.)*
   a. Pain over the cheek radiating to the teeth.
   b. Tenderness to percussion over the sinuses.
   c. Generalized musculoskeletal achiness.
   d. General facial pain when bending forward.
   e. Referred pain to the temple or back of the head.

5. To reduce the spread of colds, which teaching points must the nurse include when teaching patients? *(Select all that apply.)*
   a. Stay home from work, school, or other places where people gather.
   b. Seek medical attention at the first sign of an oncoming cold.
   c. Cover both mouth and nose when coughing or sneezing.
   d. Always dispose of used tissues properly.
   e. Thorough handwashing is essential.

6. A patient reports throat soreness and dryness, throat pain, pain on swallowing (odynophagia), and difficulty swallowing. Which disorder does the nurse suspect?
   a. Pharyngitis
   b. Tonsillitis
   c. Rhinosinusitis
   d. Pneumonia

7. An older adult patient residing in a long-term care facility demonstrates new onset of coughing and sneezing with rhinorrhea after his grandchildren came to visit him. He denies pain or fever. Which infection control procedures does the nurse instruct the LPN to initiate in order to protect the other residents?
   a. Initiate the use of standard precautions when caring for the patient.
   b. Place the patient on droplet precautions for the first 2 to 3 days.
   c. Use gown and gloves when entering the room and perform hand hygiene.
   d. Instruct the patient to wash his hands after coughing or sneezing.

8. The nurse is assessing an older adult who has been diagnosed with bacterial pharyngitis. Which assessment finding is typically associated with this medical diagnosis, but may not be present in the older adult patient?
   a. Cough and rash
   b. High fever and elevated white blood cell (WBC) count
   c. Pain with speaking or swallowing
   d. Erythema of tonsils with yellow exudate

9. Which factors can contribute to acute pharyngitis? *(Select all that apply.)*
   a. Viruses
   b. Coughing
   c. Irritants
   d. Bacteria
   e. Alcohol

10. A patient reporting a "sore throat" also has a temperature of 101.4° F, scarlatiniform rash, and a positive rapid test throat culture. This patient will most likely be treated for which type of bacterial infection?
    a. Staphylococcus
    b. Pneumococcus
    c. Streptococcus
    d. Epstein-Barr virus

11. A patient reporting soreness in the throat is diagnosed with "strep throat." To prevent complications such as rheumatic heart disease, this patient should receive which intervention?
    a. Humidification of the air
    b. Saline gargles 4 to 6 times a day
    c. Increased fluid intake of 3 to 4 L/day
    d. Oral antibiotics such as penicillin

12. A child is diagnosed with a group B streptococcus throat infection. In teaching the parents about treatment of the infection, what does the nurse instruct the parents?
    a. Need to complete entire course of penicillin or penicillin-like antibiotics
    b. Gradual return to activities until there are no physical complaints
    c. Purpose of a clear liquid diet until infection subsides
    d. Signs and symptoms of meningitis, which is a common complication

13. Which patients are at risk for developing health-care acquired pneumonia? *(Select all that apply.)*
    a. Confused patient
    b. Patient with atrial fibrillation who is alert and oriented
    c. Patient with gram-negative colonization of the mouth
    d. Patient with hyperthyroid disease
    e. Malnourished patient

14. The nurse is teaching the patient and family about care of a peritonsillar abscess at home. For what symptoms does the nurse indicate the need for the patient to go to the emergency department (ED) immediately? *(Select all that apply.)*
    a. Persistent cough
    b. Hoarseness
    c. Stridor
    d. Drooling
    e. Nausea and vomiting

15. A 35-year-old male patient with no health problems states that he had a flu shot last year and asks if it is necessary to have it again this year. What is the best response by the nurse?
    a. "No, because once you get a flu shot, it lasts for several years and is effective against many different viruses."
    b. "Yes, because the immunity against the virus wears off, increasing your chances of getting the flu."
    c. "Yes, because the vaccine guards against a specific virus and reduces your chances of acquiring flu and is only effective for one year."
    d. "No, flu shots are only for high-risk patients and you are not considered to be high risk."

16. An active 45-year-old schoolteacher with chronic obstructive pulmonary disease (COPD) taking prednisone asks if it is necessary to get a flu shot. What is the best response by the nurse?
    a. "Yes, flu shots are highly recommended for patients with chronic illness and/or patients who are receiving immunotherapy."
    b. "No, flu shots are only recommended for patients 50 years old and older."
    c. "Yes, it will help minimize the risk of triggering an exacerbation of COPD."
    d. "No, patients who are active, not living in a nursing home, and not health care providers do not need a flu shot."

17. A patient who had sinus surgery has a surgical incision under the upper lip. The nurse intervenes when a well-intentioned family member performs which action in attempting to make the patient feel better?
    a. Uses the bed controls to move the patient to a semi-Fowler's position
    b. Hands the patient a tissue to blow the nose
    c. Brings the patient a special custard dessert from a nearby restaurant
    d. Gently helps the patient with oral hygiene during morning care

18. The nurse is giving discharge instructions to a patient diagnosed with a viral pharyngitis. Which statement by the patient indicates the need for further teaching?
    a. "I should try to rest, increase my fluid intake, and get a humidifier for the house."
    b. "I will wait for my test results, then I can get a prescription for antibiotics."
    c. "Over-the-counter analgesics, like Tylenol or ibuprofen, can be used for pain."
    d. "I should gargle several times a day with warm salt water and use throat lozenges."

19. A patient with COPD needs instruction in measures to prevent pneumonia. What information does the nurse include? (Select all that apply.)
    a. Avoid going outside.
    b. Clean all respiratory equipment you have at home.
    c. Avoid indoor pollutants such as dust and aerosols.
    d. Get plenty of rest and sleep daily.
    e. Limit alcoholic beverages to 4 to 5 per week.

20. The nurse is taking a history on a patient who presents with symptoms of pharyngitis: sore throat with dry sensation, pain on swallowing, and low-grade fever. The patient mentions plans to take an overseas trip. Which immunization does the nurse suggest the patient should have, if not already received, before leaving?
    a. Tetanus toxoid
    b. Hepatitis B
    c. Diphtheria
    d. Yellow fever

21. A patient with a history of frequent and recurrent episodes of tonsillitis now reports a severe sore throat with pain that radiates behind the ear and difficulty swallowing. The nurse suspects the patient may have a peritonsillar abscess. On physical assessment, which deviated structure supports the nurse's supposition?
    a. Uvula
    b. Trachea
    c. Tongue
    d. Mucous membranes

22. A parent calls the ED about her child who reports a severe sore throat and refuses to drink fluids or to take liquid pain medication. What is the most important question for the nurse to ask in order to determine the need to seek immediate medical attention?
    a. "Does the child seem to be refusing fluids and medications because of the sore throat?"
    b. "Is the child drooling or do you hear stridor, a raspy rough sound when the child breathes?"
    c. "When did the symptoms start and how long have you been encouraging fluids?"
    d. "Is the throat red or do you see any white patches in the back of the throat?"

23. In a long-term care facility for older adults and immunocompromised patients, one employee and several patients have been diagnosed with influenza (flu). What does the supervising nurse do to decrease risk of infection to other patients?
    a. Ask employees who have flu to stay at home for at least 24 hours.
    b. Place any patient with a sore throat, cough, or rhinorrhea into isolation for 1 to 2 weeks.
    c. Ask employees with flu symptoms to stay at home for up to 5 days after onset of symptoms.
    d. Recommend that all patients and employees be immediately vaccinated for flu.

24. The nurse is giving discharge instructions to an adult patient diagnosed with the flu. The patient says, "I am generally pretty healthy, but I am concerned because my wife has several serious chronic health problems. What can I do to protect her from getting my flu?" What does the nurse instruct the patient to do? *(Select all that apply.)*
    a. Wash hands thoroughly after sneezing, coughing, or blowing nose.
    b. Avoid kissing, hugging, close face-to-face proximity, or hand-holding.
    c. If there is no tissue immediately available, cough or sneeze into your upper sleeve.
    d. Have the wife wear a respiratory filter mask until coughing stops.
    e. Use disposable tissues rather than cloth handkerchiefs, and immediately dispose of tissues.

25. The patient developed flu symptoms less than 24 hours ago. Which drug therapy does the nurse expect the health care provider to order at this time?
    a. Penicillin therapy
    b. Amantadine (Symmetrel)
    c. Oseltamivir (Tamiflu)
    d. IV steroid therapy

26. Which patient is at highest risk for developing pneumonia?
    a. Any hospitalized patient between the ages of 18 and 65 years
    b. 32-year-old trauma patient on a mechanical ventilator
    c. Disabled 54-year-old with osteoporosis; discharged to home
    d. Any patient who has not received the vaccine for pneumonia

27. Which statement best describes pneumonia?
    a. An infection of just the "windpipe" because the lungs are "clear" of any problems
    b. A serious inflammation of the bronchioles from various causes
    c. Only an infection of the lungs with mild to severe effects on breathing
    d. An inflammation resulting from lung damage caused by long-term smoking

28. A patient is seen in the health care provider's office and is diagnosed with community-acquired pneumonia. What are the most common symptoms the patient will have? *(Select all that apply.)*
    a. Dyspnea
    b. Abdominal pain
    c. Back pain
    d. Hypoxemia
    e. Chest discomfort

29. Which diagnostic tests are most likely to be done for a patient suspected of having community-acquired pneumonia? *(Select all that apply.)*
    a. Sputum gram stain
    b. Pulmonary function test
    c. Fluorescein bronchoscopy
    d. Peak flowmeter measurement
    e. Chest x-ray

30. The nurse is reviewing laboratory results for a patient who has pneumonia. Which laboratory value does the nurse expect to see for this patient?
    a. Decreased hemoglobin
    b. Increased red blood cells (RBCs)
    c. Decreased neutrophils
    d. Increased white blood cells (WBCs)

31. A patient is diagnosed with pneumonia. During auscultation of the lower lung fields, the nurse hears coarse crackles and identifies the patient problem of impaired oxygenation. What is the underlying physiologic condition associated with the patient's condition?
    a. Hypoxemia
    b. Hyperemia
    c. Hypocapnia
    d. Hypercapnia

32. Which patient is the least likely to be at risk for developing pneumonia?
    a. Patient with a 5-year history of smoking
    b. Renal transplant patient
    c. Postoperative patient with a bedside commode
    d. Postoperative patient with a hip replacement

33. A patient is admitted to the hospital with pneumonia. What does the nurse expect the chest x-ray results to reveal?
    a. Patchy areas of increased density
    b. Tension pneumothorax
    c. Thick secretions causing airway obstruction
    d. Large hyperinflated airways

34. What nursing intervention may help to prevent the complication of pneumonia for a surgical patient?
    a. Monitoring chest x-rays and WBC counts for early signs of infection
    b. Monitoring lung sounds every shift and encouraging fluids
    c. Teaching coughing, deep-breathing exercises, and use of incentive spirometry
    d. Encouraging hand hygiene among all caregivers, patients, and visitors

35. The nurse is conducting an in-service for the hospital staff about practices that help prevent pneumonia among at-risk patients. Which nursing intervention is encouraged as standard practice?
    a. Administering vaccines to patients at risk
    b. Implementing isolation for debilitated patients
    c. Restricting foods from home in immunosuppressed patients
    d. Decontaminating respiratory therapy equipment weekly

36. A patient hospitalized for pneumonia has the priority patient problem of ineffective airway clearance related to fatigue, chest pain, excessive secretions, and muscle weakness. What nursing intervention helps to correct this problem?
    a. Administer oxygen to prevent hypoxemia and atelectasis.
    b. Push fluids to greater than 3000 mL/day to ensure adequate hydration.
    c. Administer bronchodilator therapy in a timely manner to decrease bronchospasms.
    d. Maintain semi-Fowler's position to facilitate breathing and prevent further fatigue.

37. A patient is admitted to the hospital for treatment of pneumonia. Which nursing assessment finding best indicates that the patient is responding to antibiotics?
    a. Wheezing, oxygen at 2 L/min, respiratory rate 26, no shortness of breath or chills
    b. Temperature 99° F, lung sounds clear, pulse oximetry on 2 L/min at 98%, cough with yellow sputum
    c. Cough, clear sputum, temperature 99° F, pulse oximetry at 96% on room air
    d. Feeling tired, respiratory rate 28 on 2 L/min of oxygen, audible breath sounds

38. The nurse is reviewing the laboratory results for an older adult patient with pneumonia. Which laboratory value frequently seen in patients with pneumonia may not be seen in this patient?
    a. RBC 4.0 to 5.0
    b. Hgb 12 to 16
    c. Hct 36 to 48
    d. WBC 12 to 18

39. A patient is admitted to the hospital to rule out pneumonia. Which infection control technique does the nurse maintain?
    a. Strict respiratory isolation and use of a specially designed facemask
    b. Respiratory isolation and contact isolation for sputum
    c. Respiratory isolation with a stock surgical mask
    d. Standard precautions and no respiratory isolation

40. A critical concern for a patient returning to the unit after a surgical procedure is related to impaired oxygenation caused by inadequate ventilation. Which arterial blood gas value and assessment finding indicates to the nurse that oxygen and incentive spirometry must be administered?
    a. Pao_2 is 90 mm Hg with crackles.
    b. Pao_2 is 90 mm Hg with wheezing.
    c. Pco_2 is 38 mm Hg with clear lung sounds.
    d. Pco_2 is 45 mm Hg with atelectasis.

41. The nurse has identified the priority patient problem of ineffective airway clearance with bronchospasms for a patient with pneumonia. The patient has no previous history of chronic respiratory disorders. The nurse obtains an order for which nursing intervention?
    a. Increased liters of humidified oxygen via facemask
    b. Scheduled and prn (as-needed) aerosol nebulizer bronchodilator treatments
    c. Handheld bronchodilator inhaler as needed
    d. Corticosteroid via inhaler or IV to reduce the inflammation

42. An older adult patient asks the nurse how often one should receive the pneumococcal vaccine for pneumonia prevention. What is the nurse's best response?
    a. Every year, when the patient is receiving the 'flu shot.'
    b. The standard is vaccination every 3 years.
    c. It is usually given once, but some older adults may need a second vaccination after 5 years.
    d. There is no set schedule; it depends on the patient's history and risk factors.

43. The nurse is providing discharge instructions about pneumonia to a patient and family. Which discharge information must the nurse be sure to include?
    a. Complete antibiotics as prescribed, rest, drink fluids, and minimize contact with crowds.
    b. Take all antibiotics as ordered, resume diet and all activities as before hospitalization.
    c. No restrictions regarding activities, diet, and rest because the patient is fully recovered when discharged.
    d. Continue antibiotics only until no further signs of pneumonia are present; avoid exposing immunosuppressed individuals.

44. A patient is admitted to the hospital with cough, purulent sputum production, temperature of 37.9° C (100.3° F), and reports of shortness of breath. Which intervention does the nurse provide first?
    a. Set up oxygen equipment and administer oxygen.
    b. Instruct the patient about the importance of keeping the oxygen delivery device on.
    c. Monitor the effectiveness of oxygen therapy (pulse oximetry, ABGs) as appropriate.
    d. Monitor the patient's anxiety related to the need for oxygen delivery.

45. A patient has been treated for pneumonia and the nurse is preparing discharge instructions. The patient is capable of performing self-care and is anxious to return to his job at the construction site. Which instructions does the nurse give to this patient?
    a. "You are not contagious to others, so you can return to work as soon as you like."
    b. "You will continue to feel tired and will fatigue easily for the next several weeks."
    c. "Try to drink 4 quarts of water per day, especially if you are very physically active."
    d. "You should be able to return to work full-time in 2 weeks when your energy returns."

46. Which complication of pneumonia creates pain that increases on inspiration because of inflammation of the parietal pleura?
    a. Pleuritic chest pain
    b. Pulmonary emboli
    c. Pleural effusion
    d. Meningitis

47. Which conditions may cause patients to be at risk for aspiration pneumonia? *(Select all that apply.)*
    a. Continuous tube feedings
    b. Bronchoscopy procedure
    c. Magnetic resonance imaging (MRI) procedure
    d. Decreased level of consciousness
    e. Stroke
    f. Chest tube

48. An older adult patient often coughs and chokes while eating or trying to take medication. The patient insists that he is okay, but the nurse identifies the priority patient problem of risk for aspiration. Which nursing interventions are used to prevent aspiration pneumonia? *(Select all that apply.)*
    a. Head of bed should always be elevated during feeding.
    b. Monitor the patient's ability to swallow small bites.
    c. Give thin liquids to drink in small, frequent amounts.
    d. Consult a nutritionist and obtain swallowing studies.
    e. Monitor the patient's ability to swallow saliva.
    f. Place the patient on NPO (nothing by mouth) status until swallowing is normal.

49. Which condition causes a patient to have the greatest risk for community-acquired pneumonia?
    a. Tube feedings
    b. History of tobacco use
    c. Poor nutritional status
    d. Altered mental status

50. In the event of a new severe acute respiratory syndrome (SARS) outbreak, what is the nurse's primary role?
    a. Immediately report new cases of SARS to the Centers for Disease Control and Prevention (CDC).
    b. Administer oxygen, standard antibiotics, and supportive therapies to patients.
    c. Prevent the spread of infection to other employees and patients.
    d. Initiate and strictly enforce contact isolation procedures.

51. The nurse is preparing a community information packet about "bird flu." What information does the nurse include for public dissemination? *(Select all that apply.)*
    a. In the event of an outbreak, do not eat any cooked or uncooked poultry products.
    b. Prepare a minimum of 2 weeks supply of food, water, and routine prescription drugs.
    c. Listen to public health announcements and early warning signs for disease outbreaks.
    d. Avoid traveling to areas where there has been a suspected outbreak of disease.
    e. Obtain a supply of antiviral drugs such as oseltamivir (Tamiflu).
    f. In the event of an outbreak, avoid going to public areas such as churches or schools.

52. A patient reports experiencing mild fatigue and a dry, harsh cough. There is a possibility of exposure to inhalation anthrax, but the patient currently reports feeling much better. What does the nurse advise the patient to do?
    a. Have a complete blood count to rule out the disease.
    b. Monitor for and immediately seek attention for respiratory symptoms.
    c. Consult a provider for diagnostic testing and antibiotic therapy.
    d. Stay at home, rest, increase fluid intake, and avoid public places.

53. A patient with human immunodeficiency virus (HIV) is admitted to the hospital with a temperature of 99.6° F, and reports of bloody sputum, night sweats, feeling of tiredness, and shortness of breath. What are these assessment findings consistent with?
    a. *Pneumocystis jiroveci* pneumonia (PJP)
    b. Tuberculosis
    c. Superinfection as a result of a low CD4 count
    d. Severe bronchitis

54. Which statements about the precautions of caring for a hospitalized patient with tuberculosis (TB) are true? *(Select all that apply.)*
    a. Health care workers must wear a mask that covers the face and mouth.
    b. Negative airflow rooms are required for these patients.
    c. Health care workers must wear an N95 or high-efficiency particulate air (HEPA) mask.
    d. Gown and gloves are included in appropriate barrier protection.
    e. Strict contact precautions must be maintained.

55. Which people are at greatest risk for developing TB in the United States? *(Select all that apply.)*
    a. An alcoholic homeless man who occasionally stays in a shelter
    b. A college student sharing a room in a dormitory
    c. A person with immune dysfunction or HIV
    d. A homemaker who does volunteer work at a homeless shelter
    e. Foreign immigrants (especially those from the Philippines and Mexico)

56. After several weeks of "not feeling well," a patient is seen in the provider's office for possible TB. If TB is present, which assessment findings does the nurse expect to observe? *(Select all that apply.)*
    a. Fatigue
    b. Weight gain
    c. Night sweats
    d. Chest soreness
    e. Low-grade fever

57. Which test result indicates a patient has clinically active TB?
    a. Induration of 12 mm and positive sputum
    b. Positive chest x-ray for TB
    c. Positive chest x-ray and clinical symptoms
    d. Sputum tests positive for blood

58. After receiving the subcutaneous Mantoux skin test, a patient with no risk factors returns to the clinic in the required 48 to 72 hours for the test results. Which assessment finding indicates a positive result?
    a. Test area is red, warm, and tender to touch
    b. Induration or a hard nodule of any size at the site
    c. Induration/hardened area measures 5 mm or greater
    d. Induration/hardened area measures 10 mm or greater

59. A patient has a positive skin test result for TB. What explanation does the nurse give to the patient?
    a. "There is active disease, but you are not yet infectious to others."
    b. "There is active disease and you need immediate treatment."
    c. "You have been infected but this does not mean active disease is present."
    d. "A repeat skin test is necessary because the test could give a false-positive result."

60. A patient has been compliant with drug therapy for TB and has returned as instructed for follow-up. Which result indicates that the patient is no longer infectious/communicable?
    a. Negative chest x-ray
    b. No clinical symptoms
    c. Negative skin test
    d. Three negative sputum cultures

61. A patient diagnosed with TB agrees to take the medication as instructed and to complete the therapy. When does the nurse tell the patient is the best time to take the medication?
    a. Before breakfast
    b. After breakfast
    c. Midday
    d. Bedtime

62. A patient has an HIV infection, but the TB skin test shows an induration of less than 10 mm and no clinical symptoms of TB are present. Which medication does the patient receive for a period of 12 months to prevent TB?
    a. Bacille Calmette-Guérin (BCG) vaccine
    b. Isoniazid (INH)
    c. Ethambutol
    d. Streptomycin

63. The nurse is teaching a patient about the combination drug therapy that is used in the treatment of TB. Which patient statement indicates the nurse's instruction was effective?
    a. "I will take three drugs: isoniazid, rifampin, and pyrazinamide, then ethambutol may be added later."
    b. "Combining the drugs in one pill is a convenient way for me to take all the medications."
    c. "The isoniazid combines with the TB bacteria. I can take the rifampin and pyrazinamide if I continue to have symptoms."
    d. "Combining the medications means to take the isoniazid, rifampin, and pyrazinamide all at the same time."

64. A patient diagnosed with TB has been receiving treatment for 3 weeks and has clinically shown improvement. The family asks the nurse if the patient is still infectious. What is the nurse's reply?
    a. "The patient is still infectious until the entire treatment is completed."
    b. "The patient is not infectious but needs to continue treatment for at least 6 months."
    c. "The patient is infectious until there is a negative chest x-ray."
    d. "The patient may or may not be infectious; a purified protein derivative test (PPD) must be done."

65. The patient is receiving isoniazid (INH) to treat TB. Which nursing teaching points are essential when giving this drug? *(Select all that apply.)*
    a. Teach the patient not to take medications such as Maalox with this medication.
    b. Avoid drinking alcoholic beverages.
    c. Teach the patient that urine will be orange in color.
    d. Take a multivitamin with B complex.
    e. If going out in the sun, be sure to wear protective clothing and sunscreen.
    f. Teach women that this drug reduces the effectiveness of oral contraceptives.

66. A patient with suspected TB is admitted to the hospital. Along with a private room, which nursing intervention is appropriate related to isolation procedures?
    a. Respiratory isolation and contact isolation for sputum only
    b. Strict respiratory isolation and use of specially designed facemasks
    c. Respiratory isolation with surgical masks until diagnosis is confirmed
    d. No respiratory isolation necessary until diagnosis is confirmed

67. A patient is admitted to the hospital to rule out TB. What type of mask does the nurse wear when caring for this patient?
    a. Surgical facemask
    b. Surgical facemask with eye shield
    c. HEPA respirator mask
    d. Any type of mask that covers the nose and mouth

68. After being discharged from the hospital, a patient is diagnosed with TB at the outpatient clinic. What is the correct procedure regarding public health policy in this case?
    a. Contact the infection control nurse at the hospital because the hospital is responsible for follow-up of this case.
    b. There are no regulations because the patient was diagnosed at the clinic and not during hospitalization.
    c. Contact the public health nurse so that all individuals who have come in contact with the patient can be screened.
    d. Have the patient sign a waiver regarding the hospital and clinic's liability for treatment.

69. Patients who are at high risk for TB would be asked which questions upon assessment? *(Select all that apply.)*
    a. "What does your diet normally consist of?"
    b. "Do you have an immune dysfunction or HIV?"
    c. "Do you use alcohol or inject recreational drugs?"
    d. "Where do you live in the United States?"
    e. "Do you work in a crowded area such as a prison or mental health facility?"

70. The nurse is making home visits to an older adult recovering from a hip fracture and identifies the priority patient problem of risk for respiratory infection. Which condition represents a factor of normal aging that would contribute to this increased risk?
    a. Inability to force a cough
    b. Decreased strength of respiratory muscles
    c. Increased elastic recoil of alveoli
    d. Increased macrophages in alveoli

32 CHAPTER

Care of Critically Ill Patients with Respiratory Problems

1. Which are the risk factors for pulmonary embolism (PE) and deep vein thrombosis (DVT)? *(Select all that apply.)*
   a. Trauma
   b. Swimming activity
   c. Heart failure
   d. Chronic obstructive pulmonary disease (COPD)
   e. Cancer (particularly lung or prostate)

2. What is the most common site of origin for a clot to occur, causing a PE?
   a. Right side of the heart
   b. Deep veins of the legs and pelvis
   c. Antecubital vein in upper extremities
   d. Subclavian veins

3. What is the most common cause of embolism?
   a. Amniotic fluid
   b. Air bolus
   c. Blood clot
   d. Arterial plaque

4. Which conditions define respiratory failure? *(Select all that apply.)*
   a. Ventilatory failure
   b. Circulatory failure
   c. Oxygenation failure
   d. Severe anemia
   e. Combination of ventilatory and oxygenation failure

5. A patient in the hospital being treated for a PE is receiving a continuous infusion of heparin. When the nurse comes to take vital signs, the patient has blood on the front of his chest and nose, and is holding a tissue saturated with blood to his nose. What is the first priority action the nurse must take?
   a. Have the patient sit up and lean forward, pinching the nostrils.
   b. Have a patient care technician set up oral suctioning to suction excess blood from patient's mouth.
   c. Stop the heparin IV infusion.
   d. Obtain laboratory results for prothrombin time and complete blood count.

6. The nurse's young neighbor who smokes is going on an overseas flight. The neighbor knows he is at risk for DVT and PE, and asks the nurse for advice. What does the nurse suggest?
   a. Exercise regularly and walk around before boarding the flight.
   b. Get a prescription for heparin therapy and take it before the flight.
   c. Drink water and get up every hour for at least 5 minutes during the flight.
   d. Elevate the legs as much as possible during and after the flight.

7. The nurse is caring for several postoperative patients at risk for developing PE. Which interventions does the nurse use to help prevent the development of PE in these patients? *(Select all that apply.)*
   a. Start passive and active range-of-motion exercises for the extremities.
   b. Ambulate postoperative patients soon after surgery.
   c. Use antiembolism devices postoperatively.
   d. Elevate legs in an extended position.
   e. Change patient position every 4 to 6 hours.
   f. Administer drugs to prevent episodes of Valsalva maneuver.

8. The nurse suspects a patient has a PE and notifies the provider who orders an arterial blood gas. The provider is en route to the facility. The nurse anticipates and prepares the patient for which additional diagnostic test?
   a. Ultrasound
   b. Pulmonary angiography
   c. 12-lead ECG
   d. Ventilation and perfusion scan

9. The provider orders heparin therapy for a patient with a relatively small PE. The patient states, "I didn't tell the doctor my complete medical history." Which condition may affect the provider's decision to immediately start heparin therapy?
   a. Type 2 diabetes mellitus
   b. Recent cerebral hemorrhage
   c. Newly diagnosed osteoarthritis
   d. Asthma since childhood

10. A patient with a PE asks for an explanation of heparin therapy. What is the nurse's best response?
   a. "It keeps the clot from getting larger by preventing platelets from sticking together to improve blood flow."
   b. "It will improve your breathing and decrease chest pain by dissolving the clot in your lung."
   c. "It promotes the absorption of the clot in your leg that originally caused the PE."
   d. "It increases the time it takes for blood to clot, therefore preventing further clotting and improving blood flow."

11. A patient is being treated with heparin therapy for a PE. The patient has the potential for bleeding with the administration of heparin. What does the nurse monitor in relation to the heparin therapy?
   a. Lab values for any elevation of prothrombin time (PT) or partial thromboplastin time (PTT) value
   b. PTT values for greater than 2.5 times the control and/or the patient for bleeding
   c. Occurrence of a pulmonary infarction by blood in sputum
   d. PT values for International Normalized Ratio (INR) for a therapeutic range of 2 to 3 and/or the patient for bleeding

12. Acute respiratory failure is classified by which critical values of $Paco_2$? *(Select all that apply.)*
   a. 39 mm Hg
   b. 52 mm Hg
   c. < 60 mm Hg
   d. 77 mm Hg
   e. >50 mm Hg with a pH value of < 7.3

13. Upon diagnosis of a PE, the nurse expects to perform which therapeutic intervention for the patient?
   a. Oral anticoagulant therapy
   b. Bedrest in the supine position
   c. Oxygen therapy via mechanical ventilator
   d. Parenteral anticoagulant therapy

14. The nurse is caring for a patient with a postoperative complication of PE. The patient has been receiving treatment for several days. Which factors are indicators of adequate perfusion in the patient? *(Select all that apply.)*
   a. Pulse oximetry of 95%
   b. Arterial blood gas, pH of 7.28
   c. Patient's subjective desire to go home
   d. Absence of pallor or cyanosis
   e. Mental status at patient's baseline

15. Which are extrapulmonary causes of ventilatory failure? *(Select all that apply.)*
   a. Stroke
   b. Use of opioid analgesics
   c. Pulmonary edema
   d. Chronic obstructive pulmonary disease
   e. Morbid obesity

16. The nurse is caring for several postoperative patients with high risk for a PE. All of these patients have preexisting chronic respiratory problems. What is a unique assessment finding for a clot in the lung?
    a. Dyspnea
    b. Sudden dry cough
    c. Pursed-lip breathing
    d. Audible wheezing

17. The nurse is caring for several patients at risk for DVT and PE. Which condition causes the patient to be a candidate for placement of a vena cava filter?
    a. Massive PE causing the patient to experience shock symptoms
    b. Multiple emboli with deteriorating cardiopulmonary status
    c. Recurrent bleeding while receiving anticoagulants
    d. No response to oxygen therapy and conservative management

18. A patient with a massive PE has hypotension and shock, and is receiving IV crystalloids. However, the patient's cardiac output is not improving. The nurse anticipates an order for which drug?
    a. Hydromorphone (Dilaudid)
    b. Alteplase (Activase, tPA)
    c. Diltiazem (Cardizem)
    d. Dobutamine (Dobutrex)

19. An older adult patient on anticoagulation therapy for a PE is somewhat confused and requires assistance with activities of daily living (ADLs). Which instruction specific to this therapy does the nurse give to the unlicensed assistive personnel (UAP)?
    a. Count and report episodes of urinary incontinence.
    b. Use a lift sheet when moving or turning the patient in bed.
    c. Assist with ambulation because the patient is likely to have dizziness.
    d. Give the patient an extra blanket, because the patient is likely to feel cold.

20. A patient with a PE is receiving anticoagulant therapy. Which assessment related to the therapy does the nurse perform?
    a. Measure abdominal girth because the medication causes fluid retention.
    b. Check skin turgor because dehydration contributes to anticoagulation.
    c. Monitor for nausea, vomiting, and diarrhea.
    d. Examine skin every 2 hours for evidence of bleeding.

21. What does the nurse monitor for in a patient with a PE? *(Select all that apply.)*
    a. Nausea and vomiting
    b. Cyanosis
    c. Rapid heart rate
    d. Dyspnea
    e. Paradoxical chest movement
    f. Crackles in the lung fields

22. After receiving IV heparin anticoagulant therapy, patients are generally not discharged from the hospital without a prescription and instructions for which drug?
    a. Protamine sulfate
    b. Prednisone (Deltasone)
    c. Warfarin (Coumadin)
    d. Oral heparin

23. A patient is following up on a postoperative complication of PE. The patient must have blood drawn to determine the therapeutic range for Coumadin. Which lab test determines this therapeutic range?
    a. PTT level
    b. Platelets
    c. PT and INR
    d. Coumadin peak and trough

24. The nurse is reviewing lab results for a patient with a new-onset PE. What is the INR therapeutic range?
    a. 1.0 to 1.5
    b. 2.0 to 3.0
    c. 3.0 to 4.5
    d. 5

25. A patient demonstrates chest pain, dyspnea, dry cough, and change in level of consciousness. The nurse suspects PE and notifies the health care provider who orders an arterial blood gas (ABG). In the early stage of a PE, what would ABG results probably indicate?
    a. Respiratory alkalosis
    b. Respiratory acidosis
    c. Metabolic acidosis
    d. Metabolic alkalosis

26. A patient recently received anticoagulant therapy for complications of PE after knee surgery. The patient is now in a rehabilitation facility and is receiving warfarin (Coumadin). What is the nursing responsibility related to Coumadin?
    a. Having protamine sulfate available as an antidote
    b. Administering NSAIDs or aspirin for pain related to the knee
    c. Teaching the patient about foods high in vitamin K
    d. Monitoring platelets for thrombocytopenia

27. Ventilatory failure is the result of what processes? *(Select all that apply.)*
    a. Hematologic disease
    b. Defect in the respiratory control center of the brain
    c. Physical problem of the lungs
    d. Poor function of the diaphragm
    e. Physical problem of the chest wall

28. Which conditions are related to acute respiratory distress syndrome (ARDS)? *(Select all that apply.)*
    a. Lung fluid increases.
    b. A systemic inflammatory response occurs.
    c. The lungs dry out and become stiff.
    d. Lung volume is decreased.
    e. Hypoxemia results.

29. The nurse is reviewing the ABG results for a patient. The latest ABGs show pH 7.48, HCO_3^- 23 mEq/L, $Paco_2$ 25 mm Hg, Pao_2 98 mm Hg. What is the correct interpretation of these lab findings?
    a. Chronic respiratory alkalosis with compensation
    b. Acute respiratory alkalosis and hyperventilation
    c. Acute respiratory acidosis and hypoventilation
    d. Chronic respiratory acidosis and hypoventilation

30. The nurse is caring for a patient with acute hypoxemia. Which nursing interventions are best for the care of this patient? *(Select all that apply.)*
    a. Minimal self-care
    b. Sedatives prn
    c. Upright position
    d. Oxygen therapy
    e. Keep NPO while dyspneic
    f. Prescribed metered-dose inhalers

31. A patient reports pain with inspiration after falling off a skateboard. The provider makes the diagnosis of rib fracture. The nurse prepares to do patient teaching for which treatment?
    a. Mechanical ventilation
    b. Tight bandage around chest
    c. Coughing and deep-breathing
    d. Opioid analgesics for pain

32. The nurse is assessing a patient who sustained significant chest trauma during a motor vehicle accident. What significant assessment finding suggests tension pneumothorax?
    a. Tracheal deviation to the unaffected side
    b. Inspiratory stridor and respiratory distress
    c. Diminished breath sounds over the affected hemothorax
    d. Hyperresonant percussion note over the affected side

33. The nurse is assessing a patient with a hemothorax. When the nurse performs percussion of the chest on the affected side, what type of sound is expected?
    a. Hypertympanic
    b. Dull
    c. Hyperresonant
    d. Crackles

34. On arrival to the emergency department (ED), the patient develops extreme respiratory distress and the provider identifies a tension pneumothorax. The nurse prepares to assist with which initial urgent procedure?
    a. Endotracheal intubation with mechanical ventilation
    b. Placement of a chest tube to reduce pneumothorax on the affected side
    c. Insertion of a 8-inch (20.3-cm), 16- or 18-gauge pericardial needle
    d. Insertion of a large-bore needle into the second intercostal space on the affected side

35. The nurse is performing patient teaching for a patient who will be taking anticoagulants at home. What does the nurse include in the instructions? (Select all that apply.)
    a. Use a soft-bristled toothbrush and floss frequently.
    b. Do not take aspirin or any aspirin-containing products.
    c. Do not participate in activities that will cause bumps, scratches, or scrapes.
    d. If you are bumped, apply ice to the site for at least 24 hours.
    e. Eat warm, cool, or cold foods to avoid burning your mouth.
    f. If you must blow your nose, do so gently without blocking either nasal passage.

36. Which patient has the greatest risk for developing ARDS?
    a. 74-year-old who aspirates a tube feeding
    b. 34-year-old with chronic renal failure
    c. 56-year-old with uncontrolled diabetes mellitus
    d. 18-year-old with a fractured femur

37. Which assessment finding is considered an early sign of ARDS?
    a. Adventitious lung sounds
    b. Hyperthermia and hot, dry skin
    c. Intercostal and suprasternal retractions
    d. Heightened mental acuity and surveillance

38. A patient with which condition is a potential candidate for autotransfusion, should the need arise?
    a. Tension pneumothorax
    b. Hemothorax
    c. Abdominal bleeding
    d. Esophageal bleeding

39. A patient sustained a chest injury resulting from a motor vehicle accident. The patient is asymptomatic at first, but slowly develops decreased breath sounds, crackles, wheezing, and blood in the sputum. The mechanism of injury and physical findings are consistent with which condition?
    a. Flail chest
    b. Rib fractures
    c. Pneumothorax
    d. Pulmonary contusion

40. A patient is admitted after a near-drowning and develops ARDS, which is confirmed by the provider. The nurse prepares equipment for which treatment?
    a. Oxygen therapy via continuous positive airway pressure (CPAP)
    b. Mechanical ventilation and endotracheal tube
    c. High-flow oxygen via facemask
    d. Tracheostomy tube

41. A 19-year-old patient was seen in the ED after a motorcycle accident for multiple rib fractures that resulted in free-floating ribs, paradoxical breathing, and inadequate oxygenation. What is this condition called?
    a. Tension pneumothorax
    b. Flail chest
    c. Pulmonary contusion
    d. Subcutaneous emphysema

42. The high-pressure alarm of a patient's mechanical ventilator goes off. What are the potential causes for this? *(Select all that apply.)*
    a. Mucus plug
    b. Endotracheal tube cuff has air leak
    c. Patient is fighting the ventilator
    d. Bronchospasm
    e. Patient is coughing

43. The low-pressure alarm of a patient's mechanical ventilator goes off. What are potential causes for this? *(Select all that apply.)*
    a. Blockage in the circuit
    b. Cuff leak in the endotracheal or tracheostomy tube
    c. Patient has stopped breathing
    d. Cuff of the endotracheal or tracheostomy tube is overinflated
    e. Leak in the circuit

44. A patient with ARDS is currently in the exudative management stage. What is the focus of the nursing assessment?
    a. Monitor closely for progressive hypoxemia.
    b. Note early changes in dyspnea and tachypnea.
    c. Review the x-ray reports for evidence of patchy infiltrates.
    d. Monitor for multiple organ dysfunction syndrome.

45. The nurse is caring for a patient at risk for pulmonary contusion. Why is this a potentially lethal chest injury?
    a. The patient could have broken ribs.
    b. The patient could develop laryngospasm.
    c. Respiratory failure develops over time.
    d. There is a risk of infection from chest tubes.

46. A patient has been successfully intubated by the provider, and the nurse and respiratory therapist are securing the tube in place. What does the nurse include in the documentation regarding the intubation procedure? *(Select all that apply.)*
    a. Presence of bilateral and equal breath sounds
    b. Level of the tube
    c. Changes in vital signs during the procedure
    d. Rate of the IV fluids
    e. Presence (or absence) of dysrhythmias
    f. Placement verification by end-tidal carbon dioxide levels

47. The nurse is assisting with an emergency intubation for a patient in severe respiratory distress. Although the provider is experienced, the procedure is difficult because the patient has severe kyphosis. At what point does the nurse intervene?
    a. First intubation attempt lasts longer than 15 seconds.
    b. First intubation attempt lasts longer than 30 seconds.
    c. Second intubation attempt is unsuccessful.
    d. Second intubation attempt causes the patient to struggle.

48. A patient in the ED required emergency intubation for status asthmaticus. Immediately after the insertion of an endotracheal (ET) tube, what is the most accurate method for the nurse and/or provider to use to verify correct placement?
    a. Observe for chest excursion.
    b. Listen for expired air from the ET tube.
    c. Check end-tidal CO_2 level.
    d. Wait for the results of the chest x-ray.

49. The nurse is caring for several patients on the medical-surgical unit who are experiencing acute respiratory problems. Which conditions may eventually require a patient to be intubated? *(Select all that apply.)*
    a. Trouble maintaining a patent airway because of mucosal swelling
    b. History of congestive heart failure and demonstrating orthopnea
    c. Copious secretions and lacking muscular strength to cough
    d. Pulse oximetry of 93% with a high-flow oxygen facemask
    e. Increasing fatigue because of the work of breathing

50. The nurse receives report on a patient with ARDS who has been intubated for 6 days and has progressive hypoxemia that responds poorly to high levels of oxygen. This patient is in which phase of ARDS case management?
    a. Exudative phase
    b. Fibroproliferative phase
    c. Resolution phase
    d. Recovery phase

51. A postoperative patient reports sudden onset of shortness of breath and pleuritic chest pain. Assessment findings include diaphoresis, hypotension, crackles in the left lower lobe, and pulse oximetry of 85%. What does the nurse suspect has occurred with this patient?
    a. Atelectasis
    b. Pneumothorax
    c. Pulmonary embolism
    d. Flail chest

52. The nurse hears in shift report that a patient has been agitated and pulling at the ET. Soft restraints have recently been ordered and placed, but the patient continues to move his head and chew at the tube. What does the nurse do to ensure proper placement of the ET tube?
    a. Suction the patient frequently through the oral airway.
    b. Talk to the patient and tell him to calm down.
    c. Mark the tube where it touches the patient's teeth.
    d. Auscultate for breath sounds every 4 hours.

53. The nurse is caring for a patient on a mechanical ventilator. What does the nurse monitor to assess for the most likely cardiac problem associated with this therapy?
    a. Check blood pressure.
    b. Check for ventricular dysrhythmias.
    c. Take an apical pulse before giving medications.
    d. Ask the patient about chest pain.

54. A patient in the critical care unit requires an emergency ET intubation. The nurse immediately obtains and prepares which supplies to perform this procedure? *(Select all that apply.)*
    a. Tracheostomy tube or kit
    b. Resuscitation Ambu bag
    c. Source for 100% oxygen
    d. Suction equipment
    e. Airway equipment box (e.g., laryngoscope)
    f. Oral airway
    g. Bronchodilator inhaler

55. A patient on a ventilator is biting and chewing at the ET tube. Which nursing intervention is used for ET management?
    a. Reassure the patient that everything is okay.
    b. Administer a paralyzing agent.
    c. Insert an oral airway.
    d. Frequently suction the mouth.

56. The nurse is performing a check of the ventilator equipment. What is included during the equipment check?
    a. Drain the condensed moisture back into the humidifier.
    b. Empty the humidifier and the drainage tubing.
    c. Note the prescribed and actual settings.
    d. Turn off the alarms during the system check.

57. The nursing student is assisting in the care of a critically ill patient on a ventilator. Which action by the student nurse requires intervention by the supervising nurse?
    a. Deflates the cuff on the ET tube to check placement.
    b. Applies soft wrist restraints as ordered.
    c. Suctions the patient for 10 seconds at a time.
    d. Maintains the correct placement of the ET tube.

58. A patient has a history of COPD and had to be intubated for respiratory failure. The patient is currently on a mechanical ventilator. The nurse obtains an order for which type of dietary therapy for this patient?
    a. High-fat nutritional supplement
    b. High-protein nutritional supplement
    c. High-carbohydrate nutritional supplement
    d. High-calorie nutritional supplement

59. The nursing student is assisting in the care of a patient on a mechanical ventilator. Which action by the student contributes to the prevention of ventilator-assisted pneumonia?
    a. Suctions the patient frequently
    b. Performs oral care every 2 hours
    c. Encourages visitors to wear masks
    d. Obtains a sputum specimen for culture

60. The nurse is caring for a patient on a mechanical ventilator. During the shift, the nurse hears the patient talking to himself. What does the nurse do next?
    a. See if the patient has a change of mental status.
    b. Check the inflation of the pilot balloon.
    c. Assess the pulse oximetry for saturation level.
    d. Evaluate the patient's readiness to be weaned.

61. The nurse notices that a patient has a gradual increase in peak inspiratory pressure over the last several days. What is the best nursing intervention for this patient?
    a. Assess for a reason such as ARDS or pneumonia.
    b. Continue to increase peak airway pressure as needed.
    c. Change to another mode such as intermittent mandatory ventilation (IMV).
    d. Make arrangements for permanent ventilatory support.

62. A patient is intubated and has mechanical ventilation with positive end-expiratory pressure (PEEP). Because this patient is at risk for a tension pneumothorax, what is the nurse's priority action?
    a. Assess lung sounds every 30 to 60 minutes.
    b. Obtain an order for an arterial blood gas.
    c. Have chest tube equipment on standby.
    d. Direct the unlicensed assistive personnel to turn the patient every 2 hours.

63. The nurse is caring for a patient on a mechanical ventilator. Which assessments does the nurse perform for this patient? *(Select all that apply.)*
    a. Observe the patient's mouth around the tube for pressure ulcers.
    b. Auscultate the lungs for crackles, wheezes, equal breath sounds, and decreased or absent breath sounds.
    c. Assess the placement of the ET.
    d. Check at least every 24 hours to be sure the ventilator settings are as prescribed.
    e. Check to be sure alarms are set.
    f. Observe the patient's need for tracheal, oral, or nasal suctioning every 2 hours.

64. What are the characteristics of a mechanical ventilator that is pressure-cycled? *(Select all that apply.)*
    a. Preset inspiration and expiration rate is programmed with possible variation of tidal volume and pressure.
    b. It is a positive-pressure ventilator.
    c. It pushes air into the lungs until a preset airway pressure is reached.
    d. There is no need for an artificial airway such as a tracheostomy or ET.
    e. Tidal volumes and inspiratory times are varied.

65. What are the characteristics of a mechanical ventilator that is time-cycled? *(Select all that apply.)*
    a. It needs an artificial airway such as a tracheostomy or ET.
    b. It is a positive-pressure ventilator.
    c. Its tidal volumes are variable.
    d. Preset inspiration and expiration rate can be set with possible variation of tidal volume.
    e. Inspiratory time is variable.

66. What are the characteristics of a noninvasive pressure support (Bi-PAP)? *(Select all that apply.)*
    a. It provides noninvasive pressure support ventilation by nasal mask or facemask.
    b. It takes over most of the work of breathing for the patient.
    c. It is most often used for patients with sleep apnea.
    d. It delivers a breath when a patient does not breathe.
    e. It may be used for patients with respiratory muscle fatigue.

67. Which statement about a microprocessor ventilator is true?
    a. Positive pressure is maintained throughout the entire respiratory cycle to prevent alveolar collapse.
    b. Positive pressure is exerted during expiration to keep lungs partially inflated.
    c. Noninvasive pressure support ventilation is provided by nasal mask or facemask.
    d. A computer monitors ventilatory functions, alarms, and patient condition.

68. The nurse hears an alarm go off on a mechanical ventilator that signals the ventilator is not able to give the patient a breath. What are the possible reasons that would make this alarm go off? *(Select all that apply.)*
    a. The tubing has become disconnected.
    b. The patient is not breathing on his or her own.
    c. The pulse oximetry reading is below 90%.
    d. The patient has become disconnected from the ventilator.
    e. The patient needs to be suctioned.

69. A patient with a tracheostomy who is on a mechanical ventilator is beginning to take spontaneous breaths at his own rate and tidal volume between set ventilator breaths. Which mode is the ventilator on?
    a. Assist-control (AC) ventilation
    b. Bi-PAP
    c. SIMV (synchronized intermittent ventilation)
    d. Continuous flow (flow-by)

70. A patient who is on a mechanical ventilator needs a set volume and set rate delivered because the patient is not able to do the work of breathing. To what mode must the ventilator be set?
    a. PEEP
    b. CPAP
    c. Bi-PAP
    d. AC

71. The provider instructs the nurse to watch for and report signs and symptoms of improvement so the patient can be weaned from the ventilator. Which assessment finding indicates the patient is ready to be weaned?
    a. Indications that respiratory infection is resolving
    b. Showing signs of becoming ventilator-dependent
    c. Maintaining blood gases within normal limits
    d. Patient is receiving only 1-2 mechanical ventilator breaths per minute

72. An older adult patient arrives in the ED after falling off a roof. The nurse observes "sucking inward" of the loose chest area during inspiration and a "puffing out" of the same area during expiration. ABG results show severe hypoxemia and hypercarbia. Which procedure does the nurse prepare for?
    a. Chest tube insertion
    b. Endotracheal intubation
    c. Needle thoracotomy
    d. Tracheostomy

73. The charge nurse in the intensive care unit is reviewing the patient census and caseload to identify staffing needs and potential transfers. Which patient might take the longest time to wean from a ventilator?
    a. 54-year-old man with metastatic colon cancer who has been intubated for 6 days
    b. 32-year-old woman recovering from a general anesthetic following a tubal ligation
    c. 25-year-old man intubated for 28 hours after an anaphylactic reaction
    d. 49-year-old man with a gunshot wound to the chest who was intubated for 8 hours

74. A patient is being extubated and the nurse has emergency equipment at the bedside. Which intervention is implemented during extubation?
    a. Ensure that the cuff is inflated at all times.
    b. Remove the tube during expiration.
    c. Instruct the patient to pant while the tube is removed.
    d. Instruct the patient to cough after tube is removed.

75. The nurse is caring for a patient who was recently extubated. What is an expected assessment finding for this patient?
    a. Stridor
    b. Dyspnea
    c. Restlessness
    d. Hoarseness

76. The patient is to be extubated. What action does the nurse perform first?
    a. Hyperoxygenate the patient.
    b. Rapidly deflate the cuff of the ET tube.
    c. Thoroughly suction both the ET tube and the oral cavity.
    d. Explain the procedure.

77. Which patients on mechanical ventilators are at high risk for barotraumas? *(Select all that apply.)*
    a. Patient with ARDS
    b. Patient with underlying chronic airflow limitation
    c. Patient on Bi-PAP
    d. Patient on PEEP
    e. Patient on SIMV

78. The nurse is caring for a patient who has just been extubated. What interventions does the nurse use in caring for this patient? *(Select all that apply.)*
    a. Monitor vital signs every 30 minutes at first.
    b. Assess the ventilatory pattern for manifestations of respiratory distress.
    c. Place the patient in a recumbent position.
    d. Instruct the patient to take deep breaths every half hour.
    e. Encourage use of an incentive spirometer every 2 hours.
    f. Advise the patient to limit speaking right after extubation.

79. The nurse is assessing a patient who was extubated several hours ago. Which patient finding warrants notification of the Rapid Response Team?
    a. Hoarseness
    b. Report of sore throat
    c. Inability to expectorate secretions
    d. 90% saturation on room air

80. A patient is admitted to the trauma unit following a front-end motor vehicle collision. The patient is currently asymptomatic, but the provider advises the nurse that the patient has a high risk for pulmonary contusion. What does the nurse carefully monitor for?
    a. Tracheal deviation
    b. Paradoxical chest movements
    c. Progressive chest pain
    d. Decreased breath sounds

81. Which finding might delay weaning a patient from mechanical ventilation support?
    a. Hematocrit = 42%
    b. Arterial Po_2 = 70 mm Hg on a 40% Fio_2
    c. Apical heart rate = 72 beats per minute
    d. Oral temperature = 101° F

82. A patient in respiratory failure is diagnosed with a flail chest. After the patient is intubated, which treatment does the nurse expect to be implemented?
    a. PEEP
    b. SIMV
    c. Bi-PAP
    d. PIP

83. A patient in a motor vehicle accident was unrestrained and appears to have hit the front dashboard. The patient has severe respiratory distress, inspiratory stridor, and extensive subcutaneous emphysema. The ED physician identifies tracheobronchial trauma. Which procedure does the nurse immediately prepare for?
    a. Cricothyroidotomy
    b. Chest tube insertion
    c. Cardiopulmonary resuscitation
    d. Pericardiocentesis

84. What causes the potential cardiac problems that can result from mechanical ventilation?
    a. Negative pressure increases in the chest.
    b. Positive pressure increases in the chest.
    c. Positive pressure decreases in the heart.
    d. Negative pressure increases in the heart.

85. What is the cardiac problem that can occur from mechanical ventilation?
    a. Hypotension
    b. Dehydration
    c. Bradycardia
    d. Hypertension

86. Which clinical manifestations can occur from cardiac problems due to mechanical ventilation? *(Select all that apply.)*
    a. Decreased cardiac output
    b. Diuresis
    c. Bradycardia
    d. Fluid retention
    e. Tachycardia

33 CHAPTER

Assessment of the Cardiovascular System

1. Which description best defines the cardiovascular concept afterload?
   a. Degree of myocardial fiber stretch at end of diastole and just before heart contracts
   b. Amount of pressure or resistance that the ventricles must overcome to eject blood through the semilunar valves and into the peripheral blood vessels
   c. Pressure that ventricle must overcome to open aortic valve
   d. Force of contraction independent of preload

2. Which are risk factors for cardiovascular disease (CVD) in women? *(Select all that apply.)*
   a. Waist and abdominal obesity
   b. Excess fat in the buttocks, hips, and thighs
   c. Postmenopausal
   d. Diabetes mellitus
   e. Asian ethnicity

3. The nurse is assessing a patient's nicotine dependency. Which questions does the nurse ask for an accurate assessment? *(Select all that apply.)*
   a. "How soon after you wake up in the morning do you smoke?"
   b. "What kind of cigarettes do you smoke?"
   c. "Do you inhale deeply when you smoke?"
   d. "Do you find it difficult not to smoke in places where smoking is prohibited?"
   e. "Do you smoke when you are ill?"
   f. "What happened the last time you tried to quit smoking?"

4. The nurse is talking to a patient who has been trying to quit smoking. Which statement by the patient indicates an understanding of cigarette usage as it relates to reducing cardiovascular risks?
   a. "I need to be completely cigarette-free for at least 3 years."
   b. "I don't smoke as much as I used to; I'm down to one pack a day."
   c. "I started smoking a while ago, but I'll quit in a couple of years."
   d. "I only smoke to relax, when I drink, or when I go out with friends."

5. The nurse is providing health teaching for a patient at risk for heart disease. Which factor is the most modifiable, controllable risk factor?
   a. Obesity
   b. Diabetes mellitus
   c. Ethnic background
   d. Family history of cardiovascular disease

6. The nurse is giving a community presentation about heart disease in women. What information does the nurse include in the presentation? *(Select all that apply.)*
   a. Dyspnea on exertion may be the first and only symptom of heart failure.
   b. Symptoms are subtle or atypical.
   c. Pain is often relieved by rest.
   d. Having waist and abdominal obesity is a higher risk factor than having fat in buttocks and thighs.
   e. Pain always responds to nitroglycerin.
   f. Common symptoms include back pain, indigestion, nausea, vomiting, and anorexia.

7. Which blood pressure readings require further assessment? *(Select all that apply.)*
   a. 90 mm Hg systolic
   b. 139 mm Hg systolic
   c. 115 mm Hg systolic
   d. 66 mm Hg diastolic
   e. 100 mm Hg diastolic

8. The nurse working in the public health department is reviewing data for populations at risk for CVD. Which group has the greatest need for intervention to reduce CVD risk?
   a. Government employees who make approximately $40,000 a year
   b. Part-time fast-food workers who make approximately $9,000 a year
   c. Hospital-employed nurses who make approximately $52,000 a year
   d. Chain retail employees who make approximately $18,000 a year

9. Which category of cardiovascular drugs increases heart rate and contractility?
   a. Diuretics
   b. Beta blockers
   c. Catecholamines
   d. Benzodiazepines

10. Which category of cardiovascular drugs blocks the sympathetic stimulation to the heart and decreases the heart rate?
    a. Beta blockers
    b. Catecholamines
    c. Steroids
    d. Benzodiazepines

11. What different pathophysiologic conditions can the healthy heart adapt to? *(Select all that apply.)*
    a. Menses
    b. Stress
    c. Gastroesophageal reflux disease
    d. Infection
    e. Hemorrhage

12. Which statements about blood pressure are accurate? *(Select all that apply.)*
    a. Pulse pressure is the difference between the systolic and diastolic pressures.
    b. The right ventricle of the heart generates the greatest amount of blood pressure.
    c. Diastolic blood pressure is primarily determined by the amount of peripheral vasoconstriction.
    d. To maintain adequate blood flow through the coronary arteries, mean arterial pressure (MAP) must be at least 60 mm Hg.
    e. Diastolic blood pressure is the highest pressure during contraction of the ventricles.

13. The nurse is assessing a 62-year-old native Hawaiian woman. She is postmenopausal, diabetic for 10 years, smokes 1 pack a day of cigarettes for 20 years, walks twice a week for 30 minutes, is an administrator, and describes her lifestyle as sedentary. For her weight and height she has a body mass index of 32. Which risk factors for this patient are controllable for CVD? *(Select all that apply.)*
    a. Ethnic background
    b. Smoking
    c. Age
    d. Obesity
    e. Postmenopausal
    f. Sedentary lifestyle

14. The health care provider orders orthostatic vital signs on a patient who experienced dizziness and feeling lightheaded. What is the nurse's first action?
    a. Patient changes position to sitting or standing.
    b. Measure the blood pressure when the patient is supine.
    c. Place the patient in supine position for at least 3 minutes.
    d. Wait for at least 1 minute before auscultating blood pressure and counting the radial pulse.

15. In a hypovolemic patient, stretch receptors in the blood vessels sense a reduced volume or pressure and send fewer impulses to the central nervous system. As a result, which signs/symptoms does the nurse expect to observe in the patient?
    a. Reddish mottling to skin and a blood pressure elevation
    b. Cool, pale skin and tachycardia
    c. Warm, flushed skin with low blood pressure
    d. Pale pink skin with bradycardia

16. What term describes the difference between systolic and diastolic values, which is an indirect measure of cardiac output?
    a. Paradoxical blood pressure
    b. Pulse pressure
    c. Ankle-brachial index
    d. Normal blood pressure

17. The nurse is performing a dietary assessment on a 45-year-old business executive at risk for CVD. Which assessment method used by the nurse is the most reliable and accurate?
    a. Ask the patient to identify foods he or she eats that contain sodium, sugar, cholesterol, fiber, and fat.
    b. Ask the patient's spouse, who does the cooking and shopping, to identify the types of foods that are consumed.
    c. Ask the patient how cultural beliefs and economic status influence the choice of food items.
    d. Ask the patient to recall the intake of food, fluids, and alcohol during a typical 24-hour period.

18. Based on the physiologic force that propels blood forward in the veins, which patient has the greatest risk for venous stasis?
    a. Older adult patient with hypertension who rides a bicycle daily
    b. Middle-aged construction worker taking Coumadin
    c. Bedridden patient in the end stage of Alzheimer's disease
    d. Teenage patient with a broken leg who sits and plays videogames

19. Which statement about the peripheral vascular system is true?
    a. Veins are equipped with valves that direct blood flow to the heart and prevent backflow.
    b. The velocity of blood flow depends on the diameter of the vessel lumen.
    c. Blood flow decreases and blood tends to clot as the viscosity decreases.
    d. The parasympathetic nervous system has the largest effect on blood flow to organs.

20. A patient comes to the clinic stating "my right foot turns a darkish red color when I sit too long, and when I put my foot up, it turns pale." Which conditions does the nurse suspect?
    a. Central cyanosis
    b. Peripheral cyanosis
    c. Arterial insufficiency
    d. Venous insufficiency

21. Which exercise regimen for an older adult meets the recommended guidelines for physical fitness to promote heart health?
    a. 6-hour bike ride every Saturday
    b. Golfing for 4 hours two times a week
    c. Running for 15 minutes three times a week
    d. Brisk walk 30 minutes every day

22. The patient has smoked half a pack of cigarettes per day for 2 years. How many pack-years has this patient smoked?
    a. 1/2 pack year
    b. 1 pack year
    c. 1 1/5 pack years
    d. 2 pack years

23. In assessing a patient who has come to the clinic for a physical exam, the nurse sees that the patient has pallor. What is this finding most indicative of?
    a. Anemia
    b. Thrombophlebitis
    c. Heart disease
    d. Stroke

24. Emergency personnel discovered a patient lying outside in the cool evening air for an unknown length of time. The patient is in a hypothermic state and the metabolic needs of the tissues are decreased. What other assessment finding does the nurse expect to see?
    a. Blood pressure and heart rate lower than normal
    b. Heart rate and respiratory rate higher than normal
    c. Normal vital signs due to compensatory mechanisms
    d. Gradually improved vital signs with enteral nutrition

25. The advanced-practice nurse is assessing the vascular status of a patient's lower extremities using the ankle-brachial index. What is the correct technique for this assessment method?
    a. A blood pressure cuff is applied to the lower extremities and the systolic pressure is measured by Doppler ultrasound at both the dorsalis pedis and posterior tibial pulses.
    b. The dorsalis pedis and posterior tibial pulses are manually palpated and compared bilaterally for strength and equality and compared to the standard index.
    c. A blood pressure cuff is applied to the lower extremities to observe for an exaggerated decrease in systolic pressure by more than 10 mm Hg during inspiration.
    d. Measure blood pressure on the legs when the patient is supine; then have the patient stand for several minutes and repeat blood pressure measurement in the arms.

26. What is the correct technique for assessing a patient with arterial insufficiency in the right lower leg?
    a. Use the Doppler to find the dorsalis pedis and posterior tibial pulses on the right leg.
    b. Palpate the peripheral arteries in a head-to-toe approach with a side-to-side comparison.
    c. Check all the pulse points in the right leg in dependent and supine positions.
    d. Palpate the major arteries, such as the radial and femoral, and observe for pallor.

27. The nurse is performing a cardiac assessment on an older adult. What is a common assessment finding for this patient?
    a. S_4 heart sound
    b. Leg edema
    c. Pericardial friction rubs
    d. Change in point of maximum impulse location

28. A patient's chart notes that the examiner has heard S_1 and S_2 on auscultation of the heart. What does this documentation refer to?
    a. First and second heart sounds
    b. Pericardial friction rub
    c. Murmur
    d. Gallop

29. The nurse is taking report on a patient who will be transferred from the cardiac intensive care unit to the general medical-surgical unit. The reporting nurse states that S_4 is heard on auscultation of the heart. This indicates that the patient has which condition?
    a. Heart murmur
    b. Pericardial friction rub
    c. Ventricular hypertrophy
    d. Normal heart sounds

30. Which patient has an abnormal heart sound?
    a. S_1 in a 45-year-old patient
    b. S_2 in a 30-year-old patient
    c. S_3 in a 15-year-old patient
    d. S_3 in a 54-year-old patient

31. The nurse is caring for a patient at risk for heart problems. What are normal findings for the cardiovascular assessment of this patient? *(Select all that apply.)*
    a. Presence of a thrill
    b. Splitting of S_2; decreases with expiration
    c. Jugular venous distention to level of the mandible
    d. Point of maximal impulse (PMI) in fifth intercostal space at midclavicular line
    e. Paradoxical chest movement with inspiration and expiration

32. The nurse practitioner reads in a patient's chart that a carotid bruit was heard during the last two annual checkups. Today on auscultation, the bruit is not present. How does the nurse practitioner evaluate this data?
    a. The problem has resolved spontaneously.
    b. There may have been an anomaly in previous findings.
    c. The occlusion of the vessel may have progressed past 90%.
    d. The antiplatelet therapy is working.

33. The nurse is assessing a patient with suspected CVD. When assessing the precordium, which assessment technique does the nurse begin?
    a. Percussion
    b. Palpation
    c. Auscultation
    d. Inspection

34. In assessing a patient, the nurse finds that the PMI appears in more than one intercostal space, and has shifted lateral to the midclavicular line. How does the nurse interpret this data?
    a. Left ventricular hypertrophy
    b. Superior vena cava obstruction
    c. Pulmonary hypertension
    d. Constrictive pericarditis

35. When the nurse assesses a patient with CVD, there is difficulty auscultating the first heart sound (S_1). What is the nurse's best action?
    a. Ask the patient to lean forward or roll to his or her left side.
    b. Instruct the patient to take a deep breath and hold it.
    c. Auscultate with the bell instead of the diaphragm.
    d. Ask the unlicensed assistive personnel (UAP) to complete a 12-lead electrocardiogram (ECG) immediately.

36. While listening to a patient's heart sounds, the nurse detects a murmur. What does the nurse understand about the cause of murmurs?
    a. A murmur is caused by the closing of the aortic and pulmonic valves.
    b. A murmur is caused when blood flows from the atrium to a noncompliant ventricle.
    c. A murmur is caused by anemia, hypertension, or ventricular hypertrophy.
    d. A murmur is caused when there is turbulent blood flow through normal or abnormal valves.

37. The patient has a diagnosis of angina. Which assessment findings would the nurse expect to find? *(Select all that apply.)*
    a. Sudden onset of pain
    b. Intermittent pain relieved with sitting upright
    c. Substernal pain which may spread across chest, back, arms
    d. Pain usually lasts less than 15 minutes
    e. Sharp, stabbing pain which is moderate to severe

38. The nurse working in a women's health clinic is reviewing the risk factors for several patients for stroke and myocardial infarction (MI). Which patient has the highest risk for MI?
    a. 49-year-old on estrogen replacement therapy
    b. 40-year-old taking oral contraceptives who smokes
    c. 23-year-old with diabetes that is currently not well-controlled
    d. 60-year-old with well-controlled hypertension

39. A patient comes to the emergency department (ED) reporting chest pain. In evaluating the patient's pain, which questions does the nurse ask the patient? *(Select all that apply.)*
    a. "How long does the pain last and how often does it occur?"
    b. "How do you feel about the pain?"
    c. "Is the pain different from any other episodes of pain you've had?"
    d. "What activities were you doing when the pain first occurred?"
    e. "Where is the chest pain? What does it feel like?"
    f. "Have you had other signs and symptoms that occur at the same time?"

40. The nurse is instructing a patient with congestive heart failure (CHF) on what signs to look for when experiencing an exacerbation of CHF. Which are appropriate teaching points for this patient? *(Select all that apply.)*
    a. "It is possible to gain up to 10 or 15 lbs before edema develops."
    b. "Notify the provider of a weight loss of 3 to 5 lbs within 2 weeks."
    c. "Notify the provider of a weight gain of 2 lbs within 1 to 2 days."
    d. "Notify the provider if you notice that your shoes or rings feel tight."
    e. "Notify the provider if your skin becomes dry and scaly."

41. A 65-year-old patient comes to the clinic reporting fatigue. The patient would like to start an exercise program, but thinks "anemia might be causing the fatigue." What is the nurse's first action?
    a. Advise the patient to start out slowly and gradually build strength and endurance.
    b. Obtain an order for a complete blood count and nutritional profile.
    c. Assess the onset, duration, and circumstances associated with the fatigue.
    d. Perform a physical assessment to include testing of muscle strength and tone.

42. A young patient reports having frequent episodes of palpitations but denies having chest pain. Which follow-up question does the nurse ask to assess the patient's symptom of palpitations?
    a. "Have you noticed a worsening of shortness of breath when you are lying flat?"
    b. "Do your shoes feel unusually tight, or are your rings tighter than usual?"
    c. "Do you feel dizzy or have you lost consciousness with the palpitations?"
    d. "Does anyone in your family have a history of palpitations?"

43. Syncope in the aging person can likely occur with which actions by the patient? *(Select all that apply.)*
    a. Laughing
    b. Turning the head
    c. Performing a Valsalva maneuver
    d. Walking briskly for 20 to 30 minutes
    e. Shrugging the shoulders

44. The nurse performing a physical assessment on a patient with a history of CVD observes that the patient has ascites, jaundice, and anasarca. How does the nurse interpret these findings?
    a. Late signs of severe right-sided heart failure
    b. Early signs of mild right-sided heart failure
    c. Late signs of mild left-sided heart failure
    d. Early signs of left- and right-sided heart failure

45. The nurse is performing an assessment on a patient brought in by emergency personnel. The nurse immediately observes that the patient has spontaneous respirations and the skin is cool, pale, and moist. What is the priority patient problem?
    a. Abnormal body temperature
    b. Impaired oxygenation
    c. Altered skin integrity
    d. Potential for peripheral neurovascular dysfunction

46. The nurse is caring for a patient at risk for MI. For what primary reason does the nurse plan interventions to prevent anxiety or overexertion?
    a. An increase in heart rate increases myocardial oxygen demand.
    b. A release of epinephrine and norepinephrine causes MI.
    c. An increase in activity or emotion effects preload and afterload.
    d. Cardiac output is decreased by anxiety or physical stress.

47. The nurse is caring for a patient with the priority problem of decreased cardiac output. Which situation may result in decreased myocardial contractility that will further lower cardiac output?
    a. Administration of a positive inotropic medication
    b. Hyperventilation to correct respiratory acidosis
    c. Frequent endotracheal suctioning that results in hypoxemia
    d. Administration of IV fluids to correct underlying hypovolemia

48. A patient reports severe cramping in the legs while attempting to walk for exercise. The provider diagnoses the patient with intermittent claudication. What does the nurse advise the patient to do?
    a. Elevate the legs on a pillow.
    b. Buy and wear supportive shoes.
    c. Massage the legs before walking.
    d. Rest the legs in a dependent position.

49. A patient entering the cardiac rehabilitation unit seems optimistic and at times unexpectedly cheerful and upbeat. Which statement by the patient causes the nurse to suspect a maladaptive use of denial in the patient?
    a. "I am sick and tired of talking about these dietary restrictions. Could we talk about it tomorrow?"
    b. "Oh, I don't really need that medication information. I'm sure that I'll soon be able to get by without it."
    c. "This whole episode of heart problems has been an eye-opener for me, but I really can't wait to get out of here."
    d. "That doctor is really driving me crazy with all his instructions. Could you put all that information away in my suitcase?"

50. The nurse taking a medical history of a patient makes a special notation to follow up on valvular abnormalities of the heart. Which recurrent condition in the patient's history causes the nurse to make this notation?
    a. Streptococcal infections of the throat
    b. Staphylococcal infections of the skin
    c. Vaginal yeast infections
    d. Fungal infections of the feet or inner thighs

51. The nurse interprets a patient's serum lipid tests. Which results suggest an increased risk for CVD? *(Select all that apply.)*
    a. LDL 160 mg/dL
    b. HDL 60 mg/dL
    c. Total cholesterol 180 mg/dL
    d. Triglycerides 175 mg/dL
    e. Lp(a) 45 mg/dL

52. What is the most significant laboratory cardiac marker in a patient who has had an MI?
    a. Presence of troponin T and I
    b. Elevation of myoglobin levels
    c. Creatine kinase levels
    d. Elevation of the white blood cell count

53. A patient in the ED with chest pain has a possible MI. Which laboratory test is done to determine this diagnosis?
   a. Troponin T and I
   b. Serum potassium
   c. Homocysteine
   d. Highly sensitive C-reactive protein

54. Which laboratory tests are used to predict a patient's risk for coronary artery disease (CAD)? *(Select all that apply.)*
   a. Cholesterol level
   b. Triglyceride level
   c. Prothrombin time
   d. Low-density lipoprotein level
   e. Albumin level

55. The patient with a history of allergy to iodine-based contrast dyes is scheduled for a cardiac catheterization. What action does the nurse expect with regard to the scheduled test?
   a. Delay the test for a week or more.
   b. Administer an antihistamine and/or steroid before the test.
   c. The test will be performed without administration of contrast dye.
   d. The patient will receive anticoagulation therapy before the test.

56. A patient is undergoing diagnostic testing for reports of chest pain. Which test is done to determine the location and extent of CAD?
   a. ECG
   b. Echocardiogram
   c. Cardiac catheterization
   d. Chest x-ray

57. Which medications will the nurse be sure to hold until after a patient's cardiac catheterization?
   a. Daily vitamin and enteric coated aspirin
   b. Atenolol and IV antibiotic
   c. Potassium and folic acid
   d. Digoxin and furosemide

58. Which interventions and actions does the nurse perform to detect and prevent kidney toxicity when caring for a patient after cardiac catheterization? *(Select all that apply.)*
   a. Provide IV and oral fluids for 12 to 24 hours.
   b. Monitor intake and output.
   c. Check the catheterization site every hour.
   d. Administer acetylcysteine if ordered
   e. Keep the catheterized extremity straight for 6 hours.

59. Microalbuminuria has been shown to be a clear marker of widespread endothelial dysfunction in CVD. Which conditions should prompt patients to be tested annually for microalbuminuria? *(Select all that apply.)*
   a. Hypertension
   b. Metabolic syndrome
   c. Smoker
   d. Diabetes mellitus
   e. Use of anticoagulant therapy

60. A patient is being discharged with a prescription for warfarin (Coumadin). Which test does the nurse instruct the patient to routinely have done for follow-up monitoring?
   a. Prothrombin time (PT) and International Normalized Ratio (INR)
   b. Partial thromboplastin time (PTT)
   c. Complete blood count and platelet count
   d. Sodium and potassium levels

61. What is the significance of a sodium level of 130 mEq/L for a patient with heart failure?
   a. Increased risk for ventricular dysrhythmias
   b. Dilutional hyponatremia and fluid retention
   c. Potential for electrical instability of the heart
   d. Slowed conduction of impulse through the heart

62. Which test is performed to determine valve disease of the mitral valve, left atrium, or aortic arch?
    a. Transesophageal echocardiogram
    b. ECG
    c. Myocardial nuclear perfusion imaging (MNPI)
    d. Phonocardiography

63. A patient is scheduled to have an exercise electrocardiography test. What instruction does the nurse provide to the patient before the procedure takes place?
    a. "Have nothing to eat or drink after midnight."
    b. "Avoid smoking or drinking alcohol for at least 2 weeks before the test."
    c. "Wear comfortable, loose clothing and rubber-soled, supportive shoes."
    d. "Someone must drive you home because of possible sedative effects of the medications."

64. A nurse is monitoring the patient's blood pressure and ECG during a stress test. Which parameter indicates the patient should stop exercising?
    a. Increase in heart rate
    b. Increase in blood pressure
    c. ECG showing the PQRS complex
    d. ECG showing ST-segment depression

65. What measures are taken to prepare a patient for a pharmacologic stress echocardiogram? *(Select all that apply.)*
    a. Patient can eat his/her diet as ordered.
    b. IV access needs to be present.
    c. Oxygen at 2 L per nasal cannula is placed on patient 3 hours prior to test.
    d. An oral laxative is given the day before the test.
    e. Patient is to be NPO for 3 to 6 hours before the test.

66. What are the purposes of angiography? *(Select all that apply.)*
    a. Determine an abnormal structure of the heart
    b. Identify an arterial obstruction
    c. Assess the cardiovascular response to increased workload
    d. Identify an arterial narrowing
    e. Identify an aneurysm

67. What is included in postprocedural care of a patient after a cardiac catheterization? *(Select all that apply.)*
    a. Patient remains on bedrest for 12 to 24 hours.
    b. Patient is placed in a high-Fowler's position.
    c. Dressing is assessed for bloody drainage or hematoma.
    d. Peripheral pulses in the affected extremity, as well as skin temperature and color, are monitored with every vital sign check.
    e. Adequate oral and IV fluids are provided for hydration.
    f. Vital signs are monitored every hour for 24 hours.

68. Which assessment finding in a patient who has had a cardiac catheterization does the nurse report immediately to the provider?
    a. Pain at the catheter insertion site
    b. Catheterized extremity dusky with decreased peripheral pulses
    c. Small hematoma at the catheter insertion site
    d. Pulse pressure of 40 mm Hg with a slow, bounding pulse

69. The nurse is providing discharge instructions for a patient who had a cardiac catheterization. Which instructions must the nurse include? *(Select all that apply.)*
    a. Notify the health care provider for increased swelling, redness, warmth, or pain.
    b. Leave the dressing in place for the first day.
    c. Limit activity for at least 2 to 3 weeks.
    d. Avoid lifting and exercise for a few days.
    e. Report any bruise or hematoma to the health care provider.

70. The patient is scheduled for an exercise stress test. Which medications does the nurse expect the cardiologist will want held before the procedure?
   a. Atenolol and Cardizem
   b. Vitamins and potassium
   c. Colace and enteric-coated aspirin
   d. Acetaminophen and metered-dose bronchodilator

34 CHAPTER

Care of Patients with Dysrhythmias

1. What does stimulation of the sympathetic nervous system produce?
   a. Delayed electrical impulse that causes hypotension and bradypnea
   b. Contractility and dilation of coronary vessels and increased heart rate
   c. Virtually no effect on the ventricles of the heart or vital signs
   d. A slowed atrioventricular (AV) conduction time that results in a slow heart rate

2. The primary pacemaker of the heart, the sinoatrial (SA) node, is functional if a patient's pulse is at what regular rate?
   a. Fewer than 60 beats/min
   b. 60 to 100 beats/min
   c. 80 to 100 beats/min
   d. Greater than 100 beats/min

3. The nurse is taking vital signs and reviewing the electrocardiogram (ECG) of a patient who is training for a marathon. The heart rate is 45 beats/min and the ECG shows sinus bradycardia. How does the nurse interpret this data?
   a. A rapid filling rate that lengthens diastolic filling time and leads to decreased cardiac output
   b. The body's attempt to compensate for a decreased stroke volume by decreasing the heart rate
   c. An adequate stroke volume that is associated with cardiac conditioning
   d. A common finding in the healthy adult that would be considered normal

4. The nurse is performing the shift assessment on a cardiac patient. In order to determine if the patient has a pulse deficit, what does the nurse do?
   a. Take the patient's blood pressure and subtract the diastolic from the systolic pressure.
   b. Take the patient's pulse in a supine position and then in a standing position.
   c. Assess the apical and radial pulses for a full minute and observe for differences.
   d. Take the radial pulse, have the patient rest for 15 minutes, and then retake the pulse.

5. What does the P wave in an ECG represent?
   a. Atrial depolarization
   b. Atrial repolarization
   c. Ventricular depolarization
   d. Ventricular repolarization

6. What is the normal measurement of the PR interval in an ECG?
   a. Less than 0.11 second
   b. 0.06 to 0.10 second
   c. 0.12 to 0.20 second
   d. 0.16 to 0.26 second

7. What is the QRS complex in an ECG normally?
   a. Less than 0.12 second
   b. 0.10 to 0.16 second
   c. 0.12 to 0.20 second
   d. 0.16 to 0.24 second

8. What is the ST segment in an ECG normally?
   a. Isoelectric
   b. Elevated
   c. Depressed
   d. Biphasic

9. What is the total time required for ventricular depolarization and repolarization as represented on the ECG?
   a. PR interval
   b. QRS complex
   c. ST segment
   d. QT interval

10. The nurse is performing a 12-lead ECG on a patient with chest pain. Because the positioning of the electrodes is crucial, how does the nurse place the ECG components?
    a. Four leads are placed on the limbs and six are placed on the chest.
    b. The negative electrode is placed on the left arm and the positive electrode is placed on the right leg.
    c. Four leads are placed on the limbs and four are placed on the chest.
    d. The negative electrode is placed on the right arm and the positive electrode is placed on the left leg.

11. Cardiac dysrhythmias are abnormal rhythms of the heart's electrical system. How does this affect the heart's function?
    a. It cannot oxygenate the blood throughout the body.
    b. It cannot remove carbon dioxide from the body.
    c. It cannot effectively pump oxygenated blood throughout the body.
    d. It cannot effectively conduct impulses with increased activity.

12. The nurse is caring for several patients in the telemetry unit who are being remotely watched by a monitor technician. What is the nurse's primary responsibility in the monitoring process of these patients?
    a. Watching the bank of monitors on the unit
    b. Printing ECG rhythm strips routinely and as needed
    c. Interpreting rhythms
    d. Assessment and management

13. A patient in the telemetry unit is having continuous ECG monitoring. The patient is scheduled for a test in the radiology department. Who is responsible for determining when monitoring can be suspended?
    a. Telemetry technician
    b. Charge nurse
    c. Health care provider
    d. Primary nurse

14. The nurse is reviewing preliminary ECG results of a patient admitted for mental status changes. The nurse alerts the health care provider about ST elevation or depression in the patient because it is an indication of which condition?
    a. Myocardial injury or ischemia
    b. Ventricular irritability
    c. Subarachnoid hemorrhage
    d. Prinzmetal's angina

15. The nurse is reviewing ECG results of a patient admitted for fluid and electrolyte imbalances. The T waves are tall and peaked. The nurse reports this finding to the provider and obtains an order for which serum level test?
    a. Sodium
    b. Glucose
    c. Potassium
    d. Phosphorus

16. Which actions are the responsibilities of the monitor tech? (Select all that apply.)
    a. Watch the bank of monitors on a unit.
    b. Notify the health care provider of any changes.
    c. Print routine ECG strips.
    d. Apply battery-operated transmitter leads to patients.
    e. Interpret the rhythms.

17. The nurse is notified by the telemetry monitor technician about a patient's heart rate. Which method does the nurse use to confirm the technician's report?
    a. Count QRS complexes in a 6-second strip and multiply by 10.
    b. Analyze an ECG rhythm strip by using an ECG caliper.
    c. Run an ECG rhythm strip and use the memory method.
    d. Assess the patient's heart rate directly by taking an apical pulse.

18. The nurse has four patients on telemetry monitors and is analyzing the ECG rhythm strips. What is the nurse's first action?
    a. Analyze the P waves.
    b. Determine the heart rate.
    c. Measure the QRS duration.
    d. Measure the PR interval.

19. A patient's ECG rhythm strip is irregular. Which method does the nurse use for an accurate assessment?
    a. 6-second strip method
    b. Memory method
    c. Big block method
    d. Commercial ECG rate ruler

20. The nurse is assessing a patient's ECG rhythm strip and checking the regularity of the atrial rhythm. What is the correct technique?
    a. Place one caliper point on a QRS complex; place the other point on the precise spot on the next QRS complex.
    b. Place one caliper point on a P wave; place the other point on the precise spot on the next P wave.
    c. Place one caliper point at the beginning of the P wave; place the other point at the end of the P-R segment.
    d. Place one caliper point at the beginning of the QRS complex; place and the other point where the S-T segment begins.

21. The nurse is assessing a patient's ECG rhythm strip and analyzing the P waves. Which questions does the nurse use to evaluate the P waves? *(Select all that apply.)*
    a. Are P waves present?
    b. Are the P waves occurring regularly?
    c. Does one P wave follow each QRS complex?
    d. Are the P waves greater than 0.20 second?
    e. Do all the P waves look similar?
    f. Are the P waves smooth, rounded, and upright in appearance?

22. The nurse is assessing a patient's ECG rhythm strip and notes that occasionally the QRS complex is missing. How does the nurse interpret this finding?
    a. A junctional impulse
    b. A supraventricular impulse
    c. Ventricular tachycardia
    d. A dysrhythmia

23. The student nurse is looking at a patient's ECG rhythm strip and suspects a normal sinus rhythm (NSR). Which ECG criteria are included for NSR? *(Select all that apply.)*
    a. Rate: Atrial and ventricular rates of 40 to 120 beats/min
    b. Rhythm: Atrial and ventricular rhythms regular
    c. P waves: Present, consistent configuration, one P wave before each QRS complex
    d. P-R interval 0.24 second
    e. QRS duration: 0.04 to 0.10 second and constant

24. The heart monitor of a patient shows a rhythm that appears as a wandering or fuzzy baseline. What is the priority action for the nurse?
    a. Immediately obtain a 12-lead ECG to assess the actual rhythm.
    b. Assess the patient to differentiate artifact from actual lethal rhythms.
    c. Check to see if the patient has a do-not-resuscitate order.
    d. Ask the patient care technician to take vital signs on the patient.

25. What does the T wave on an ECG represent?
    a. Ventricular depolarization
    b. Atrial repolarization
    c. Atrial depolarization
    d. Ventricular repolarization

26. The remote telemetry technician calls the nurse to report that a patient's ECG signal transmission is not very clear. What does the nurse do to enhance the transmission?
    a. Clean the skin with povidone-iodine solution before applying the electrodes.
    b. Ensure that the area for electrode placement is dry and nonhairy.
    c. Apply tincture of benzoin to the electrode sites and allow it to dry.
    d. Abrade the skin by rubbing briskly with a rough washcloth.

27. With the speed set for 25 mm/second, the segment between the dark lines on a monitor ECG strip represents how many seconds?
    a. 3
    b. 6
    c. 10
    d. 20

28. Which components measure ECG waveforms?
    a. Blood pressure (BP) and cardiac output (CO)
    b. Seconds (sec) and minutes (min)
    c. Heart rate per minute (HR/min)
    d. Amplitude (voltage) and duration (time)

29. What is the heart rate from an ECG strip when there are 25 small blocks from one R wave to the next R wave?
    a. 50/minute
    b. 60/minute
    c. 70/minute
    d. 80/minute

30. What is the heart rate shown on a 6-second ECG strip when the number of R-R intervals is 5? What is this rhythm?
    a. 30/minute bradycardia
    b. 40/minute bradycardia
    c. 50/minute bradycardia
    d. 60/minute normal

31. How does the nurse interpret the measurement of the P-R interval when the interval to be measured is six small boxes on the ECG strip?
    a. Atrium is taking longer to repolarize.
    b. Longer-than-normal impulse time from the SA node to the ventricles is shown.
    c. There is a problem with the length of time the ventricles are depolarizing.
    d. This is the normal length of time for the P-R interval.

32. The nurse is reviewing a patient's ECG and interprets a wide distorted QRS complex of 0.14 second followed by a P wave. What does this finding indicate?
    a. Wide but normal complex, and no cause for concern
    b. Premature ventricular contraction
    c. Problem with the speed set on the ECG machine
    d. Delayed time of the electrical impulse through the ventricles

33. Which clinical manifestations are reflections of sustained tachydysrhythmias and bradydysrhythmias? *(Select all that apply.)*
    a. Weakness and fatigue
    b. Warm, dry skin
    c. Dyspnea
    d. Hypertension
    e. Decreased urine output

34. Which dysrhythmia results in asynchrony of atrial contraction and decreased cardiac output?
    a. Sinus tachycardia
    b. Atrial flutter
    c. Atrial fibrillation
    d. First-degree atrioventricular block

35. Which dysrhythmia causes the ventricles to quiver, resulting in absence of cardiac output?
    a. Ventricular tachycardia
    b. Ventricular fibrillation
    c. Asystole
    d. Third-degree heart block

36. The nurse hears in report that a patient has sinus arrhythmia. In order to validate that this is associated with the changes in intrathoracic pressure, what does the nurse do next?
    a. Count the respiratory and pulse rate at rest and then count both rates after moderate exertion.
    b. Observe that the heart rate increases slightly during inspiration and decreases slightly during exhalation.
    c. Ask the patient to hold the breath and take an apical pulse; then have the patient resume normal breathing.
    d. Have the patient take a deep breath and count the patient's apical pulse rate while the patient slowly exhales.

37. The nurse is caring for a patient with coronary artery disease (CAD). The patient reports palpitations and chest discomfort and the nurse notes a tachydysrhythmia on the ECG monitor. What does the nurse do next?
    a. Analyze the ECG strip.
    b. Notify the health care provider.
    c. Give supplemental oxygen.
    d. Administer a narcotic analgesic.

38. The nurse is taking the initial history and vital signs on a patient with fatigue. The nurse notes a regular apical pulse of 130 beats/min. Which contributing factors does the nurse assess for? *(Select all that apply.)*
    a. Anxiety or stress
    b. Fever
    c. Hypovolemia
    d. Anemia or hypoxemia
    e. Hypothyroidism
    f. Constipation

39. The nurse is taking a history and vital signs on a patient who has come to the clinic for a routine checkup. The patient has a pulse rate of 50 beats/min, but denies any distress. What does the nurse do next?
    a. Give supplemental oxygen.
    b. Establish IV access.
    c. Complete the health history.
    d. Check the blood pressure.

40. The nurse is reviewing the monitored rhythms of several patients in the cardiac stepdown unit. The patient with which cardiac anomaly has the greatest need of immediate attention?
    a. Chronic atrial fibrillation
    b. Paroxysmal supraventricular tachycardia (SVT) that is suddenly terminated
    c. Sustained rapid ventricular response
    d. Sinus tachycardia with premature atrial complexes

41. A patient is diagnosed with recurrent SVT. What does the nurse do in order to accomplish the preferred treatment?
    a. Place the patient on the cardiac monitor and perform carotid massage.
    b. Give oxygen and establish IV access for antidysrhythmic drugs.
    c. Assist the provider in attempting atrial overdrive pacing.
    d. Provide information about radiofrequency catheter ablation therapy.

42. The patient has sustained SVT and the health care provider orders IV adenosine. Which important actions must the nurse perform when this drug is given? *(Select all that apply.)*
    a. Inject the drug slowly over one minute.
    b. Have emergency equipment at the bedside.
    c. Follow the drug injection with a normal saline bolus.
    d. Have injectable beta blocker drugs at the bedside.
    e. Monitor the patient for bradycardia, nausea, and vomiting.

43. Based on the prevalence and risk factors for atrial fibrillation (AF), which patient group is at highest risk for AF?
    a. Older adults
    b. Diabetics
    c. Substance abusers
    d. Pediatric cardiology patients

44. What are the risk factors for AF? *(Select all that apply.)*
    a. Chronic obstructive pulmonary disease (COPD)
    b. Hypertension
    c. Peripheral vascular disease
    d. Diabetes mellitus
    e. Valvular disease

45. A patient with AF suddenly develops shortness of breath, chest pain, hemoptysis, and a feeling of impending doom. The nurse recognizes these symptoms as which complication?
    a. Pulmonary embolism
    b. Embolic stroke
    c. Absence of atrial kick
    d. Increased cardiac output

46. A patient scheduled to have elective cardioversion for AF will receive drug therapy for about 6 weeks before the procedure. What information about the drug therapy does the nurse teach the patient?
    a. Managing orthostatic hypotension
    b. Watching for bleeding signs
    c. Eating potassium-rich food sources
    d. Reporting muscle weakness or tremors

47. The bedside cardiac monitor of a postoperative patient who becomes confused shows sinus rhythm, but there is no palpable pulse. How does the nurse interpret these findings?
    a. ECG monitor artifact or dysfunction
    b. Pulseless electrical activity with inadequate perfusion
    c. A paced rhythm with hypotension
    d. Idioventricular rhythm as seen in the dying heart

48. The remote telemetry technician alerts the nurse to the presence of premature ventricular contractions (PVCs) in a newly admitted patient. How does the nurse assess whether the premature complexes perfuse to the extremities?
    a. Palpate peripheral arteries while observing the monitor for widened complexes.
    b. Auscultate for the apical heart sounds and listen for irregularities or pauses.
    c. Check the color and temperature of extremities, and capillary refill of fingers and toes.
    d. Assess the ECG strip for regularity and width of QRS complexes.

49. What is the primary significance of ventricular tachycardia (VT) in a cardiac patient?
    a. It increases the ventricular filling time, therefore increasing cardiac output.
    b. It signals that the patient needs potassium supplement for replacement.
    c. It warrants immediate initiation of cardiopulmonary resuscitation.
    d. It is commonly the initial rhythm before deterioration into ventricular fibrillation (VF).

50. The nurse is interviewing a patient who suddenly becomes faint, immediately loses consciousness, and becomes pulseless and apneic. There is no blood pressure, and heart sounds are absent. What does the nurse do next?
    a. Begin compressions.
    b. Defibrillate the patient.
    c. Establish or ensure IV access.
    d. Give supplemental oxygen.

51. A patient is in full cardiac arrest and CPR is in progress. The ECG monitor shows ventricular asystole. What does the nurse do next?
    a. Assist with or administer defibrillation.
    b. Assess another ECG lead to ensure the rhythm is asystole and not fine VF.
    c. Assist the provider with noninvasive pacing or invasive transvenous pacing.
    d. Encourage the family's presence during the resuscitation.

52. Traditionally, what medications will most likely be ordered for a patient with AF? *(Select all that apply.)*
    a. Diltiazem hydrochloride (Cardizem)
    b. Furosemide (Lasix)
    c. Heparin
    d. Enoxaparin (Lovenox)
    e. Sodium warfarin (Coumadin)

53. A patient is diagnosed with torsades de pointes. The nurse prepares to administer which emergency medication?
    a. Magnesium sulfate
    b. Epinephrine (Adrenalin)
    c. Adenosine (Adenocard)
    d. Calcium chloride

54. In a patient's record, the nurse notes frequent episodes of bradycardia and hypotension related to unintended vagal stimulation. Which instruction for this patient's care does the nurse relay to the unlicensed assistive personnel (UAP)?
    a. Avoid raising the patient's arms above the head during hygiene.
    b. Ambulate the patient slowly and stop frequently for brief rests.
    c. Generously lubricate rectal thermometer probes and insert very cautiously.
    d. Monitor the heart rate and rhythm if the patient is vomiting.

55. Excessive vagal stimulation can result from which activities? *(Select all that apply.)*
    a. Jogging
    b. Carotid sinus massage
    c. Suctioning
    d. Voiding
    e. Valsalva maneuver

56. The nurse is caring for several patients who have a dysrhythmia. What does the nurse instruct these patients to do?
    a. Stay at least 4 feet away from a microwave oven that is operating.
    b. Avoid electronic metal detectors, such as those at airports.
    c. Learn the procedure for assessing the pulse.
    d. Purchase an automatic external defibrillator (AED) for home use.

57. A patient reports chest pain and dizziness after exertion, and the family reports a concurrent new onset of mild confusion in the patient, as well as difficulty concentrating. What is the priority problem for this patient?
    a. Activity intolerance
    b. Decreased cardiac output
    c. Acute confusion
    d. Inadequate oxygenation

58. According to the Vaughn-Williams classification of antidysrhythmics, which class II drug controls dysrhythmias associated with excessive beta-adrenergic stimulation?
    a. Amiodarone hydrochloride (Cordarone)
    b. Propranolol hydrochloride (Inderal)
    c. Diltiazem (Cardizem)
    d. Verapamil hydrochloride (Calan)

59. Which drug for symptomatic bradycardia does the nurse prepare to administer to a patient with a bradydysrhythmia?
    a. Epinephrine
    b. Atropine
    c. Calcium
    d. Lidocaine

60. Which medication does an adult patient with VF or pulseless VT receive?
    a. Propranolol (Inderal)
    b. Adenosine (Adenocard)
    c. Diltiazem hydrochloride (Cardizem)
    d. Epinephrine (Adrenalin chloride)

61. The respiratory therapist (RT) and the medical student are ventilating a patient in cardiac arrest, while the nurse and provider are preparing the patient and equipment for intubation. At which point does the nurse intervene?
    a. The RT inserts an oropharyngeal airway.
    b. The medical student sets the oxygen flow meter at 2 L/min.
    c. The RT ventilates with a manual resuscitation bag and mask.
    d. The medical student uses the chin-lift position on the patient.

62. After advanced cardiac life support (ACLS) is performed, a patient who experienced VF has a return of spontaneous circulation. To protect the patient's nervous system, which intervention does the nurse anticipate will be performed?
    a. Neurologic checks every 4 hours
    b. Administration of IV mannitol
    c. Application of a cooling blanket
    d. Continuous ECG monitoring

63. The nurse discovers a patient is unconscious and without palpable pulses and immediately initiates CPR. For what reason is CPR started on this patient?
    a. To identify the underlying heart rhythm
    b. For the rapid return of a pulse, blood pressure, and consciousness
    c. To prevent rib fractures or lacerations of the liver and spleen
    d. To mimic cardiac function until the defibrillator arrives

64. AED electrodes are placed on a patient who is unconscious and pulseless. The nurse prepares to immediately defibrillate if the monitor shows which cardiac anomaly?
    a. Third-degree heart block
    b. Pulseless electrical activity
    c. VF
    d. Idioventricular rhythm

65. A patient is found pulseless and the cardiac monitor shows a rhythm that has no recognizable deflections, but instead has coarse "waves" of varying amplitudes. What is the priority ACLS intervention for this rhythm?
    a. Immediate defibrillation
    b. Administration of epinephrine IVP
    c. Administration of lidocaine IVP
    d. Noninvasive temporary pacing

66. What other actions are essential interventions for the patient in question 65? (Select all that apply.)
    a. Providing effective CPR
    b. Supplying a temporary pacemaker
    c. Administrating epinephrine, vasopressin, and atropine, as appropriate
    d. Identifying and correcting the cause of the pulseless rhythm
    e. Providing continuous ECG monitoring

67. A patient has no pulse and the cardiac monitor shows VF. Which drugs does the nurse prepare to administer during the resuscitation? (Select all that apply.)
    a. Lidocaine
    b. Epinephrine
    c. Calcium chloride
    d. Amiodarone hydrochloride (Cordarone)
    e. Dopamine hydrochloride (Intropin)
    f. Magnesium sulfate

68. The nurse is placing the electrodes on a patient for cardioversion. What is the correct placement for the electrodes?
    a. One electrode is placed on the upper left chest and the other is placed on the lower left chest in a midaxillary line.
    b. One electrode is placed the upper right chest below the clavicle and the other is placed on the back.
    c. One electrode is placed to the left of the precordium, and the other is placed on the right next to the sternum and below the clavicle.
    d. One electrode is placed on the sternum and the other is placed on the lower left chest in a midaxillary line.

69. A patient is in VF. The nurse sets the biphasic defibrillator to deliver how many joules?
    a. 100
    b. 200
    c. 300
    d. 360

70. A patient is about to undergo elective cardioversion. The nurse sets the defibrillator for synchronized mode so that the electrical shock is not delivered on the T wave. This is done to avoid which complication?
    a. Electrical burns to the skin
    b. Ventricular standstill
    c. Arcing from the electrodes
    d. VF

71. The nurse is performing external defibrillation. Which step is most vital this procedure?
    a. Place the gel pads anterior over the apex and posterior for better conduction.
    b. Do not administer a second shock for 1 minute to allow for recharging.
    c. No-one must touch the patient at the time a shock is delivered.
    d. Continuously ventilate the patient via endotracheal tube during the defibrillation.

72. Which definition best describes the synchronous (demand) pacing mode?
    a. The pacemaker continues to fire at a fixed rate as set on the generator.
    b. The pacemaker's sensitivity is set to sense the patient's own beats.
    c. Electrical pulses are transmitted through two large external electrodes then transcutaneously to stimulate ventricular depolarization.
    d. External battery-operated pulse generator on one end and wires in contact with the heart on the other end.

73. The nurse is assisting the provider to perform temporary pacing for a patient who has atropine-refractory symptomatic bradycardia. What is the desired outcome for this patient as evidenced by the cardiac monitor?
    a. No spike, but a complete QRS complex indicating atrial depolarization
    b. A spike followed by a QRS complex indicating ventricular depolarization
    c. Two spikes, followed by a QRS complex indicating ventricular depolarization
    d. A spike before and after a QRS complex indicating atrial depolarization

74. The provider has completed the placement of lead wires for the invasive temporary pacemaker in a patient who is asystolic. In turning on the pacing unit, which setting does the nurse use?
    a. Synchronous pacing mode
    b. Demand pacing mode
    c. Asynchronous pacing mode
    d. Temporary pacing mode

75. The nurse in the telemetry unit must perform transcutaneous pacing. How does the nurse position the electrodes?
    a. One over breast tissue on the right side and one over breast tissue on left side
    b. One on the upper chest to the left of the sternum and one beneath the left scapula
    c. One on the upper chest to the right of the sternum and one over the heart apex
    d. One over the sternum and one on the left anterior lateral chest

76. A patient has an invasive temporary pacemaker. In what ways does the nurse ensure the patient's safety related to electrical issues with the pacemaker? *(Select all that apply.)*
    a. Ensure that external ends of the lead wires are insulated with rubber gloves.
    b. Loop the wire ends and cover with non-conductive tape.
    c. Ensure that no electrical equipment is used in the patient's room.
    d. Report frayed wire to the biomedical engineering department.
    e. Wash hands before touching any of the wires.

77. What effects does dobutamine (Dobutrex) have on the heart? *(Select all that apply.)*
    a. Decreases myocardial contractility
    b. Stimulates beta-adrenergic receptors
    c. Improves myocardial contractility
    d. Depresses stimulation of beta-adrenergic receptors
    e. May cause dysrhythmias

78. Which descriptions are characteristic of a class III antidysrhythmic? *(Select all that apply.)*
    a. Lengthens the absolute refractory period
    b. Is a beta blocker
    c. Includes hypertension as a side effect
    d. Prolongs repolarization
    e. Includes bradycardia as a side effect

79. A patient has an implantable cardioverter defibrillator (ICD). In cardioversion shock, the defibrillator is set in the synchronized mode to do what?
    a. Avoid discharging the shock during the T wave
    b. Discharge the shock during the R wave
    c. Discharge the shock during the T wave
    d. Avoid discharging the shock during the Q wave

80. A patient with atrial fibrillation is scheduled to have an elective cardioversion. The nurse ensures that the patient has a prescription for a 4-6 week supply of which type of medication?
    a. Anticoagulants
    b. Digitalis
    c. Diuretics
    d. Potassium supplements

81. The nurse is teaching a patient with an ICD. What instruction does the nurse emphasize to the patient?
    a. Rest for several hours after an internal defibrillator shock before resuming activities.
    b. Have family members step away during the internal defibrillator shock for safety.
    c. Expect that the shock may feel like a thud or a painful kick in the chest.
    d. Report any pulse rate higher than what is set on the pacemaker.

82. A patient has had synchronized cardioversion for unstable VT. Which interventions does the nurse include in this patient's care after the procedure? *(Select all that apply.)*
    a. Administer therapeutic hypothermia.
    b. Assess vital signs and the level of consciousness.
    c. Administer antidysrhythmic drug therapy.
    d. Monitor for dysrhythmias.
    e. Monitor for loss of capture.
    f. Assess for chest burns from electrodes.

83. The nurse is teaching a community group how to use an AED. What is the first step for using the AED that the nurse teaches?
    a. Rescuer presses the "analyze" button on the machine.
    b. Place the patient on a firm, dry surface.
    c. Rescuer stops CPR and directs anyone present to move away.
    d. Place two large adhesive-patch electrodes on the patient's chest.

84. A patient has had a permanent pacemaker surgically implanted. What are the nursing responsibilities for the care of this patient related to the surgery? *(Select all that apply.)*
    a. Administer short-acting sedatives.
    b. Assess the implantation site for bleeding, swelling, redness, tenderness, or infection.
    c. Teach about and monitor for the initial activity restrictions.
    d. Observe for overstimulation of the chest wall, which could lead to pneumothorax.
    e. Monitor the ECG rhythm to check that the pacemaker is working correctly.

85. The nurse is interviewing a patient with spontaneous VT who may be a possible candidate for an ICD. The nurse senses that the patient is anxious. What is the nurse's most therapeutic response?
   a. "Your feelings are natural; patients report psychological distress related to ICD."
   b. "ICD is similar to defibrillation, which saved your life during the last episode."
   c. "You seem anxious. What are your concerns about having this treatment?"
   d. "Would you like to talk to the doctor about the details of the procedure?"

86. The nurse is teaching a patient with a permanent pacemaker. What information about the pacemaker does the nurse tell the patient? *(Select all that apply.)*
   a. Report any pulse rate lower than what is set on the pacemaker.
   b. If the surgical incision is near the shoulder, avoid overextending the joint.
   c. Keep handheld cellular phones at least 6 inches away from the generator.
   d. Avoid sources of strong electromagnetic fields, such as magnets.
   e. Avoid strenuous activities that may cause the device to discharge inappropriately.
   f. Carry a pacemaker identification card and wear a medical alert bracelet.

Interpret each ECG strip below. Write your answers in the blanks provided.

87. _____

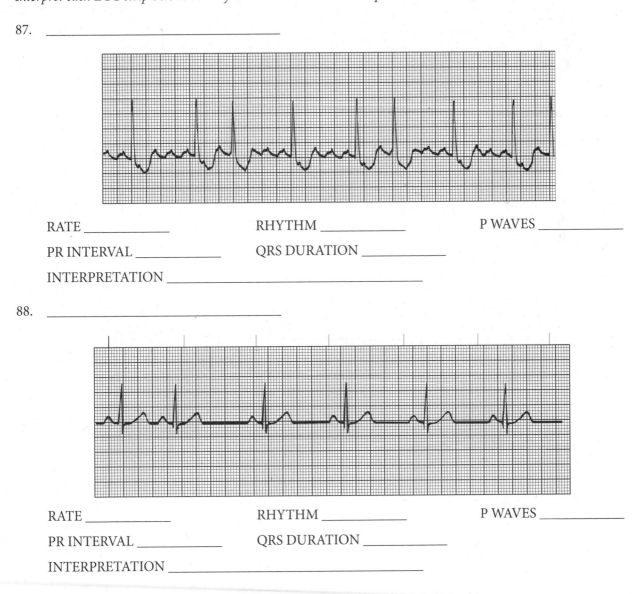

RATE _____   RHYTHM _____   P WAVES _____

PR INTERVAL _____   QRS DURATION _____

INTERPRETATION _____

88. _____

RATE _____   RHYTHM _____   P WAVES _____

PR INTERVAL _____   QRS DURATION _____

INTERPRETATION _____

89.   _____

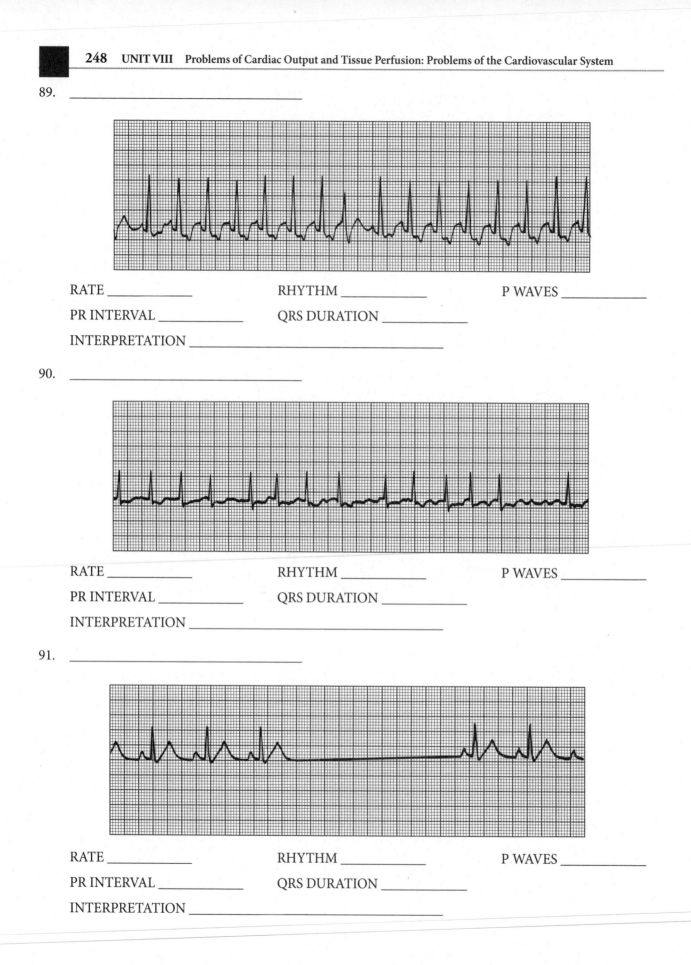

RATE _____   RHYTHM _____   P WAVES _____

PR INTERVAL _____   QRS DURATION _____

INTERPRETATION _____

90.   _____

RATE _____   RHYTHM _____   P WAVES _____

PR INTERVAL _____   QRS DURATION _____

INTERPRETATION _____

91.   _____

RATE _____   RHYTHM _____   P WAVES _____

PR INTERVAL _____   QRS DURATION _____

INTERPRETATION _____

92. _____

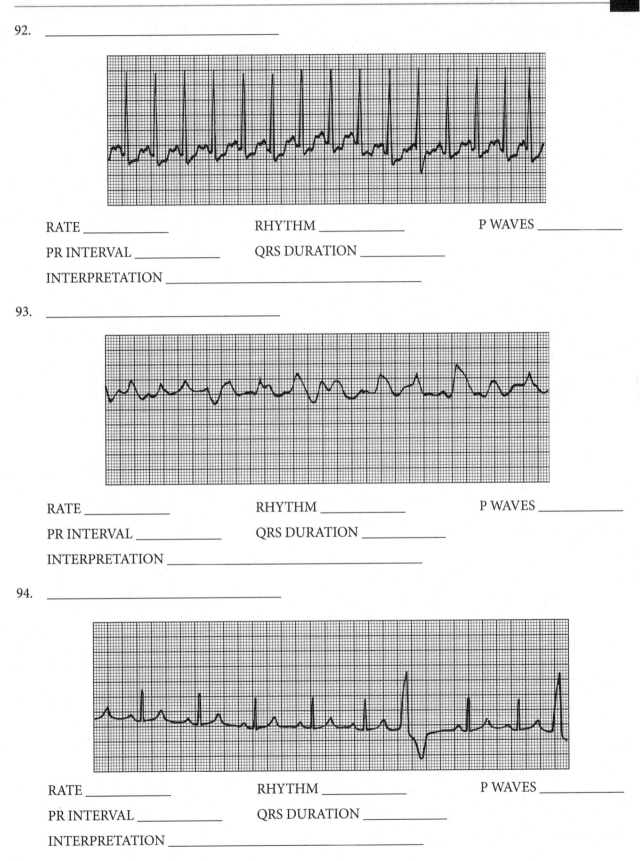

RATE _____   RHYTHM _____   P WAVES _____

PR INTERVAL _____   QRS DURATION _____

INTERPRETATION _____

93. _____

RATE _____   RHYTHM _____   P WAVES _____

PR INTERVAL _____   QRS DURATION _____

INTERPRETATION _____

94. _____

RATE _____   RHYTHM _____   P WAVES _____

PR INTERVAL _____   QRS DURATION _____

INTERPRETATION _____

95. _____

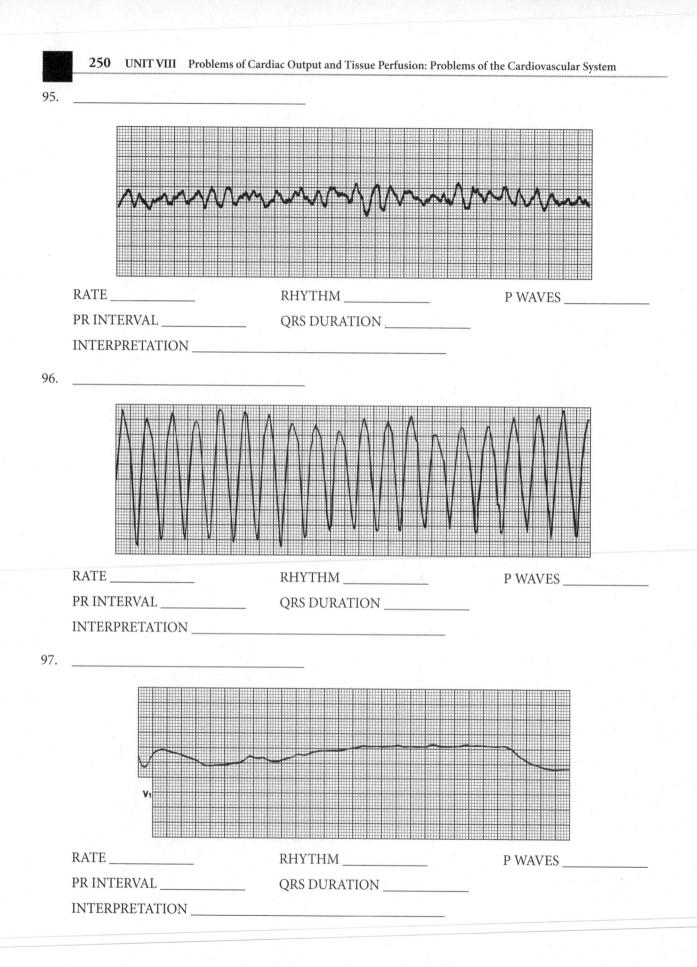

RATE _____ RHYTHM _____ P WAVES _____

PR INTERVAL _____ QRS DURATION _____

INTERPRETATION _____

96. _____

RATE _____ RHYTHM _____ P WAVES _____

PR INTERVAL _____ QRS DURATION _____

INTERPRETATION _____

97. _____

V₁

RATE _____ RHYTHM _____ P WAVES _____

PR INTERVAL _____ QRS DURATION _____

INTERPRETATION _____

98. _____

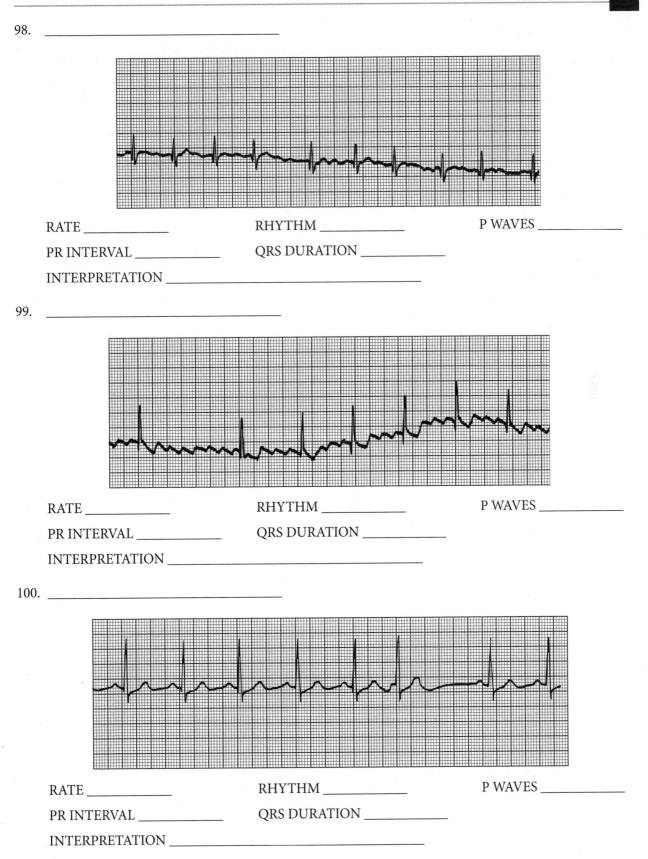

RATE _____   RHYTHM _____   P WAVES _____

PR INTERVAL _____   QRS DURATION _____

INTERPRETATION _____

99. _____

RATE _____   RHYTHM _____   P WAVES _____

PR INTERVAL _____   QRS DURATION _____

INTERPRETATION _____

100. _____

RATE _____   RHYTHM _____   P WAVES _____

PR INTERVAL _____   QRS DURATION _____

INTERPRETATION _____

101. _____

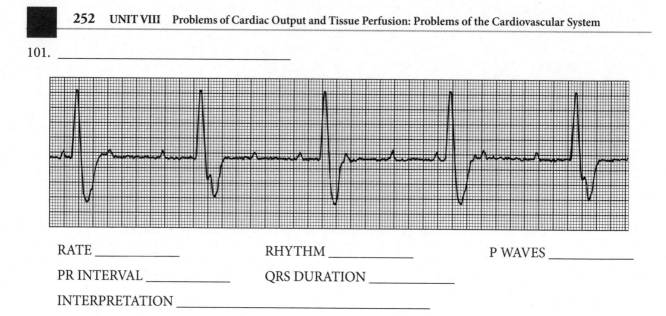

RATE _____   RHYTHM _____   P WAVES _____

PR INTERVAL _____   QRS DURATION _____

INTERPRETATION _____

35 CHAPTER

Care of Patients with Cardiac Problems

1. Which definition best describes left-sided heart failure?
   a. Increased volume and pressure develop and result in peripheral edema.
   b. Can occur when cardiac output remains normal or above normal.
   c. Decreased tissue perfusion from poor cardiac output and pulmonary congestion from increased pressure in the pulmonary vessels.
   d. Percentage of blood ejected from the heart during systole.

2. During assessment of a patient with heart failure, the nurse notes that the patient's pulses alternate in strength. What does this assessment indicate to the nurse?
   a. Pulsus paradoxus
   b. Orthostatic hypotension
   c. Hypotension
   d. Pulsus alternans

3. When heart failure develops, what is the initial compensatory mechanism of the heart that maintains cardiac output?
   a. Sympathetic stimulation
   b. Parasympathetic stimulation
   c. Renin-angiotensin activation system (RAAS)
   d. Myocardial hypertrophy

4. When is B-type natriuretic peptide (BNP) produced and released for a patient with heart failure?
   a. When a patient has an enlarged liver
   b. When a patient has fluid overload
   c. When a patient's ejection fraction is lower than normal
   d. When a patient has ventricular hypertrophy

5. The nurse is taking a history on a patient recently diagnosed with heart failure. The patient admits to "sometimes having trouble catching my breath," but is unable to provide more specific details. What question does the nurse ask to gather more data about the patient's symptoms?
   a. "Do you have any medical problems, such as high blood pressure?"
   b. "What did your doctor tell you about your diagnosis?"
   c. "What was your most strenuous activity in the past week?"
   d. "How do you feel about being told that you have heart failure?"

6. The night shift nurse is listening to report and hears that a patient has paroxysmal nocturnal dyspnea. What does the nurse plan to do next?
   a. Instruct the patient to sleep in a side-lying position and then check on the patient every 2 hours to help with switching sides.
   b. Make the patient comfortable in a bedside recliner with several pillows to keep the patient more upright throughout the night.
   c. Check on the patient several hours after bedtime and assist the patient to sit upright and dangle the feet when dyspnea occurs.
   d. Check the patient frequently because the patient has insomnia due to a fear of suffocation.

7. The nurse is assessing a patient with right-sided heart failure. Which assessment findings does the nurse expect to see in this patient? *(Select all that apply.)*
   a. Dependent edema
   b. Weight loss
   c. Polyuria at night
   d. Hypotension
   e. Hepatomegaly
   f. Angina

8. The nurse is assessing a patient with left-sided heart failure. Which assessment findings does the nurse expect to see in this patient? *(Select all that apply.)*
   a. Displacement of the apical impulse to the left
   b. S_3 heart sound
   c. Paroxysmal nocturnal dyspnea
   d. Jugular venous distention
   e. Oliguria during the day
   f. Wheezes or crackles

9. Based on the etiology and the main cause of heart failure, which patient has the greatest need for health promotion measures to prevent heart failure?
   a. Alzheimer's patient
   b. Patient with cystitis
   c. Patient with asthma
   d. Patient with hypertension

10. What is an early sign of left ventricular failure that a patient is most likely to report?
    a. Nocturia
    b. Weight gain
    c. Swollen legs
    d. Nocturnal coughing

11. The nurse is reviewing diagnostic test results for a patient who is hypertensive. Which laboratory result is an early warning sign of decreased heart compliance, and prompts the nurse to immediately notify the health care provider?
    a. Normal B-type natriuretic peptide
    b. Decreased hemoglobin and hematocrit
    c. Elevated thyroxine (T_4)
    d. Presence of microalbuminuria

12. The nurse is interviewing a patient with a history of high blood pressure and heart problems. Which statement by the patient causes the nurse to suspect the patient may have heart failure?
    a. "I noticed a very fine red rash on my chest."
    b. "I had to take off my wedding ring last week."
    c. "I've had fever quite frequently."
    d. "I have pain in my shoulder when I cough."

13. A patient who was admitted for newly diagnosed heart failure is now being discharged. The nurse instructs the patient and family on how to manage heart failure at home. What major self-management categories should the nurse include? *(Select all that apply.)*
    a. Medications
    b. Weight
    c. Heart transplants
    d. Activity
    e. Diet

14. A patient's bilateral radial pulses are occasionally weak and irregular. Which assessment technique does the nurse use first to investigate this finding?
    a. Check the color and the capillary refill in the upper extremities.
    b. Check the peripheral pulses in the lower extremities.
    c. Take the apical pulse for 1 minute, noting any irregularity in heart rhythm.
    d. Check the cardiac monitor for irregularities in rhythm.

15. A patient is at risk for heart failure, but currently has no official medical diagnosis. While assessing the patient's lungs, the nurse hears profuse fine crackles. What does the nurse do next?
    a. Report the finding to the health care provider.
    b. Document the finding as a baseline for later comparison.
    c. Give the patient low-flow supplemental oxygen.
    d. Ask the patient to cough and reauscultate the lungs.

16. A patient is admitted for heart failure and has edema, neck vein distention, and ascites. What is the most reliable way to monitor fluid gain or loss in this patient?
    a. Check for pitting edema in the dependent body parts.
    b. Auscultate the lungs for crackles or wheezing.
    c. Assess skin turgor and the condition of mucous membranes.
    d. Weigh the patient daily at the same time with the same scale.

17. The home health nurse is evaluating a patient being treated for heart failure. Which statement by the patient is the best indicator of hope and well-being as a desired psychological outcome?
    a. "I'm taking the medication and following the doctor's orders."
    b. "I'm looking forward to dancing with my wife on our wedding anniversary."
    c. "I'm planning to go on a long trip; I'll never go back to the hospital again."
    d. "I want to thank you for all that you have done. I know you did your best."

18. The nurse is reviewing the laboratory results for a patient whose chief complaint is dyspnea. Which diagnostic test best differentiates between heart failure and lung dysfunction?
    a. Arterial blood gas
    b. B-type natriuretic peptide
    c. Hemoglobin and hematocrit
    d. Serum electrolytes

19. The nursing student is assisting in the care of a patient with advanced right-sided heart failure. In addition to bringing a stethoscope, what additional piece of equipment does the student bring in order to assess this patient?
    a. Tape measure
    b. Glasgow coma scale
    c. Portable Doppler
    d. Bladder ultrasound scanner

20. Which test is the best tool for diagnosing heart failure?
    a. Echocardiography
    b. Pulmonary artery catheter
    c. Radionuclide studies
    d. Multigated angiographic (MUGA) scan

21. A patient with heart failure has inadequate tissue perfusion. Which nursing interventions are included in the plan of care for this patient? *(Select all that apply.)*
    a. Monitor respiratory rate, rhythm, and quality every 1 to 4 hours.
    b. Auscultate breath sounds every 4 to 8 hours.
    c. Provide supplemental oxygen to maintain oxygen saturation at 90% or greater.
    d. Place the patient in a supine position with pillows under each leg.
    e. Assist the patient in performing coughing and deep-breathing exercises every 2 hours.

22. Which interventions are effective for a patient with a potential for pulmonary edema caused by heart failure? *(Select all that apply.)*
    a. Sodium and fluid restriction
    b. Slow infusion of hypotonic saline
    c. Administration of potassium
    d. Administration of loop diuretics
    e. Position in semi-Fowler's to high-Fowler's position
    f. Weekly weight monitoring

23. An older adult patient with heart failure is volume-depleted and has a low sodium level. The health care provider has ordered valsartan (Diovan), an angiotensin-receptor blocker (ARB). After the initial dose, for what complication does the nurse carefully monitor in this patient?
    a. Hypotension
    b. Cough
    c. Fluid retention
    d. Chest pain

24. The health care provider has ordered an ARB for a patient with heart failure. The parameters are to maintain a systolic blood pressure ranging from 90 to 110 mm Hg. Today the patient has a blood pressure of 110/80 mm Hg, but shows acute confusion. What is the nurse's first priority action?
    a. Give the medication because blood pressure is within the parameters.
    b. Call the health care provider about the new onset of confusion.
    c. Hold the medication and document the new findings.
    d. Assess the patient for other symptoms of decreased tissue perfusion.

25. A patient with heart failure has excessive aldosterone secretion and is therefore experiencing thirst and continuously asking for water. What instruction does the nurse give the unlicensed assistive personnel (UAP)?
    a. Severely restrict fluid to 500 mL plus output from the previous 24 hours.
    b. Give the patient as much water as desired to prevent dehydration.
    c. Restrict fluid to a normal 2 L daily, with accurate intake and output.
    d. Frequently offer the patient ice chips and moistened toothettes.

26. A patient is prescribed diuretics for treatment of heart failure. Because of this therapy, the nurse pays particular attention to which laboratory test level?
    a. Peak and trough of medication
    b. Serum potassium
    c. Serum sodium
    d. Prothrombin time (PT) and partial thromboplastin time (PTT)

27. An older adult patient is taking digoxin for treatment of heart failure. What is the priority nursing action for this patient related to the medication therapy?
    a. Give the medication in conjunction with an antacid.
    b. Keep the patient on the cardiac monitor and observe for ventricular dysrhythmias.
    c. Check that the dose is in the lowest possible range for therapeutic effect.
    d. Advise the patient that there is increased mortality related to toxicity.

28. A patient is receiving digoxin therapy for heart failure. What assessment does the nurse perform before administering the medication?
    a. Auscultate the apical pulse rate and heart rhythm.
    b. Assess for nausea and abdominal distention.
    c. Auscultate the lungs for crackles.
    d. Check for increased urine output.

29. The nurse is reviewing the ECG of a patient on digoxin therapy. What early sign of digitalis toxicity does the nurse look for?
    a. Tachycardia
    b. Peaked T wave
    c. Atrial fibrillation
    d. Loss of P wave

30. Which laboratory test does the nurse monitor for potential cardiac problems and digoxin toxicity?
    a. Complete blood count
    b. BUN and creatinine level
    c. Serum potassium level
    d. PT and International Normalized Ratio (INR)

31. A patient is receiving an infusion of nesiritide (Natrecor) for treatment of heart failure. What is the priority nursing assessment while administering this medication?
    a. Monitor for hypotension.
    b. Assess for cardiac dysrhythmias.
    c. Observe for respiratory depression.
    d. Monitor for peripheral vasoconstriction.

32. A patient has recently been diagnosed with acute heart failure. Which medication order does the nurse question?
    a. Dobutamine (Dobutrex), a beta-adrenergic agonist
    b. Milrinone (Primacor), a phosphodiesterase inhibitor
    c. Levosimendan (Simdax), a positive inotropic
    d. Carvedilol (Coreg), a beta blocker

33. A patient has an ejection fraction of less than 30%. The nurse prepares to provide patient education about which potential treatment?
    a. Automatic implantable cardio-defibrillator
    b. Heart transplant
    c. Mechanical implanted pump
    d. Ventricular reconstructive procedures

34. The nurse identifies a priority problem of fatigue and weakness for the patient with heart failure. After ambulating 200 feet down the hall, the patient's blood pressure change is more than 20 mm Hg. How does the nurse interpret this data?
    a. The patient is building endurance.
    b. The activity is too stressful.
    c. The patient could walk farther.
    d. The activity is appropriate.

35. A patient with heart failure is anxious to recover quickly. After ambulating with the UAP, the nurse observes that the patient has dyspnea. The nurse asks the patient to rate her exertion on a scale of 1 to 20 and the patient says, "I can keep going. It's only about a 15." What is the nurse's best response?
    a. "Slow down a bit; ideally you should be less than 12."
    b. "As long as you are less than 18, you can keep going."
    c. "Stop right now; you should not tax your heart beyond 5."
    d. "You should go slower; you cannot reach level 0 in one day."

36. Why does the nurse document the precise location of crackles auscultated in the lungs of a patient with heart failure?
    a. Crackles will eventually change to wheezes as the pulmonary edema worsens.
    b. The level of the fluid spreads laterally as the pulmonary edema worsens.
    c. The level of the fluid ascends as the pulmonary edema worsens.
    d. Crackles will eventually diminish as the pulmonary edema worsens.

37. A patient comes to the ED extremely anxious, tachycardic, struggling for air, and with a moist cough productive of frothy, blood-tinged sputum. What is the priority nursing intervention?
    a. Apply a pulse oximeter and cardiac monitor.
    b. Administer high-flow oxygen therapy via facemask.
    c. Prepare for continuous positive airway pressure ventilation.
    d. Prepare for intubation and mechanical ventilation.

38. A patient is treated for acute pulmonary edema. Which medications does the nurse prepare to administer to this patient? *(Select all that apply.)*
    a. Sublingual nitroglycerin
    b. IV Lasix
    c. IV morphine sulfate
    d. IV beta blocker
    e. IV nitroglycerin

39. What is the expected outcome for the collaborative problem potential for pulmonary edema?
    a. No dysrhythmias
    b. Clear lung sounds
    c. Less fatigue
    d. No disorientation

40. The nurse is teaching a patient with heart failure about signs and symptoms that suggest a return or worsening of heart failure. What does the nurse include in the teaching? *(Select all that apply.)*
    a. Rapid weight loss of 3 lbs in a week
    b. Increase in exercise tolerance lasting 2 to 3 days
    c. Cold symptoms (cough) lasting more than 3 to 5 days
    d. Excessive awakening at night to urinate
    e. Development of dyspnea or angina at rest or worsening angina
    f. Increased swelling in the feet, ankles, or hands

41. A patient is prescribed bumetanide (Bumex). What is an important teaching point for the nurse to include about this medication?
    a. Caution to move slowly when changing positions, especially from lying to sitting
    b. Information about potassium-rich foods to include in the diet
    c. Written instructions on how to count the radial pulse rate
    d. Information about low-sodium diets and reading food labels for sodium content

42. The nurse is teaching a patient about the treatment regimen for heart failure. Which statement by the patient indicates a need for further instruction?
    a. "I must weigh myself once a month and watch for fluid retention."
    b. "If my heart feels like it is racing, I should call the doctor."
    c. "I'll need to consider my activities for the day and rest as needed."
    d. "I'll need periods of rest and activity, and I should avoid activity after meals."

43. Which characteristics describe mitral valve stenosis? (Select all that apply.)
    a. Classic signs of dyspnea, angina, and syncope
    b. Rumbling apical diastolic murmur
    c. S_3 often present due to severe regurgitation
    d. Right-sided failure results in neck vein distention
    e. The patient may experience palpitations while lying on left side

44. Which characteristic describes mitral valve prolapse? (Select all that apply.)
    a. Hepatomegaly is a late sign.
    b. Leaflets enlarge and fall back into left atrium during systole.
    c. Most patients are asymptomatic.
    d. Patients have normal heart rate and blood pressure.
    e. Mitral valve prolapse is becoming a disorder of aging populations.

45. A patient is diagnosed with moderate mitral valve stenosis. Which findings is the nurse most likely to encounter during the physical assessment of this patient? (Select all that apply.)
    a. Dyspnea on exertion
    b. Orthopnea
    c. Palpitations
    d. Asymptomatic
    e. Neck vein distention

46. The nurse hears in report that a patient has been diagnosed with mitral insufficiency. Which early symptom is most likely to be first reported by the patient?
    a. Atypical chest pain
    b. Chronic weakness
    c. Anxiety
    d. Dyspnea

47. A patient is diagnosed with mitral valve stenosis. Which finding warrants immediate notification of the health care provider because of potential for decompensation?
    a. Irregularly irregular heart rhythm signifying atrial fibrillation
    b. Slow, bounding peripheral pulses associated with bradycardia
    c. An increase and decrease in pulse rate that follows inspiration and expiration
    d. An increase in pulse rate and blood pressure after exertion

48. The nurse is assessing the pulses of a patient with valvular disease and finds "bounding" arterial pulses. What is this finding most characteristic of?
    a. Aortic regurgitation
    b. Aortic stenosis
    c. Mitral valve prolapse
    d. Mitral insufficiency

49. A patient with a history of valvular heart disease requires a routine colonoscopy. The nurse notifies the health care provider to obtain a patient prescription for which type of medication?
    a. Anticoagulants
    b. Antihypertensives
    c. Antibiotics
    d. Antianginals

50. What is the most common preventable cause of valvular heart disease?
    a. Congenital disease or malformation
    b. Calcium deposits and thrombus formation
    c. Beta-hemolytic streptococcal infection
    d. Hypertension or Marfan syndrome

51. The nurse is assessing a patient at risk for valvular disease and finds pitting edema. This finding is a sign for which type of valvular disease?
    a. Mitral valve stenosis and insufficiency
    b. Aortic valve stenosis and insufficiency
    c. Tricuspid valve prolapse
    d. Mitral valve prolapse

52. The health care provider recommends to a patient that diagnostic testing be performed to assess for valvular heart disease. The nurse teaches the patient about which test that is commonly used for this purpose?
    a. Echocardiography
    b. Electrocardiography
    c. Exercise testing
    d. Thallium scanning

53. Long-term anticoagulant therapy for a patient with valvular heart disease and chronic atrial fibrillation includes which drug?
    a. Heparin sodium
    b. Warfarin sodium (Coumadin)
    c. Diltiazem (Cardizem)
    d. Enoxaparin (Lovenox)

54. The surgical noninvasive intervention of a balloon valvuloplasty is often used for which type of patient?
    a. Young adults with a genetic valve defect
    b. Older adults who are nonsurgical candidates
    c. Adults whose open-heart surgery failed
    d. Older adults who need replacement valves

55. The nurse is caring for a patient who had a valvuloplasty. The nurse monitors for which common complication in the postprocedural period?
    a. Myocardial infarction
    b. Angina
    c. Bleeding and emboli
    d. Infection

56. A patient with a prosthetic valve replacement must understand that postoperative care will include lifelong therapy with which type of medication?
    a. Antibiotics
    b. Anticoagulants
    c. Immunosuppressants
    d. Pain medication

57. A patient is a candidate for a xenograft valve. The nurse emphasizes that this type of valve does not require anticoagulant therapy, but will require which intervention?
    a. Replacement in about 7 to 10 years
    b. An exercise program to develop collateral circulation
    c. Daily temperature checks to watch for signs of rejection
    d. Frequent monitoring for pulmonary edema

58. A patient is scheduled for valve surgery. Which medication does the nurse advise the patient to discontinue for several days before the procedure?
    a. Antihypertensives
    b. Diuretics
    c. Anticoagulants
    d. Antibiotics

59. What is the most common problem for the patient with valvular heart disease?
    a. Reduced cardiac output
    b. Difficulty coping
    c. Shortness of breath
    d. Altered body image

60. The nurse is giving discharge instructions to a patient who had valve surgery. Which home care instructions does the nurse include in the teaching plan? *(Select all that apply.)*
    a. Increase consumption of foods high in vitamin K.
    b. Use an electric razor to avoid skin cuts.
    c. Report any bleeding or excessive bruising.
    d. Watch for and report any fever, drainage, or redness at the site.
    e. Avoid heavy lifting for 3 to 6 months.
    f. Report dyspnea, syncope, dizziness, edema, and palpitations.

61. The nurse assesses a patient and notes red, flat, pinpoint spots on the mucous membranes. Which finding has the nurse assessed?
    a. Pericardial friction rub
    b. Splinter hemorrhages
    c. Petechiae
    d. Systemic emboli

62. The patient has excess fluid in the pericardial cavity seen on echocardiogram. For which complication is the patient at increased risk?
    a. Pericardial friction rub
    b. Pulsus paradoxus
    c. Cardiac tamponade
    d. Systemic emboli

63. The patient has endocarditis. Which findings does the nurse expect when assessing this patient? *(Select all that apply.)*
    a. Pericardial friction rub
    b. Osler's nodes
    c. Petechiae
    d. A new regurgitant murmur
    e. Grating pain that is aggravated by breathing

64. Which patients are at greatest risk of developing infective endocarditis? *(Select all that apply.)*
    a. IV drug user
    b. Patient with a myocardial infarction
    c. Patient with a prosthetic mitral valve replacement, postoperative
    d. Patient with mitral stenosis who recently had an abscessed tooth removed
    e. Older adult patient with urinary tract infection and valve damage
    f. Patient with cardiac dysrhythmias

65. A patient with aortic valve endocarditis reports fatigue and shortness of breath. Crackles are heard on lung auscultation. What do these assessment findings most likely indicate?
    a. Emboli to the lung
    b. Valve incompetence resulting in heart failure
    c. Valve stenosis resulting in increased chamber size
    d. Coronary artery disease

66. A patient is admitted for possible infective endocarditis. Which test does the nurse anticipate will be performed to confirm a positive diagnosis?
    a. CT scan
    b. MRI
    c. Blood cultures
    d. Echocardiogram

67. A patient is diagnosed with new-onset infective endocarditis. Which recent procedure is the patient most likely to report?
    a. Teeth cleaning
    b. Urinary bladder catheterization
    c. Chest radiography
    d. ECG

68. In what way does arterial embolization to the brain manifest itself in a patient with infective endocarditis?
    a. Dysarthria
    b. Dysphagia
    c. Atelectasis
    d. Electrolyte imbalances

69. Which treatment intervention applies to a patient with infective endocarditis?
    a. Administration of oral penicillin for 6 weeks or more
    b. Hospitalization for initial IV antibiotics, possibly with a central line
    c. Complete bedrest for the duration of treatment
    d. Long-term anticoagulation therapy with heparin

70. What is the definitive treatment for a patient with chronic constrictive pericarditis?
    a. Antibiotic therapy
    b. Surgical excision of the pericardium
    c. Administration of beta blockers and corticosteroids
    d. Pericardiocentesis

71. A patient is admitted to the unit with assessment findings that include substernal pain that radiates to the left shoulder. The pain is described by the patient as grating, and is worse with inspiration and coughing. What likely is the cause of this patient's symptoms?
    a. Chronic constrictive pericarditis
    b. Cardiac tamponade
    c. Hypertrophic cardiomyopathy
    d. Acute pericarditis

72. Which signs/symptoms occur with chronic constrictive pericarditis? *(Select all that apply.)*
    a. Pericardium becomes rigid
    b. Heart valves stiffen
    c. Ventricles inadequately fill
    d. Signs of left-sided heart failure appear
    e. Heart failure eventually occurs

73. The nurse is assessing a patient with pericarditis. In order to hear a pericardial friction rub, which technique does the nurse use?
    a. Place the diaphragm at the apex of the heart.
    b. Place the diaphragm at the left lower sternal border.
    c. Place the bell just below the left clavicle.
    d. Place the bell at several points while the patient holds his or her breath.

74. A patient is admitted for pericarditis. In order to assist the patient to feel more comfortable, what does the nurse instruct the patient to do?
    a. Sit in a semi-Fowler's position with pillows under the arms.
    b. Lie on the side in a fetal position.
    c. Sit up and lean forward.
    d. Lie down and bend the legs at the knees.

75. The nurse is reviewing the ECG of a patient admitted for acute pericarditis. Which ECG change does the nurse anticipate?
    a. Normal ECG
    b. ST-T spiking
    c. Peaked T waves
    d. Wide QRS complexes

76. A patient is admitted for pericarditis. How will the patient likely describe his pain?
    a. Grating substernal pain that is aggravated by inspiration.
    b. Sharp pain that radiates down the left arm.
    c. Dull ache that feels vaguely like indigestion.
    d. Continuous boring pain that is relieved with rest.

77. Which patient is at greatest risk for developing viral pericarditis?
    a. 35-year-old woman with tuberculosis
    b. 45-year-old man who has had radiation therapy for lung cancer
    c. 30-year-old man with a respiratory infection
    d. 50-year-old woman with chest trauma

78. What is the common treatment for rheumatic carditis?
    a. Pericardiocentesis
    b. Antibiotics for 10 days
    c. Pain medication for substernal pain control
    d. Rest with observation for further necessary treatment

79. Which medication is used to treat rheumatic carditis?
    a. Antibiotic (penicillin)
    b. NSAIDs
    c. Pain medications (opioids)
    d. Steroids

80. Assessment findings for a patient with acute pericarditis indicate neck vein distention, clear lungs, muffled heart sounds, tachycardia, tachypnea, and a greater than 10 mm Hg difference in systolic pressure on inspiration than on expiration. What is the nurse's first response to these assessment findings?
    a. Continue to monitor the patient; these are normal signs of pericarditis.
    b. Administer oxygen and immediately report the findings to the health care provider.
    c. Monitor oxygen saturation and seek order for pain medication to control symptoms.
    d. Check ECG, administer morphine for pain, and administer diuretics.

81. A patient had an emergency pericardiocentesis for cardiac tamponade. Which nursing interventions are included in the postprocedural care of this patient? *(Select all that apply.)*
    a. Closely monitor for the recurrence of tamponade.
    b. Be prepared to provide adequate fluid volumes to increase cardiac output.
    c. Be prepared to assist in emergency sternotomy if tamponade recurs.
    d. Administer diuretics to decrease fluid volumes around the heart.
    e. Send the pericardial effusion specimen to the laboratory for culture.

82. Which is a characteristic of dilated cardiomyopathy?
    a. Results from replacement of myocardial tissue with fibrous tissue
    b. Causes stiff ventricles that restrict filling during diastole
    c. Causes symptoms of left ventricular failure
    d. Causes a stiff left ventricle

83. Which type of cardiomyopathy results from replacement of myocardial tissue with fibrous and fatty tissue?
    a. Hypertrophic cardiomyopathy
    b. Arrhythmogenic right ventricular cardiomyopathy
    c. Dilated cardiomyopathy
    d. Restrictive cardiomyopathy

84. A patient may die without any symptoms from which type of cardiomyopathy?
    a. Dilated cardiomyopathy
    b. Arrhythmogenic right ventricular cardiomyopathy
    c. Restrictive cardiomyopathy
    d. Hypertrophic cardiomyopathy

85. The cause of dilated cardiomyopathy may include which factors? *(Select all that apply.)*
    a. Alcohol abuse
    b. Sedentary lifestyle
    c. Infection
    d. Chemotherapy
    e. Poor nutrition

86. Which descriptions accurately characterize restrictive cardiomyopathy? *(Select all that apply.)*
    a. Prognosis is poor.
    b. Symptoms are similar to left- or right-sided heart failure.
    c. Some patients die without any symptoms.
    d. It is the most common type of cardiomyopathy.
    e. It is the rarest of cardiomyopathies.

87. A patient who reports having a sore throat 2 weeks ago now reports chest pain. On physical assessment, the nurse hears a new murmur, pericardial friction rub, and tachycardia. ECG shows a prolonged P-R interval. What condition does the nurse suspect in this patient?
    a. Rheumatic carditis
    b. Heart failure
    c. Cardiomyopathy
    d. Aortic stenosis

88. A patient has received a heart transplant for dilated cardiomyopathy. Because the patient has a high risk for cardiac tamponade, of which sign/symptoms does the nurse immediately notify the provider?
    a. Crackles and wheezes of the lungs
    b. Pulsus paradoxus and muffled heart sounds
    c. Hepatomegaly and ascites
    d. Dependent edema and fluid retention

89. The nurse is assessing a patient who has received a heart transplant. Which clinical manifestations suggest transplant rejection? *(Select all that apply.)*
    a. Shortness of breath
    b. Depression
    c. Severe abdominal pain
    d. New bradycardia
    e. Hypotension
    f. Decreased ejection fraction

36 CHAPTER

Care of Patients with Vascular Problems

1. Atherosclerosis affects which larger arteries? *(Select all that apply.)*
   a. Renal
   b. Femoral
   c. Coronary
   d. Brachial cephalic
   e. Aorta

2. An African-American man is being seen for a right toe blister. What factors increase this patient's risk for developing atherosclerosis? *(Select all that apply.)*
   a. 20 year history of type 1 diabetes
   b. Sedentary lifestyle
   c. Father with history of colon cancer
   d. 35 pounds overweight
   e. Grandmother who died after myocardial infarction

3. Which factors can increase systemic arterial pressure? *(Select all that apply.)*
   a. Decreased cardiac output
   b. Increased heart rate
   c. Increased peripheral vascular resistance
   d. Increased stroke volume
   e. Decreased blood pressure

4. The effects of hyperglycemia in diabetes can result in which conditions? *(Select all that apply.)*
   a. Intimal arterial damage
   b. Severe atherosclerosis
   c. Decreased cardiac output
   d. Premature atherosclerosis
   e. Decreased total peripheral vascular resistance

5. A patient is admitted with a vascular problem. Based on the pathophysiology of systemic arterial pressure, what is the systemic arterial pressure a product of? *(Select all that apply.)*
   a. Cardiac output
   b. Peripheral vascular volume
   c. Preload
   d. Peripheral vascular resistance
   e. Diastolic blood pressure

6. A patient's cholesterol screening shows a high-density lipoprotein (HDL) value greater than 40, and a total serum cholesterol level of 188. The patient has no other cardiac or vascular risk factors. What does the nurse advise the patient to do?
   a. Modify the diet to exclude fats and increase fiber, then repeat tests.
   b. Contact the physician for a prescription of antilipemic medication.
   c. Repeat total and HDL cholesterol testing in 6 to 12 weeks.
   d. Repeat total and HDL cholesterol testing during the next routine exam.

7. The nurse is counseling a group of women about triglyceride levels. For women, what is a normal triglyceride level?
   a. Over 150 mg/dL
   b. Under 135 mg/dL
   c. Over 100 mg/dL
   d. Under 70 mg/dL

8. The nurse is conducting dietary teaching with a patient. Which statement by the patient indicates an understanding of fat sources and the need to limit saturated fats?
   a. "Coconut oil has a rich flavor and is a good cooking oil."
   b. "Sunflower oil is high in saturated fats, so I should avoid it."
   c. "Meat and eggs mostly contain unsaturated fats."
   d. "Canola oil has monounsaturated fat and is recommended."

9. The nurse educates and advises a patient to follow the National Cholesterol Education Program (NCEP) Therapeutic Lifestyle Changes (TLC) diet. Which instruction does the nurse give to the patient?
   a. Review the literature and see what aspects of the program fit into the patient's current lifestyle.
   b. Return for serum cholesterol levels at 6 and 12 weeks after starting the diet.
   c. Record dietary intake and weight for 12 weeks and then call the physician.
   d. Weigh self once a week for 6 weeks and consult the physician if not losing weight.

10. A patient is prescribed atorvastatin (Lipitor). The nurse instructs the patient to watch for and report which side effect?
    a. Nausea and vomiting
    b. Cough
    c. Headaches
    d. Muscle cramps

11. A patient gets a new prescription for Pravigard for treatment of high cholesterol. Because this is a combination drug, the nurse alerts the physician when the patient discloses an allergy to which drug?
    a. Sulfa
    b. Aspirin
    c. Some calcium channel blockers
    d. Some diuretics

12. A patient is prescribed niacin (Niaspan) to lower low-density lipoprotein cholesterol (LDL-C) and very-low-density lipoprotein (VLDL). Why are lower doses prescribed to the patient?
    a. To reduce side effects of flushing and feeling warm
    b. To prevent muscle myopathies
    c. To prevent elevation of blood pressure
    d. To prevent undesirable hypokalemia

13. The nurse is conducting an initial cardiovascular assessment on a middle-aged patient. What techniques does the nurse include in the assessment? *(Select all that apply.)*
    a. Take blood pressure on the dominant arm.
    b. Palpate pulses at all of the major sites.
    c. Palpate for temperature differences in the lower extremities.
    d. Perform bilateral but separate palpation on the carotid arteries.
    e. Auscultate for bruits in the radial and brachial arteries.

14. The nurse is performing blood pressure screening at a community center. Which patients are referred for evaluation of their blood pressure? *(Select all that apply.)*
    a. Diabetic patient with a blood pressure of 118/78 mm Hg
    b. Patient with heart disease with a blood pressure of 134/90 mm Hg
    c. Patient with no known health problems who has a blood pressure of 125/86 mm Hg
    d. Diabetic patient with a blood pressure of 180/80 mm Hg
    e. Patient with no known health problems who has a blood pressure of 106/70 mm Hg

15. The home health nurse is making the initial visit to an older adult patient with hypertension. The nurse recommends that the patient obtain which item for home use?
    a. Ambulatory blood pressure monitoring device
    b. Exercise bicycle
    c. Blood glucose monitor scale
    d. Food scale

16. The nurse is evaluating the blood pressure of a 75-year-old woman. Based on current research, which finding is the better indicator of heart disease risk for this patient?
    a. Diastolic of 86 mm Hg
    b. Systolic of 160 mm Hg
    c. Blood pressure of 138/68 mm Hg
    d. Blood pressure of 110/90 mm Hg

17. A 32-year-old patient with diabetes reports sudden onset of headaches, blurred vision, and dyspnea. The patient's blood pressure is normally 120/80 mm Hg, but today is 200/130 mm Hg. What condition does the nurse suspect?
    a. Sustained hypertension
    b. Malignant hypertension
    c. Primary hypertension
    d. Secondary hypertension

18. Which are risk factors for hypertension? *(Select all that apply.)*
    a. Age greater than 40 years
    b. Family history of hypertension
    c. Excessive calorie consumption
    d. Physical inactivity
    e. Excessive alcohol intake
    f. Hypolipidemia

19. The nurse is reviewing the laboratory results of urine tests for a patient with a medical diagnosis of essential hypertension. The presence of catecholamines in the urine is evidence of which disorder?
    a. Renal failure
    b. Primary aldosteronism
    c. Cushing's syndrome
    d. Pheochromocytoma

20. The nurse is reviewing the electrocardiogram (ECG) for a patient with a medical diagnosis of essential hypertension. What is the first ECG sign of heart disease resulting from hypertension?
    a. Left atrial and ventricular hypertrophy
    b. Right atrial and ventricular atrophy
    c. Malfunction of the sinoatrial (SA) node
    d. Malfunction of the atrioventricular (AV) node

21. Which blood pressure finding for a 55-year-old adult patient with no other medical problems is evaluated further for hypertension?
    a. 118/78 mm Hg
    b. 124/80 mm Hg
    c. 138/78 mm Hg
    d. 140/86 mm Hg

22. A middle-aged patient with no health insurance has tried lifestyle modifications to control uncomplicated hypertension, but continues to struggle. What is considered a first drug of choice for this patient?
    a. Calcium channel blocker
    b. Alpha blocker
    c. Thiazide-type diuretic
    d. Angiotensin-converting enzyme (ACE) inhibitor

23. The nurse is reviewing the medication schedule for an older adult patient who needs medication for hypertension. The patient lives alone, but is able to manage self-care. What frequency of drug therapy does the nurse advocate for this patient?
    a. Once a day
    b. Two times a day
    c. Three times a day
    d. Four times a day

24. The nurse is reviewing prescriptions for a patient recently diagnosed with hypertension. The nurse questions a prescription for which type of drug?
    a. Aldosterone receptor antagonist
    b. Alpha blocker
    c. Thiazide-type diuretic
    d. ACE inhibitor

25. For which patient does the nurse question the use of hydrochlorothiazide (HydroDIURIL)?
    a. Asthmatic patient
    b. Patient with chronic airway limitation
    c. Patient with hyperkalemia
    d. Patient with hypokalemia

26. The nurse is teaching a patient about taking hydrochlorothiazide (HydroDIURIL). Which food does the nurse instruct the patient to eat in conjunction with the use of this drug?
    a. Bananas and oranges
    b. Milk and cheese
    c. Cranberries and prunes
    d. Cabbage and cauliflower

27. A patient reports dizziness when she changes positions from sitting to standing and a sudden cough after starting a prescription for captopril (Capoten). Which nursing intervention is most useful for this patient?
    a. Instruct the patient to change positions slowly and take an over-the-counter cough syrup.
    b. Tell the patient to take the medication at bedtime and use over-the-counter throat lozenges.
    c. Notify the prescribing physician because the medication should be discontinued.
    d. Teach the patient to increase her fluid intake.

28. Which intervention renders angiotensin II receptor blockers (ARBs) and ACE inhibitors effective in African Americans?
    a. Take with diuretics, a beta blocker, or calcium channel blocker.
    b. Give at a much higher dosage than for other ethnic groups.
    c. Combine with rigorous lifestyle modification.
    d. Take around the clock on a very individualized schedule.

29. The nurse is reviewing antihypertensive medication orders for a patient with asthma. The nurse questions the use of which type of medication?
    a. Cardioselective beta blockers because they reduce cardiac output
    b. Noncardioselective beta blockers because they may cause bronchoconstriction
    c. ACE inhibitors because they cause a nagging cough
    d. Thiazide diuretics because they promote potassium excretion

30. The nurse prepares to teach a patient recovering from a myocardial infarction (MI) about combination drug therapy based on "best practice" for controlling hypertension. Which drugs does the nurse include in the teaching plan? *(Select all that apply.)*
    a. Beta blockers
    b. ACE inhibitors or ARBs
    c. Aldosterone antagonists
    d. Central alpha agonists
    e. NSAIDs
    f. Aspirin

31. The student nurse is giving a patient with benign prostatic hyperplasia a morning dose of terazosin (Hytrin). The student says, "This is your blood pressure medicine," but the patient responds, "I don't have high blood pressure." What does the student nurse do next?
    a. Explain to the patient that his blood pressure is not high because the drug is controlling it.
    b. Stop and recheck the medication administration record and then do additional drug research.
    c. Recheck the blood pressure, then hold the drug if blood pressure is not elevated.
    d. Contact the charge nurse for advice about how to handle the patient's refusal.

32. A patient admits difficulty with long-term adherence to antihypertensive therapy. Which nursing interventions promote compliance for this patient? *(Select all that apply.)*
    a. Carefully review all medication instructions with the patient.
    b. Give the patient a list of resources for finding information on the medications.
    c. Reinforce the fact that damage to organs occurs even if there are no symptoms.
    d. Teach the patient about the continuous ambulatory blood pressure monitoring device.
    e. Assess the patient's resources to obtain medications.

33. The nurse is reviewing medical records for several patients with kidney problems and actual or potential for hypertension. Which patient does the nurse expect to be screened for renal artery stenosis?
    a. Patient with a history of kidney stones
    b. Patient taking three categories of antihypertensive drugs at high doses
    c. Patient with newly diagnosed hypertension
    d. Patient with a history of frequent urinary tract infections

34. The nurse assesses a patient and documents the following findings: "edema 2+ bilateral ankles, brown pigmentation of lower extremities skin, aching pain of lower extremities when standing that is relieved with elevation." What condition does the patient likely have?
    a. Deep vein thrombosis
    b. Venous insufficiency
    c. Peripheral arterial disease (PAD)
    d. Raynaud's syndrome

35. The nurse assesses a patient and documents the following findings: "decreased pedal and posterior tibial pulses bilateral (1+), skin is cool-to-cold to touch, loss of hair on lower extremities, patient reports that lower extremity pain is reproducible when walking and relieved by rest, and also noted are thickened toenails." What condition does the patient likely have?
    a. Peripheral vascular disease
    b. Deep vein thrombosis
    c. Raynaud's syndrome
    d. Peripheral arterial disease

36. Which patients are at risk for PAD? *(Select all that apply.)*
    a. Hypertensive patient
    b. Patient with diabetes mellitus
    c. Patient who is a cigarette smoker
    d. Anemic patient
    e. Patient who is very thin
    f. African-American patient

37. Which symptom is the most common initial manifestation of PAD?
    a. Intermittent claudication
    b. Pain at rest
    c. Redness in the extremity
    d. Muscle atrophy

38. The nurse is caring for a patient with a medical diagnosis of inflow PAD. Which symptom does the nurse expect the patient to report?
    a. Very frequent episodes of rest pain
    b. Discomfort in the lower back, buttocks, or thighs after walking
    c. Burning or cramping in the calves, ankles, feet, or toes after walking
    d. Waking frequently at night to hang the feet off the bed

39. The nurse is assessing the lower extremity of a patient with PAD. What does the nurse palpate?
    a. Posterior tibial pulse of the affected leg
    b. Pedal pulses in both feet
    c. All pulses in both legs
    d. Strength of the pulses in the affected leg

40. While assessing a patient, the nurse sees a small, round ulcer with a "punched out" appearance and well-defined borders on the great toe. The patient reports the ulcer is painful. How does the nurse interpret this finding?
    a. Venous stasis ulcer
    b. Diabetic ulcer
    c. Gangrenous ulcer
    d. Arterial ulcer

41. A patient is undergoing diagnostic testing for pain and burning sensation in the legs. What does an ankle-brachial index (ABI) of less than 0.9 in either leg indicate?
    a. Normal arterial circulation to the lower extremities
    b. Presence of peripheral arterial disease
    c. Severe venous disease of the lower extremities
    d. Need for immediate surgical intervention

42. The nurse is consulting with the physical therapist to design an exercise program for patients with peripheral vascular disease. Which patient is a candidate for an exercise program?
    a. Patient with severe rest pain
    b. Patient with intermittent claudication
    c. Patient with gangrene
    d. Patient with venous ulcers

43. A patient with PAD asks, "Why should I exercise when walking several blocks seems to make my leg cramp up?" What is the nurse's best response?
    a. "Exercise may improve blood flow to your leg because small vessels will compensate for blood vessels that are blocked off."
    b. "This type of therapy is free and you can do it by yourself to improve the muscles in your legs."
    c. "The cramping will eventually stop if you continue the exercise routine. If you have too much pain, just rest for a while."
    d. "Exercise is a noninvasive nonsurgical technique that is used to increase arterial flow to the affected limb."

44. The nurse is teaching a patient with PAD about positioning and position changes. What suggestion does the nurse give to the patient?
    a. Sit upright in a chair if legs are not swollen.
    b. Sleep with legs above the heart level if legs are swollen.
    c. Avoid crossing the legs at all times.
    d. Change positions slowly when getting out of bed.

45. The nurse is instructing a patient with PAD about ways to promote vasodilation. What information does the nurse include? *(Select all that apply.)*
    a. Maintain a warm environment at home.
    b. Wear socks or insulated shoes at all times.
    c. Apply direct heat to the limb by using a heating pad.
    d. Prevent cold exposure of the affected limb.
    e. Limit fluids to prevent increased blood viscosity.
    f. Completely abstain from smoking or chewing tobacco.

46. The nurse is assessing a patient at risk for peripheral vascular disease. Which assessment finding indicates arterial ulcers rather than diabetic or venous ulcers?
    a. Ulcer located over the pressure points of the feet
    b. Ulcer of deep, pale color with even edges and little granulation tissue
    c. Severe pain or discomfort occurring at the ulcer site
    d. Associated ankle discoloration and edema

47. Which are complications that can result from severe PAD? *(Select all that apply.)*
    a. Gangrene
    b. Varicose veins
    c. Aneurysm
    d. Amputation
    e. Ulcer formation

48. Which drugs are used to promote circulation in a patient with chronic PAD? *(Select all that apply.)*
    a. Pentoxifylline (Trental)
    b. Propranolol hydrochloride (Inderal)
    c. Aspirin
    d. Clopidogrel (Plavix)
    e. Ezetimibe (Zetia)

49. Which statements pertaining to a percutaneous transluminal balloon angioplasty are correct? *(Select all that apply.)*
    a. One or more arteries are dilated with a balloon catheter to open the vessel.
    b. It is a minor surgical procedure.
    c. Stents may be placed to ensure adequate blood flow.
    d. Placement of stents results in a longer hospital stay.
    e. Some patients are occlusion-free for 3 to 5 years.

50. A patient with PAD is scheduled to have percutaneous transluminal angioplasty (PTA). What information does the nurse give the patient about this procedure?
    a. It is usually used when amputation is inevitable.
    b. Reocclusion may occur afterwards and the procedure may be repeated.
    c. Most patients are occlusion-free afterwards, particularly if stents are placed.
    d. It is painless and there are very few risks or dangers.

51. A patient has returned to the unit after having PTA. What nursing actions are included in the routine postprocedural care of this patient? *(Select all that apply.)*
    a. Observe for bleeding at the puncture site.
    b. Observe vital signs frequently.
    c. Perform frequent checks of the distal pulses in both limbs.
    d. Encourage bedrest with the limb straight for about 1 to 2 hours.
    e. Administer anticoagulant therapy such as heparin.
    f. Provide supplemental oxygen via nasal cannula.

52. A patient has returned to the unit after surgery for arterial revascularization with graft placement. The nurse monitors for graft occlusion, which is most likely to occur within which time frame?
    a. First 2 hours
    b. First 24 hours
    c. Next 2 days
    d. First week

53. A patient is in the postanesthesia care unit (PACU) after surgery for arterial revascularization with graft placement. Which procedure does the nurse use to check the patency of the graft?
    a. Check the extremity every 15 minutes for the first hour, then hourly, for changes in color, temperature, and pulse intensity.
    b. Check the dorsalis pedis pulse every 15 minutes for the first hour, then hourly.
    c. Ask the patient if there is any pain or loss of sensation anywhere in the extremity, and withhold patient-controlled analgesia.
    d. Gently palpate the site every 15 minutes for the first hour and assess for warmth, redness, and edema.

54. A patient has returned to the unit after a PTA. What is the postprocedural nursing priority?
    a. Pain management
    b. Check the distal pulses
    c. Early ambulation to prevent complications
    d. Monitoring for bleeding at the puncture site

55. The student nurse is assisting in the care of a patient returning from the PACU after aortofemoral bypass. The nurse intervenes when the student performs which action?
    a. Offers to obtain a meal tray for the patient
    b. Demonstrates to the patient how to use the incentive spirometer
    c. Encourages the patient to deep-breathe every 1 to 2 hours
    d. Explains to the patient the purpose of 24-hour bedrest

56. A patient has had surgery for arterial revascularization with graft placement. The nurse notes swelling, tenseness of the skin tissue, and the patient reports an increasing pain with numbness and tingling, as well as a decrease in the ability to wiggle toes and ankles. What does the nurse suspect is occurring with this patient?
    a. Graft infection
    b. Compartment syndrome
    c. Graft occlusion
    d. Reaction to thrombolytic therapy

57. A patient has had aortoiliac bypass surgery with graft placement. The nurse notes induration, erythema, tenderness, warmth, edema, and drainage at the site. Before calling the physician, what additional assessment does the nurse perform?
    a. Palpates the patient's abdomen and checks for the last bowel movement
    b. Auscultates the patient's lung sounds and checks the pulse oximeter reading
    c. Assesses the patient for signs of occult bleeding and looks at the PT results
    d. Checks the patient's temperature and looks at the white blood cell results

58. A patient is admitted with a medical diagnosis of acute arterial occlusion. What documentation does the nurse expect to see in this patient's medical record?
    a. Acute MI and/or atrial fibrillation within the previous weeks
    b. History of chronic venous stasis disease treated with débridement and wound care
    c. History of Marfan syndrome or Ehlers-Danlos syndrome
    d. Episode of blunt trauma that occurred several months ago

59. A patient with an acute arterial occlusion requires abciximab (ReoPro). What nursing responsibilities are associated with the administration of this platelet inhibitor?
    a. Platelet counts must be monitored at 3, 6, and 12 hours after the start of the infusion.
    b. For platelet counts over 100,000/mm³, infusion must be readjusted or discontinued.
    c. Monitor for manifestations of rash, itching, or swelling.
    d. Monitor for edema, pain on passive movement, or poor capillary refill.

60. Which is a postoperative nursing intervention for a patient with arterial revascularization?
    a. Promote graft patency by limiting IV fluid infusion.
    b. Instruct the patient to avoid bending at the hips or knees.
    c. Resume regular diet immediately after surgery.
    d. Avoid coughing and deep-breathing exercises.

61. Which statements are accurate about true aneurysms? *(Select all that apply.)*
    a. Permanent dilatation of an artery
    b. Enlarged artery to at least 2 times the normal diameter
    c. Formed when blood accumulates in the wall of the artery
    d. Is a result of arterial injury or trauma
    e. Arterial wall is congenitally weakened

62. The nurse is reviewing a patient's abdominal CT scan and notes that the patient has a berry-shaped segment coming off of his abdominal aorta. What is the nurse's best interpretation of these results?
    a. Dissecting aneurysm
    b. Saccular aneurysm
    c. Fusiform aneurysm
    d. False aneurysm

63. What is the most common location for an aneurysm?
    a. Abdominal aorta
    b. Thoracic aorta
    c. Femoral arteries
    d. Popliteal arteries

64. What is the most common cause of an aneurysm?
    a. Emboli
    b. Trauma
    c. Atherosclerosis
    d. Thrombus formation

65. A patient is suspected to have an abdominal aortic aneurysm (AAA). What does the nurse assess for?
    a. Abdominal, flank, or back pain
    b. Chest pain and shortness of breath
    c. Hoarseness and difficulty swallowing
    d. Disruption of bowel and bladder patterns

66. A 75-year-old man with a history of atherosclerosis comes to the emergency department (ED) with abdominal pain. What findings indicate a possible AAA? *(Select all that apply.)*
   a. Left-sided chest pain
   b. Abdominal, flank, or back pain
   c. Visible pulsation on the upper abdominal wall
   d. Hoarseness
   e. Difficulty swallowing

67. A patient with an AAA is admitted to the hospital. Which tests does the physician order to confirm an accurate diagnosis as well as to determine the size and location of the AAA? *(Select all that apply.)*
   a. Abdominal x-rays
   b. Ultrasound
   c. Electrocardiogram
   d. Magnetic resonance imaging
   e. Computed tomography

68. A patient is diagnosed with a small 3-cm AAA. What is the best nonsurgical intervention to decrease the risk of rupture of an aneurysm and to slow the rate of enlargement?
   a. Maintenance of normal blood pressure and avoidance of hypertension
   b. Bedrest until there is shrinkage of the aneurysm
   c. Heparin and Coumadin therapy to decrease clotting
   d. Intraarterial thrombolytic therapy

69. A patient with a ruptured aneurysm may exhibit which symptoms? *(Select all that apply.)*
   a. Bradypnea
   b. Tachycardia
   c. Increased systolic pressure
   d. Decreased blood pressure
   e. Severe pain
   f. Decreased level of consciousness

70. Which action does the nurse take first if a patient has a suspected aneurysm rupture?
   a. Start an IV infusion with a large-bore needle.
   b. Assess baseline measurements of blood pressure and pulse rate.
   c. Palpate the pulsating abdominal mass to determine its size.
   d. Assess all peripheral pulses to use as a baseline for comparison.

71. A patient has had a repair of an AAA. For what reason is this patient being monitored postoperatively for urinary output and renal function studies (creatinine and BUN)?
   a. The patient was probably in shock preoperatively, and there may be glomerular damage.
   b. The patient is usually in a critical care nursing unit where this is done routinely.
   c. The aorta was clamped during the surgery and the kidneys may have been inadvertently damaged.
   d. Repair of the aneurysm improves renal perfusion and the urinary output should increase.

72. A patient has had an aneurysm repair. Which activity does the nurse suggest as an example of appropriate exercise during the recovery period?
   a. Playing golf
   b. Washing dishes
   c. Raking leaves
   d. Driving a car

73. A patient is admitted for a medical diagnosis of detectable AAA. What does the nurse expect to find documented in the patient's description of symptoms?
   a. Hematuria and painful urination that started very suddenly
   b. Steady and gnawing abdominal pain unaffected by movement and lasting for days
   c. No subjective complaints of pain, but episodes of dizziness
   d. Pain in the lower extremities exacerbated by walking and relieved by rest

74. While assessing a patient with AAA, the nurse notes a pulsation in the upper abdomen slightly to the left of the midline between the xiphoid process and the umbilicus. What does the nurse do next?
    a. Measure the mass with a ruler.
    b. Palpate the mass for tenderness.
    c. Percuss the mass to determine the borders.
    d. Auscultate for a bruit over the mass.

75. A patient was admitted for AAA with a pulsating abdominal mass. The nurse notes a sudden onset of diaphoresis, decreased level of consciousness, a blood pressure of 88/60 mm Hg, and an irregular apical pulse. Oxygen is in place via mask. What is the priority nursing action at this time?
    a. Establish IV access.
    b. Alert the Rapid Response Team.
    c. Auscultate for a bruit and assess the mass.
    d. Place the patient on the cardiac monitor.

76. The nurse is reviewing the radiologist's report of the abdominal x-ray of a patient suspected of having AAA. The report notes an "eggshell" appearance. How does the nurse interpret this data?
    a. Validates the presence of an aneurysm
    b. Suggests an artifact; therefore, the x-ray must be repeated
    c. Indicates a congenital anomaly that will obscure the aneurysm
    d. Indicates the aneurysm is the size of an egg

77. The nurse is designing a teaching plan for a patient with a small 4-cm AAA. The patient is currently asymptomatic. What is the nurse's goal for nonsurgical management of this patient?
    a. Teach lifestyle modifications that will minimize the growth of the aneurysm.
    b. Monitor the growth of the aneurysm and follow the antihypertensive medication regimen.
    c. Encourage compliance with anticoagulant drugs and laboratory follow-up appointments.
    d. Stabilize the patient's condition and improve overall health so surgery can be safely performed.

78. The nurse is performing preoperative teaching for a patient who is having an elective endovascular stent graft repair for an AAA. What key points are included in teaching for this patient? *(Select all that apply.)*
    a. "This type of repair has decreased hospital stays."
    b. "The stents are inserted through the skin into the femoral artery."
    c. "You will be receiving general anesthesia."
    d. "In the OR you will receive a large volume of IV fluids."
    e. "This procedure has resulted in improved mortality for AAA repairs."
    f. "After the procedure you will be in the surgical ICU for at least 1-2 days."

79. Which are common complications of endovascular stent graft repair of an AAA? *(Select all that apply.)*
    a. Myocardial infarction
    b. Misplacement of the graft
    c. Bleeding
    d. Paralytic ileus
    e. Peripheral embolization
    f. Conversion to open surgical repair

80. The nurse notes a change in pulses, a cool extremity below the graft, bluish discoloration to the flanks, and abdominal distention in a patient who has had AAA open surgical repair. These symptoms are consistent with which postoperative complication?
    a. Ischemic colitis
    b. Cerebral and spinal cord ischemia
    c. Graft occlusion or rupture
    d. Thoracic outlet syndrome

81. A patient is admitted through the ED for emergency surgery of a ruptured aneurysm. Why does the nurse monitor the patient for renal failure?
    a. A urinary catheter was inserted under potentially nonsterile conditions.
    b. Aggressive fluid management in the ED could overload the kidneys.
    c. Hypovolemia associated with rupture can result in acute tubular necrosis.
    d. Medications used in the emergency procedure are nephrotoxic.

82. A patient who had open surgical repair for an AAA was just extubated. What does the nurse do in caring for this patient for the next 24 hours?
    a. Assess respiratory rate and depth every hour.
    b. Turn and suction the patient every 2 hours.
    c. Discourage coughing and deep-breathing.
    d. Assist the patient to a bedside chair.

83. The nurse is assessing a patient with a suspected thoracic aortic aneurysm. Which assessment finding is most likely to be present?
    a. Loss of pulses distal to the aneurysm
    b. Decreased level of consciousness
    c. Hoarseness and difficulty swallowing
    d. Disruption of bowel and bladder patterns

84. A patient who had a thoracic aortic aneurysm repair has been progressing well for several days after the surgery, but today tells the nurse, "My toes and lower legs feel a little numb and tingly." What is the nurse's best first action?
    a. Encourage the patient to do active range-of-motion exercises in bed.
    b. Help the patient get up, dangle the legs, and then ambulate.
    c. Assess extremities for sensation, movement, or pulse changes.
    d. Instruct unlicensed assistive personnel (UAP) to assist the patient in elevating the legs.

85. Which actions does the nurse instruct the patient to avoid after discharge with an AAA repair? *(Select all that apply.)*
    a. Lifting heavy objects
    b. Going up stairs
    c. Using the bathroom
    d. Sitting in a chair for meals
    e. Driving a car

86. A patient has had an open repair of a thoracic aortic aneurysm. What does the nurse monitor for in this patient and immediately report to the surgeon?
    a. Productive cough when using the incentive spirometer
    b. Increased drainage from chest tubes
    c. Sternal pain with coughing and deep-breathing
    d. Increased urinary output from the indwelling catheter

87. A patient is considering endovascular stent grafts. What is one of the advantages of this procedure?
    a. Decreased length of hospital stay
    b. Less risk for hemorrhage
    c. Decreased incidence of postprocedural rupture
    d. Use of local, rather than general, anesthesia

88. The home health nurse is making the first visit to a patient who had an open surgical aneurysm repair. In evaluating the home situation, what does the nurse observe that is cause for concern?
    a. The patient has been having groceries delivered for several weeks.
    b. There is a calendar hanging on the refrigerator with medication times.
    c. The patient's bedroom and bathroom access are on the ground floor.
    d. The patient decides to vacuum the house and clean out the garage.

89. A patient comes to the ED with anterior chest pain described as a "tearing" sensation. The patient is diaphoretic, nauseated, faint, apprehensive, and blood pressure is 200/130 mm Hg. Which medication is most likely to be ordered for this patient?
    a. Antianginal such as nitroglycerin (Nitrobid)
    b. Antihypertensive such as sodium nitroprusside (Nipride)
    c. Calcium channel antagonist such as amlodipine (Norvasc)
    d. Beta blocker such as propranolol (Inderal)

90. Which are characteristics of Raynaud's disease? *(Select all that apply.)*
    a. Occurs In smokers, often in young men
    b. Claudication in feet and lower extremities
    c. Occurs mostly in young women
    d. Episodic, causing white, then blue, fingers
    e. Cold intolerance

91. A young male patient is diagnosed with early stage Buerger's disease. What assessment finding does the nurse expect to find in the patient's record?
    a. Claudication of the arch of the foot
    b. Intolerance of warm environments
    c. Dizziness and lightheadedness
    d. Pain in the lower back with ambulation

92. The nurse is teaching a patient with Buerger's disease about self-care. What is the most important point that the nurse emphasizes?
    a. Lower intake of fat and reducing cholesterol to reverse the disease process.
    b. Perform daily exercise of fingers or toes to slow the progress of the disease.
    c. Limit exposure to extreme or prolonged cold temperatures because of vasoconstriction.
    d. Cease cigarette smoking and tobacco use to arrest the disease process.

93. A patient reports tiredness in the arm with exertion, paresthesia, dizziness, and exercise-induced pain in the forearm when the arms are elevated. The nurse suspects subclavian steal. What physical assessment does the nurse perform?
    a. Check blood pressure in both arms.
    b. Auscultate for a carotid bruit.
    c. Check for orthostatic hypotension.
    d. Observe the arm for redness or edema.

94. A patient who is an avid golfer is diagnosed with thoracic outlet syndrome. What does the nurse advise the patient that is specific to this syndrome?
    a. Rest if shortness of breath occurs.
    b. Avoid walking long distances.
    c. Avoid elevating the arms.
    d. Perform deep-breathing exercises.

95. A 25-year-old woman reports bilateral blanching of both upper extremities that occurs in cold temperatures. She reports numbness and cold sensation, and afterwards the arms become very red. Which condition are these symptoms most consistent with?
    a. Raynaud's disease
    b. Buerger's disease
    c. Subclavian steal
    d. Raynaud's phenomenon

96. Which medication is a patient with Raynaud's disease most likely to be prescribed?
    a. Lovastatin (Mevacor)
    b. Coumadin (Warfarin)
    c. Nifedipine (Procardia)
    d. Captopril (Capoten)

97. A patient has been on bedrest following a motor vehicle accident. The nurse notes on assessment that the patient's left lower extremity has edema and is warm to the touch. The patient reports the calf of the left leg is slightly painful. The nurse suspects that this assessment may indicate which disorder?
    a. Raynaud's syndrome
    b. Cellulitis
    c. Aneurysm
    d. Venous thromboembolism

98. A patient is admitted to the hospital with deep vein thrombosis (DVT). Which drug therapy does the nurse expect the health care provider to order?
    a. Heparin 5000 units subcutaneously twice a day
    b. Loading high dose of warfarin (Coumadin), then smaller doses on following days
    c. Alternate heparin and warfarin (Coumadin) depending on the laboratory values
    d. Heparin via IV infusion, with warfarin (Coumadin) therapy started at the same time

99. The patients with which conditions are candidates for an inferior vena cava filter placement? *(Select all that apply.)*
   a. Abdominal aortic aneurysm
   b. Chronic obstructive pulmonary disease
   c. Recurrent deep vein thrombosis
   d. No response to medical treatment
   e. Intolerance to anticoagulation drug therapy

100. What is the recommended therapeutic range for the International Normalized Ratio (INR) that is done along with prothrombin time in a patient receiving warfarin sodium (Coumadin)?
   a. 0.5 to 1.0
   b. 1.0 to 1.5
   c. 1.5 to 2.0
   d. 2.0 to 2.5

101. A patient prescribed warfarin sodium (Coumadin) is instructed that certain foods decrease the effect of the drug. Which foods, if eaten, must be consumed in consistent and small amounts each day?
   a. Fresh fruits
   b. Chicken and beef
   c. Spinach and asparagus
   d. Milk and cheese

102. The nurse is teaching a patient who is at risk for venous thromboembolism (VTE). The patient is currently asymptomatic and is living in the community. What interventions does the nurse instruct the patient to do to minimize the risk of VTE? *(Select all that apply.)*
   a. Avoid oral contraceptives.
   b. Drink adequate fluids to avoid dehydration.
   c. Exercise the legs during long periods of bedrest or sitting.
   d. Arise early in the morning for ambulation.
   e. Use a venous plexus foot pump.

103. The nurse is reviewing the diagnostic test results for a patient suspected of having a DVT. The results show a negative D-dimer test. How does the nurse interpret this data?
   a. The test excludes DVT.
   b. Venous duplex ultrasonography is needed.
   c. The patient has arterial disease.
   d. Impedance plethysmography is needed.

104. The health care provider has ordered unfractionated heparin (UFH) for a patient with DVT. Before administering the drug, the nurse ensures that which laboratory tests were obtained for baseline measurement? *(Select all that apply.)*
   a. Prothrombin time (PT)
   b. Activated partial thromboplastin time (APTT or aPTT)
   c. INR
   d. Complete blood count (CBC) with platelet count
   e. Arterial blood gas
   f. Urinalysis

105. The nurse notes that the platelet count for a patient who is to receive UFH is 100,000/mm³. How does the nurse interpret this result?
   a. It is slightly lowered and worth monitoring for trends.
   b. It is significantly low, so the health care provider should be notified.
   c. It is insignificant unless other values such as PT or APTT are abnormal.
   d. It is higher than expected, but within normal limits for therapy.

106. The medication order for UFH is for 80 units/kg of body weight. How does the nurse interpret this order?
   a. Appropriate dose for the continuous IV infusion
   b. Higher than expected dose for the initial IV bolus
   c. Appropriate dose for the initial IV bolus
   d. Appropriate dose for maintenance therapy

107. A patient is receiving UFH therapy. The nurse instructs the UAP in which task related to the UFH therapy?
    a. Observe the skin for ecchymosis, bruising, and petechiae during AM hygiene.
    b. Replace the antiembolism devices after bathing or ambulating.
    c. Check on the patient every 2 hours and report changes in mental status.
    d. Watch for and report blood in the stool when assisting the patient with toileting.

108. A patient receiving UFH therapy is ordered to discontinue the therapy and begin low–molecular-weight heparin (LMWH) with enoxaparin (Lovenox). What is the priority nursing intervention?
    a. Discontinue the UFH at least 30 minutes before the first LMWH injection.
    b. Check the APTT results after giving the first LMWH injection.
    c. Assess the patient's IV site before starting the LMWH.
    d. Check the PT and INR results before giving the first LMWH injection.

109. What are the contraindications for thrombolytic therapy for DVT? (Select all that apply.)
    a. Recent surgery
    b. Trauma
    c. Stroke
    d. Diabetes mellitus
    e. Spinal injury

110. A patient is receiving thrombolytic therapy. How does the nurse monitor for the most serious complication from thrombolytic therapy?
    a. Performing neurologic checks and monitoring for level of consciousness
    b. Auscultating for breath sounds and counting respiratory rates
    c. Assessing the IV site and watching for infiltration and swelling
    d. Checking patency of the Foley catheter and monitoring urinary output

111. The nurse is teaching a patient about the side effects and potential problems associated with taking warfarin sodium (Coumadin). Which statement by the patient indicates a correct understanding of the nurse's instruction?
    a. "If I notice bleeding of the gums, I should skip one or two doses of the medication."
    b. "I should eat a lot of cabbage, cauliflower, and broccoli to prevent bleeding."
    c. "For injury and bleeding, I should apply direct pressure and seek medical assistance."
    d. "I should avoid going to the dentist while I am taking this medication."

112. A patient with a history of vascular disease as a result of diabetes has developed a peripheral neuropathy. This patient is at risk for which problem?
    a. Fatigue
    b. Severe pain
    c. Injury
    d. Poor circulation

113. The nurse is instructing a patient and caregiver on warfarin (Coumadin) therapy at home. Which items does the nurse include in the teaching plan? (Select all that apply.)
    a. "Eat small amounts of broccoli and spinach."
    b. "Avoid beta-blockers and ACE inhibitors."
    c. "Inform your dentist of taking warfarin prior to treatment."
    d. "Eat small amounts of oranges and bananas."
    e. "Avoid NSAIDs and birth control pills."

114. Which statements pertaining to the use of the Unna boot are correct? (Select all that apply.)
    a. It is used to heal peripheral arterial disease ulcers.
    b. It is applied from the toes to the knee.
    c. The patient is instructed on the signs and symptoms of arterial occlusion.
    d. It is changed by a health care provider every 3 to 4 days.
    e. It is used to heal venous stasis ulcers.

115. The nurse is assessing an obese patient's lower leg and notes a small irregular-shaped ulcer over the medial malleolus with brownish discoloration. The patient reports that the "leg has been that way for a long time." What do these findings suggest to the nurse?
    a. Varicose vein
    b. Venous stasis ulcer
    c. Phlebitis
    d. Raynaud's phenomenon

116. The nurse is consulting with the registered dietitian about diet therapy for a patient with chronic venous stasis ulcers. What are the dietary recommendations to help this patient promote wound healing?
    a. High-protein foods
    b. Vitamin D and B supplements
    c. Low-fat foods
    d. High-calcium foods

117. A patient has a venous stasis ulcer that requires a dressing. Which dressing materials are selected for this type of wound? *(Select all that apply.)*
    a. Oxygen-permeable polyethylene film
    b. Oxygen-impermeable hydrocolloid dressing
    c. Dry gauze dressings
    d. Artificial skin products
    e. Unna boot
    f. Vacuum-assisted wound closure

118. The nurse is assessing a patient with distended, protruding veins. In order to assess for varicose veins, what technique does the nurse use?
    a. Place the patient in a supine position with elevated legs; as the patient sits up, observe the veins filling from the proximal end.
    b. Place the patient in the Trendelenburg position and observe the distention and protruding of the veins.
    c. Ask the patient to stand and observe the leg veins; then ask the patient to sit or lie down and observe the veins.
    d. Ask the patient to walk around the room and observe the veins; then have the patient rest for several minutes and reassess the veins.

119. A patient with varicose veins asks the nurse to provide a list of all available treatment options. Which options does the nurse include on the list for the patient? *(Select all that apply.)*
    a. Elastic stockings and elevation of the extremities
    b. Vein stripping
    c. Application of radiofrequency (RF) energy
    d. Endovenous laser treatment
    e. Anticoagulant therapy

120. The nurse is assessing the IV site of a patient who has been receiving a normal saline infusion. There is redness and warmth radiating up the arm with pain, soreness, and swelling. What does the nurse do next?
    a. Discontinue the IV and apply warm, moist soaks.
    b. Slow the infusion rate and reassess within 1 hour.
    c. Discontinue the IV and apply a cold pack.
    d. Contact the health care provider for an order for an antidote.

121. Which patient has the greatest risk for a pulmonary embolus related to a venous disorder?
    a. Patient with bilateral varicose veins
    b. Patient with phlebitis of superficial veins
    c. Patient with thrombophlebitis in a deep vein of the lower extremity
    d. Patient with venous insufficiency throughout the leg

122. What information does the nurse include when teaching a patient with chronic venous stasis? *(Select all that apply.)*
    a. Elevate the legs when sitting.
    b. Avoid crossing the legs.
    c. Wear antiembolic stockings at night during sleep.
    d. Avoid standing still for any length of time.
    e. Avoid wearing tight girdles, tight pants, and narrow-banded knee-high socks.

123. Which patient is at greatest risk for developing varicose veins?
    a. 37-year-old mail carrier
    b. 19-year-old retail store clerk
    c. 40-year-old operating room scrub technician
    d. 25-year-old pregnant woman in the first trimester

124. What is the preferred treatment for phlebitis?
    a. Dry heat
    b. Ice packs
    c. Warm, moist packs
    d. Massage and elevation

125. Which type of vascular injury is most likely to result from blunt trauma?
    a. Arteriovenous fistula
    b. Hematoma
    c. Dissection
    d. Incompetent valves

126. Which patient with vascular trauma is a candidate for immediate emergency surgery?
    a. 54-year-old with fractured humerus
    b. 36-year-old with a ruptured renal artery
    c. 18-year-old with a contusion of the pelvis
    d. 67-year-old with a chronic subdural hematoma

127. The nurse observes diminished pulses, cold skin, and a pulsatile mass over the femoral artery in a patient reporting pain in the right leg. What condition does the nurse suspect in this patient?
    a. Venous thromboembolism
    b. Buerger's disease
    c. Femoral aneurysm
    d. Popliteal entrapment

37 CHAPTER

Care of Patients with Shock

1. Which statements about shock are true? *(Select all that apply.)*
   a. Shock is a whole-body response to tissues not receiving enough oxygen.
   b. Shock is widespread abnormal cellular metabolism.
   c. Shock only occurs in the acute care setting.
   d. Shock may occur in older adults in response to urinary tract infections.
   e. Shock is mostly classified as a disease.

2. Which hormones are released in response to decreased mean arterial pressure (MAP)? *(Select all that apply.)*
   a. Insulin
   b. Renin
   c. Antidiuretic hormone (ADH)
   d. Epinephrine
   e. Aldosterone
   f. Serotonin

3. The patient has decreased oxygenation and impaired tissue perfusion. Which clinical manifestations are evidence of onset of the non-progressive or compensatory stages of shock? *(Select all that apply.)*
   a. Decreased urine output
   b. Low-grade fever
   c. Narrowing pulse pressure
   d. Decreased heart rate
   e. Increased heart rate

4. Which statement about the systemic effects of shock is correct?
   a. The liver is essentially unaffected, but liver enzymes may be lower than normal.
   b. The current heart rate and blood pressure indicate cardiac system is at baseline.
   c. The brain and neurologic system can withstand 10 to 15 minutes of severe hypoperfusion.
   d. The kidneys can tolerate hypoxia and anoxia up to 1 hour without permanent damage.

5. Which patients are at risk for shock related to fluid shifts? *(Select all that apply.)*
   a. Hypoglycemic patient
   b. Severely malnourished patient
   c. Patient with paralytic ileus
   d. Patient with kidney disease
   e. Patient with minor burns
   f. Patient with large wounds

6. A young woman comes to the emergency department (ED) with lightheadedness and "a feeling of impending doom." Pulse is 110 beats/min; respirations 30/min; blood pressure 140/90 mm Hg. Which factors does the nurse ask about that could contribute to shock? *(Select all that apply.)*
   a. Recent accident or trauma
   b. Prolonged diarrhea or vomiting
   c. History of depression or anxiety
   d. Possibility of pregnancy
   e. Use of over-the-counter medications

7. Which are specific causes or risk factors for cardiogenic shock? *(Select all that apply.)*
   a. Anesthesia
   b. Myocardial infarction
   c. Cardiac tamponade
   d. Ventricular dysrhythmias
   e. Constrictive pericarditis

8. Which patient is at risk for obstructive shock?
   a. Patient with a history of angina
   b. Patient with chronic atrial fibrillation
   c. Patient with a pulmonary embolus
   d. Patient with a history of heart failure

9. A patient has cardiac dysrhythmias and pulmonary problems as a result of receiving an IV antibiotic. What type of shock does the nurse recognize this represents?
   a. Hypovolemic
   b. Cardiogenic
   c. Anaphylactic
   d. Septic

10. A patient with a head injury was treated for a cerebral hematoma. After surgery, this patient is at risk for what type of shock?
    a. Obstructive
    b. Cardiogenic
    c. Chemical-induced distributive
    d. Neural-induced distributive

11. The nurse is performing a morning shift assessment on several patients. For which patient is the nurse immediately concerned about decreased tissue perfusion if the capillary refill time was delayed?
    a. Patient with diabetes mellitus
    b. Anemic patient
    c. Patient with peripheral vascular disease
    d. Asthmatic patient

12. The nursing student takes the morning blood pressure of a postoperative patient and the reading is 90/50 mm Hg. What does the student do next? *(Select all that apply.)*
    a. Report the reading to the primary nurse as a possible sign of hypovolemia.
    b. Assess the patient for subjective feelings of dizziness or shortness of breath.
    c. Check the patient's chart for trends of morning vital sign readings.
    d. Notify the instructor to verify the significance of the finding.
    e. Call a "code blue."

13. A patient at risk for shock has had some small, subtle changes in behavior within the past hour. How does the nurse evaluate the patient's mental status throughout the night?
    a. Assess the patient while he or she is awake, and then allow him or her to sleep until morning.
    b. Ask the patient and family to describe the patient's normal sleep and behavioral patterns.
    c. Periodically attempt to awaken the patient and document how easily he or she is aroused.
    d. Allow the patient to sleep, but assess respiratory effort and skin temperature.

14. For which indications would the nurse be prepared to administer a colloid product? *(Select all that apply.)*
    a. Hemorrhagic shock
    b. Dehydration
    c. Peripheral tissue hypoxia
    d. Fluid replacement
    e. Restore osmotic pressure

15. The nurse is caring for a patient at risk for hypovolemic shock. For which indicators of shock does the nurse monitor? *(Select all that apply.)*
    a. Elevated body temperature
    b. Increased peristalsis
    c. Decreasing urine output
    d. Vasodilation
    e. Increasing heart rate

16. Assessment findings of a patient with trauma injuries reveal cool, pale skin; reported thirst, urine output 100 mL/8 hr, blood pressure 122/78 mm Hg, pulse 102 beats/min, respirations 24/min with decreased breath sounds. This patient is in what phase of shock?
    a. Compensatory/nonprogressive
    b. Progressive
    c. Refractory
    d. Multiple organ dysfunction

17. A patient with blunt trauma to the abdomen has been NPO for several hours in preparation for a procedure and now reports subjective thirst. What is the nurse's first priority action?
    a. Get the patient a few ice chips or a moistened swab.
    b. Obtain an order for a stat hematocrit and hemoglobin.
    c. Take the patient's vital signs and compare to baseline.
    d. Obtain an order to increase the IV rate.

18. A patient is brought to the ED with a gunshot wound. For which early signs of hypovolemic shock does the nurse monitor? *(Select all that apply.)*
    a. Elevated serum potassium level
    b. Increase in heart rate
    c. Decrease in oxygen saturation
    d. Marked decrease in blood pressure
    e. Increase in respiratory rate

19. The unlicensed assistive personnel (UAP) reports repeatedly and unsuccessfully trying to take a patient's blood pressure with the electronic and manual devices. The nurse notes that the patient's apical pulse is elevated and the patient is at risk for hypovolemic shock. The patient begins to deteriorate. What is the best method for the nurse to determine the systolic blood pressure?
    a. Apply the electronic device to a lower extremity.
    b. Instruct the UAP to immediately get the Doppler.
    c. Apply the manual cuff and palpate for the systolic.
    d. Tell the UAP to try the electronic device on the other arm.

20. The nurse identifies signs and symptoms of internal hemorrhage in a postoperative patient. What is included in the care of this patient for hypovolemic shock? *(Select all that apply.)*
    a. Elevate the feet with the head flat or elevated 30 degrees.
    b. Monitor vital signs every 5 minutes until they are stable.
    c. Administer clotting factors or plasma.
    d. Provide oxygen therapy.
    e. Ensure IV access.
    f. Notify the Rapid Response Team.

21. A young trauma patient is at risk for hypovolemic shock related to occult hemorrhage. What baseline indicator allows the nurse to recognize the early signs of shock?
    a. Urine output
    b. Pulse rate
    c. Fluid intake
    d. Skin color

22. Which patient is most likely to show elevated hemoglobin and hematocrit during shock?
    a. Patient with severe vomiting and large amounts of watery diarrheal stools
    b. Patient with a large wound with copious drainage
    c. Patient who was stable after surgery, but is now decompensating
    d. Patient with a hemothorax and chest tube

23. A patient in hypovolemic shock is receiving sodium nitroprusside (Nitropress) to enhance myocardial perfusion. What is an important nursing implication for administering this drug?
    a. Assess the patient for headache because it is an early symptom of drug excess.
    b. Assess blood pressure at least every 15 minutes because hypertension is a symptom of overdose.
    c. Assess blood pressure at least every 15 minutes because systemic vasodilation can cause hypotension.
    d. Assess the patient every 30 minutes for extravasation because nitroprusside can cause severe vasoconstriction and tissue ischemia.

24. A patient is at risk for hypovolemia secondary to large amounts of watery diarrhea and vomiting. The patient reports feeling a little thirsty and a slightly lightheaded. What does the nurse do next?
    a. Take the blood pressure and pulse and compare results to the patient's baseline.
    b. Obtain an order to start a sodium nitroprusside (Nipride) IV infusion.
    c. Have the patient rest in bed and take small frequent sips of water.
    d. Compare the patient's intake to the urinary output.

25. A patient with hypovolemia is restless and anxious. The skin is cool and pale, pulse is thready at a rate of 135 beats/min; blood pressure is 92/50 mm Hg; respirations are 32/min. What actions must the nurse take? *(Select all that apply.)*
    a. Obtain a stat order for an IV normal saline bolus.
    b. Administer supplemental oxygen.
    c. Notify the Rapid Response Team.
    d. Place the patient in a semi-Fowler's position.
    e. Call a "code blue."

26. A patient is showing early clinical manifestations of hypovolemic shock. The provider orders an arterial blood gas (ABG). Which ABG values does the nurse expect to see in hypovolemic shock?
    a. Increased pH with decreased Pao_2 and increased $Paco_2$
    b. Decreased pH with decreased Pao_2 and increased $Paco_2$
    c. Normal pH with decreased Pao_2 and normal $Paco_2$
    d. Normal pH with decreased Pao_2 and decreased $Paco_2$

27. The nurse finds a patient on the bathroom floor. There is a large amount of blood on the floor and on the patient's hospital gown. Which actions must the nurse take? *(Select all that apply.)*
    a. Elevate the patient's legs.
    b. Establish large-bore IV access.
    c. Look for the source of the bleeding.
    d. Ensure a patent airway.
    e. Begin a nitroprusside (Nitropress) infusion.

28. The nurse is caring for a postoperative patient who had major abdominal surgery. Which assessment finding is consistent with hypovolemic shock?
    a. Pulse pressure of 40 mm Hg
    b. A rapid, weak, thready pulse
    c. Warm, flushed skin
    d. Increased urinary output

29. Which IV therapy results in the greatest increase in oxygen-carrying capacity for a patient with hypovolemic shock?
    a. Lactated Ringer's solution
    b. Hetastarch
    c. Fresh frozen plasma (FFP)
    d. Packed red cells

30. A patient comes to the ED with severe injury and significant blood loss. The nurse anticipates that resuscitation will begin with which fluid?
    a. Whole blood
    b. 0.5% dextrose in water
    c. 0.9% sodium chloride
    d. Plasma protein fractions

31. Which change in the skin is an early indication of hypovolemic shock?
    a. Pallor or cyanosis in the mucous membranes
    b. Color changes in the trunk area
    c. Axilla and groin feel moist or clammy
    d. Generalized mottling of skin

32. A patient is in hypovolemic shock related to hemorrhage from a large gunshot wound. Which order must the nurse question?
    a. Establish a large-bore peripheral IV and give crystalloid bolus.
    b. Give furosemide (Lasix) 20 mg slow IVP.
    c. Insert a Foley catheter and monitor intake and output.
    d. Give high-flow oxygen via mask at 10 L/min.

33. The nurse is performing a psychosocial assessment on a patient who is at risk for shock. Which statement made by the patient is of greatest concern to the nurse?
    a. "Do you have any idea when I might go home? No one is feeding my cat."
    b. "Something feels wrong, but I'm not sure what is causing me to feel this way."
    c. "I live alone in my house and my family lives in a different state."
    d. "I would usually go golfing with my friends today. I hope they're not worried about me."

34. A patient has a systemic infection with a fever, increased respiratory rate, and change in mental status. Which laboratory values does the nurse seek out that are considered "hallmark" of sepsis?
    a. Increased white blood count and increased glucose level
    b. Increased serum lactate level and rising band neutrophils
    c. Increased oxygen saturation and decreased clotting times
    d. Decreased white blood count with increased hematocrit

35. The nurse is caring for an older adult patient at risk for shock. What is an early sign of shock in this patient?
    a. Cool, clammy skin
    b. Decreased urinary output
    c. Restlessness
    d. Hypotension

36. The nurse is caring for a patient with sepsis. At the beginning of the shift, the patient is in a hypodynamic state. Several hours later, the patient's blood pressure is elevated and pulse is bounding. How does the nurse interpret this change?
    a. A positive response and a signal of recovery
    b. Temporary situation that is likely to normalize
    c. Worsening of the condition rather than improvement
    d. Expected response to standard therapies

37. The nurse is caring for a patient with sepsis. What is a late clinical manifestation of shock?
    a. Drop in blood pressure
    b. MAP is decreased by less than 10 mm Hg
    c. Tachycardia with a bounding pulse
    d. Increased urine output

38. The nurse is caring for a patient at risk for sepsis. Why does the nurse closely monitor the patient for early signs of shock?
    a. The patient is unable to self-identify or report these early signs.
    b. Distributive shock usually begins as a bacterial or fungal infection.
    c. Prevention of septic shock is easier to achieve in the early phase.
    d. There is widespread vasodilation and pooling of blood in some tissues.

39. A patient has a localized infection. What assessment findings are considered evidence of a beneficial inflammatory response?
    a. Decreased urine output which normalizes after fluid bolus
    b. Pulse rate of 120 beats/min related to increased metabolic activity
    c. Decreased oxygen saturation which responds to supplemental O_2
    d. Redness and edema that appear but subside in several days

40. The student nurse is assessing a patient's mental status because of the patient's risk for decreased tissue perfusion. The supervising nurse intervenes when the student nurse asks the patient which question?
    a. "What is today's date?"
    b. "Who is the president of this country?"
    c. "Where are we right now?"
    d. "Is your name Mr. John Smith?"

41. The nurse is caring for a patient at risk for septic shock from a wound infection. In order to prevent systemic inflammatory response syndrome, the nurse's priority is to monitor which factor?
    a. Patient's pulse rate and quality
    b. Patient's electrolyte imbalance
    c. Localized infected area
    d. Patient's intake and output

42. The nurse is evaluating the care and treatment for a patient in shock. Which finding indicates that the patient is having an appropriate response to the treatment?
    a. Blood pH of 7.28
    b. Arterial Po_2 of 65 mm Hg
    c. Distended neck veins
    d. Increased urinary output

43. The nurse is caring for a patient with septic shock. Which therapy specific to the management of septic shock for this patient does the nurse anticipate will be used?
    a. Inotropics
    b. Antibiotics
    c. Colloids
    d. Antidysrhythmics

44. A patient receives dopamine 20 mcg/kg/min IV for the treatment of shock. What does the nurse assess for while administering this drug?
    a. Decreased urine output and decreased blood pressure
    b. Increased respiratory rate and increased urine output
    c. Chest pain and hypertension
    d. Bradycardia and headache

45. When administering norepinephrine (Levophed), what does the nurse monitor for in the patient? *(Select all that apply.)*
    a. Extravasation
    b. Headache
    c. High-output renal failure
    d. Chest pain
    e. Hypertension

46. The nurse is caring for a patient in septic shock. The nurse notes that the rate and depth of respirations is markedly increased. The nurse interprets this as a possible manifestation of the respiratory system compensating for which condition?
    a. Metabolic acidosis
    b. Metabolic alkalosis
    c. Respiratory acidosis
    d. Respiratory alkalosis

47. The ICU nurse observes petechiae, ecchymoses, and blood oozing from gums and other mucous membranes of a patient with septic shock. How does the nurse interpret this finding?
    a. Pulmonary emboli (PE)
    b. Acute respiratory distress syndrome (ARDS)
    c. Systemic inflammatory response syndrome (SIRS)
    d. Disseminated intravascular coagulation (DIC)

48. The nurse is reviewing the laboratory results of a patient with a systemic infection. What is the significance of a "left shift" in the differential leukocyte count?
    a. Expected finding because the patient has a serious infection.
    b. Indication that the infection is progressing toward resolution.
    c. Indication that the infection is outpacing the white cell production.
    d. Important to watch for trends, but otherwise not urgently significant.

49. The ICU nurse is caring for a patient with septic shock. Which IV infusion order for this patient does the nurse question?
    a. Antibiotics
    b. Insulin
    c. 10% dextrose in water
    d. Synthetic activated C protein

50. The nurse is preparing a teaching session for a patient at risk for septic shock. Which topics does the nurse include in this teaching? *(Select all that apply.)*
    a. Wash hands frequently using antimicrobial soap.
    b. Avoid aspirin and aspirin-containing products.
    c. Avoid large crowds or gatherings where people might be ill.
    d. Do not share utensils; wash toothbrushes in a dishwasher.
    e. Take temperature once a week.
    f. Do not change pet litter boxes.

51. A patient is at risk for sepsis. Which assessment finding is most indicative of the hyperdynamic activity that occurs in septic shock?
    a. Crackles in lung bases
    b. Weak, rapid peripheral pulses
    c. Cool, clammy, cyanotic skin
    d. Increased pulse rate with warm, pink skin

52. The home health nurse is visiting a frail older adult patient at risk for sepsis because of failure to thrive and immunosuppression. What does the nurse assess this patient for? *(Select all that apply.)*
    a. Signs of skin breakdown and presence of redness or swelling
    b. Cough or any other symptoms of a cold or the flu
    c. Appearance and odor of urine, and pain or burning during urination
    d. Patient's and family's understanding of isolation precautions
    e. Availability and type of facilities for handwashing

53. A postoperative hospitalized patient has a decrease in MAP of greater than 20 mm Hg from baseline value; elevated, thready pulse; decreased blood pressure; shallow respirations of 26/min; pale skin; moderate acidosis; and moderate hyperkalemia. The nurse recognizes that this patient is in what phase of shock?
    a. Compensatory/nonprogressive
    b. Progressive
    c. Refractory
    d. Multiple organ dysfunction

54. A 70-year-old man is admitted to the hospital with an infected finger of several days' duration. He is lethargic, confused, and has a temperature of 101.3° F. Other assessment findings include blood pressure of 94/50 mm Hg, pulse 105 beats/min, respirations 40, and shallow breathing. Pulmonary arterial wedge pressure (PAWP) is 4 mm Hg. These assessment findings indicate what type of shock?
    a. Hypovolemic
    b. Cardiogenic
    c. Anaphylactic
    d. Septic

55. The clinical manifestations in the first phase of sepsis-induced distributive shock results from the body's reaction to which factor?
    a. Leukocytes
    b. Infectious microorganisms
    c. Hemorrhage
    d. Hypovolemia

56. What factor increases an older adult's risk for distributive (septic) shock?
    a. Reduced skin integrity
    b. Diuretic therapy
    c. Cardiomyopathy
    d. Musculoskeletal weakness

57. The nurse on a medical unit is presenting an in-service program on how to recognize sepsis. Which patients are at risk for distributive septic shock? *(Select all that apply.)*
    a. Older adult with urinary tract infection
    b. Patient with ruptured aortic aneurysm
    c. Patient with pneumonia
    d. Patient receiving heparin therapy
    e. Older adult with sacral pressure ulcers

58. The nurse is caring for a patient in septic shock with a serum glucose level of 280 mg/dL. What is the nurse's best interpretation of this finding?
    a. The patient is developing type 2 diabetes.
    b. The patient is developing type 1 diabetes.
    c. This finding is associated with a poor outcome.
    d. This finding is unexpected in septic shock.

59. The patient has been diagnosed with sepsis. Following the sepsis resuscitation bundle, which interventions should the nurse expect within the first 3 hours? *(Select all that apply.)*
    a. Obtain serum lactate level.
    b. Begin administering vasopressor drugs.
    c. Draw blood cultures.
    d. Administer broad-spectrum antibiotics.
    e. Assist with insertion of a central venous pressure line.

60. The UAP working under supervision of an RN is checking vital signs on the patient at risk for hypovolemic shock. Which instruction must the nurse give the UAP?
    a. Report any increase in heart rate because it is an early sign of shock.
    b. Report any increased systolic pressure, which is an early sign of shock.
    c. Report any changes in body temperature, which may indicate sepsis.
    d. Report any increase in respiratory rate because of acid-base changes.

38 CHAPTER

Care of Patients with Acute Coronary Syndromes

1. The nurse is interviewing a patient reporting chest discomfort that occurs with moderate to prolonged exertion. The patient describes the pain as being "about the same over the past several months and going away with nitroglycerin or rest." Based on the patient's description of symptoms, what does the nurse suspect in this patient? *(Select all that apply.)*
   a. Chronic stable angina (CSA)
   b. Unstable angina
   c. Acute coronary syndrome (ACS)
   d. Acute myocardial infarction (MI)
   e. Coronary artery disease (CAD)

2. A patient with a history of angina is admitted for surgery. The patient reports nausea, pressure in the chest radiating to the left arm, appears anxious, skin is cool and clammy, blood pressure is 150/90 mm Hg, pulse is 100, and respiratory rate is 32. What are the priorities of nursing care for this patient? *(Select all that apply.)*
   a. Relieve nausea
   b. Maintain NPO status
   c. Improve coronary perfusion
   d. Improve coronary oxygenation
   e. Relieve chest pain

3. A patient has been admitted for acute angina. Which diagnostic test identifies if the patient will benefit from further invasive management after acute angina or an MI?
   a. Exercise tolerance test
   b. Cardiac catheterization
   c. Thallium scan
   d. Multigated angiogram (MUGA) scan

4. The nurse is talking to a patient with angina about resuming sexual activity. Which statement by the patient indicates a correct understanding about the effects of angina on sexual activity?
   a. "I won't be able to resume the same level of physical exertion as I did before I had chest pain."
   b. "I will discuss alternative methods with my partner since I will no longer be able to have sexual intercourse."
   c. "If I cannot walk a mile, I am not strong enough to resume intercourse."
   d. "With approval from my health care provider, I should resume sexual activity in the mornings or after a rest period."

5. A patient with angina is prescribed nitroglycerin tablets. What information does the nurse include when teaching the patient about this drug? *(Select all that apply.)*
   a. "If one tablet does not relieve the angina after 5 minutes, take two pills."
   b. "You can tell the pills are active when your tongue feels a tingling sensation."
   c. "Keep your nitroglycerin with you at all times."
   d. "The prescription should last about 6 months before a refill is necessary."
   e. "If pain doesn't go away, just wait; the medication will eventually take effect."
   f. "The medication can cause a temporary headache."

6. A patient reports chest pain that is unrelieved with a sublingual nitroglycerin tablet. What does the nurse administer next to this patient?
   a. Valium intramuscularly
   b. Morphine sulfate IV
   c. Supplemental oxygen
   d. Chewable aspirin

7. A patient is hypertensive and continues to have angina despite therapy with beta blockers. The nurse anticipates which type of drug will be prescribed for this patient?
   a. Calcium channel blocker
   b. Digoxin
   c. Angiotensin-converting enzyme (ACE) inhibitor
   d. Dopamine

8. The nurse has just given a patient two doses of sublingual nitroglycerin for anginal pain. The patient's blood pressure is typically 130/80 mm Hg. Which finding warrants immediate notification of the health care provider?
   a. Patient reports a headache.
   b. Systolic pressure is 140 mm Hg.
   c. Systolic pressure is 90 mm Hg.
   d. Anginal pain continues but is somewhat relieved.

9. A patient is admitted for unstable angina. The patient is currently asymptomatic and all vital signs are stable. Which position does the nurse place the patient in?
   a. Any position of comfort
   b. Supine
   c. Sitting in a chair
   d. Fowler's

10. Which are characteristics of angina? *(Select all that apply.)*
    a. Pain is precipitated by exertion or stress.
    b. Pain occurs without cause, usually in the morning.
    c. Pain is relieved only by opioids.
    d. Pain is relieved by nitroglycerin or rest.
    e. Nausea, diaphoresis, feelings of fear, and dyspnea may occur.
    f. Pain lasts less than 15 minutes.

11. Which statement about CAD is accurate?
    a. Ischemia that occurs with angina lasts more than 30 minutes and does not cause permanent damage of myocardial tissue.
    b. Postmenopausal women in their 70s have the same incidence of MI as men.
    c. Many patients suffering sudden cardiac arrest die before reaching the hospital due to atrial fibrillation.
    d. Studies have shown that CAD in women manifests with the same symptoms as with men.

12. A patient is admitted for acute MI, but the nurse notes that the traditional manifestation of ST elevation myocardial infarction (STEMI) is not occurring. What other evidence for acute MI does the nurse expect to find in the patient? *(Select all that apply.)*
    a. Positive troponin markers
    b. Chronic stable angina
    c. Non-ST elevation MI (non-STEMI) on ECG
    d. Cardiac dysrhythmia
    e. Heart failure

13. People should seek treatment for symptoms of MI rather than delay because physical changes will occur approximately how many hours after an infarction?
    a. 3 hours
    b. 6 hours
    c. 12 hours
    d. 24 hours

14. The nurse is caring for a patient admitted with unstable angina and elevated lipid levels. What does the nurse include in teaching this patient about his or her elevated lipid levels? *(Select all that apply.)*
    a. Begin a vigorous exercise program.
    b. Avoid trans-fatty acids.
    c. Reduce intake of saturated fats.
    d. Monitor the amount of cholesterol ingested, staying below 200 mg/day.
    e. Consider a weight loss program.

15. The nurse is auscultating the heart of a patient who had an MI. Which finding most strongly indicates heart failure?
    a. Murmur
    b. S₃ gallop
    c. Split S₁ and S₂
    d. Pericardial friction rub

16. The nurse administers sublingual nitroglycerine to a patient experiencing an angina episode. How soon does the nurse expect the pain to begin to subside?
    a. 1-2 minutes
    b. 5-6 minutes
    c. 10-12 minutes
    d. 15-20 minutes

17. Which diagnostic tests are used to assess myocardial damage caused by an MI? *(Select all that apply.)*
    a. Positive chest x-ray
    b. Creatine kinase (CK) elevation
    c. ECG: ST depression
    d. CK-MB isoenzymes elevation
    e. Troponin I isoenzyme elevation

18. A patient has heart failure related to MI. What intervention does the nurse plan for this patient's care?
    a. Administering digoxin (Lanoxin) 1.0 mg as a loading dose and then daily
    b. Infusing IV fluids to maintain a urinary output of 60 mL/hr
    c. Titrating vasoactive drugs to maintain a sufficient cardiac output
    d. Observing for such complications as hypertension and flushed, hot skin

19. Which patient has the highest risk for death because of ventricular failure and dysrhythmias related to damage to the left ventricle?
    a. Patient with an anterior wall MI (AWMI)
    b. Patient with a posterior wall MI (PWMI)
    c. Patient with a lateral wall MI (LWMI)
    d. Patient with an inferior wall MI (IWMI)

20. A patient had an IWMI. The nurse closely monitors the patient for which dysrhythmia associated with IWMI?
    a. Bradycardia and second-degree heart block
    b. Premature ventricular contractions
    c. Supraventricular tachycardia
    d. Atrial fibrillation

21. The nurse is giving a community presentation about heart disease. Because many sudden cardiac arrest victims die of ventricular fibrillation before reaching the hospital, which teaching point does the nurse emphasize?
    a. Controlling alcohol consumption and quitting cigarette smoking
    b. Modifying risk factors such as diet and weight, and blood pressure medication compliance
    c. Recognizing the difference between chronic stable angina and unstable angina
    d. Learning to operate the automatic external defibrillators (AEDs) in the workplace

22. Metabolic syndrome increases the risk for coronary heart disease. Which are indicators of this syndrome? *(Select all that apply.)*
    a. Triglyceride level of 170 mg/dL
    b. HDL cholesterol level of 45 mg/dL in a male
    c. HDL cholesterol level of 45 mg/dL in a female
    d. Blood pressure of 130/86 mm Hg while taking a beta blocker
    e. Fasting blood sugar level of 120 mg/dL

23. Which early reaction is most common in patients with the chest discomfort associated with unstable angina or MI?
    a. Depression
    b. Anger
    c. Fear
    d. Denial

24. A patient is trying to make dietary modifications to reduce lipid levels. The patient would like information about omega-3 fatty acid food sources. What best source does the nurse recommend?
    a. Flaxseed
    b. Flaxseed oil
    c. Fish
    d. Walnuts

25. A patient comes to the walk-in clinic reporting left anterior chest discomfort with mild shortness of breath. The patient is alert, oriented, diaphoretic, and anxious. What is the priority action for the nurse?
    a. Obtain a complete cardiac history to include a full description of the presenting symptoms.
    b. Place the patient in Fowler's position and start supplemental oxygen.
    c. Instruct the patient to go immediately to the closest full-service hospital.
    d. Immediately alert the physician and establish IV access.

26. A patient reports having chest discomfort that started during exercise. The patient is currently pain-free, but is "concerned." What questions must the nurse ask to assess the patient's pain episode? (Select all that apply.)
    a. "When did the pain start and how long did it last?"
    b. "What were you doing when the pain started?"
    c. "What did you do to alleviate the pain?"
    d. "How did you feel about the pain?"
    e. "Did the pain radiate to other locations?"
    f. "On a scale of 0 to 10 with 10 as the worst pain, what number would you use to categorize the pain?"

27. A patient is currently pain- and symptom-free, but reports having intermittent episodes of chest pain over the past week. The nurse asks about which associated symptoms? (Select all that apply.)
    a. Nausea
    b. Diarrhea
    c. Diaphoresis
    d. Dizziness
    e. Joint pain
    f. Shortness of breath

28. The emergency department (ED) nurse is assessing an 86-year-old patient with acute confusion, increased respiratory rate, anxiety, and chest pain. The nurse finds a respiratory rate of 36/min with crackles and wheezes on auscultation. How does the nurse interpret these findings?
    a. Left ventricular heart failure
    b. Atypical angina
    c. CAD
    d. Unstable angina

29. The nurse is assessing a middle-aged woman with diabetes who denies any history of known heart problems. However, on auscultation of the heart the nurse hears an S_4 heart sound. The nurse alerts the physician and obtains an order for which diagnostic test?
    a. Blood glucose level
    b. Electrocardiogram
    c. Chest x-ray
    d. Echocardiogram

30. A middle-aged patient with no known medical problems has acute-onset chest pain and dyspnea. In order to rule out acute MI, the nurse obtains orders for which diagnostic tests? (Select all that apply.)
    a. Triglyceride levels and C-reactive protein
    b. Chest x-ray
    c. Total serum cholesterol, low-density lipoprotein, high-density lipoprotein
    d. Troponin T and I
    e. Creatine kinase-MB
    f. Arterial blood gases

31. A patient had severe chest pain several hours ago but is currently pain-free and has a normal ECG. Which statement by the patient indicates a correct understanding of the significance of the ECG results?
    a. "I'll go home and make an appointment to see my family doctor next week."
    b. "The ECG could be normal since I am currently pain-free."
    c. "A normal ECG means I am okay."
    d. "I have always had a strong heart, low blood pressure, and a normal ECG."

32. Which statement about silent MI is correct?
    a. In a silent MI, the patient does not have any pain, so there is less myocardial damage.
    b. Diabetic patients are prone to silent MI that goes undiagnosed without complications.
    c. Silent MI increases the incidence of new coronary events.
    d. In silent MI, the myocardium is oxygenated by increased collateral circulation.

33. The ED nurse is caring for a patient with acute pain associated with MI. What are the purposes of collaborative management that address the patient's pain? (Select all that apply.)
    a. Return the vital signs and cardiac rhythm to baseline, so the patient can resume activities of daily living.
    b. Prevent further damage to the cardiac muscle by decreasing myocardial oxygen demand and increasing myocardial oxygen supply.
    c. Aggressively diagnose and treat life-threatening cardiac dysrhythmias and restore pulmonary wedge pressure.
    d. Closely monitor the patient for accompanying symptoms such as nausea and vomiting or indigestion.
    e. Eliminate discomfort by providing pain relief modalities, decrease myocardial oxygen demand, and increase myocardial oxygen supply.

34. The ED nurse, caring for a patient with severe chest pain and ECG changes, gives supplemental oxygen to the patient as ordered. Which other medications does the nurse anticipate giving to this patient? (Select all that apply.)
    a. IV nitroglycerin
    b. Beta blocker
    c. IV morphine
    d. Oral aspirin
    e. ACE inhibitor

35. The nurse is caring for a hospitalized patient being treated initially with IV nitroglycerin. What intervention must the nurse include in this patient's care?
    a. Increase the dose rapidly to achieve pain relief.
    b. Restrict the patient to bedrest with bedpan use.
    c. Monitor blood pressure continuously.
    d. Elevate the head of the bed to 90 degrees.

36. During an annual physical exam, a patient receives an ECG and has an abnormal Q wave in several leads. What is the nurse's best interpretation of this result?
    a. The patient is experiencing a silent MI.
    b. The patient has experienced an MI in the past.
    c. The patient is having an acute MI at the moment.
    d. The patient is experiencing ischemia at the moment.

37. The home health nurse receives a call from a patient with CAD who reports having new onset of chest pain and shortness of breath. What does the nurse instruct the patient to do?
    a. Rest quietly until the nurse can arrive at the house to check the patient.
    b. Chew 325 mg of aspirin and immediately call 911.
    c. Use supplemental home oxygen until symptoms resolve.
    d. Take three nitroglycerin tablets and have family drive the patient to the hospital.

38. A patient is newly diagnosed with cardiovascular disease. What psychosocial reactions does the nurse assess for? *(Select all that apply.)*
    a. Fear
    b. Anxiety
    c. Anger
    d. Suspicion
    e. Denial
    f. Depression

39. Which drug is given within 1 to 2 hours of an MI when the patient is hemodynamically stable, to help the heart to perform more work without ischemia?
    a. Vasodilators, such as sublingual or spray nitroglycerin (NTG)
    b. Beta-adrenergic blocking agents, such as metoprolol (Lopressor)
    c. Antiplatelet agents, such as clopidogrel (Plavix)
    d. Calcium channel blockers, such as diltiazem (Cardizem)

40. Which statements are true about the use of thrombolytic agents for a patient with an acute MI? *(Select all that apply.)*
    a. A patient who has received a thrombolytic agent must be continuously monitored before and after the medication is given.
    b. Thrombolytic therapy is indicated for chest pain of longer than 30 minutes duration that is unrelieved by other medications.
    c. There are no contraindications to thrombolytic therapy if the patient is having an acute MI as evidenced by cardiac enzymes and ECG.
    d. Bleeding is a risk for patients receiving thrombolytic therapy.
    e. The nurse need only monitor clotting studies of the patient who has received thrombolytic therapy. No further assessment is needed.

41. The health care provider is considering use of thrombolytic therapy for a patient. What is the criterion for this therapy?
    a. Chest pain of greater than 15 minutes duration that is unrelieved by nitroglycerin
    b. Indications of transmural ischemia and injury as shown by the ECG
    c. Ventricular dysrhythmias shown on the cardiac monitor
    d. History of chronic, severe, poorly controlled hypertension

42. A patient is being evaluated for thrombolytic therapy. What are absolute contraindications for this procedure? *(Select all that apply.)*
    a. Ischemic stroke within 3 months
    b. Pregnancy
    c. Suspected aortic aneurysm
    d. Major trauma in the last 12 months
    e. Intracranial hemorrhage
    f. Malignant intracranial neoplasm

43. The health care provider is considering treating a 125-pound 76-year-old MI patient with thrombolytic therapy. What action does the nurse expect regarding this therapy for this patient?
    a. Due to her age, the patient will not receive this therapy.
    b. The thrombolytic therapy dosage may be decreased to decrease risk of bleeding.
    c. Heparin by continuous IV is the best choice after antiplatelet therapy with an aspirin.
    d. Because the MI is recent, the patient will receive the usual dosage of thrombolytic drug.

44. A patient has received thrombolytic therapy for treatment of acute MI. What are postadministration nursing responsibilities for this treatment? *(Select all that apply.)*
    a. Document the patient's neurologic status.
    b. Observe all IV sites for bleeding and patency.
    c. Monitor white blood cell (WBC) count and differential.
    d. Monitor clotting studies.
    e. Monitor hemoglobin and hematocrit.
    f. Test stools, urine, and emesis for occult blood.

45. A patient is receiving beta-blocker therapy for treatment of MI. What does the nurse monitor for in relation to this therapy? *(Select all that apply.)*
    a. Tachycardia
    b. Hypotension
    c. Decreased level of consciousness
    d. Chest discomfort
    e. Increased urinary output

46. A patient is being treated with medication therapy following an acute MI. The nurse questions the order for which type of drug?
    a. Calcium channel blocker
    b. Beta-blocker
    c. ACE inhibitor
    d. Angiotensin receptor blocker (ARB)

47. A patient with angina is taking calcium channel blockers. For which complication does the nurse monitor with this patient?
    a. Wheezes
    b. Hypotension
    c. Bradycardia
    d. Forgetfulness

48. Which diagnostic test is performed after angina or MI to determine cardiac changes that are consistent with ischemia, to evaluate medical interventions, and to determine whether invasive intervention is necessary?
    a. Stress test
    b. ECG
    c. Echocardiography
    d. Chest x-ray

49. The nurse is monitoring a patient who received fibrinolytics and percutaneous coronary intervention (PCI). What is an indication that the clot has lysed and the artery reperfused?
    a. Abrupt increase of pain or discomfort
    b. Sudden onset of ventricular dysrhythmias
    c. Appearance of ST-segment depression
    d. Obvious T wave inversion

50. A patient has had an MI. The nurse anticipates which type of drug will be prescribed within 48 hours to prevent the development of heart failure?
    a. Calcium channel blockers
    b. ACE inhibitor
    c. Beta blockers
    d. Digoxin

51. The nurse has identified the priority problem of activity intolerance for a patient who had an acute MI. What is the best expected outcome for this patient?
    a. Patient will walk at least 200 feet four times a day without chest discomfort or shortness of breath.
    b. Patient will name three or four activities that will not cause shortness of breath or chest pain.
    c. Nurse will teach the patient to exercise and to take the pulse if symptoms of shortness of breath or pain occur.
    d. Nurse will assist the patient with ADLs until shortness of breath or pain resolves.

52. A patient is in the acute phase (phase 1) of cardiac rehabilitation. Which task is best to delegate to the unlicensed assistive personnel (UAP)?
    a. Assist the patient to ambulate approximately 200 feet three times a day.
    b. Assist the patient with ambulation to the bathroom.
    c. Assess heart rate, blood pressure, respiratory rate, and fatigue with each higher level of activity.
    d. Assist the patient into the bathtub.

53. A patient in the cardiac rehabilitation facility is having difficulty coping with the changes in her health status. Which statement by the patient is the strongest indicator of ineffective or harmful coping?
    a. "I don't mind going to therapy, but I'm not sure if I'm getting any benefit from it."
    b. "I'll take the pills and just do whatever you want me to do."
    c. "I don't want to go to therapy; I had a bad experience yesterday with the therapist."
    d. "I know I need to talk about going home soon, but could we discuss it later?"

54. A post-MI patient in phase 1 cardiac rehabilitation is encouraged to perform which activity?
    a. Range-of-motion exercises
    b. Modified weight training
    c. Stair climbing
    d. Jogging

55. The nurse is caring for a patient admitted for an IWMI. The patient develops heart block with bradycardia. Because the patient's pulse rate is low and the blood pressure is unstable, which procedure is the nurse prepared to assist with?
    a. Temporary pacemaker
    b. Defibrillation
    c. 16-lead ECG
    d. Percutaneous intervention

56. The nurse is contacted by the cardiac monitoring technician who says a patient is having a dysrhythmia. What does the nurse do first?
    a. Notify the Rapid Response Team.
    b. Administer antidysrhythmic medication.
    c. Evaluate the patient for chest pain or discomfort.
    d. Double-check the lead placement.

57. The nurse is evaluating a patient with CAD. What is an expected patient outcome that demonstrates hemodynamic stability?
    a. Blood pressure and pulse are within range and adequate for metabolic demands.
    b. Urine output increases from 15 to 30 mL per hour.
    c. P waves are regular and there are no abnormal heart sounds.
    d. Patient expresses verbal understanding of risk factors and need for compliance.

58. The nurse is assessing a patient at risk for left ventricular failure and inadequate organ perfusion. Which signs and symptoms signal decreased cardiac output? *(Select all that apply.)*
    a. Change in orientation or mental status
    b. Urine output less than 1 mL/kg (2.2 lbs)/hr or less than 30 mL/hr
    c. Hot, dry skin with flushed appearance
    d. Cool, clammy extremities with decreased or absent pulses
    e. Unusual fatigue
    f. Recurrent chest pain

59. The nurse is reviewing medication orders for several cardiac patients. There is an order for beta-adrenergic blocking agent metoprolol XL (Toprol XR) once a day. This drug order is most appropriate for which class of patients, according to the Killip classification system?
    a. All classes
    b. Class I only
    c. Class II and III
    d. Class IV only

60. The nurse is caring for a patient with an AWMI. The patient develops tachycardia, hypotension, urine output of 10 mL/hr, cold and clammy skin with poor peripheral pulses, and agitation. What does the nurse suspect in this patient?
    a. Ventricular dysrhythmia
    b. Cardiogenic shock
    c. Postpericardiotomy syndrome
    d. Acute coronary syndrome

61. The nurse is assessing a cardiac patient and finds a paradoxical pulse, clear lungs, and jugular venous distention that occurs when the patient is in a semi-Fowler's position. What are these findings consistent with?
    a. Right ventricle failure
    b. Unstable angina
    c. CAD
    d. Valvular disease

62. The intensive care nurse is monitoring a patient with a right ventricular MI. The pulmonary artery wedge pressure (PAWP) reading is 30 mm Hg. What does the nurse do next?
    a. Increase the IV fluid rate to 200 mL/hour.
    b. Auscultate the lungs to assess for left-sided heart failure.
    c. Perform an ECG using right-sided precordial leads.
    d. Place the patient in semi-Fowler's position.

63. A patient continues to have chest pain despite compliance with medical therapy. The nurse teaches the patient about which diagnostic test?
    a. Left-sided cardiac catheterization with coronary angiogram
    b. Percutaneous transluminary coronary angioplasty (PTCA)
    c. Coronary artery bypass grafting (CABG)
    d. Stent placement in coronary artery

64. Immediate reperfusion is an invasive intervention that shows some promise for managing which disorder?
    a. Right ventricular failure
    b. Metabolic syndrome
    c. Cardiogenic shock
    d. Acute coronary syndrome

65. A patient is scheduled to have PCI. The nurse anticipates that an initial dose of which medication will be given before the procedure?
    a. Clopidogrel (Plavix)
    b. Nitroglycerin (Nitrostat)
    c. Isosorbide mononitrate (Imdur)
    d. Carvedilol (Coreg)

66. A patient has angina and is scheduled for PCI. Based on negative outcomes of the PCI, the nurse prepares the patient for immediate transfer to undergo which procedure?
    a. Intraaortic balloon pump
    b. CABG
    c. Cardiac catheterization
    d. Carotid endarterectomy

67. The nurse is caring for a patient who had PCI. Which symptom indicates acute closure of the vessel and therefore warrants immediate notification of the health care provider?
    a. Chest pain
    b. Hyperkalemia
    c. Bleeding at the insertion site
    d. Cough and shortness of breath

68. Which patients may be potential candidates for CABG? *(Select all that apply.)*
    a. Patient with angina and greater than 50% occlusion of left main coronary artery that cannot be stented
    b. Patient with unstable angina with moderate vessel disease appropriate for stenting
    c. Patient with valvular disease
    d. Patient with coronary vessels unsuitable for PTCA
    e. Patient with acute MI responding to therapy
    f. Patient with signs of ischemia or impending MI after angiography or PTCA

69. The ICU patient with left ventricular failure has not responded to drug therapy to improve tissue perfusion. What intervention does the nurse expect may be tried next?
    a. CABG surgery
    b. Percutaneous insertion of an intraaortic balloon pump
    c. Intravenous infusion of a thrombolytic agent
    d. Insertion of a pulmonary artery catheter

70. A patient is having an elective CABG with a minimally invasive surgical technique. What does the nurse include in the preoperative teaching?
    a. Prevention of edema and scarring at the harvest site
    b. Protection and splinting of the chest incision while coughing
    c. Availability of analgesics if needed, but probably unnecessary
    d. Limitation of ambulation for several days after the procedure

71. A patient is having a CABG with the traditional surgical procedure. What does the nurse include in the preoperative teaching? *(Select all that apply.)*
    a. Coughing will be avoided to keep stress off the sternal incision.
    b. There will be a sternal incision.
    c. Expect one, two, or three chest tubes.
    d. An indwelling urinary catheter will be placed.
    e. An endotracheal tube will prevent talking.

72. The intensive care nurse is caring for a patient who has just had a CABG. The nurse notes that the patient has edema. In order to adjust fluid administration, the nurse collects which additional information and then consults the health care provider? *(Select all that apply.)*
    a. Blood pressure
    b. PAWP
    c. Skin turgor
    d. Cardiac output
    e. Blood loss
    f. Urine output

73. A potassium bolus of 80 mEq mixed in 100 mL of IV solution at a rate of 40 mEq/hr is ordered for a patient in the critical care unit. What does the nurse do next?
    a. Contact the health care provider because the order exceeds the recommended amount.
    b. Give the infusion; the order exceeds the recommended amount, but is within acceptable standards of practice for critical care patients.
    c. Contact the health care provider because even though the dosage is acceptable, the rate is too fast.
    d. Consult with the pharmacist because even though the rate is acceptable, the mixture is too concentrated.

74. The intensive care nurse is caring for a patient who has just had CABG surgery. The patient has a systolic blood pressure of 80 mm Hg. What is the primary concern related to this patient's hypotension?
    a. It is associated with warm cardioplegia.
    b. It may result in the collapse of the graft.
    c. It will result in acute tubular necrosis.
    d. It is related to mechanical ventilation.

75. Following CABG surgery, a patient has a body temperature below 96.8° F (36° C). What measures should be used to rewarm the patient?
    a. Infuse warm IV fluids.
    b. Do not rewarm; cold cardioplegia is protective.
    c. Place the patient in a warm fluid bath.
    d. Use lights or thermal blankets.

76. The intensive care nurse is caring for a patient who has just had CABG surgery. What does the nurse do to assess for postoperative bleeding?
    a. Measure mediastinal and pleural chest tube drainage at least hourly and report drainage amounts over 150 mL/hr to the surgeon.
    b. Measure mediastinal and pleural chest tube drainage at least once a shift and report drainage amounts over 50 mL/hr to the surgeon.
    c. Assess the dressing over the sternal site every 4 hours and reinforce the dressing with sterile gauze as needed.
    d. Assess the donor site every 4 hours and report serous drainage and increasing pain to the surgeon.

77. Following CABG surgery, a patient in the ICU on a mechanical ventilator suddenly decompensates. The health care provider makes a diagnosis of cardiac tamponade. The nurse prepares the patient for which emergency procedure?
    a. Chest tube
    b. Sternotomy
    c. Pericardiocentesis
    d. Thoracentesis

78. The nurse is assessing a patient who had CABG surgery. Which finding is a permanent deficit that is associated with an intraoperative stroke?
    a. Decreased level of consciousness that resolves when body temperature is normal
    b. Arousal from anesthesia takes several hours
    c. Inability to speak clearly and coherently immediately after surgery
    d. Generalized seizure activity

79. A patient reports pain after CABG surgery. Which statement by the patient suggests that the pain is related to the sternotomy and not anginal in origin?
    a. "The pain goes down my arm or sometimes into my jaw."
    b. "My pain increases when I cough or take a deep breath."
    c. "The nitroglycerin helped to relieve the pain."
    d. "I feel nausea and shortness of breath when the pain occurs."

80. A patient with CABG surgery is transferred from the ICU to the intermediate care unit. Which activity does the nurse assist the patient with?
    a. Ambulating 25 to 100 feet three times a day as tolerated
    b. Turning the patient every 2 hours for the first 48 hours
    c. Dangling and turning every 2 hours for at least 24 hours
    d. Coughing and deep-breathing three times a day

81. A patient had CABG surgery with the radial artery used as a graft. The nurse performs which assessment specific to this patient?
    a. Check the blood pressure every hour on the unaffected arm or use the legs.
    b. Check the fingertips, hand, and arm for sensation and mobility every shift.
    c. Assess hand color, temperature, ulnar/radial pulses, and capillary refill every hour initially.
    d. Note edema, bleeding, and swelling at the donor site, which are expected.

82. A patient with CABG surgery has been diagnosed with mediastinitis. What information does the nurse expect to find in the patient's assessment documentation? *(Select all that apply.)*
    a. Fever continuing beyond the first 4 days after CABG
    b. Bogginess of the sternum
    c. Redness and drainage from suture sites
    d. Decreased white blood cell count
    e. Induration or swelling at the suture sites
    f. Anginal-type chest pain

83. A patient had CABG surgery with a vein graft. To help prevent collapse of the graft, what assessment does the nurse perform?
    a. Auscultate lung sounds.
    b. Monitor for hypotension.
    c. Assess for motion and sensation.
    d. Observe for generalized hypothermia.

84. The nurse is caring for a patient who had CABG surgery. The nurse pays close attention to which electrolyte levels for this postoperative patient? *(Select all that apply.)*
    a. Sodium
    b. Potassium
    c. Calcium
    d. Magnesium
    e. Phosphorus

85. After a CABG surgery, a postoperative patient suddenly has a decrease in mediastinal drainage, jugular vein distention with clear lung sounds, pulsus paradoxus, and equalizing PAWP and right atrial pressure. What do these signs suggest to the nurse?
    a. Acute MI
    b. Occlusion at the donor site
    c. Cardiac tamponade
    d. Prinzmetal's angina

86. The nurse coming on duty receives the change of shift report. Which patient must be assessed first by the nurse?
    a. Patient with anxiety, nausea, diaphoresis, and shortness of breath
    b. Patient with diabetes mellitus and elevated serum lipid levels
    c. Patient with a friction rub and elevated temperature
    d. Patient with fever, instability of sternum, and increased white blood cell count

87. The nurse is caring for a patient who had a minimally invasive direct coronary artery bypass (MIDCAB). Which sign/symptom prompts the nurse to immediately contact the health care provider?
    a. Acute incisional pain
    b. ST-segment changes in the V leads
    c. Drainage from the chest tubes
    d. Problems with coughing

88. A patient has discrete, proximal, noncalcified lesions of only one or two vessels. Which procedure is most likely to be recommended for this patient?
    a. Percutaneous coronary intervention (PCI)
    b. Stress test with pharmacologic agent
    c. Immediate thrombolytic reperfusion therapy
    d. Minimally invasive bypass surgery

89. The nurse is caring for a patient who had a PCI. Which postoperative interventions are included in the care for this patient? (Select all that apply.)
    a. Monitor for acute closure of the vessel.
    b. Observe for bleeding from the insertion site.
    c. Maintain bedrest for 48 hours.
    d. Observe for hypotension, hypokalemia, and dysrhythmias.
    e. Teach about medications such as aspirin and beta blockers or ACE inhibitors.
    f. Instruct about lifestyle changes relating to CAD.

90. Treatment of hypothermia, a common problem after CABG surgery, is necessary because this condition may cause a patient to be at risk for which condition?
    a. Hypotension
    b. Hypertension
    c. Heart failure
    d. Loss of consciousness

91. Which statement is true about postpericardiotomy syndrome?
    a. It is a psychological disorder for which the patient needs emotional support.
    b. It is generally mild and self-limiting.
    c. It places the patient at high risk for cardiac tamponade.
    d. It can be prophylactically managed with antibiotics.

92. The patient is scheduled to have robotic heart surgery. Which advantages of this type of surgery does the nurse teach the patient about? (Select all that apply.)
    a. Shorter (2-3 day) hospital stay
    b. Shorter surgical time than with traditional heart surgery
    c. Less pain due to smaller incisions
    d. Shorter time on heart-lung bypass machine
    e. Chest tubes are never needed

39 Assessment of the Hematologic System

CHAPTER

1. The nurse is performing a hematologic assessment of an older adult patient. Which findings does the nurse identify as normal changes in the older adult? *(Select all that apply.)*
   a. Progressive loss of body hair
   b. Thickened or discolored nails
   c. Yellowing of the skin
   d. Dryness of the skin
   e. Ecchymosis

2. Which statement about hematologic changes associated with aging is true?
   a. The older adult has increased blood volume.
   b. The older adult has increased levels of plasma proteins.
   c. Platelet counts decrease with age.
   d. Antibody levels and responses are lower and slower in older adults.

3. For a patient who has a dysfunction of the bone marrow, which sign/symptom is the nurse most likely to observe?
   a. Long bone pain
   b. Fatigue
   c. Loss of appetite
   d. Weight gain

4. In the bone marrow of an older adult, what would be considered a normal physiologic change related to aging?
   a. Fatty tissue replaces bone marrow.
   b. Bone marrow cells become smaller.
   c. Weakened bones absorb bone marrow.
   d. Bone marrow cells fail to function.

5. The nurse knows that erythropoietin is a growth factor that is required for stem cells specialization. Which sign/symptom would the nurse observe if erythropoietin is lacking or not performing its role?
   a. Elevated body temperature
   b. Bruising and ecchymosis
   c. Swelling of lymph nodes
   d. Easily fatigued

6. Based on knowledge of albumin's role in maintaining osmotic pressure of the blood, which sign/symptom would the nurse observe for if the patient has low albumin levels?
   a. Fever
   b. Edema
   c. Dizziness
   d. Pain

7. The nurse is interviewing a patient who reports dizziness and lightheadedness, and bleeding gums every time she brushes her teeth. Which questions does the nurse ask the patient in order to focus in on the problem? *(Select all that apply.)*
   a. "How often do you take aspirin or any other nonsteroidal antiinflammatory drug?"
   b. "Do you have swollen glands or a sore throat?"
   c. "How much meat do you eat in a week?"
   d. "Are you having trouble swallowing?"
   e. "Does your heart ever seem to pound?"

8. Which drug disrupts platelet action?
   a. Vitamin K
   b. Ibuprofen
   c. Methyldopa
   d. Azathioprine

9. The nurse is interviewing a patient who has iron deficiency anemia. Which symptom is the patient most likely to report?
   a. Fatigue
   b. Nights sweats
   c. Calf pain
   d. Blood in urine

10. When assessing the patient with darker skin for pallor and cyanosis, which area would the nurse examine?
   a. Chest and abdomen
   b. General appearance of face
   c. Fingertips and toes
   d. Oral mucous membranes

11. Which laboratory result would indicate that the prescription for Epogen is having the desired therapeutic effect?
   a. Increase in platelet count
   b. Increase in white blood cell (WBC) count
   c. Increase in red blood cell (RBC) count
   d. Increase in iron level

12. Based on knowledge of physiologic triggers for RBC production, the nurse would anticipate which chronic health condition to be associated with an increase in RBC production?
   a. Diabetes mellitus
   b. Osteoarthritis
   c. Chronic obstructive pulmonary disease
   d. Chronic kidney disease

13. The patient reports a history of splenectomy. Based on this information, what is the nurse most likely to assess for?
   a. Signs of bleeding
   b. Signs of infection
   c. Digestive problems
   d. Jaundice of the skin

14. The patient is admitted for a chronic liver disorder and will be receiving vitamin K to address one of the problems associated with the disorder. Which clinical manifestation is the nurse most likely to observe before the vitamin K therapy is initiated?
   a. Sore throat and a smooth tongue
   b. Bruising and bleeding at venipuncture sites
   c. Fever and increase in WBC count
   d. Calf swelling due to deep vein thrombosis

15. Venous stasis is considered an intrinsic factor that could result in activating which physiologic process?
   a. Increased RBC production
   b. Adjustment of osmotic fluid pressure
   c. Initiation of anticlotting forces
   d. Initiation of blood clotting cascade

16. A deficiency in any of the anticlotting factors, such as protein C, protein S, and antithrombin III increases the patient's risk for which disorder(s)? *(Select all that apply.)*
   a. Pulmonary embolism
   b. Myocardial infarction
   c. Sepsis
   d. Pernicious anemia
   e. Stroke

17. Severe anemia could cause enlargement of which organ?
   a. Gallbladder
   b. Kidneys
   c. Colon
   d. Liver

18. The nurse sees that a 45-year-old woman has a low hemoglobin level. The nurse would perform a dietary assessment to identify a possible deficiency in which nutrient?
   a. Calcium
   b. Vitamin K
   c. Iron
   d. Vitamin D

19. In assessing the patient's hematologic status, which questions would the nurse include? *(Select all that apply.)*
   a. "Have you had unusual or increased fatigue?"
   b. "Have you ever had any radiation therapy?"
   c. "Have you ever had a job that exposed you to chemicals?"
   d. "Do you have a personal or family history of blood disorders?"
   e. "What drugs have you used in the past 3 days?"

20. The nurse is reviewing the patient's medication list and sees that the patient is receiving parenteral enoxaparin (Lovenox). Which outcome statement is the target of the enoxaparin therapy?
    a. Patient will not develop signs/symptoms of a blood clot.
    b. Patient will report a decrease in fatigue and dizziness.
    c. Patient will not develop signs/symptoms of infection.
    d. Patient will demonstrate no shortness of breath on exertion.

21. To assist the health care provider in determining whether a patient is a candidate for fibrinolytic therapy, the nurse is interviewing the patient diagnosed with a myocardial infarction. Why is determining the time of symptom onset essential in decision-making?
    a. Fibrinolytic drugs will not dissolve clots that are older than 6 hours.
    b. Clots that are older than 6 hours are too large and tightly meshed.
    c. Tissue that is anoxic for more than 6 hours is unlikely to benefit.
    d. After 6 hours, the patient is more likely to have excessive bleeding.

22. The home health nurse is reviewing the patient's medication list and sees that new medications were added during a recent hospitalization. In addition, the patient reports he takes a daily low dose of aspirin, but aspirin is not on the final discharge list. Because of the aspirin usage, the nurse is most likely to call the prescribing health care provider for clarification of which type of medication?
    a. Vitamin supplement
    b. Platelet inhibitor
    c. Antihypertensive
    d. Erythrocyte stimulating agent

23. A patient has a suspected hematologic problem. Which instruction is the nurse most likely to give to the UAP?
    a. Record urine output for the shift.
    b. Take the vital signs every 2 hours.
    c. Assess the patient for fatigue after exertion.
    d. Handle the patient gently to avoid bruising.

24. A patient is diagnosed with iron deficiency anemia. Which assessment finding is the nurse most likely to observe in this patient?
    a. Neck veins are distended and edema is present.
    b. Lower extremities show signs of phlebitis.
    c. Systolic blood pressure is lower than normal.
    d. Palpation of ribs or sternum elicits tenderness.

25. An experienced nurse is supervising a new nurse who is assessing a patient with a suspected hematologic problem. The experienced nurse would intervene if the new nurse performed which action?
    a. Palpated the edge of the liver in the right upper quadrant
    b. Auscultated the heart for abnormal heart sounds or irregular rhythms
    c. Used the fingertips to firmly press over the ribs or sternum
    d. Palpated the left upper quadrant to locate an enlarged spleen

Care of Patients with Hematologic Problems

1. The nurse is interviewing a patient who is newly admitted to the unit with a diagnosis of anemia. Which assessment findings does the nurse expect? *(Select all that apply.)*
   a. Dyspnea on exertion
   b. Systolic hypertension
   c. Intolerance to heat
   d. Concave appearance of the nails
   e. Pallor of the ears
   f. Headache

2. A patient with sickle cell crisis is admitted to the hospital. Which questions does the nurse ask the patient to elicit information about the cause of the current crisis? *(Select all that apply.)*
   a. "Have you recently traveled on an airplane?"
   b. "Have you ever had radiation therapy?"
   c. "In the past 24 hours, has any activity made you short of breath?"
   d. "Have you recently consumed alcohol or used recreational drugs?"
   e. "Have you had any symptoms of infection, such as fever?"

3. A patient is scheduled to undergo diagnostic testing for sickle cell anemia. For which diagnostic test does the nurse provide patient teaching?
   a. Bone marrow biopsy
   b. Platelet count
   c. Philadelphia chromosome analysis
   d. Hemoglobin S

4. The student nurse is caring for a patient in sickle cell crisis. Which action by the student nurse warrants intervention by the supervising nurse?
   a. Keeping the patient's room cool
   b. Using distraction and relaxation techniques
   c. Positioning painful areas of the patient with support
   d. Using therapeutic touch

5. The nurse has taught the patient about dietary modifications for his vitamin B_{12} deficiency anemia. Which statement by the patient indicates that additional teaching is needed?
   a. "Dairy products are a good source of vitamin B_{12}."
   b. "Dried beans taste okay if they are prepared correctly."
   c. "Leafy green vegetables interfere with my therapy."
   d. "I like nuts and I will gladly eat them."

6. Which patient is most likely to have severe manifestations of sickle cell disease even when triggering conditions are mild?
   a. Both parents have hemoglobin S gene alleles
   b. Mother has hemoglobin S gene alleles and father has hemoglobin A gene alleles
   c. Mother has sickle cell trait and father has hemoglobin A gene alleles
   d. Both parents have hemoglobin A gene alleles

7. The nurse is caring for a patient in sickle cell crisis. What are priority interventions for this patient? *(Select all that apply.)*
   a. Managing pain
   b. Managing nutrition
   c. Ensuring hydration
   d. Administering platelets
   e. Assessing oxygen saturation

8. The unlicensed assistive personnel (UAP) is providing care to a patient in sickle cell crisis. Which action by the UAP requires intervention by the supervising nurse?
   a. Elevating the head of the bed to 25 degrees
   b. Assisting to remove any restrictive clothing
   c. Obtaining the blood pressure with an external cuff
   d. Offering the patient her beverage of choice

9. A patient admitted for sickle cell crisis is being discharged home. Which statement by the patient indicates the need for further postdischarge instruction?
   a. "I will stop running 2 miles every morning."
   b. "I will visit my friends in Denver."
   c. "I will avoid the sauna at the gym."
   d. "I will not drink alcoholic beverages."

10. A patient has polycythemia vera. Which action by the UAP requires intervention by the supervising nurse?
    a. Assisting the patient to floss his teeth
    b. Using an electric shaver on the patient
    c. Using a soft-bristled toothbrush on the patient
    d. Assisting the patient to don support hose

11. A patient with a low white blood cell count is being discharged home. In which situations will the patient be instructed by the nurse to contact his or her health care provider? *(Select all that apply.)*
    a. When temperature goes over 102° F (38.9° C)
    b. A persistent cough develops with or without sputum
    c. Pus or foul-smelling drainage develops from open skin or a body opening
    d. Whenever exposed to fresh fruit or vegetables or live plants
    e. Urine is cloudy or foul-smelling, or if burning on urination is experienced

12. Which food should a patient with a low white blood cell count be encouraged to eat?
    a. Fresh strawberries
    b. Raw carrots
    c. Green leaf lettuce
    d. Well-done poultry

13. The nurse is caring for a patient with acute leukemia. Which signs/symptoms is the nurse most likely to observe during the assessment? *(Select all that apply.)*
    a. Hematuria
    b. Orthostatic hypotension
    c. Bone pain
    d. Joint swelling
    e. Fatigue
    f. Weight gain

14. In caring for a patient with acute leukemia, what is the priority collaborative problem?
    a. Protecting the patient from infection
    b. Minimizing the side effects of chemotherapy
    c. Controlling the patient's pain
    d. Assisting the patient to cope with fatigue

15. The nurse is helping a patient prepare for induction therapy for acute leukemia. What information will the nurse give to the patient?
    a. A donor is needed for hematopoietic stem cell transplantation.
    b. Prolonged hospitalization is common to protect against infection.
    c. The therapy may last from months to years to maintain remission.
    d. Success of the therapy results in remission and the intent is to cure.

16. Which factors are associated with an increased risk for lymphoma? *(Select all that apply.)*
    a. Immunosuppressive disorders
    b. Chronic infection from *Helicobacter pylori*
    c. Epstein-Barr viral infection
    d. Chronic alcoholism
    e. Pesticides and insecticides

17. Which disorder creates the highest risk for the patient to develop infection?
    a. Sickle cell crisis
    b. Vitamin B_{12} deficiency anemia
    c. Polycythemia vera
    d. Thrombocytopenia

18. Which medication increases the risk for the patient to develop infection?
    a. Steroids
    b. Aspirin
    c. Iron solutions
    d. Heparin

19. The nurse is caring for a patient with thrombocytopenia. Which order does the nurse question?
    a. Test all urine and stool for occult blood.
    b. Avoid IM injections.
    c. Administer enemas.
    d. Apply ice to areas of trauma.

20. A patient undergoing hematopoietic stem cell transplantation reports severe fatigue. To assist the patient with energy management, what does the nurse encourage the patient to do? *(Select all that apply.)*
    a. Verbalize feelings about limitations.
    b. Monitor nutritional intake to ensure adequate energy resources.
    c. Avoid napping throughout the day.
    d. Limit the number of visitors as appropriate.
    e. Plan activities for periods when the patient has the most energy.
    f. Monitor overall response to self-care activities.

21. The home care nurse is visiting a patient who had a stem cell transplant. Which observation by the nurse requires immediate action?
    a. The patient's grandson is visiting after receiving a MMR vaccine.
    b. The patient bumps his toe on a chair and applies pressure to the toe for 10 minutes.
    c. The patient with a platelet count of 48,000/mm^3 follows platelet precautions.
    d. The patient avoids going out to grocery shop in the winter months.

22. A patient has been taught how to care for his central venous catheter at home. Which statements by the patient indicate that further instruction is necessary? *(Select all that apply.)*
    a. "I will flush the catheter with heparin three times a day."
    b. "I will change the Luer-Lok cap on each catheter daily."
    c. "I will tape the catheter to my skin."
    d. "If the catheter lumen breaks or punctures, I will immediately clamp the catheter between myself and the opening."
    e. "I will wash my hands before working with the catheter."

23. The nurse has instructed a patient at risk for bleeding about techniques to manage this condition. Which statements by the patient indicate that teaching has been successful? *(Select all that apply.)*
    a. "I will take a stool softener to prevent straining during a bowel movement."
    b. "I won't take aspirin or aspirin-containing products."
    c. "I won't participate in any contact sports."
    d. "I will report a headache that is not responsive to acetaminophen."
    e. "I will avoid bending over at the waist."
    f. "If I am bumped, I will apply ice to the site for at least 10 minutes."

24. The new registered nurse is giving a blood transfusion to a patient. Which statement by the new nurse indicates the need for action by the supervising nurse?
    a. "I will complete red blood cell transfusion within 6 hours."
    b. "I will check the patient verification with another registered nurse."
    c. "I will use normal saline solution to dilute the blood."
    d. "I will remain with the patient for the first 15 to 30 minutes of the infusion."

25. The new registered nurse is identifying a patient for blood transfusion. Which action by the new nurse warrants intervention by the supervising nurse?
    a. Checks the health care provider's order before the blood transfusion
    b. Compares the hospital identification band name and number to those on the blood component tag
    c. Uses the patient's room number as a form of identification
    d. Examines blood bag tag and attached tag to ensure that the ABO and Rh types are compatible

26. A patient with lymphoma requires a hematopoietic stem cell transplant and a donor is being sought. Which type of transplant is likely to yield the best results?
    a. Synthetic human leukocyte antigen (HLA)
    b. HLA-identical twin sibling
    c. HLA-matched first-degree relative
    d. HLA-matched stem cells from an umbilical cord of a related donor

27. Patients with sickle cell disease are more susceptible to infections. Which actions help prevent infection? *(Select all that apply.)*
    a. Perform consistent thorough handwashing
    b. Encourage yearly flu vaccination
    c. Administer twice-daily oral penicillin
    d. Administer NSAIDs three times a day
    e. Monitor CBC and differential white cell count
    f. Assess vital signs at least every 4 hours

28. The nurse is caring for a patient who has donated bone marrow. In addition to having the aspiration sites monitored, the nurse will anticipate the need for which interventions? *(Select all that apply.)*
    a. Fluid for hydration
    b. Pain management
    c. Possible RBC infusion
    d. Prophylactic antibiotic therapy
    e. Assessment for complications of anesthesia

29. When caring for a patient after bone marrow stem cell transplantation, when does the nurse expect engraftment (the settling in of stem cells and the start of producing new cells) to occur?
    a. 8 to 12 hours after infusion
    b. 7 days after infusion
    c. 21 days after infusion
    d. 6 weeks after infusion

30. A patient is at high risk for the development of venoocclusive disease (VOD). What assessments does the nurse perform for early detection of this disorder? *(Select all that apply.)*
    a. Jaundice
    b. Weight loss
    c. Hepatomegaly
    d. Right upper quadrant abdominal pain
    e. Ascites

31. While being interviewed for admission, a patient tells the nurse that he has Christmas disease. What does the nurse document this as?
    a. Hemophilia A
    b. Hemophilia B
    c. Thrombocytopenia
    d. Sickle cell disease

32. Which hematologic disorder is most likely to cause the patient to have joint problems?
    a. Thrombocytopenia
    b. Aplastic anemia
    c. Hemophilia
    d. Warm antibody anemia

33. The nurse is inserting an intravenous needle into an older patient for the purpose of administering a blood transfusion. Which size needle should the nurse select?
    a. 22-gauge needle
    b. 20-gauge needle
    c. 19-gauge needle
    d. 23-gauge butterfly needle

34. A patient is receiving a blood transfusion. Which solution does the nurse administer with the blood?
    a. Ringer's lactate
    b. Normal saline
    c. Dextrose in water
    d. Dextrose in saline

35. A nursing student asks the registered nurse why D_5W is contraindicated when transfusing blood. How does the nurse respond?
    a. "It causes hemolysis of blood cells."
    b. "It dilutes the cells."
    c. "It shrinks the blood cells."
    d. "It is in the procedure manual."

36. A patient is receiving a blood transfusion through a single-lumen peripherally inserted central catheter. The patient has two other peripheral IVs: one is capped and the other has $D_5/.45$ NS running at a rate of 50 mL/hr. What can be given concurrently through the line that is selected for the blood product?
    a. Normal saline
    b. Piggyback of 10 mEq potassium chloride
    c. Total parenteral nutrition
    d. Furosemide (Lasix) 5 mg IV push

37. To avoid transfusion reaction, the nurse is carefully monitoring the patient during a blood transfusion. When are hemolytic reactions to blood transfusion most likely to occur?
    a. 1 mL is sufficient
    b. 5 mL is typical
    c. Within the first 50 mL
    d. Occurs after 100 mL

38. Which type of medication is used for patients receiving a platelet transfusion as premedication to prevent a reaction?
    a. Vitamin K and a diuretic
    b. Aspirin and hydroxyurea
    c. Diphenhydramine and acetaminophen
    d. Hydrocortisone and an antihypertensive

39. An older patient has been receiving frequent blood transfusions without any complications or adverse reactions; however, the nurse carefully monitors the patient during the current transfusion. Which signs/symptoms suggest that the patient is experiencing circulatory overload?
    a. Hypertension, bounding pulse, and distended neck veins
    b. Fever, chills, and tachycardia
    c. Urticaria, itching, and bronchospasm
    d. Headache, chest pain, and hemoglobinuria

40. The nurse is performing the immediate post-procedure care for a bone marrow donor. What is the priority assessment that the nurse will perform?
    a. Monitoring for activity intolerance
    b. Monitoring for infection
    c. Monitoring for fluid loss
    d. Monitoring CBC and platelet counts

41. Experienced nurse A is supervising new nurse B. In which circumstance would nurse A intervene?
    a. Nurse B prepares to use blood administration tubing to infuse stems cells.
    b. Nurse B obtains Y-tubing with a blood filter to administer packed red blood cells.
    c. Nurse B uses a special shorter tubing with a smaller filter to deliver platelets.
    d. Nurse B rapidly delivers fresh frozen plasma through regular straight filtered tubing.

42. Which outcome indicates that engraftment of transplanted cells in the patient's bone marrow has been successful?
    a. There is no evidence of graft-versus-host disease.
    b. WBC, RBC, and platelet counts begin to rise.
    c. Laboratory results indicate probable regressive chimerism.
    d. Laboratory results show decreasing percentage of donor cells.

43. The nurse would measure abdominal girth to monitor for which complication of hematopoietic stem cell transplantation?
    a. Failure to engraft
    b. Graft-versus-host disease
    c. Venoocclusive disease
    d. Septic shock

44. A patient reports fatigue, bone pain, and frequent bacterial infections. Further investigation reveals anemia, hypercalcemia, and x-ray findings show bone thinning with areas of bone loss that resemble Swiss cheese. The signs/symptoms and diagnostic findings are consistent with which disorder?
    a. Acute leukemia
    b. Multiple myeloma
    c. Non-Hodgkin's lymphoma
    d. Sickle cell anemia

45. A patient with acute leukemia has been receiving an erythropoiesis-stimulating agent. When would the nurse call the health care provider to have this order discontinued?
    a. Hemoglobin level is 6 mg/dL.
    b. Hematocrit is 20%.
    c. Hemoglobin level is 10.5 mg/dL.
    d. Platelet count is 50,000/mm^3.

41 CHAPTER

Assessment of the Nervous System

1. Which areas of the brain are responsible for speech and processing of language? *(Select all that apply.)*
    a. Motor cortex of the frontal lobe
    b. Broca's area
    c. Occipital lobe
    d. Parietal lobe
    e. Limbic lobe
    f. Wernicke's area

2. The nurse is performing a mental status examination on a patient. Which question best assesses recall memory?
    a. "How did you get to the hospital?"
    b. "What city were you born in?"
    c. "What is your mother's maiden name?"
    d. "How many children do you have?"

3. Which type of stroke or stroke damage is most likely to cause problems with respiratory distress related to neurologic function?
    a. Frontal lobe damage
    b. Thalamic stroke
    c. Affected temporal lobe
    d. Involvement of medulla and pons

4. With what will a patient with a cerebellar dysfunction most likely need assistance?
    a. Orientation to place and time
    b. Buttoning the shirt
    c. Verbal communication
    d. Mood and pain control

5. Which substances can pass through the blood-brain barrier? *(Select all that apply.)*
    a. Oxygen
    b. Albumin
    c. Water
    d. Anesthetics
    e. Many antibiotics
    f. Carbon dioxide

6. Which spinal tract has the function of voluntary movement?
    a. Spinothalamic
    b. Spinocerebellar
    c. Fasciculus gracilis or cuneatus
    d. Corticospinal

7. Which descriptors describe the sympathetic nervous system (SNS)? *(Select all that apply.)*
    a. Has cell bodies in the gray matter of the spinal cord from S2 to S4
    b. "Fight or flight" system
    c. Has some sensory function
    d. Is part of cranial nerves III, VII, IX, and X
    e. Causes the heart to pump faster

8. The nurse is teaching an older adult patient about medication and healthy lifestyle. Which teaching strategy is the best to use with this patient?
    a. Give limited and simplified information.
    b. Do the teaching late in the afternoon.
    c. Relate the information to recent events.
    d. Allow extra time for teaching and questions.

9. The nurse is caring for an older adult patient who is at risk for falling related to altered balance and decreased coordination. Which initial interventions will the nurse employ for this patient? *(Select all that apply.)*
   a. Instruct the patient to move slowly when changing positions.
   b. Instruct the patient to call for assistance before getting out of bed.
   c. Put up all the side rails and place the bed in the lowest position.
   d. Place the call bell and personal items within the patient's reach.
   e. Store personal items out of sight and instruct the patient to call for help.
   f. Assign a sitter to stay with the patient and assist as needed.

10. The nurse is obtaining baseline information from an older adult patient at risk for a neurologic disorder about his ability to perform activities of daily living (ADLs). Why does the nurse ask whether the patient is right- or left-handed?
    a. The patient may be somewhat stronger on the dominant side, which is expected.
    b. Effects of a neurologic event will be worse if the nondominant side is involved.
    c. This information is part of any standardized database for patients with neurologic disorders.
    d. The patient should be encouraged to strengthen and rely on the dominant side.

11. The nurse is assessing the mental status of a patient in the emergency department. Which finding is an early and reliable indication that central neurologic function has declined?
    a. Pupils are equal but not reactive to light.
    b. Level of consciousness has decreased.
    c. Cannot be aroused.
    d. Drowsy but easily arousable.

12. The nurse on the neurologic unit is evaluating several patients using the Glasgow coma scale (GCS). Which findings must be reported to the health care provider immediately? *(Select all that apply.)*
    a. A GCS decrease of 3 points
    b. Fixed nonreactive pupils
    c. Drowsy but arousable
    d. Extreme flexion of upper extremities
    e. Patient unable to state where he is located

13. When performing a neurologic examination, which method is best used to assess attention?
    a. Ask the patient to respond to questions about name, date of birth, today's date, time, and location.
    b. State 3 unrelated words to a patient and after 5 minutes ask the patient to repeat those words.
    c. Ask the patient to repeat 3 numbers then add a number with each repetition until 7 or 8 digits are remembered.
    d. Give the patient a 3-step set of commands such as pick up the pencil, fold the paper, and draw a circle on the paper then observe whether the commands are carried out.

14. An older adult patient is brought to the clinic by the family who reports that "Dad doesn't seem to be quite like himself." Which behavior is an early sign of a neurologic problem?
    a. Inability to remember a trip that he took last week
    b. Failure to remember his mother's maiden name
    c. Failure to recall where he went to high school
    d. Inability to describe his favorite hobby

15. In performing a mental status examination on a patient, the nurse asks, "What would you do if you saw a fire in the wastebasket?" What is the nurse assessing with this question?
    a. Executive function
    b. Level of consciousness
    c. Remote memory
    d. Orientation

16. The emergency department nurse detects sudden one-sided loss of function and sensation while completing a neurologic assessment on a patient. What is the nurse's first priority action at this time?
    a. Apply oxygen at 2 L/min by nasal cannula.
    b. Order a stat computed tomography (CT) scan.
    c. Immediately notify the health care provider.
    d. Place the patient in semi-Fowler's position.

17. Which sensory assessment technique is correct?
    a. Separate assessments for pain and temperature
    b. Assessment of only the affected or injured side
    c. Assessment of the proximal and distal areas of extremities
    d. Assessment of sharp and dull senses by using a paper clip

18. The nurse is caring for several older adult patients in a long-term care facility. In planning care with consideration for the sensory changes related to aging, which intervention does the nurse implement?
    a. Controls environmental odors because older adults have a heightened sense of smell
    b. Plans simple teaching sessions because of the decline in intellectual ability
    c. Increases the ambient lighting because of the decrease in pupil size
    d. Limits physical contact because the touch sensation increases

19. The nurse instructs the patient to close his eyes and hold the arms perpendicular to the body with the palms up for 15-30 seconds. Which reaction indicated to the nurse that the patient has a cerebral or brainstem reason for muscle weakness?
    a. The arm on the patient's weak side starts to drift with the palm turning inward.
    b. The patient's arms, wrists, and fingers are flexed with internal rotation.
    c. There is abnormal movement with rigidity characterized by extension of the arms.
    d. Dorsiflexion of the thumb and spreading of the other fingers occur.

20. An older adult patient is admitted to a long-term care facility and the nurse performs a baseline physical assessment that includes neurologic and sensory function. What is the purpose of the assessment?
    a. Determine a level of function for later comparison
    b. Show the family what problems the older adult has
    c. Gain information on past sensory changes
    d. Determine rehabilitation potential

21. Which question would the nurse ask to best assess a patient's remote (long-term) memory?
    a. "Can you tell me about your hobbies?"
    b. "What health care providers have you seen during the past six months?"
    c. "What is your date of birth?"
    d. "What is your usual bowel and bladder pattern?"

22. The nurse is assessing the sensory functions of a patient with Guillain-Barré syndrome (GBS). The nurse makes a clinical judgment to forgo assessing for light touch discrimination. Why does the nurse make this decision?
    a. The patient's pain and temperature sensations are intact.
    b. Sensory testing is done routinely every 4 hours.
    c. Only patients with spinal trauma require this assessment.
    d. The patient with GBS will be too confused to respond appropriately.

23. The nurse is testing a patient for touch discrimination by touching the patient on both shoulders. What is a normal finding for this assessment?
    a. Pointing to where each shoulder was touched
    b. Moving the shoulders against resistance
    c. Describing the touch as sharp or dull
    d. Sensing touch on the unaffected side

24. During a nurse's neurologic assessment, which test demonstrates coordination?
    a. Patient walks across the room, and returns.
    b. With arms out to the side, the patient touches the nose two to three times.
    c. Patient holds the arms perpendicular to the body with eyes closed.
    d. Patient grasps and squeezes the nurse's fingers.

25. The nursing student is performing a neurologic assessment on a patient who sustained a stroke (brain attack). The nurse observes the student evaluating grip and hand strength only on the affected side. What is the nurse's first action?
    a. Give the student positive feedback for performing the assessment correctly.
    b. Remind the student that strength testing needs to be done bilaterally.
    c. Redo the entire assessment and instruct the student to watch the process.
    d. Suggest to the instructor that the student needs remediation for assessment.

26. A patient is admitted to a rehabilitation center following a stroke that has left him with residual weakness on his left side. The nurse has completed the physical and neurologic assessment. Which documentation note best communicates the patient's progress?
    a. Shows progress and 3+ strength in left leg
    b. Demonstrates 5/5 in left leg and 5/5 in right leg against resistance
    c. Demonstrates 30-degree abduction of left leg
    d. Able to push against resistance with equal power in both legs

27. While assessing a patient's gait and equilibrium, the nurse observes that the patient has the Romberg sign. What is the priority patient problem associated with this objective data?
    a. Potential for falls related to dysfunction in awareness of body position
    b. Inability to perform ADLs related to decreased muscle strength
    c. Incontinence related to inability to ambulate to bathroom
    d. Potential for falls related to unsteady gait

28. Which statement about the GCS is correct?
    a. It is a thorough neurologic assessment tool.
    b. It establishes a baseline for eye-opening and motor and verbal response.
    c. It establishes a baseline cognitive function.
    d. A score of 15 indicates serious neurologic impairment with poor prognosis.

29. The nurse is attempting to assess a coma patient's response to pain. Which technique does the nurse try first?
    a. Gently shake the patient, similar to attempting to wake a sleeping child.
    b. Speak to the patient and call his or her name using a normal tone of voice.
    c. Face the patient and speak loudly and clearly, similar as with a hearing-impaired patient.
    d. Apply supraorbital pressure by placing the thumb under the orbital rim.

30. The nurse is assessing response to painful stimuli in a patient. What is the maximum length of time to apply the stimulus in the comatose patient?
    a. 1 to 2 seconds
    b. 5 to 10 seconds
    c. 20 to 30 seconds
    d. 40 to 60 seconds

31. Which neurologic disorder is most likely to require hourly sensory assessments of a patient?
    a. Parkinson disease
    b. Alzheimer's disease
    c. Guillain-Barré syndrome
    d. Huntington disease

32. The nurse is assessing several patients using the GCS. Which factors indicate the most serious neurologic presentation based on the GCS information?
    a. Eye opening to sound, localizes pain, confused conversation
    b. Eye opening to sound, obeys commands, inappropriate words
    c. Eye opening spontaneous, obeys commands, confused conversation
    d. Eye opening to pain, abnormal flexion, incomprehensible sounds

33. The nurse is performing neurologic checks every 4 hours for a patient who sustained a head injury. Which early sign indicates a decline in neurologic status?
    a. Nonreactive, dilated pupils
    b. Change in level of consciousness
    c. Decorticate posturing
    d. Loss of remote memory

34. The nursing student is talking to the patient and family about diagnostic testing. Which statement by the nursing student indicates the need for further study about the understanding of diagnostic procedures?
    a. "You are scheduled for a magnetic resonance imaging (MRI). Do you have a cardiac pacemaker?"
    b. "You are scheduled for a CT of the head. Are you wearing hairpins?"
    c. "You are to have x-rays of the skull. Are you allergic to iodine?"
    d. "You are to have a cerebral angiography. Do you take medication for diabetes?"

35. Which statement about lumbar puncture is accurate?
    a. It is indicated for patients with infections at or near the puncture site.
    b. It is done at the T1 to T3 spinal level.
    c. It requires the patient to lie flat for 24 to 48 hours after the procedure.
    d. It is done with the patient in the "fetal" position.

36. The nurse is reviewing the results of a lumbar puncture test. Which cerebrospinal fluid result does the nurse inform the health care provider about as a significant abnormal finding?
    a. Protein 500-700 mg/100 mL
    b. Cells 0-5 small lymphocytes/mm³
    c. Color straw-yellow
    d. Glucose 50 to 75 mg/100 mL

37. A patient is scheduled for an electroencephalogram (EEG). How does the nurse prepare the patient for this diagnostic test?
    a. Giving a sedative before bedtime
    b. Having the patient drink extra fluids before the test
    c. Keeping the patient NPO after midnight
    d. Ensuring that the hair is clean

38. A patient arrives on the unit alert and oriented after undergoing cerebral angiography. The report from the radiology nurse indicates the catheter was inserted into the left femoral artery. For which postprocedural order does the nurse call for clarification?
    a. Keep the left leg straight and immobilized.
    b. Maintain an ice pack and pressure dressing to the insertion site x 2 hours.
    c. IV and oral fluid restrictions for a total of 1000 mL/24 hours.
    d. Neurocirculation checks every 15 minutes x 2 hours; then every hour x 4 hours.

39. A patient is scheduled to have a CT with contrast media and the nurse is reviewing the patient's laboratory results. Which laboratory result could impact the procedure, prompting the nurse to notify the radiology department and the health care provider?
    a. Creatinine level
    b. White blood cell count
    c. Blood glucose
    d. Urobilinogen level

40. The nurse has instructed the patient and family on information about positron emission tomography (PET). However, the patient is suspected of having early signs of Alzheimer's disease. Which statement by the patient indicates he did not understand the information?
    a. "I may be asked to add or subtract numbers or to remember things during the test."
    b. "I am a little bit nervous about the idea of being blindfolded. Could you tell me about that?"
    c. "They will not give me my insulin shot on the morning of the test."
    d. "I will be asleep during most of the test; I will get a mild medication to help me relax."

41. Which factors are potential contraindications for having an MRI? *(Select all that apply.)*
    a. Cardiac pacemaker
    b. Implanted infusion pump
    c. Confusion or agitation
    d. Pregnancy
    e. Vascular stent
    f. Recent tattoo

42. A patient is scheduled for a cerebral blood flow evaluation with use of radioactive substance. Which medications does the nurse anticipate the physician will likely withhold from the patient for 24 hours before the test?
    a. Central nervous system depressants and stimulants
    b. Insulin or oral hypoglycemics
    c. Antihypertensives and diuretics
    d. Anticoagulants and antiplatelets

43. For which reasons would a neurologist order a patient to receive single-photon emission computed tomography (SPECT)? *(Select all that apply.)*
    a. The patient has amnesia
    b. To study cerebral blood flow
    c. The patient has type 2 diabetes
    d. Patient in a persistent vegetative state
    e. Breastfeeding woman with suspected brain tumor

44. The neurologic patient has documented severely increased intracranial pressure (ICP). Which diagnostic test would the neurologist avoid?
    a. MRI
    b. EEG
    c. CT scan with contrast
    d. Lumbar puncture

45. The nurse is performing a Glasgow coma scale on a traumatic neurologically injured patient. The patient does not follow commands and is unresponsive to voice. Which assessment does the nurse complete next?
    a. Instruct the patient to open his eyes and squeeze the nurse's hand.
    b. Check light touch at multiple points on the body bilaterally.
    c. In a loud voice, ask if the patient knows his name and where he is located.
    d. Pinch or squeeze the trapezius muscle at the angle of the shoulder and neck muscle.

42

CHAPTER

Care of Patients with Problems of the Central Nervous System: The Brain

1. Which pathophysiologic changes can lead to cluster headache? *(Select all that apply.)*
   a. Increase in hypothalamic size
   b. Release of the vasoconstrictor serotonin
   c. Overactive hypothalamus
   d. Spasm in the arteries at the base of the brain
   e. Vasoreactivity and neurogenic inflammation
   f. Decrease in cerebral blood flow

2. Which are characteristics of migraine headache? *(Select all that apply.)*
   a. Occurs more often in men
   b. Familial disorder
   c. Associated with runny nose and ptosis
   d. May last from hours to several days
   e. Occurs at regular intervals with long remission periods
   f. Occurs more often in women

3. A patient arrives at the clinic with a chief complaint of headache. He is irritable and impatient to receive treatment, but he is alert and oriented, his speech is clear, and he is able and willing to answer the nurse's questions. Which questions will the nurse ask to solicit additional relevant information about this patient's headache? *(Select all that apply.)*
   a. "When do the headaches occur?"
   b. "How often do the headaches occur?"
   c. "Why do you have headaches?"
   d. "Did you eat an unusually large meal just before your headache?"
   e. "Do you experience other symptoms with the headache?"
   f. "Have there been any recent changes in your headaches?"

4. A patient with a history of migraine headaches reports his current headache as "my usual throbbing pain, but today it is behind my left eye." Which question does the nurse ask to elicit information about trigger factors?
   a. "Do you have a history of illicit substance abuse?"
   b. "Do you smoke cigars or cigarettes?"
   c. "Are you having any trouble with your vision?"
   d. "Did you drink wine or coffee before the headache occurred?"

5. Which medication can be used to prevent migraines?
   a. Lamotrigine (Lamictal)
   b. Metoclopramide (Reglan)
   c. Sumatriptan (Imitrex)
   d. Propranolol (Inderal)

6. During a patient's last visit, the nurse instructed the patient about headaches and techniques to manage this condition. Which statement by the patient indicates teaching has been successful?
   a. "I have been keeping track of when my headaches occur."
   b. "My doctor told me that my headaches were not very serious."
   c. "My spouse knows the instructions that you gave me."
   d. "I have not had any headaches since we last talked."

7. A patient with a history of migraine headaches reports that noise makes her "head hurt worse." How does the nurse document this subjective finding?
   a. "Patient reports photophobia."
   b. "Patient reports phonophobia."
   c. "Patient reports vertigo."
   d. "Patient reports diplopia."

8. A patient is prescribed ergotamine with caffeine for migraine headaches. Which statement by the patient indicates the patient is experiencing a side effect of this drug?
   a. "My headache is initially relieved by the medication, but then it returns."
   b. "I seem to be gaining weight since I started taking this medication."
   c. "My headache seems worse in the morning when I take the medication."
   d. "I notice that I bruise more easily and my skin seems fragile and dry."

9. A patient has received a prescription for sumatriptan (Imitrex) for the treatment of migraine headaches. The patient tells the nurse that she elected not to tell the physician about all of her health conditions "because I just wanted treatment for my headaches and I didn't want to go into everything else." What is the nurse's response?
   a. The drug is contraindicated for patients who have glaucoma.
   b. It is necessary to monitor laboratory values such as prothrombin time (PT) and electrolytes.
   c. The drug is contraindicated in actual or suspected ischemic heart disease.
   d. The dosage is calculated by using relevant factors from the health history.

10. The patient tells the nurse she is interested in exploring the possible usefulness of complementary/alternative therapies for treatment of the pain from her migraine headaches. Which therapy would the nurse recommend?
    a. Meditation
    b. Massage
    c. Yoga
    d. Acupressure

11. A patient with migraine headaches tells the nurse that with his headaches he experiences an aura of flashing lights. During which phase of migraine headache would the nurse expect this to occur?
    a. First or prodrome phase
    b. Second phase
    c. Third phase
    d. After the headache subsides

12. Which foods or drinks are common triggers of migraine headaches? *(Select all that apply.)*
    a. Smoked fish
    b. Milk
    c. Coffee
    d. Aged cheese
    e. Fresh fruit
    f. Chocolate

13. Which definition best describes myoclonic seizures?
    a. Brief jerking of extremities, singly or in groups
    b. Brief period of staring or loss of consciousness
    c. Rigidity followed by rhythmic jerking
    d. Sudden loss of body tone

14. An elementary school teacher has just been informed that her student's brother has absence seizures. The teacher is fearful that her student may have the same type of seizures and is unsure what to expect. Which signs does the school nurse advise the teacher to look for?
    a. Brief jerking or stiffening of muscles that lasts only a few seconds
    b. Loss of consciousness and rhythmic jerking of extremities
    c. Brief loss of consciousness that may appear as daydreaming or blank staring
    d. "Blackout" that lasts 10 to 30 minutes with loss of memory and disorientation

15. What is the priority patient problem for atonic (akinetic) seizures?
    a. Potential for injury related to falls
    b. Organ ischemia related to neuromuscular dysfunction
    c. Confusion related to postictal state
    d. Limited mobility related to atonicity of muscles

16. Which tests does the nurse anticipate will be ordered for a patient to confirm a suspected diagnosis of epilepsy?
    a. Electrocardiogram (ECG) and positron emission tomography (PET)
    b. Electroencephalogram (EEG) and computed tomography (CT)
    c. Lumbar puncture (LP) and magnetic resonance imaging (MRI)
    d. Complete series of skull x-rays and neuroimaging

17. The nursing student is caring for a patient with clonic seizures. Which statement by the student indicates an understanding of clonic seizures?
    a. "The patient should be placed in a vest when sitting in a chair."
    b. "There is no medical treatment for clonic seizures."
    c. "I should have a padded tongue blade at the bedside."
    d. "The patient will have several minutes of muscle contraction followed by relaxation."

18. An older adult patient is brought to the emergency department from the local mall after bystanders saw her "having a seizure." The patient is currently responsive to voice, but is lethargic, confused, and unable to give an accurate history. Which aspect of this patient's health history is the most important to verify with the family?
    a. History of acute or chronic respiratory problems
    b. General ability to answer questions accurately
    c. Likelihood of the patient shopping at the mall alone
    d. Patient's doctor's name

19. Which order from the health care provider would the nurse clarify before administering an antiepileptic drug (AED)?
    a. Warfarin for a patient taking phenytoin
    b. Carbamazepine for a patient with tonic-clonic seizures
    c. Diastat for a patient in status epilepticus
    d. Gabapentin for a patient with partial seizures

20. A patient is treated in the emergency department for status epilepticus and is admitted to the hospital. The physician has ordered seizure precautions. What equipment does the nurse place in the room before the patient's arrival?
    a. Cardiac monitor and a pulse oximeter
    b. Penlight and a neurologic assessment flow sheet
    c. Padded tongue blades and padding for side rails
    d. Oxygen and suction equipment

21. Which factors are associated with viral meningitis? *(Select all that apply.)*
    a. Condition is usually self-limiting; full recovery is expected.
    b. Manifestations vary according to the state of the immune system.
    c. Cerebrospinal fluid (CSF) is hazy.
    d. No organisms grow from the CSF.
    e. Outbreaks occur in crowded conditions such as dormitories.

22. The nurse is caring for a patient who was admitted for a diagnosis of meningococcal meningitis. Which nursing action is specific to this type of meningitis?
    a. Administer an antifungal agent such as amphotericin B as ordered.
    b. Observe the patient for genital lesions.
    c. Place the patient in isolation per hospital procedure.
    d. Check to see if the patient is HIV-positive.

23. The nurse is reviewing the electrolyte values for a patient with bacterial meningitis and notes that the serum sodium is 126 mEq/L. How does the nurse interpret this finding?
    a. Within normal limits considering the diagnosis of bacterial meningitis
    b. Evidence of syndrome of inappropriate antidiuretic hormone (SIADH), which is a complication of bacterial meningitis
    c. A protective measure that causes increased urination and therefore reduces the risk of increased intracranial pressure (ICP)
    d. An early warning sign that the electrolyte imbalances will potentiate an acute myocardial infarction (AMI) or shock

24. A patient with meningitis reports a headache, and the nurse gives the appropriate IV push prn medication. Several hours later, the patient reports pain in the left hand; the radial pulse is very weak, the hand feels cool, and capillary refill is sluggish compared to the left. What does the nurse suspect is occurring in this patient?
    a. Stroke secondary to increased ICP resulting from meningitis
    b. Sickle cell crisis associated with an increased risk of meningitis
    c. Septic emboli causing vascular compromise
    d. Local phlebitis from the IV push pain medication that was given

25. A patient arrives in the emergency department reporting headache, fever, nausea, and photosensitivity. The patient has been living in close proximity with two people who were diagnosed with meningitis. Which diagnostic test does the nurse anticipate the physician will order to rule out meningitis?
    a. X-rays of the skull
    b. Lumbar puncture
    c. Myelography
    d. Cerebral angiogram

26. The nurse is caring for a patient who has symptoms and risk factors for bacterial meningitis. For which symptom must the nurse alert the physician?
    a. Capillary refill of 3 seconds
    b. Headache with nausea and vomiting
    c. Inability to move eyes laterally
    d. Oral temperature of 101.6° F

27. The nurse is carefully monitoring a patient with a severe case of encephalitis for signs of increased ICP. What vital sign changes are associated with increased ICP?
    a. Tachycardia and shallow, rapid respirations
    b. Increased core temperature and bradycardia
    c. Decreased pulse pressure and tachypnea
    d. Widened pulse pressure and bradycardia

28. The student nurse is caring for a patient with encephalitis. Which action by the student nurse warrants intervention by the supervising nurse?
    a. Performs deep suctioning for copious secretions
    b. Elevates the head of bed to 30 degrees after a lumbar puncture
    c. Turns the patient every 2 hours
    d. Performs a neurologic assessment every 2 hours

29. The nurse is assessing a patient with Parkinson disease. Which cardinal findings does the nurse expect to observe? *(Select all that apply.)*
    a. Tremors
    b. Rigidity
    c. Dementia
    d. Aphasia
    e. Postural instability
    f. Slow movements

30. A patient with Parkinson disease is being discharged on selegiline (Eldepryl), which is a selective monoamine oxidase type B (MAO-B) inhibitor. What information does the nurse include for safe medication administration?
    a. Take the medication with meals.
    b. Avoid driving or operating heavy machinery for several hours after taking the medication.
    c. Avoid tyramine-rich foods such as aged or cured foods.
    d. Take the medication daily at bedtime.

31. During the nurse's assessment of a patient with Parkinson disease, the nurse notes that the patient has a masklike facies. What functional assessment is now a priority?
    a. Ability to hear normal voice tones
    b. Ability to chew and swallow
    c. Ability to sense pain in the facial area
    d. Visual acuity

32. The home health nurse is visiting an older adult patient with Stage 1 Parkinson disease. He demonstrates some trembling and weakness in his right hand and arm, and reports he occasionally gets dizzy when he first stands up. The patient is currently living by himself and has no family in the immediate area. What is the priority patient problem?
    a. Decreased ability to perform activities of daily living (ADLs)
    b. Feeling of isolation
    c. Potential for falls
    d. Decreased nutritional status

33. A patient is on long-term medication therapy for Parkinson disease. What sign indicates that the patient may be having drug toxicity associated with these drugs?
    a. Acute confusion
    b. Tremors and rigidity
    c. Choreiform movements
    d. Seizure activity

34. A patient has moderate Parkinson disease with an impaired ability to communicate related to psychomotor deficit. Which nursing intervention is the best to use with this patient?
    a. Speaking clearly and slowly
    b. Watching the patient's lips when he speaks
    c. Giving step-by-step instructions to the patient
    d. Providing visual cues when trying to explain

35. The nurse is assessing an older adult patient who was brought to the clinic by her husband after she went out to do some gardening, but several hours later was spotted walking down the street by a neighbor. She is currently "just like herself," but the patient cannot explain what she was doing or where she was going. Which questions will the nurse ask to assess cognitive changes in this patient? *(Select all that apply.)*
    a. "Have you noticed any forgetfulness, for example misplacing your keys?"
    b. "Has there been any memory loss, such as not remembering a recent conversation?"
    c. "Are there any changes in ability to make judgments, such as taking a medication?"
    d. "Have you noticed any weakness; for example, in the arms or legs?"
    e. "Are there any changes in abilities to do a task like balancing your checkbook?"
    f. "Has there been any incontinence; for example, wetting the bed at night?"

36. The nurse observes a patient with Alzheimer's disease pushing at the food on her tray with her eyeglasses. This is documented as an example of what condition?
    a. Apraxia
    b. Aphasia
    c. Agnosia
    d. Anomia

37. The nurse is assessing an older adult patient with Alzheimer's disease using the Mini Mental State Examination (MMSE). What does this exam measure?
    a. Level of intelligence
    b. Functional ability
    c. Severity of the patient's dementia
    d. Alterations in ability to communicate

38. A patient has advanced Alzheimer's disease and is staying in a long-term care facility. Which intervention is the best to use with this patient?
    a. Reality orientation
    b. Cognitive training
    c. Memory training
    d. Validation therapy

39. A patient is experiencing mild memory loss and the patient and family are hoping the nurse can offer suggestions to help stimulate and strengthen the patient's current abilities. What is the nurse's first action?
    a. Show the family how to stimulate the memory by repeating what the patient just said.
    b. Discuss with the family and patient any practical memory problems that are occurring.
    c. Suggest that the patient identify and reminisce about pleasant past experiences.
    d. Provide name tags for the patient, family, and friends for use during group gatherings.

40. The daughter of an older adult patient with Alzheimer's disease has heard that there is a genetic disposition for Alzheimer's, and asks the nurse if there are preventive measures she can take. What does the nurse tell her about the current research on Alzheimer's disease?
    a. There is no evidence that first-degree relatives have an increased risk for this disease.
    b. Eating dark-colored fruits and vegetables has been associated with decreased risk.
    c. Use of NSAIDs such as ibuprofen increases the risk for the disease.
    d. Cessation of all tobacco products has been associated with decreased risk.

41. The patient with mild Alzheimer's disease lives at home with her daughter who is the primary caregiver and who works part-time. Which home safety precaution is appropriate for this patient?
    a. Puzzles and board games are provided for the patient.
    b. A geri-chair with a waist belt is in the patient's bedroom.
    c. The patient is wearing an identification bracelet with the daughter's address.
    d. The patient's medications are carefully organized in the bathroom cabinet.

42. The nurse is caring for several patients with Alzheimer's disease in a long-term care facility. Which task is best to delegate to the unlicensed assistive personnel (UAP)?
    a. Give hygienic care to the patient who is currently exhibiting sundowning.
    b. Assist the patient who has incontinence with toileting every 2 hours.
    c. Calm the agitated patient by using soft voice tones and distraction.
    d. Follow the patient and observe for hoarding or rummaging.

43. The patient with Alzheimer's disease does not recognize herself or other members of her family. The nurse knows this is an example of which phenomenon?
    a. Agnosia
    b. Prosopagnosia
    c. Delusions
    d. Hallucinations

44. The patient with dementia was just admitted to the hospital. Which strategies should the nurse use to protect the patient? *(Select all that apply.)*
    a. Soft restraints especially at night
    b. Frequent surveillance
    c. Toileting every 2 hours
    d. Side rails up at all times
    e. Sitters at the bedside
    f. Keep a clear path between the bed and bathroom

45. The nurse is assessing a patient with Huntington disease and observes jerky movements of the face, limbs, and trunk. How does the nurse document this assessment finding?
    a. Partial seizure
    b. Chorea
    c. Akinesia
    d. Nuchal rigidity

43 CHAPTER

Care of Patients with Problems of the Central Nervous System: The Spinal Cord

1. The nurse is taking a history on an older adult patient who reports chronic back pain. The nurse seeks to identify factors that are contributing to the pain. Which question is the most useful in eliciting this information?
   a. "Have you had any recent falls or have you been in an accident?"
   b. "Do you have a history of osteoarthritis?"
   c. "Do you have a history of diabetes mellitus?"
   d. "Are you having pain that radiates down your leg or into the buttocks?"

2. The nurse is preparing to physically assess a patient's subjective report of paresthesia in the lower extremities. In order to accomplish this assessment, which assessment technique does the nurse use?
   a. Use a Doppler to locate the pedal pulse, the dorsalis pedis pulse, or the popliteal pulse.
   b. Ask the patient to identify sharp and dull sensation by using a paper clip and cotton ball.
   c. Use a reflex hammer to test for deep tendon patellar or Achilles reflexes.
   d. Ask the patient to walk across the room and observe his gait and equilibrium.

3. Which position is therapeutic and comfortable for a patient with lower back pain?
   a. Semi-Fowler's position with a pillow under the knees to keep them flexed
   b. Supine position with arms and legs in a correct anatomical position
   c. Orthopneic position; sitting with trunk slightly forward; arms supported on a pillow
   d. Modified Sims' position with upper arm and leg supported by pillows

4. A patient has been talking to his physician about drugs that could potentially be used in the treatment of acute low back pain. Which statement by the patient indicates a need for additional teaching?
   a. "The doctor may prescribe an antiseizure drug such as oxcarbazepine; therefore, I would need to have blood tests to check my sodium level."
   b. "The doctor may suggest over-the-counter ibuprofen; therefore, I should watch for and report dark or tarry stools."
   c. "The doctor may prescribe an oral steroid such as prednisone; this would be short-term therapy and the dose would gradually taper off."
   d. "The doctor may prescribe hydromorphone and it may cause drowsiness; I should not drive or drink alcohol when I take it."

5. A patient is scheduled for lumbar surgery. Which key points must the nurse include in a preoperative teaching plan for this patient? *(Select all that apply.)*
   a. Techniques for getting in and out of bed
   b. Expectations for turning and moving in bed
   c. Limitations and restrictions for home activities
   d. Restriction of bedrest for at least 48 hours
   e. Report any numbness and tingling to the nurse immediately

6. The nurse is assessing a patient who presented to the emergency department (ED) reporting acute onset of numbness and tingling in the right leg. How does the nurse document this subjective finding?
   a. Paraparesis
   b. Paresthesia
   c. Ataxia
   d. Quadriparesis

7. A patient has just undergone a spinal fusion and a laminectomy and has returned from the operating room. Which assessments are done in the first 24 hours? *(Select all that apply.)*
   a. Take vital signs every 4 hours and assess for fever and hypotension.
   b. Perform a neurologic assessment every 4 hours with attention to movement and sensation.
   c. Monitor intake and output and assess for urinary retention.
   d. Assess for ability and independence in ambulating and moving in bed.
   e. Observe for clear fluid on or around the dressing.

8. A patient has a long history of chronic back pain and has undergone several back surgeries in the past. At this point, the surgeon is recommending a surgical procedure for spine stabilization. Which procedure does the nurse anticipate this patient will need?
   a. Laparoscopic diskectomy
   b. Spinal fusion
   c. Laminectomy
   d. Traditional diskectomy

9. A patient has just undergone a laminectomy and returned from surgery at 1300 hours. At 1530 hours, the nurse is performing the change of shift assessment. Which postoperative findings are reported to the surgeon immediately? *(Select all that apply.)*
   a. Minimal serosanguineous drainage in the surgical drain
   b. Pain at the operative site
   c. Swelling or bulging at the operative site
   d. Reluctance or refusal to cough and deep-breathe
   e. Moderate clear drainage on the postoperative dressing

10. A patient has just undergone spinal fusion surgery and returned from the operating room 12 hours ago. Which task is best to delegate to the unlicensed assistive personnel (UAP)?
    a. Log-roll the patient every 2 hours.
    b. Help the patient dangle the legs on the evening of surgery.
    c. Assist the patient to put on a brace so he can get out of bed.
    d. Help the patient ambulate to the bathroom as needed.

11. The nurse reviews the discharge and home care instructions with a patient who had back surgery. Which statement by the patient indicates further teaching is needed?
    a. "I will drive myself to my doctor's office next week."
    b. "I will put a piece of plywood under my mattress."
    c. "I will try to increase fruits and vegetables and decrease fat intake."
    d. "I plan to get a new ergonomic chair at work."

12. A patient has had an anterior cervical diskectomy with fusion and has returned from the recovery room. What is the priority assessment?
    a. Assess for the gag reflex and ability to swallow own secretions.
    b. Check for bleeding and drainage at the incision site.
    c. Monitor vital signs and check neurologic status.
    d. Assess for patency of airway and respiratory effort.

13. The patient with chronic back pain is receiving ziconotide (Prialt) by intrathecal (spinal) infusion with a surgically implanted pump. The patient develops hallucinations. What is the nurse's best first action?
    a. Request a psychiatric evaluation
    b. Notify the health care provider
    c. Perform an assessment of level of consciousness
    d. Decrease the dose of the medication

14. Which statements about spinal shock are accurate? *(Select all that apply.)*
    a. It lasts for from less than 48 hours up to a few weeks.
    b. There is temporary loss of motor and sensory function.
    c. There is permanent loss of motor and sensory function.
    d. There is temporary loss of reflex and autonomic function.
    e. There is permanent loss of reflex and autonomic function.

15. The nurse is caring for a patient with a spinal cord injury who is experiencing neurogenic shock. The patient's systolic blood pressure is 88 mm/Hg despite starting a dopamine drip 2 hours earlier. There is a new order to infuse 500 mL of Dextran-40 over 4 hours. At what rate does the nurse set the infusion pump?
    a. 75 mL/hr
    b. 100 mL/hr
    c. 125 mL/hr
    d. 150 mL/hr

16. A patient involved in a high-speed motor vehicle accident with sustained multiple injuries and active bleeding is transported to the emergency department by ambulance with immobilization devices in place. There is a high probability of cervical spine fracture; the patient has altered mental status and extremities are flaccid. What is the priority assessment for this patient?
    a. Check the mental status using the Glasgow coma scale.
    b. Assess the respiratory pattern and ensure a patent airway.
    c. Observe for intraabdominal bleeding and hemorrhage.
    d. Assess for loss of motor function and sensation.

17. Because the patient is at risk for spinal shock, what does the nurse monitor for?
    a. Decreased blood pressure, bradycardia, and decreased bowel sounds
    b. Tachycardia and a change in the level of consciousness
    c. Decreased respiratory rate and loss of sensation to pain and touch
    d. Paralytic ileus and loss of bowel and bladder function

18. Which neurologic assessment technique does the nurse use to test a patient for sensory function?
    a. Touch the skin with a clean paper clip and ask whether it is a sharp or dull sensation.
    b. Ask the patient to elevate both arms off the bed and extend wrists and fingers.
    c. Have the patient close the eyes and move the toes up or down; the patient identifies the positions.
    d. Have the patient sit with the legs dangling; use a reflex hammer to test reflex responses.

19. Assessment of a patient with a lower spinal cord injury confirms that the patient has paralysis of the bilateral lower extremities. How does the nurse document this finding?
    a. Paraparesis
    b. Paraplegia
    c. Quadriparesis
    d. Quadriplegia

20. Which symptoms indicate that a patient with a spinal cord injury is experiencing autonomic dysreflexia? *(Select all that apply.)*
    a. Flaccid paralysis
    b. Hypertension
    c. Hypotension
    d. Severe headache
    e. Blurred vision
    f. Loss of reflexes below the injury

21. The nurse is assessing a patient with a spinal cord injury and recognizes that the patient is experiencing autonomic dysreflexia. What is the nurse's first priority action?
    a. Check for bladder distention.
    b. Raise the head of the bed.
    c. Administer an antihypertensive medication.
    d. Notify the primary health care provider.

22. The nurse is providing discharge teaching for a patient with a spinal cord injury who will be performing intermittent self-catheterizations at home. Which signs and symptoms will the nurse instruct the patient to report immediately to the primary health care provider? *(Select all that apply.)*
    a. Dysuria
    b. Retention
    c. Fever
    d. Urgency
    e. Foul-smelling urine
    f. Back pain

23. The nurse is preparing a quadriplegic patient for discharge and has taught the patient's spouse to assist the patient with a "quad cough" to prevent respiratory complications. Which observation indicates that the spouse has understood what has been taught?
    a. The spouse assists the patient to the side of bed to encourage deep breaths.
    b. The spouse places her hands below the patient's diaphragm and pushes upward as the patient exhales.
    c. The spouse places her hands above the patient's diaphragm and pushes upward as the patient inhales.
    d. The spouse places the patient in an upright sitting position to encourage deep breaths.

24. The nurse is caring for a patient with a recent spinal cord injury (SCI). Which intervention does the nurse use to target and prevent the potential SCI complication of autonomic dysreflexia? *(Select all that apply.)*
    a. Frequently perform passive ROM exercises.
    b. Loosen or remove any tight clothing.
    c. Monitor stool output and maintain a bowel program.
    d. Keep the patient immobilized with neck or back braces.
    e. Monitor urinary output and check for bladder distention.

25. What is a potential adverse outcome of autonomic dysreflexia in a patient with a spinal cord injury?
    a. Heatstroke
    b. Paralytic ileus
    c. Hypertensive stroke
    d. Aspiration and pneumonia

26. After suffering an SCI, a patient develops autonomic dysfunction, including a neurogenic bladder. What is the priority patient problem for this condition?
    a. Risk for urinary tract infection
    b. Risk for dehydration
    c. Risk for urinary retention
    d. Risk for urinary incontinence

27. The nurse and the nursing student are working together to bathe and reposition a patient who is in a halo fixator device. Which action by the nursing student causes the supervising nurse to intervene?
    a. Uses the log-roll technique to clean the patient's back and buttocks
    b. Turns the patient by pulling on the top of the halo device
    c. Positions the patient with the head and neck in alignment
    d. Supports the head and neck area during the repositioning

28. The nurse is caring for several patients with SCIs. Which task is best to delegate to the UAP?
    a. Encourage use of incentive spirometry; evaluate the patient's ability to use it correctly.
    b. Log-roll the patient; maintain proper body alignment and place a bedpan for toileting.
    c. Check for skin breakdown under the immobilization devices during bathing.
    d. Insert a Foley catheter and report the amount and color of the urine.

29. A patient with an SCI has paraplegia and paraparesis. The nurse has identified a priority patient problem of inability to ambulate. The nurse assesses the calf area of both legs for swelling, tenderness, redness, or possible complaints of pain. This assessment is specific to the patient's increased risk for which condition?
    a. Contractures of joints
    b. Bone fractures
    c. Pressure ulcers
    d. Deep vein thrombosis

30. The nurse is caring for a patient who has been in a long-term care facility for several months following an SCI. The patient has had problems with urinary retention and subsequent overflow incontinence, and a bladder retraining program was recently initiated. Which are expected outcomes of the training program? *(Select all that apply.)*
    a. Demonstrates a predictable pattern of voiding
    b. Is able to independently catheterize himself
    c. Pours warm water over perineum to stimulate voiding
    d. Takes bethanechol chloride (Urecholine) 1 hour before voiding
    e. Is able to empty the bladder completely
    f. Does not experience a urinary tract infection

31. The patient with a spinal cord injury has a heart rate of 42/minute. Which drug does the nurse expect to administer?
    a. Methylprednisolone
    b. Dextran
    c. Atropine
    d. Dopamine

32. What key points does the nurse include in teaching an SCI patient about bowel and bladder retraining? *(Select all that apply.)*
    a. Ensure the patient gets a sufficient quantity of fluid each day.
    b. Instruct the patient about the purpose of stool softeners.
    c. Teach the patient about high-fiber foods.
    d. Teach the patient that continence is dependent upon spinal cord healing.
    e. Digital rectal stimulation is essential for regular bowel movements.

33. The patient is an adolescent who is quadriplegic as a result of a diving accident. The nursing assistant reports that the patient started yelling and spitting at her while she was trying to bathe him. He is angry and hostile, stating "Nobody is going to do anything else to me! I'm going to get out of this place!" What is the priority patient problem?
    a. Noncompliance
    b. Cognitive limitations
    c. Inability to cope with the situation
    d. Feelings of hopelessness

34. The nurse is giving home care instructions to a patient who will be discharged with a halo device. What does the nurse instruct the patient to avoid? *(Select all that apply.)*
    a. Going out in the cold
    b. Swimming or contact sports
    c. Sexual activity
    d. Bathing in the bathtub
    e. Driving

35. During the morning assessment of a patient with a spinal cord tumor, the nurse observes decreased sensation in the lower extremities and the linen is smeared with feces and smells of urine. The patient reports low back pain and appears to be having trouble moving his legs. The nurse suspects the tumor to be in which area of the spine?
    a. Upper cervical
    b. Lower cervical
    c. Thoracic
    d. Lumbosacral

36. A patient is hospitalized for a spinal cord tumor and is receiving medication for pain. The patient is having problems with constipation and urinary retention, and in addition, has limited mobility related to site of the tumor. Which task is best to delegate to the UAP?
    a. Measure and record intake and output.
    b. Check for blanching over reddened skin areas.
    c. Report the patient's relief of pain after using PCA morphine.
    d. Manually disimpact fecal matter.

37. The patient with a spinal cord tumor has developed a sudden rapid loss of motor and sensory function with a loss of bladder and bowel control. What does the nurse teach the patient about and prepare the patient for?
    a. Need for insertion of a urinary catheter
    b. Complete neurologic assessment
    c. Surgical decompression of the tumor
    d. Use of adult diapers

38. A patient reports increased fatigue and stiffness of the extremities. These symptoms have occurred in the past, but resolved and no medical attention was sought. Which questions does the nurse ask to assess whether the symptoms may be associated with multiple sclerosis? *(Select all that apply.)*
    a. "Do you feel unsteady or unbalanced when you walk?"
    b. "Do you have a persistent sensitivity to cold?"
    c. "Do you ever have slurred speech or trouble swallowing?"
    d. "Do you wake at night and then have trouble getting back to sleep?"
    e. "Has anyone in your family been diagnosed with multiple sclerosis?"

39. A patient with multiple sclerosis (MS) is prescribed oral fingolimod (Gilenya). Which key point must the nurse teach the patient about this drug?
    a. "You must be carefully monitored for allergic or anaphylactic reaction because the drug tends to build up in the body."
    b. "We need to teach you how to monitor your pulse rate because this drug can cause a slow heart rate."
    c. "This drug will decrease the frequency of clinical relapses that you will have with MS."
    d. "It will improve your ability to walk but also puts you are increased risk for seizure activity."

40. The patient is a woman in her early 30s who has recently been diagnosed with multiple sclerosis. The nurse has taught the patient's husband about the course of the illness and what problems might occur in the future. Which statement by her husband indicates the need for additional teaching?
    a. "She could fall because she may lose her balance and have poor coordination."
    b. "Eventually she will not be able to drive because of vision problems."
    c. "She will probably have a decreased libido and diminished orgasm."
    d. "Later on she could have intermittent short-term memory loss."

41. The nurse is teaching a patient with MS and her family about her exercise program. Which points must the nurse include? *(Select all that apply.)*
    a. Range-of-motion (ROM) exercises are an important component.
    b. Rigorous activity should follow stretching exercises.
    c. Increased body temperature can lead to increased fatigue.
    d. Progressive increased walking distances can lead to jogging.
    e. Stretching and strengthening exercises will be part of your program.

42. The patient with MS has dysarthria (slurred speech). For which complication must the nurse monitor in this patient?
    a. Dysmetria
    b. Dysphagia
    c. Ataxia
    d. Vertigo

43. The patient with MS states she is bothered by diplopia (double vision). Which intervention does the nurse expect to implement?
    a. Consult for corrective lenses
    b. Teach the patient scanning techniques moving her head from side to side
    c. Application of an eye patch alternating from eye to eye every few hours
    d. Prophylactic bilateral patches to both eyes at night

44. The patient and family are referred to the nurse for education about amyotrophic lateral sclerosis (ALS). What information does the nurse include in the educational session? *(Select all that apply.)*
    a. It is a progressive disease involving the motor system.
    b. The cause of ALS is unknown.
    c. Memory loss will occur but it will be very gradual.
    d. Death typically will occur several decades after diagnosis.
    e. There is no known cure for ALS.

45. The 50-year-old patient recently diagnosed with ALS is prescribed riluzole (Rilutek). When should the nurse teach the patient to take this drug?
    a. With a meal or a snack
    b. On an empty stomach
    c. At bedtime
    d. One hour after taking an antacid

44 CHAPTER

Care of Patients with Problems of the Peripheral Nervous System

1. The nurse is assessing a patient with a diagnosis of Guillain-Barré syndrome (GBS). Which signs and symptoms are consistent with GBS? *(Select all that apply.)*
   a. Bilateral sluggish pupil response
   b. Sudden onset of weakness in the legs
   c. Muscle atrophy of the legs
   d. Change in level of consciousness
   e. Decreased deep tendon reflexes
   f. Ataxia

2. During shift report, the nurse hears that a patient with GBS has a decrease in vital capacity that is less than two-thirds of normal, and there is a progressive inability to clear and cough up secretions. The physician has been notified and is coming to evaluate the patient. What intervention is the nurse prepared to implement for this patient?
   a. Frequent oral suctioning
   b. Rigorous chest physiotherapy
   c. Elective intubation
   d. Elective tracheostomy

3. A patient with GBS is identified as having poor dietary intake secondary to dysphagia. A feeding tube is prescribed. How does the nurse monitor this patient's nutritional status? *(Select all that apply.)*
   a. Checking the patient's skin turgor and urinary output
   b. Giving the prescribed enteral feedings via feeding tube
   c. Weighing the patient three times a week
   d. Reviewing the patient's potassium and sodium levels
   e. Monitoring weekly serum prealbumin level

4. A patient with GBS has been intubated for respiratory failure. The nurse must suction the patient. In assessing the risk for vagal nerve stimulation, what does the nurse closely monitor the patient for?
   a. Thick secretions
   b. Atrial fibrillation
   c. Cyanosis
   d. Bradycardia

5. A patient is admitted for a probable diagnosis of GBS, but needs additional diagnostic testing for confirmation. Which tests does the nurse anticipate will be ordered for this patient? *(Select all that apply.)*
   a. Electroencephalography (EEG)
   b. Cerebral blood flow (CBF)
   c. Electrophysiologic studies (EPS)
   d. Electrocardiogram (ECG)
   e. Electromyography (EMG)

6. The nurse is reviewing the cerebral spinal fluid (CSF) results for a patient with probable GBS. Which abnormal finding is common in GBS?
   a. Increase in CSF protein level
   b. Increase in CSF glucose level
   c. Cloudy appearance of CSF fluid
   d. Elevation of lymphocyte count in CSF

7. An ambulatory patient has sought treatment for symptoms of GBS. IV immunoglobulin therapy has been prescribed. Which precaution does the nurse expect with this therapy?
   a. It is given concurrently with plasmapheresis.
   b. A shunt must be placed prior to beginning the therapy.
   c. IV immunoglobulin is given slowly when started.
   d. Three or four treatments are given 1 to 2 days apart.

8. The patient with GBS is at risk for aspiration. Which precautions must the nurse initiate to prevent aspiration? *(Select all that apply.)*
   a. Elevate the head of the bed at least 45 degrees.
   b. Have patient assessed for dysphagia before administering oral fluids or medications.
   c. Teach the patient coughing and deep-breathing exercises.
   d. Have suctioning equipment available at the bedside.
   e. Turn the patient from side to side at least every 2 hours.

9. Which interventions are appropriate for pain management in an older adult with GBS? *(Select all that apply.)*
   a. IV opiates
   b. Gabapentin (Neurontin)
   c. Tricyclic antidepressants
   d. Massage
   e. Music therapy

10. A patient with GBS is receiving IV immunoglobulin. The nurse monitors for which major potential complication of this drug therapy?
    a. Headache
    b. Itching
    c. Anaphylaxis
    d. Fever

11. The nurse is monitoring a patient with GBS undergoing plasmapheresis. The patient reports dizziness and has a heart rate that has dropped to 48 beats per minute. The nurse notifies the primary care provider. Which order does the nurse anticipate?
    a. Atropine IV push
    b. Epinephrine IV push
    c. Continue to monitor the patient
    d. Defibrillate the patient

12. A patient has been newly diagnosed with GBS. The nurse is teaching the patient and family about the condition. Which statement by the family indicates a need for additional teaching?
    a. "He could recover in 4 to 6 months."
    b. "He'll never be able to walk again."
    c. "He will receive medication for pain."
    d. "It usually starts with the legs and moves upward."

13. Which strategies should be incorporated in the plan of care to provide emotional support for a patient with GBS who has ascending paralysis? *(Select all that apply.)*
    a. Limit information provided to the patient and family.
    b. Encourage the patient to verbalize feelings.
    c. Teach the patient and family about the condition.
    d. Explain all procedures and tests.
    e. Allow regularly scheduled rest periods.
    f. Assess previous coping skills.

14. What is the priority expected outcome in a patient with GBS?
    a. Maintain airway patency and gas exchange.
    b. Promote communication.
    c. Manage pain.
    d. Prevent complications of immobility.

15. The nurse is reviewing the admission and history notes for a patient admitted for GBS. Which medical condition is most likely to be present before the onset of GBS?
    a. Diabetes mellitus
    b. Recent bacterial infection
    c. Peripheral vascular disease
    d. Addison's disease

16. The patient with GBS describes a chronological progression of motor weakness that started in the legs and then spread to the arms and the upper body. Which type of GBS do these symptoms indicate?
    a. Ascending
    b. Pure motor
    c. Descending
    d. Miller-Fisher variant

17. The patient with GBS is in the plateau period. Which intervention is best for the nurse to delegate to the unlicensed assistive personnel (UAP)?
    a. Perform passive range of motion every 2 to 4 hours.
    b. Turn the patient every 2 hours and assess for skin breakdown.
    c. Remove the antiembolism stockings every 24 to 48 hours and perform skin care.
    d. Make a communication board for the patient with a list of common requests.

18. The patient with GBS is immobile and shows evidence of malnutrition. What is the nurse's priority concern for this patient?
    a. Respiratory failure
    b. Inability to perform activities of daily living (ADLs)
    c. Risk for pressure ulcers
    d. Cardiac dysrhythmias

19. The nurse is assessing a patient with myasthenia gravis (MG). Which manifestations can the nurse expect to observe? *(Select all that apply.)*
    a. Ptosis
    b. Diplopia
    c. Delayed pupillary responses to light
    d. Incomplete eye closure
    e. Decreased pupillary accommodation

20. Which statements about MG are accurate? *(Select all that apply.)*
    a. It is an acquired autoimmune disease.
    b. It usually occurs in young adults.
    c. It occurs slightly more in men than women.
    d. It is often accompanied by weight gain and distal weakness.
    e. It is associated with hyperplasia of the thymus gland.
    f. It is characterized by remissions and exacerbations.

21. What is the most common electrodiagnostic test performed to detect MG?
    a. EMG
    b. Repetitive nerve stimulation (RNS)
    c. Tensilon challenge test
    d. EPS

22. What is the cause of a cholinergic crisis?
    a. Not enough anticholinesterase drugs
    b. Too many anticholinesterase drugs
    c. Some type of infection
    d. Allergic reaction to anticholinesterase drugs

23. What test is used to differentiate a cholinergic crisis from a myasthenic crisis?
    a. EPS
    b. RNS
    c. Tensilon testing
    d. CSF protein level

24. The nurse is reviewing the biographic data and history for a patient with MG. What does the nurse expect to see included in the patient's records?
    a. Muscle weakness that increases with exertion or as the day wears on
    b. Difficulty sleeping with early morning waking and restlessness
    c. Confusion and disorientation in the late afternoon
    d. Muscle pain and cramps that interfere with ADLs

25. Because the most common symptoms of MG are related to involvement of the levator palpebrae or extraocular muscles, which assessment technique does the nurse use?
    a. Use a penlight and check for pupil size and response.
    b. Observe for protrusion of the eyeballs.
    c. Check accommodation by moving the finger toward the patient's nose.
    d. Face the patient and direct him or her to open and close the eyelids.

26. A patient with MG has "bulbar involvement." What is the nurse's priority assessment for this patient?
    a. Presence of pain in the extremities
    b. Loss of bowel and bladder function
    c. Ability to chew and swallow
    d. Quality and volume of the voice

27. A patient with MG and the nurse are having a long discussion about plans for the future. After an extended conversation, what does the nurse anticipate will occur in this patient?
    a. Speech will be slurred and difficult to understand.
    b. Voice may become weaker or exhibit a nasal twang.
    c. Voice quality will become harsh and strident.
    d. Voice will become toneless and affect will be flat.

28. A patient with MG reports having difficulty climbing stairs, lifting heavy objects, and raising arms over the head. What is the pathophysiology of this patient's symptoms due to?
    a. Limb weakness is more often proximal.
    b. Spinal nerves are affected.
    c. Large muscle atrophy is occurring.
    d. Demyelination of neurons is occurring.

29. The nurse is planning activities for a patient with MG. Which factor does the nurse consider to promote self-care, yet prevent excessive fatigue?
    a. Time of day
    b. Severity of symptoms
    c. Medication times
    d. Sleep schedule

30. A patient is suspected of having MG and a Tensilon test has been ordered. What does the nurse do in order to prepare the patient for the test?
    a. Ensure that the patient has a patent IV access.
    b. Draw a blood sample and send it for baseline analysis.
    c. Keep the patient NPO after midnight.
    d. Have the patient void before the beginning of the test.

31. The nurse is caring for a patient recently diagnosed and admitted with MG. During the morning assessment, the nurse notes some abnormal findings. Which symptom does the nurse report to the physician immediately?
    a. Diarrhea
    b. Fatigue
    c. Inability to swallow
    d. Difficulty opening eyelids

32. What is considered a positive diagnostic finding of a Tensilon test?
    a. After the cholinesterase inhibitor is administered, there are no observable changes in muscle strength or tone.
    b. Within 30 to 60 seconds after receiving the cholinesterase inhibitor, there is increased muscle tone that lasts 4 to 5 minutes.
    c. Within 30 minutes of receiving the cholinesterase inhibitor, there is improved muscle strength that lasts for several weeks.
    d. After the cholinesterase inhibitor is first administered, the patient will experience muscle weakness and then return to baseline.

33. Although an adverse reaction to Tensilon is considered rare, which medication should be readily available to give as an antidote in case a patient should experience complications?
    a. Protamine sulfate
    b. Narcan
    c. Atropine sulfate
    d. Regitine

34. The nurse is caring for a patient newly diagnosed with MG. The nurse is vigilant for complications related to both myasthenic crisis and cholinergic crisis. What is the priority nursing assessment for this patient?
    a. Monitor cardiac rate and rhythm.
    b. Assess respiratory status and function.
    c. Monitor fatigue and activity levels.
    d. Perform neurologic checks every 2 to 4 hours.

35. The nurse is performing patient and family teaching about MG medication therapy. What important information does the nurse give during the teaching session? *(Select all that apply.)*
    a. If a dose of cholinesterase is missed, a double dose is taken the next day.
    b. Antibiotics such as kanamycin synergize cholinesterase inhibitors.
    c. Medications must be taken on an empty stomach with a full glass of water.
    d. Administer with a small amount of food to decrease gastrointestinal upset.
    e. If there is bulbar involvement, eat meals 45 minutes to 1 hour after taking the medication.
    f. Drugs containing morphine or sedatives can increase muscle weakness.

36. A patient with MG develops difficulty coughing. Auscultation of the lungs reveals coarse crackles throughout the lung fields. The nurse identifies the patient is unable to cough effectively enough to clear the airway of secretions. Which intervention is best for this patient?
    a. Administer oxygen 2 L per nasal cannula.
    b. Ask respiratory therapist to perform chest physiotherapy.
    c. Perform endotracheal suction.
    d. Prepare intubation equipment.

37. A patient with MG is experiencing cholinergic crisis. Interventions include IV atropine 1 mg. What is the nurse's major respiratory concern when caring for this patient?
    a. Increase heart rate
    b. Difficulty with airway clearance
    c. Copious secretions
    d. Oxygen administration

38. A patient with MG has generalized weakness and fatigue and is limited in the ability to perform ADLs. Which nursing action is best to help this patient avoid excessive fatigue?
    a. Schedule activities after medication administration.
    b. Schedule activities during the late afternoon or early evening.
    c. During periods of maximal strength, provide assistance for ambulation.
    d. Instruct UAP to assist with all ADLs and feedings.

39. The nurse is reviewing medication orders for a patient with MG. The patient is scheduled to receive pyridostigmine (Mestinon) on a daily basis. What does the nurse expect regarding this drug?
    a. Daily dosage change related to patient symptoms
    b. Administration 30 minutes after antacids such as Milk of Magnesia
    c. Immediate monitoring for decreased muscle strength
    d. Gradual tapering and weaning off of the drug

40. The nurse is caring for a patient receiving cholinesterase inhibitor drugs for MG. Which symptoms does the nurse immediately report to the physician?
    a. Increasing loss of motor function
    b. Ineffective cough
    c. Dyspnea and difficulty swallowing
    d. Gastrointestinal side effects

41. During shift report, the nurse learns that a patient with MG deteriorated toward the end of the shift and the physician was called. A Tensilon test indicated that the patient was having a myasthenic crisis. What is the priority problem for this patient?
    a. Potential for inadequate oxygenation
    b. Potential for decreased ability to perform ADLs
    c. Potential for aspiration
    d. Potential for increase in blood pressure, pulse, and respirations

42. A patient with MG has been referred to a surgeon for a procedure that may improve the patient's symptoms. Which procedure does the nurse anticipate will be recommended for this patient?
    a. Percutaneous stereotactic rhizotomy
    b. Thymectomy
    c. Resecting severed nerve ends
    d. Partial or complete severance of a nerve

43. A patient with MG experienced a cholinergic crisis and is currently being maintained on a ventilator. The patient received several 1-mg doses of atropine. What does the nurse closely monitor this patient for?
    a. Increasing muscle weakness
    b. Increased salivation
    c. Ventricular fibrillation
    d. Development of mucus plugs

44. The nurse is performing patient teaching about plasmapheresis. Which statement by the patient indicates understanding of the topic?
    a. "Plasmapheresis causes immunosuppression, so I am at risk for infection."
    b. "I will have to be admitted to the hospital for this procedure."
    c. "Two treatments are given over a 2-month period; then I must follow up on a monthly basis."
    d. "The goal of the treatment is to decrease symptoms, but it is not a cure."

45. The nurse is performing teaching for the family of a patient with MG about fatigue and ADLs. Which statement by a family member indicates a need for additional teaching?
    a. "Rest is critical because increased fatigue can precipitate a crisis."
    b. "We should do hygienic care for her to avoid undue frustration and fatigue."
    c. "Activities should be done after we give her the medication."
    d. "The physical therapist will be able to recommend some energy-saving devices."

46. A patient with MG is experiencing impaired communication related to weakness of the facial muscles. Which interventions are best in assisting the patient to communicate with the staff and family? (Select all that apply.)
    a. Instruct the patient to speak slowly.
    b. Use short, simple sentences.
    c. Ask yes or no questions.
    d. Use hand signals.
    e. Have the patient use a picture, letter, or word board.

47. A patient with MG is having difficulty maintaining an adequate intake of food and fluid because of difficulty chewing and swallowing. Which task for this patient is best to delegate to UAP?
    a. Weigh the patient daily.
    b. Monitor calorie counts.
    c. Ask the patient about food preferences.
    d. Evaluate intake and output.

48. Which interventions are appropriate to protect a patient with MG from corneal abrasions? (Select all that apply.)
    a. Instruct the patient to keep the eyes closed.
    b. Apply an eye patch to both eyes after breakfast.
    c. Administer artificial tears to keep corneas moist.
    d. Place a clean moist washcloth over the patient's eyes.
    e. Apply lubricant gel and shield to the eyes at bedtime.

49. A patient is receiving a cholinesterase (ChE) inhibitor drug for the treatment of MG. What is a nursing implication for the safe administration of this medication?
    a. Monitor for orthostatic hypotension.
    b. Take the patient's apical pulse prior to administration.
    c. Feed meals 45 to 60 minutes after administration.
    d. Drink at least 8 glasses of water each day.

50. A patient with a thymoma had surgery to relieve symptoms of MG. A single chest tube has been inserted into the patient's anterior mediastinum. The nurse notes that the patient is restless with diminished breath sounds and decreased chest wall expansion. What is the nurse's first priority action?
    a. Reposition the patient and perform chest physiotherapy.
    b. Activate the Rapid Response Team.
    c. Suction the patient and tell him to breathe deeply.
    d. Provide oxygen and elevate the head of the bed.

51. Following a thymectomy for a patient with MG, the nurse notes that the patient is restless and experiencing chest pain and shortness of breath. What are the nurse's best actions at this time? *(Select all that apply.)*
    a. Instruct the patient to use incentive spirometry.
    b. Administer oxygen.
    c. Raise the head of the bed 45 degrees.
    d. Place the patient supine to encourage rest and sleep.
    e. Notify the Rapid Response Team.
    f. Assist the patient to sit at the side of the bed.

52. The nurse is teaching the patient and family about factors that predispose the patient to episodes of exacerbation of MG. Which factors does the nurse mention? *(Select all that apply.)*
    a. Infection
    b. Stress
    c. Change in diet
    d. Any physical exercise
    e. Enemas
    f. Strong cathartics

53. A patient is admitted with a right radial nerve transsection secondary to a knife injury. The nerve distal to the injury will degenerate and retract within how many hours?
    a. 4 hours
    b. 8 hours
    c. 12 hours
    d. 24 hours

54. The nurse has provided discharge teaching for a patient who had a surgical repair for a damaged nerve in the arm. Which statement by the patient requires follow-up by the nurse?
    a. "I will keep my arm in this flexed position."
    b. "I will call the doctor immediately for numbness or coolness in my arm."
    c. "I will use a heating pad on my arm to help with the pain."
    d. "I have a follow-up appointment with the surgeon next week."

55. The nurse is assessing the skin temperature of a patient's right lower extremity. Which technique does the nurse use?
    a. Place a paper strip thermometer on the patient's skin.
    b. Palpate the extremity using the fingertips.
    c. Compare bilateral extremities using the dorsal surface of the hand.
    d. Ask the patient if the skin feels subjectively hotter or colder than usual.

56. The nurse is caring for a patient with peripheral nerve damage to the lower extremity. What does the postoperative positioning and handling of the extremity include?
    a. ROM exercises for the affected limb to maintain mobility
    b. Joint extension to keep the nerve properly aligned
    c. Joint flexion to keep tension off the suture site
    d. Abduction maintained with a wedge pillow

57. The nurse is assessing the arm of a patient with peripheral nerve damage from incorrect use of crutches which occurred several weeks ago. The nurse observes that the arm is reddish-blue and mottled. What does the nurse interpret this finding as evidence of?
    a. Warm phase
    b. Cold phase
    c. Trophic changes
    d. Plateau period

58. The nurse is teaching a patient about postsurgical care after repair of a damaged nerve in the arm that is in a cast. Which information does the nurse include?
    a. "You must protect the nerve sutures for a minimum of 2 weeks."
    b. "Physiotherapy will begin immediately within the first or second day after surgery."
    c. "The cast that is applied after surgery will remain in place for 2 to 3 days."
    d. "Discomfort, tingling, or coolness are considered abnormal and should be reported."

59. Which patient has the highest risk factors for restless leg syndrome (RLS)?
    a. Obese patient with renal failure
    b. 65-year-old woman who routinely jogs
    c. 43-year-old man with hypertension
    d. Underweight teenager who smokes

60. A patient is diagnosed with RLS. What non-pharmacologic interventions does the nurse suggest for this patient? *(Select all that apply.)*
    a. Limit caffeine intake.
    b. Smoking and alcohol cessation.
    c. Avoid strenuous activities 2 to 3 hours before bedtime.
    d. Avoid taking naps during the day.
    e. Apply ice packs and elevate legs.
    f. Walk and perform stretching exercises.

61. A patient is prescribed ropinirole (Requip) for RLS. What nursing implication is related to this medication?
    a. Teach the patient to take the medication after meals.
    b. Usual dose is between 50 and 200 mg per day.
    c. Medication should be taken at bedtime.
    d. Medication is contraindicated in Parkinson disease.

62. What is the priority in caring for a patient with trigeminal neuralgia?
    a. Pain management
    b. Promoting communication
    c. Improving mobility
    d. Providing psychosocial support

63. A patient reports "excruciating, sharp, shooting" unilateral facial pain which lasts from seconds to minutes and describes a reluctance to smile, eat, or talk because of fear of precipitating an attack. This patient's description of symptoms is consistent with the symptoms of which disorder?
    a. Peripheral nerve trauma
    b. Trigeminal neuralgia
    c. Bell's palsy
    d. Eaton-Lambert syndrome

64. A patient is diagnosed with trigeminal neuralgia. Which therapy is the first-line choice for this patient?
    a. Antiepileptic such as carbamazepine (Tegretol)
    b. Muscle relaxant such as baclofen (Lioresal)
    c. Percutaneous stereotactic rhizotomy (PSR)
    d. Microvascular decompression

65. A patient has had PSR to relieve the pain of trigeminal neuralgia. What is included in the postoperative care of this patient? *(Select all that apply.)*
    a. Apply an ice pack to the operative site on the cheek and jaw for 48 hours.
    b. Perform a focused cranial nerve assessment.
    c. Discourage the patient from chewing on the affected side until paresthesias resolve.
    d. Instruct the patient to avoid rubbing the eye on the affected side.
    e. Teach the patient that he may have enhanced pain sensation during dental procedures.
    f. Teach the patient to inspect the eye daily for redness or irritation.

66. Which strategies will the nurse teach a patient with Bell's palsy to use in managing pain and paralysis? *(Select all that apply.)*
    a. Massage
    b. Opioid pain medications
    c. Application of warm, moist heat
    d. Chew on the affected side of the mouth
    e. Facial exercises

67. A patient is diagnosed with Bell's palsy and the right side of the face is affected. Related to the patient's right eye, which nursing action is best to implement?
    a. Check the pupil size and reaction using a penlight.
    b. Check the patient's visual acuity in both eyes.
    c. Teach the patient to instill artificial tears four times a day.
    d. Teach the patient to prevent eye strain by resting eyes periodically.

45 CHAPTER

Care of Critically Ill Patients with Neurologic Problems

1. Which statement about transient ischemic attack (TIA) is accurate?
   a. TIAs do not cause permanent brain damage.
   b. TIA increases the risk of stroke.
   c. Symptoms of a TIA usually resolve in 10-15 minutes.
   d. After a TIA, a patient is prescribed a beta blocker.

2. The nurse is preparing to discharge a patient with transient ischemic attacks. What treatment areas does the nurse include in discharge teaching? *(Select all that apply.)*
   a. Reduction of high blood pressure
   b. Drug teaching for aspirin or another antiplatelet drug
   c. Lifestyle changes such as increased sleep and rest
   d. Controlling diabetes
   e. Increased risk for stroke

3. Which symptoms indicate that a patient's stroke has affected the right hemisphere? *(Select all that apply.)*
   a. Loss of depth perception
   b. Aphasia
   c. Denies illness
   d. Cannot recognize faces
   e. Loss of hearing
   f. Depression

4. The nurse is performing a neurologic assessment on a patient with a suspected stroke. In addition to the level of consciousness (LOC), what is assessed to evaluate cognitive changes that may be occurring? *(Select all that apply.)*
   a. Denial of illness
   b. Proprioceptive dysfunction
   c. Presence of flaccid paralysis
   d. Impairment of memory
   e. Decreased ability to concentrate

5. Following a left hemisphere stroke, the patient has expressive (Broca's) aphasia. Which intervention is best to use when communicating with this patient?
   a. Repeat the names of objects on a routine basis.
   b. Face the patient and speak slowly and clearly.
   c. Obtain a whiteboard with an erasable marker.
   d. Develop a picture board that has objects and activities.

6. The nurse is caring for a patient with right hemisphere damage. The patient demonstrates disorientation to time and place, he has poor depth perception, and demonstrates neglect of the left visual field. Which task is best delegated to the unlicensed assistive personnel (UAP)?
   a. Move the patient's bed so that his affected side faces the door.
   b. Teach the patient to wash both sides of his face.
   c. Ensure a safe environment by removing clutter.
   d. Suggest to the family that they bring familiar family pictures.

7. A patient with a right cerebral hemisphere stroke may have safety issues related to which factor?
   a. Poor impulse control
   b. Alexia and agraphia
   c. Loss of language and analytical skills
   d. Slow and cautious behavior

8. A stroke patient is at risk for increased intracranial pressure (ICP) and is receiving oxygen 2 L via nasal cannula. The nurse is reviewing arterial blood gas (ABG) results. Which ABG value is of greatest concern for this patient?
   a. pH 7.32
   b. $Paco_2$ of 60 mm Hg
   c. Pao_2 of 95 mm Hg
   d. HCO_3^- of 28 mEq/L

9. Which statement is true about motor changes in a patient who has had a stroke?
   a. Motor deficit is ipsilateral to the hemisphere affected.
   b. Motor deficit is contralateral to the hemisphere affected.
   c. Bowel and bladder function remain intact.
   d. Flaccid paralysis is not an expected finding and should be reported promptly.

10. The preferred administration time for recombinant tissue plasminogen activator (rtPA [Retavase]) is within how long of stroke symptom onset?
    a. 30 to 60 minutes
    b. 3 to 4.5 hours
    c. 6 to 8 hours
    d. 24 to 30 hours

11. A priority problem for a patient who was admitted for a brain attack is the potential for aspiration. Which intervention is best to delegate to the UAP?
    a. Monitor the patient for and notify the charge nurse of any occurrence of coughing, choking, or difficulty breathing.
    b. Elevate the head of the bed as appropriate and slowly feed small spoonfuls of pudding, pausing between each spoonful.
    c. Assess the swallow reflex by placing the index finger and thumb on either side of the Adam's apple.
    d. Give the patient a glass of water before feeding solid foods and have oral suction ready at the bedside.

12. A patient is diagnosed with an ischemic stroke. The UAP reports that the patient's vital signs are blood pressure 150/100 mm Hg, pulse 78 beats/min, respiratory rate of 20/min, and temperature of 98.7° F. The patient's blood pressure is normally around 120/80. What action does the nurse take first?
    a. Report the blood pressure immediately to the physician because there is a danger of rebleeding.
    b. Ask the nursing assistant to repeat the blood pressure measurement in the other extremity with a manual cuff.
    c. Check the physician's orders to see if the blood pressure is within the acceptable parameters.
    d. Nothing; an elevated blood pressure is necessary for cerebral perfusion.

13. A patient with an ischemic stroke is placed on a cardiac monitor. Which cardiac dysrhythmia places the patient at risk for emboli?
    a. Sinus bradycardia
    b. Atrial fibrillation
    c. Sinus tachycardia
    d. First-degree heart block

14. The nurse is caring for a patient receiving medication therapy to prevent recurrence of stroke. Which medication is pharmacologically appropriate for this purpose?
    a. Enteric-coated aspirin (Ecotrin)
    b. Gabapentin (Neurontin)
    c. Recombinant tissue plasminogen activator (Retavase)
    d. Bevacizumab (Avastin)

15. A patient sustained a stroke that affected the right hemisphere of the brain. The patient has visual spatial deficits and deficits of proprioception. After assessing the safety of the patient's home, the home health nurse identifies which environmental feature that represents a potential safety problem for this patient?
    a. The handrail that borders the bathtub is on the left-hand side.
    b. The patient's favorite chair faces the front door of the house.
    c. The patient's bedside table is on the right-hand side of the bed.
    d. Family has relocated the patient to a ground-floor bedroom.

16. A patient with a stroke is having some trouble swallowing. Which interventions does the nurse anticipate the speech-language pathologist to suggest after the swallowing evaluation is completed? *(Select all that apply.)*
    a. Position the patient upright while eating.
    b. Administer orange juice using a straw.
    c. Give small spoonfuls of soft foods such as custard.
    d. Add powdered thickeners to liquids.
    e. Provide liquid nutritional supplements between meals for added calories.

17. A patient presents to the emergency department with signs and symptoms of an ischemic stroke. What is the priority factor when considering fibrinolytic therapy?
    a. Age older than 80 years
    b. History of stroke
    c. Recent surgery
    d. Time since onset of symptoms

18. A patient received rtPA for the treatment of ischemic stroke and the physician ordered an IV sodium heparin infusion. In relation to the drug therapy, what does the nurse monitor for?
    a. Elevated prothrombin level
    b. Bleeding gums or bruising
    c. Nausea and vomiting
    d. Elevated hematocrit or hemoglobin

19. The nurse notices that a patient seems to be having trouble swallowing. Which intervention does the nurse employ for this patient?
    a. Limit the diet to clear liquids given through a straw.
    b. Keep the patient on NPO status until swallowing is assessed.
    c. Monitor the patient's weight and compare to baseline.
    d. Sit with the patient while the patient eats and observe for swallowing difficulties.

20. A male patient has sustained a stroke and the nurse is planning interventions to help him reestablish urinary continence. What action does the nurse take?
    a. Obtain an order for a Foley catheter.
    b. Offer the urinal to the patient every 6 hours.
    c. Check postvoid residual urine with a bladder ultrasound.
    d. Restrict fluid to 1500 mL/day.

21. A patient with increased ICP is to receive IV mannitol (Osmitrol). Which nursing actions are taken concerning this drug? *(Select all that apply.)*
    a. Draw up the drug through a filtered needle.
    b. Insert a Foley catheter for strict measurement of urine output.
    c. Monitor serum and urine osmolality on a weekly basis.
    d. Assess for acute renal failure, weakness, or edema.
    e. Administer mannitol through a filter in the IV tubing.
    f. Administer furosemide (Lasix) as an adjunctive therapy.

22. The nurse is talking to the family of a stroke patient about home care measures. Which topics does the nurse include in this discussion? *(Select all that apply.)*
    a. Need for caregivers to plan for routine respite care and protection of own health
    b. Evaluation for potential safety risks such as throw rugs or slippery floors
    c. Awareness of potential patient frustration associated with communication
    d. Avoidance of independent transfers by the patient because of safety issues
    e. Access to health resources such as publications from the American Heart Association
    f. Referral to hospice and encouragement of family discussion of advance directives

23. Which patients are at increased risk for stroke? *(Select all that apply.)*
    a. 66-year-old man with diabetes mellitus
    b. 35-year-old healthy woman who uses oral contraceptives
    c. 47-year-old woman who exercises regularly
    d. 35-year-old man with history of multiple transient ischemic attacks
    e. 25-year-old woman with Bell's palsy
    f. 53-year-old man with chronic alcoholism

24. A patient displays signs of increased ICP, confusion, slurred speech, and unilateral weakness in the upper extremity. Which diagnostic test for this patient does the nurse question?
    a. Lumbar puncture (LP)
    b. Computed tomography (CT)
    c. Positron emission tomography (PET)
    d. Magnetic resonance imaging (MRI)

25. Which interventions does the nurse use for a patient with a left hemisphere stroke? *(Select all that apply.)*
    a. Teach the patient to wash both sides of the face.
    b. Place pictures and familiar objects around the patient.
    c. Reorient the patient frequently.
    d. Repeat names of commonly used objects.
    e. Approach the patient from the unaffected side.
    f. Establish a structured routine for the patient.

26. The nurse has completed teaching a patient about carotid artery angioplasty with stenting (CAS). Which statement by the patient indicates understanding of the purpose of the procedure?
    a. "The stent opens the blockage enough to establish blood flow."
    b. "The stent occludes the abnormal artery to prevent bleeding."
    c. "The stent bypasses the blockage."
    d. "The stent catches any clot debris."

27. The nurse is caring for a patient with an ischemic stroke. Which position is the patient placed in according to current nursing practice?
    a. Head of the bed is elevated 25 to 30 degrees
    b. Head of the bed is elevated to 45 degrees
    c. Supine with hips in flexed position
    d. The best head of bed position has not been determined

28. The nurse is caring for a patient at risk for increased ICP related to ischemic stroke. For what purpose does the nurse place the patient's head in a midline neutral position?
    a. Provide comfort for the patient.
    b. Protect the cervical spine.
    c. Facilitate venous drainage from brain.
    d. Decrease pressure from cerebrospinal fluid.

29. In planning care for a patient with increased ICP, what does the nurse do to minimize ICP?
    a. Gives the bath, changes the linens, and does passive ROM exercises to hands/fingers, then allows the patient to rest.
    b. Gives the bath, allows the patient to rest, changes the linens, allows the patient to rest, and then performs passive ROM exercises to hands/fingers.
    c. Defers the bath, changes the linens, and does passive ROM exercises to extremities until the danger of increased ICP has passed.
    d. Contacts the physician for specific orders about all activities related to the care of the patient that might cause increased ICP.

30. The nurse is caring for a patient at risk for increased ICP. Which sign is most likely to be the first indication of increased ICP?
    a. Decline of level of consciousness
    b. Increase in systolic blood pressure
    c. Change in pupil size and response
    d. Abnormal posturing of extremities

31. The stroke patient is prescribed docusate (Colace) once a day in the morning. What is the purpose of this drug specific to this patient?
    a. Laxative to prevent constipation
    b. Soften the patient's stool
    c. Increase fluid content of stool
    d. Prevent increased ICP

32. Which type of hematoma occurs between the skull and the dura?
    a. Epidural hematoma
    b. Subdural hematoma
    c. Intracranial hemorrhage
    d. Contusion

33. The nurse is caring for a patient admitted with the medical diagnosis of probable epidural hematoma and decreased level of consciousness. During the shift, the patient becomes lucid and is alert and talking. The family reports this is her baseline mental status. What is the nurse's next action?
    a. Stay with the patient and have the charge nurse alert the physician because this is an ominous sign for the patient.
    b. Document the patient's exact behaviors, compare to previous nursing entries, and continue the neurologic assessments every 2 hours.
    c. Point out to the family that the dangerous period has passed, but encourage them to leave so the patient does not become overly fatigued.
    d. Monitor the patient for the next 48 hours to 2 weeks because a subacute condition may be slowly developing.

34. Blood flow to the brain remains fairly constant as a result of which process?
    a. Autostasis
    b. Automobilization
    c. Hemodynamic stasis
    d. Autoregulation

35. A patient has been diagnosed with a large lesion of the parietal lobe and demonstrates loss of sensory function. Which nursing intervention is applicable for this patient?
    a. Play music for the patient for at least 30 minutes each day.
    b. Teach the patient to test the water temperature used for bathing.
    c. Position the patient reclining in bed or in a chair for meals.
    d. Use a picture of the patient's spouse and ask the patient to state the spouse's name.

36. A patient has been diagnosed with subarachnoid hemorrhage. Which drug does the nurse anticipate will be ordered to control cerebral vasospasm?
    a. Nimodipine (Nimotop)
    b. Phenytoin (Dilantin)
    c. Dexamethasone (Decadron)
    d. Clopidogrel (Plavix)

37. Which description best defines a basilar skull fracture?
    a. A simple, clean break in the skull
    b. A direct opening to brain tissue
    c. Fragments of bone are in brain tissue
    d. Cerebrospinal fluid leaks from nose or ears

38. Which determination must be made first in assessing a patient with traumatic brain injury?
    a. Presence of spinal injury
    b. Whether the patient is hypotensive
    c. Presence of a patent airway
    d. Level of consciousness using the Glasgow coma scale

39. Which statement is true about a patient at risk for increased ICP?
    a. The appearance of abnormal posturing occurs only when the patient is not positioned for comfort.
    b. Cushing's reflex, an early sign of increased ICP, consists of severe hypertension, widening pulse pressure, and bradycardia.
    c. Dilated or pinpoint pupils that are slow to react to light or nonreactive to light are signs of increased ICP.
    d. Areas of tenderness over the scalp indicate the presence of contrecoup injuries.

40. A patient has sustained a traumatic brain injury. Which nursing intervention is best for this patient?
    a. Assess vital signs every 8 hours.
    b. Position to avoid extreme flexion.
    c. Increase fluid intake for the first 48 hours.
    d. Administer glucocorticoids.

41. The nurse is caring for a patient with a relatively minor head injury after a bump to the head. The nurse has the greatest concern about which symptom?
    a. Headache
    b. Nausea and vomiting
    c. Unequal pupils
    d. Dizziness

42. The patient with a traumatic brain injury is receiving mechanical ventilation. Why does the health care provider adjust ventilator settings to maintain a partial pressure of arterial carbon dioxide ($Paco_2$) at 35 to 38 mm Hg?
    a. Lower levels of arterial carbon dioxide are essential for gas exchange.
    b. Carbon dioxide is a potent vasodilator that can cause increased ICP.
    c. Carbon dioxide is a waste product that must be eliminated from the body.
    d. Lower levels of arterial carbon dioxide facilitate brain oxygenation.

43. Which statement is true about respiratory problems in a patient with a major head injury?
    a. Atelectasis and pneumonia can be prevented by proper pulmonary hygiene.
    b. Suctioning should be avoided because of the increase in ICP.
    c. Neurologic pulmonary edema occurs frequently.
    d. The patient should avoid breathing deeply because of increased ICP.

44. Which Glasgow coma scale (GCS) data set indicates the most severe injury for a patient with traumatic brain injury and loss of consciousness?
    a. GCS of 13 with loss of consciousness of 15 minutes
    b. GCS of 9 with loss of consciousness of 30 minutes
    c. GCS of 12 with loss of consciousness of 3 hours
    d. GCS of 8 with loss of consciousness of 6.5 hours

45. The nurse is assessing a patient who was struck in the head several times with a bat. There is clear fluid that appears to be leaking from the nose. What action does the nurse take?
    a. Hand the patient a tissue and ask him to gently blow the nose; observe the nasal discharge for blood clots.
    b. Immediately report the finding to the physician and document the observation in the nursing notes.
    c. Place a drop of the fluid on a white absorbent background and look for a yellow halo.
    d. Allow the patient to wipe his nose, but no other action is needed; he has most likely been crying.

46. Which statement is true for a patient with a basilar skull fracture?
    a. There is potential for hemorrhage caused by damage to the internal carotid artery.
    b. There is an increased risk for loss of functional abilities such as toileting.
    c. There is an increased risk for cytotoxic or cellular edema with loss of consciousness.
    d. There is potential for decorticate or decerebrate posturing with loss of motor function.

47. A patient is admitted for a closed head injury from a fall down the stairs. The patient has no history of respiratory disease and no apparent respiratory distress. However, the physician orders oxygen 2 L via nasal cannula. What is the nurse's best action?
    a. Check the pulse oximetry and apply the oxygen if the saturation level drops below 90%.
    b. Call the physician to discontinue the order because it is unnecessary.
    c. Deliver the oxygen as ordered because hypoxemia may precipitate increased ICP.
    d. Apply the nasal cannula as ordered and gradually wean the patient off the oxygen when the LOC improves.

48. The nurse is conducting a presentation to a group of students on the prevention of head injuries. Which statement by a student indicates a need for additional teaching?
    a. "Drinking, driving, and speeding contribute to the risk for injury."
    b. "Males are more likely to sustain head injury compared to females."
    c. "Young people are less likely to get injured because of faster reflexes."
    d. "Following game rules and not 'goofing around' can prevent injuries."

49. The nurse is taking a history on a teenager who was involved in a motor vehicle accident with friends. The patient has an obvious contusion of the forehead, seems confused, and is laughing loudly and yelling, "Ruby! Ruby!" What is the best question for the nurse to ask the patient's friends?
    a. "Where and why did the accident occur?"
    b. "How can we notify the family for consent for treatment?"
    c. "Was the patient using drugs or alcohol prior to the accident?"
    d. "Who is Ruby and why is the patient calling for her?"

50. The provider has prescribed barbiturate coma therapy for a patient with increased ICP. Which complication does the nurse monitor for?
    a. Decreased LOC
    b. Reduced gastric motility
    c. Decreased respiratory rate
    d. Reduced Glasgow coma scale score

51. The nurse is performing discharge teaching for the family and patient who has had prolonged hospitalization and rehabilitation therapy for severe craniocerebral trauma after a motorcycle accident. What elements of instruction does the nurse include? *(Select all that apply.)*
    a. Review seizure precautions.
    b. Stimulate the patient with frequent changes in the environment.
    c. Develop a routine of activities with consistency and structure.
    d. Attend follow-up appointments with therapists.
    e. Encourage the family to seek respite care if needed.
    f. Encourage the patient to wear a helmet when riding.

52. A patient has sustained a major head injury and the nurse is assessing the patient's neurologic status every 2 hours. What early sign of increased ICP does the nurse monitor for?
    a. Change in the LOC
    b. Cheyne-Stokes respirations
    c. Severe hypertension with widened pulse pressure (Cushing's reflex)
    d. Dilated and nonreactive pupils

53. The nurse is giving discharge instructions to the mother of a child who bumped her head on a table. Which statement by the mother indicates an understanding of the instructions?
    a. "I should not let her fall asleep."
    b. "She may have nausea or headache for the first 24 hours."
    c. "She should gently blow her nose and I'll observe for bleeding."
    d. "She can run and play as she usually does."

54. The nurse is caring for an intubated patient with increased ICP. If the patient needs to be suctioned, which nursing action does the nurse take to avoid further aggravating the increased ICP?
    a. Manually hyperventilate with 100% oxygen before passing the catheter.
    b. Maintain strict sterile technique when performing endotracheal suctioning.
    c. Perform oral suctioning frequently, but do not perform endotracheal suctioning.
    d. Obtain an order for an arterial blood gas before suctioning the patient.

55. Which are key features of a brainstem tumor? *(Select all that apply.)*
    a. Vomiting unrelated to food intake
    b. Facial pain or weakness
    c. Nystagmus
    d. Headache
    e. Hearing loss
    f. Hoarseness

56. The nurse is caring for a patient with a brain tumor. Which drug therapy does the nurse anticipate this patient will receive?
    a. Glucocorticosteroids for intracranial edema
    b. Nonsteroidal antiinflammatory drugs (NSAIDs) for pain
    c. Insulin for diabetes insipidus
    d. Ticlopidine hydrochloride (Ticlid) for platelet adhesiveness

57. Which statement is true about gamma knife therapy for brain tumors?
    a. It is used for easily reached tumors.
    b. It is noninvasive and has few complications.
    c. It is administered under general anesthesia.
    d. It replaces conventional radiation therapy.

58. A patient is scheduled for a craniotomy. What does the nurse tell the patient and family about the procedure?
    a. The head will not need to be shaved at the surgical site.
    b. There is a coma state for up to several days after surgery.
    c. Drainage of a small to moderate amount of cerebrospinal fluid after surgery is normal.
    d. The family will need to remind the patient of their names and relationships.

59. A patient has had an infratentorial craniotomy. Which position does the nurse use for this patient?
    a. High-Fowler's position, turned to the operative side
    b. Head of bed at 30 degrees, turned to the nonoperative side
    c. Flat in bed, turned to the operative side
    d. Flat in bed, may turn to either side

60. The nurse is performing discharge teaching for a patient who underwent a craniotomy for a brain tumor. What instruction does the nurse include? *(Select all that apply.)*
    a. Suggestions to make the environment safe, such as removing scatter rugs
    b. Reminder that seizures could occur frequently for the first couple of months
    c. Information about drugs such as dose, administration, and side effects
    d. Directions about how and when to contact emergency services or the physician
    e. Advice about which over-the-counter products are safe to use
    f. Referral to a resource such as the American Brain Tumor Association

61. The nurse is providing education for a patient with a brain tumor. What educational elements does the nurse include?
    a. Instructions to avoid physical activity
    b. Instructions to avoid over-the-counter drugs
    c. Advice that seizures will occur in the immediate postoperative period
    d. Information about dietary changes to prevent recurrence of the tumor

62. A patient who had a craniotomy develops the postoperative complication of syndrome of inappropriate antidiuretic hormone (SIADH). The patient's sodium level is 126 mEq/L and the serum osmolality is decreased. In light of this development, which physician order does the nurse question?
    a. Encourage oral fluids
    b. Normal saline IV at 150 mL/hr
    c. Strict intake and output
    d. Daily weights

63. The nurse is assisting a patient who had a large brain tumor removed to get positioned in bed. Which recommended position does the nurse place the patient in?
    a. Operative side to protect the unaffected side of the brain
    b. Flat and repositioned on either side to decrease tension on the incision
    c. Elevate the head of bed 30 degrees to promote venous drainage
    d. Reposition every 2 hours but do not turn the patient onto the operative side

64. A patient is admitted to the critical care unit after a craniotomy to debulk a grade 3 astrocytoma. What is the priority patient problem?
    a. Risk for infection
    b. Risk for memory loss
    c. Risk for increased intracranial pressure
    d. Potential for organ ischemia

65. The nurse observes that a patient who had surgery for a benign hemangioblastoma has bilateral periorbital edema and ecchymosis. Because this patient's care is based on the general principles of caring for the patient with a craniotomy, what is the nurse's first action?
    a. Immediately inform the surgeon.
    b. Apply cold compresses.
    c. Check the pupillary response.
    d. Perform a full neurologic assessment.

66. Which statement is true about increased ICP in a surgical patient?
    a. It is a minor postoperative complication.
    b. Diuretics such as furosemide may be given to decrease it.
    c. Cerebral edema usually subsides within 72 hours.
    d. If not contraindicated, the head of bed should be placed at 30 degrees.

67. The nurse is teaching a patient who will receive the disc-shaped Gliadel wafer as part of the treatment for a brain tumor. Which statement by the patient indicates understanding of how the wafer works?
    a. "I'll place the wafer under my tongue and allow it to dissolve."
    b. "The wafer will be taped to my chest and the drug will be absorbed."
    c. "The wafer will be placed directly into the cavity during the surgery."
    d. "The wafer is to be dissolved in water and taken with meals."

68. Which organism is commonly involved in opportunistic central nervous system infections for patients with AIDS?
    a. Streptococcus
    b. Enterobacter
    c. *Haemophilus influenzae*
    d. Toxoplasmosis

69. The nurse who is providing postoperative care for a patient who had a craniotomy immediately notifies the surgeon of which assessment finding?
    a. Drainage in the Jackson-Pratt container of 45 mL/8 hours
    b. Intracranial pressure of 15 mm Hg
    c. P_{CO_2} level of 35 mm Hg
    d. Serum sodium of 117 mEq/L

70. What is most likely to be included in the history of a patient with a brain abscess?
    a. Family history of Huntington disease
    b. History of HIV/AIDS
    c. History of osteoarthritis
    d. Vaccination against influenza

71. A patient is admitted for diagnostic testing for probable encapsulated brain abscess and risk for increased ICP. Which statement about diagnostic testing for this patient is true?
    a. WBCs may be normal, even if an infection is present.
    b. Blood cultures are the only cultures likely to grow the causative organism.
    c. MRI is useful late in the course of the disease to identify permanent lesions.
    d. The first test performed is a lumbar puncture to determine if the cerebrospinal fluid is cloudy.

72. Which are common causes of acquired hypoxic-anoxic brain injury? *(Select all that apply.)*
    a. Cardiac arrest
    b. Kidney failure
    c. Asphyxiation from attempted suicide
    d. Brain attack (stroke)
    e. Drug overdose
    f. Severe asthma

46 CHAPTER

Assessment of the Eye and Vision

1. Light waves pass through each of the eye structures listed below to reach the retina. Place them in sequence using the numbers 1 through 5, with number 1 being the outermost structure and number 5 being the innermost structure.

   _____ a. Vitreous humor

   _____ b. Aqueous humor

   _____ c. Lens

   _____ d. Cornea

   _____ e. Retina

2. A patient's intraocular pressure (IOP) has increased. Which fluids in the eye does this affect? *(Select all that apply.)*
   a. Blood
   b. Vitreous humor
   c. Lacrimal tears
   d. Aqueous humor
   e. Intracellular fluid
   f. Lymph fluid

3. If the superior rectus muscle is damaged or not functioning properly, the patient would have difficulty with which eye movement?
   a. Looking upwards
   b. Looking downwards
   c. Gazing towards the nose
   d. Gazing towards the side of the head

4. The nurse asks the patient to open and close his eyelids. Which cranial nerve is the nurse assessing?
   a. Cranial nerve II (optic)
   b. Cranial nerve III (oculomotor)
   c. Cranial nerve V (trigeminal)
   d. Cranial nerve VII (facial)

5. One of the expected changes of the eyes associated with aging is the decreased ability of iris to dilate. How will this affect the patient's eyes or vision?
   a. Difficulty with tear production resulting in dry eyes
   b. Decreased ability to see objects that are close
   c. Difficult distinguishing blues, greens, or violets
   d. Increased difficulty seeing in dark environments

6. A 29-year-old patient tells the nurse that he spends a great deal of time in the sun. In preparing a teaching plan for the patient, what information about protecting vision does the nurse include? *(Select all that apply.)*
   a. Wear sunglasses to filter ultraviolet (UV) light.
   b. UV light exposure increases the risk for cataracts.
   c. UV light exposure increases the risk for ocular melanoma.
   d. UV light exposure is only a concern with direct sunlight.
   e. Foods high in vitamin A will protect against UV damage.

7. A 45-year-old patient has diabetes mellitus. Which information about vision protection does the nurse include in the teaching plan?
   a. Diabetics have an increased incidence of ocular melanoma.
   b. Fluctuating blood glucose levels are undesirable, but do not cause vision problems.
   c. Use over-the-counter eyedrops every day to flush potential infective organisms.
   d. Annual eye examinations are recommended for patients with diabetes mellitus.

8. The nurse reads in the patient's chart that he has anisocoria. Which assessment of the eye will reveal this variation that is considered normal in 5% of the population?
   a. Corneal assessment
   b. Scleral assessment
   c. Pupillary assessment
   d. Eye movement assessment

9. A patient reports not being able to see objects in his peripheral vision. Which method is used to evaluate this symptom?
   a. Jaeger card
   b. Six cardinal positions of gaze
   c. Confrontation test
   d. Corneal light reflex test

10. A patient who works in a machine shop has a suspected metal foreign body in the eye. Which test is contraindicated for this patient?
    a. Corneal staining
    b. Computed tomography (CT) scan
    c. Magnetic resonance imaging (MRI)
    d. Ultrasonography

11. The nurse desires to assess the patient for color blindness. Which assessment tool will the nurse use?
    a. Ishihara chart
    b. Confrontation test
    c. Snellen chart
    d. Rosenberg Pocket Vision Screener

12. The nurse reads in the patient's chart that the patient's visual acuity is 20/40. What is the correct interpretation of this documentation?
    a. Patient has 50% of the ideal 20/20 visual acuity.
    b. Patent stood 40 feet from the chart rather than 20 feet from the chart.
    c. Patient sees at 20 feet from the chart what a healthy eye sees at 40 feet.
    d. Patient stood 20 feet from the chart and sees 40% of the letters.

13. When preparing the patient for a fluorescein angiography, what is included in the nurse's teaching plan? *(Select all that apply.)*
    a. Intravenous access will be necessary.
    b. Sunlight must be avoided for 2 days.
    c. Fluids are limited for the first 24 hours after the procedure.
    d. The skin may have a yellow hue for a few hours after the procedure.
    e. Mydriatic drops will be instilled 1 hour before the procedure.

14. Which are correct procedures for instilling ophthalmic drops in a patient's eyes? *(Select all that apply.)*
    a. Check the name, strength, and expiration date of the solution.
    b. Have the patient tilt the head backward and look down.
    c. Release drops into the conjunctival pocket.
    d. Avoid contaminating the tip of the bottle.
    e. After instilling the drop, instruct to squeeze the eyelids tightly.

15. Which method is used to measure IOP?
    a. Corneal staining
    b. Tonometry
    c. Slit lamp examination
    d. Electroretinography

16. What is a correct part of the procedure for using an ophthalmoscope?
    a. The nurse comes toward the patient's eye from 6 inches away.
    b. The test should be done in a brightly lit room to enhance visibility.
    c. When examining confused patients, an assistant can steady the patient.
    d. The nurse stands on the same side as the eye being examined.

17. A patient is diagnosed with arcus senilis. Which intervention will nurse use in caring for this patient?
    a. Assist the patient in activities that require near vision.
    b. Teach the patient how to instill the prescribed eyedrops.
    c. Reassure the patient that the vision is not affected.
    d. Instruct that consistent use of sunglasses prevents worsening.

18. Which assessment findings of the eye are normal? *(Select all that apply.)*
    a. Presbyopia in a 45-year-old woman
    b. Ptosis of the eyelids
    c. Yellow sclera with small pigmented dots in a dark-skinned person
    d. Pupil constriction in response to accommodation
    e. Pupil constriction within 2 seconds in response to light
    f. Nystagmus in the far lateral gaze

19. Why might the health care provider order CT to examine the eye?
    a. To validate the function of extraocular muscles
    b. To verify IOP
    c. To determine the degree of peripheral vision
    d. To detect an ocular tumor in the orbital space

20. The patient has an IOP greater than 21 mm Hg. The patient's use of which over-the-counter product should be brought to the immediate attention of the ophthalmologist?
    a. Aspirin
    b. Antihistamine
    c. Vitamin supplement
    d. Artificial tear eyedrops

21. What is the pathophysiology that underlies the development of glaucoma?
    a. Pressure on retinal vessels decreases blood flow so photoreceptors and nerve fibers become hypoxic.
    b. Decreased muscle tone reduces ability to keep the gaze focused on a single object.
    c. Cornea flattens and the surface becomes irregular with worsening of astigmatism and blurred vision.
    d. The lens hardens, shrinks, and loses elasticity and cataracts begin to form.

22. Which medications can adversely affect the eyes and vision? *(Select all that apply.)*
    a. Heparin
    b. Decongestants
    c. Oral contraceptives
    d. Acetaminophen
    e. Corticosteroids

23. Which conditions or diseases can adversely affect a patient's eyes and vision? *(Select all that apply.)*
    a. Pregnancy
    b. Inflammatory bowel disease
    c. Diabetes
    d. Hypertension
    e. Osteoarthritis

24. Which activity is most likely to be very difficult for the patient if the visual function of accommodation is not working correctly?
    a. Reading a newspaper
    b. Playing tennis
    c. Watching a sunset
    d. Walking in a dark hallway

25. Which intervention would be best to use for a patient with presbyopia?
    a. Encouragement to get a prescription for reading glasses
    b. Administration of the prescribed eye medications
    c. Reminder to wear sunglasses to protective against UV light
    d. Follow-up appointments to detect acute glaucoma

26. Which patient is advised to have yearly eye examinations because of the increased risk for cataracts?
    a. 5-year-old who was treated for an episode of conjunctivitis
    b. 10-year-old who was struck in the face by a basketball
    c. 55-year-old with no history of eye problems or vision changes
    d. 25-year-old who is pregnant with her first child

27. A neighbor calls the nurse for advice, because he thinks he may have got some metal shavings in his eye while working on a home improvement project. What advice should the nurse give?
    a. Rinse the eye with water and then don protective eye wear
    b. Immediately notify his health care provider or ophthalmologist
    c. Mention the incident during the annual eye examination
    d. Resting the eye is sufficient unless there is pain or loss of vision

28. Which food would be particularly good for eye health?
    a. Whole-grain cereal
    b. Low-fat milk
    c. Raw almonds
    d. Fresh tomatoes

29. Although the older patient denies any problems with his vision, the nurse frequently observes that he closes one eye when trying to look at his meal tray or personal items on the bedside table. What does the nurse suspect?
    a. Patient has arcus senilis.
    b. Patient has double vision.
    c. Patient has dry eye syndrome.
    d. Patient has a small cataract.

30. Which method would the nurse use to perform a corneal assessment?
    a. Inspect the corneas to determine if they equal distance from the nose.
    b. Quickly and unexpectedly bring a hand towards the patient's cornea.
    c. Use a penlight and direct the light on the cornea from the side.
    d. Ask the patient to open and close eyelids and observe the cornea.

31. The nurse reads PERRLA in the patient's chart as noted by the nurse who worked the previous shift. What does the nurse do in order to determine if the patient still displays PERRLA or if the patient's status has changed?
    a. Assesses for presence, relief, or reduction of pain
    b. Checks pulse, respiratory rate, and lung auscultation
    c. Assesses the size, shape, and reactivity of pupils
    d. Checks for signs of presbyopia or retinal detachment

32. The nurse is assessing a patient who is unable to see the 20/400 characters on the Snellen chart. Which assessment will the nurse try first?
    a. Ask the patient to detect stationary, left-right, or up-down hand movements.
    b. Ask the patient to count the number of fingers held up in front of the eyes.
    c. Ask the patient to report "on" or "off" when detecting light in a darkened room.
    d. Ask the patient to self-select a distance from Snellen chart where 20/400 is visible.

33. The home health nurse is interviewing a patient and discovers that there may be a previously undiagnosed vision problem. The nurse does not have a Jaeger card available at the patient's house to assess the suspected problem. What could the nurse use as a temporary substitute to assess the suspected problem?
    a. Flashlight
    b. Ophthalmoscope
    c. Snellen chart
    d. Newspaper

34. In assessing the corneal light reflex of the older patient's eye, the nurse notes an asymmetric reflex. What is the clinical significance of this assessment finding?
    a. This is a normal finding for an older adult.
    b. Eye is deviating because of possible muscle weakness.
    c. The reflex is asymmetrical because of a cataract.
    d. Eye strain and eye fatigue can alter the reflex.

35. For a patient who is measuring IOP at home, what is the most important teaching point to ensure accurate readings?
    a. Always wash the hands before taking the measurement.
    b. Perform the measurement in a darkened room.
    c. Take the measurement at the same time(s) of the day.
    d. Always measure and compare the pressure between eyes.

47 CHAPTER

Care of Patients with Eye and Vision Problems

1. The patient has ectropion and is scheduled for surgery to correct the problem. What does the nurse expect to find during the assessment of the patient's eye?
   a. Inflammation of the lower lid
   b. Sagging of the eyelid
   c. Turning inward of the lower lid
   d. Purulent crusting on the eyelid

2. Which complication is most likely to develop for untreated entropion?
   a. Flashes of light
   b. Central vision loss
   c. Corneal abrasion
   d. Dry eye syndrome

3. Which patient(s) has/have a factor that is associated with keratoconjunctivitis sicca? *(Select all that apply.)*
   a. Patient routinely takes an anticholinergic drug.
   b. Patient has diabetes mellitus.
   c. Patient has rheumatoid arthritis.
   d. Patient had damage to cranial nerve IV.
   e. Patient has Sjögren's syndrome.

4. For a patient with keratoconjunctivitis sicca, which intervention is the nurse most likely to implement?
   a. Administers antihistamines to stimulate tear production.
   b. Applies warm, moist compresses to moisturize the eye.
   c. Reinforces that artificial tears are used as often as necessary.
   d. Avoids transferring contamination from one eye to the other.

5. A patient is diagnosed with bacterial conjunctivitis trachoma. What is the primary focus of this patient's care?
   a. Pain control
   b. Nutrition
   c. Infection control
   d. Loss of visual function

6. A patient reports tearing, mild conjunctival edema and "pink eye." Which question could the nurse ask to assist the health care provider in distinguishing whether the patient is having an acute form of bacterial conjunctivitis or the early stages of chronic conjunctivitis?
   a. Have you had a discharge that was watery at first and is now thicker?
   b. Have you ever lived in a warm, moist climate with poor sanitary conditions?
   c. Have you recently used antihistamines or do you take a beta-adrenergic blocker?
   d. Have you had noticed blurring or double vision with difficulty focusing?

7. What are the nursing care priorities for a deceased patient who is a corneal donor?
   a. Instill saline solution into the eyes.
   b. Instill antibiotic drops into the eyes.
   c. Lay the deceased in a flat supine position.
   d. Apply loose patches moistened with saline.

8. The nurse is providing the immediate postoperative care for a patient who had a keratoplasty. Which assessment will the nurse perform to identify the most likely complication?
   a. Assess for bleeding.
   b. Assess for photosensitivity.
   c. Monitor for respiratory depression.
   d. Monitor for hypotension.

9. For a patient who had a keratoplasty, which discharge instruction will the nurse give?
   a. Sleep on the operative side to reduce intraocular pressure.
   b. Keep eye covered for 1 week with the initial dressing and shield.
   c. Wear the shield at night for the first month after surgery.
   d. Apply a small cloth-covered ice pack to reduce swelling.

10. What is an early sign/symptom of a cataract?
    a. Double vision
    b. Photophobia
    c. Decreased depth perception
    d. Decreased color perception

11. The nurse is using an ophthalmoscope to examine the lens of a patient with a cataract. Which finding does the nurse expect to see?
    a. Dilated pupil
    b. Decreased lens density
    c. Enlarged retina
    d. Opaque lens

12. What is an early sign/symptom of macular degeneration?
    a. Mild blurring
    b. Decreased tear production
    c. Loss of central vision
    d. Difficulty with activities of daily living (ADLs)

13. A 46-year-old patient calls the clinic and reports sudden "floating dark spots" in her vision. What should the nurse say to the patient?
    a. Advise the patient to immediately call her ophthalmologist.
    b. Advise the patient that this is normal for her age.
    c. Ask the patient if the spots were accompanied by pain.
    d. Tell the patient to mention this during her annual eye appointment.

14. A patient has had cataract surgery and is ready to go home. In the discharge education, what does the nurse tell the patient about activities?
    a. Driving in the daylight is okay, but do not drive at night.
    b. Meal preparation and doing dishes are acceptable activities.
    c. Vacuuming and mopping are okay, but do not bend over to scrub.
    d. Exercises, such as jogging or swimming, can be done at a slow pace.

15. Which signs and symptoms should a patient who has had cataract surgery report to the health care provider? *(Select all that apply.)*
    a. Sharp, sudden pain in the eye
    b. Decreased vision
    c. Mild eye itching
    d. Green or yellow thick discharge
    e. Flashes of light

16. In caring for a patient who was recently diagnosed with dry age-related macular degeneration, which teaching point would the nurse emphasize?
    a. Importance of adhering to the exact schedule for eyedrops
    b. Dietary modifications to slow progression of vision loss
    c. Avoiding activities that cause rapid or jerking head movements
    d. Good handwashing and keeping the tip of the eyedropper clean

17. After a scleral buckling procedure, which aspect of postoperative care is affected if gas or oil has been placed in the eye?
    a. Type of eye patch
    b. Position of the head
    c. Eyedrop schedule
    d. Effects of anesthesia

18. After a scleral buckling procedure, the patient is advised to avoid reading, writing, or close work, such as sewing. What is the rationale for avoiding these activities?
    a. They cause increased intraocular pressure.
    b. Close, fine work is likely to cause pain.
    c. They cause rapid eye movement.
    d. Close work or fine print will be blurry.

19. Which sign/symptom is the most common early clinical manifestation of retinitis pigmentosa?
    a. Cataracts
    b. Night blindness
    c. Headache
    d. Vitamin A deficiency

20. A patient with myopia tells the nurse that he forgot to bring his glasses to the hospital and that his wife will bring them later when she comes to see him. Which activity is the patient most likely to have difficulty with while he is waiting for his glasses?
    a. Eating his lunch
    b. Looking at a brochure
    c. Using his cell phone
    d. Watching television

21. A 10-year-old patient was hit in the left eye with a baseball. There is discoloration around the eye. Which treatment does the nurse expect to give for this patient?
    a. Eye patch to rest the eye
    b. Warm, moist compresses
    c. Small ice application to area
    d. Bedrest in semi-Fowler's position

22. Which traumatic injury of the eye is the most likely to cause loss of vision in the injured eye?
    a. Foreign body
    b. Contusion
    c. Laceration
    d. Penetration injury

23. The patient is wearing corrective lenses. The nurse uses a Snellen chart and the patient's visual acuity is 20/200. What is the clinical significance of this finding?
    a. Patient needs to be advised to get a new prescription for corrective lenses.
    b. Patient is considered legally blind with a visual acuity of 20/200 with corrective lenses.
    c. Patient should be assessed with other methods, such as counting fingers, or hand movements.
    d. Patient should be referred to an eye surgeon for possible vision enhancement surgery.

24. A 23-year-old athlete suffered a traumatic eye injury and enucleation was required. The nurse is trying to do discharge teaching, but the patient verbalizes anger and hopelessness, 'What's the point of learning about how to take care of this stupid empty hole in my face?' What is the nurse's best response?
    a. "Let's just take things one step at a time. I'll come back later."
    b. "Would you like information about joining a support group?"
    c. "Preventing infection will prevent further disfigurement and problems."
    d. "I know you are frustrated. Tell me how this accident will affect your life."

25. What is the priority for a patient with impaired vision?
    a. Self-care
    b. Communication
    c. Mobility
    d. Safety

26. The nurse is teaching a patient about self-medication with eyedrops for glaucoma. Which intervention does the nurse suggest to prevent systemic absorption of the medication?
    a. Wait 15 minutes between instilling different eyedrops.
    b. Place pressure on the corner of the eye near the nose.
    c. Place all eye medications in one eye, then the other.
    d. Blink rapidly after instilling drops and keep head upright.

27. The patient is diagnosed with bilateral conjunctivitis and receives a prescription for two bottles of the same antibiotic solution. What instructions should the nurse give to the patient?
    a. Obtain one bottle from the pharmacy and return for the second if the infection does not clear.
    b. Obtain and use one bottle for both eyes, the second bottle is really not necessary.
    c. Obtain both bottles and label one for the right eye and the other for the left eye.
    d. Obtain both bottles, but save the second one because the infection will probably recur.

28. The nurse hears in shift report that the patient will have phacoemulsification for treatment of an eye problem. What does the nurse anticipate in the care of this patient?
    a. Patient will be discharged within an hour of surgery.
    b. Patient is likely to mourn the loss of the body part.
    c. Patient will need opioid medication for severe pain.
    d. Patient should be closely observed for postoperative bleeding.

29. The older patient has reduced visual sensory perception and is newly admitted to the medical-surgical unit. What instructions should the nurse give to the UAP about assisting the patient with ADLs?
    a. "When entering and exiting the room, be very quiet so the patient is not disturbed."
    b. "Put personal belongings in the closet so the patient knows where they are."
    c. "During mealtimes, sit with the patient and explain how he should eat and drink."
    d. "During ambulation, let the patient hold your elbow and alert him to obstacles in the path."

30. What might the nurse notice if the patient is experiencing reduced sensory perception? *(Select all that apply.)*
    a. Patient squints or tilts the head when viewing objects or print at a distance.
    b. Patient closes one eye to read or see at a distance.
    c. Patient startles easily when a sudden move is made at the face.
    d. Pupils are equal and react to light.
    e. Patient does not make eye contact and turns head toward sounds rather than sights.

48
CHAPTER

Assessment and Care of Patients with Ear and Hearing Problems

1. Which structure is the spiral organ of hearing?
   a. Cochlea
   b. Semicircular canal
   c. Pinna
   d. Stapes

2. Which cranial nerve is the nurse testing when performing a bedside hearing test?
   a. V
   b. VI
   c. VIII
   d. IX

3. A patient who works on the tarmac at a busy airport is being seen for a routine exam. What protection measures for hearing does the nurse suggest to the patient? *(Select all that apply.)*
   a. Wear cotton ball ear inserts.
   b. Wear foam ear inserts.
   c. Wear a hat with ear covers.
   d. Wear an over-the-ear headset.
   e. Limit exposure time on tarmac.

4. Which factors can decrease blood supply to the ear in a 77-year-old patient? *(Select all that apply.)*
   a. Osteoporosis
   b. Diabetes
   c. Smoking
   d. Heart disease
   e. Hypertension

5. Identify the events in sequential order, using the numbers 1 through 6, that lead to the sense of hearing.

   _____ a. Sound waves are transferred to the malleus.

   _____ b. Sound waves are transferred to the incus and the stapes.

   _____ c. Vibrations are transmitted to the cochlea.

   _____ d. Neural impulses are conducted by the auditory nerve.

   _____ e. Sound waves strike the mastoid and the movable tympanic membrane.

   _____ f. Sound is processed and interpreted by the brain.

6. A sensorineural hearing loss results from impairment of which structure?
   a. Fused bony ossicles
   b. First cranial nerve
   c. Seventh cranial nerve
   d. Eighth cranial nerve

7. An adult patient is having problems with hearing. Which of the patient's medications is ototoxic?
   a. Vitamin B_{12}
   b. Digoxin (Lanoxin)
   c. Furosemide (Lasix)
   d. Levothyroxine (Synthroid)

8. What changes in the ear are related to aging? *(Select all that apply.)*
   a. Tympanic membrane may appear dull and retracted.
   b. Pinna becomes shorter and thickened.
   c. Cerumen is drier and impacts more easily.
   d. Bony ossicles have increased movement.
   e. Hearing of high-frequency sound increases.

9. Which technique would the nurse use to perform otoscopic assessment?
   a. The patient's head should be tilted slightly toward the nurse.
   b. The nurse holds the otoscope upside down, like a large pen.
   c. The pinna is pulled down and back.
   d. The internal canal is visualized while the speculum is slowly inserted.

10. On the figure below, locate the tympanic membrane and describe what the normal tympanic membrane looks like when assessed with an otoscope.

    _____

    _____

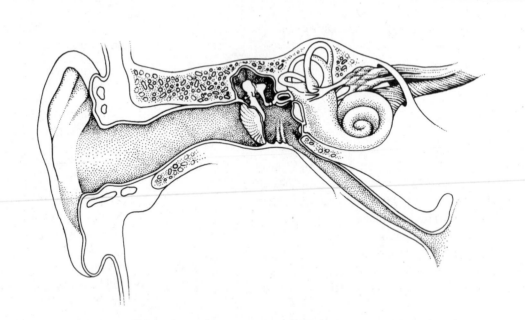

11. The nurse is on a camping trip and one of the campers reports, "I think there is an insect in my ear. I can hear it and feel it moving around inside my ear canal." What should the nurse try first?
    a. Shine a flashlight in the canal and try to coax the insect to come out.
    b. Instill cooking oil into the ear to suffocate the insect, than flush the canal with water.
    c. Apply a thin coating of antibiotic ointment to the external canal and pinna.
    d. Instruct the camper to tilt head downwards and vigorously shake the head.

12. Before performing a physical exam, what assessments related to the patient's hearing can be done while observing the patient? *(Select all that apply.)*
    a. Note how the patient is dressed.
    b. Observe body posture and position.
    c. Observe if the patient is anxious or fearful.
    d. See if the patient asks for questions to be repeated.
    e. Note whether the patient tilts the head toward the examiner.

13. The nurse gently taps over the patient's mastoid process and the patient reports tenderness. This finding may indicate which condition?
    a. Excessive cerumen
    b. Hyperacusis
    c. Ruptured eardrum
    d. Inflammatory process

14. During the physical assessment, the nurse identifies a defect of the patient's external ear. Based on knowledge of embryonic development, which question will the nurse ask to identify potential problems in a body system that developed concurrently with the external ear?
    a. "Have you ever had problems with your heart?"
    b. "Do you notice shortness of breath with minor exertion?"
    c. "Have you had any problems with your kidneys or urination?"
    d. "Do you have episodes of headaches with confusion?"

15. How would the nurse use body position and the surrounding environment when conducting an interview with a patient who may have a hearing problem?
    a. Conduct the interview in a quiet, darkened room without distractions.
    b. Sit beside the patient and speak directly into the patient's ear.
    c. Sit directly in front of the patient in a room with adequate lighting.
    d. Stand over the patient and use hand motions for emphasis.

16. Which disorder of the ear/hearing is more commonly found among men aged 20-50 years old?
    a. Ménière's disease
    b. Otosclerosis
    c. Excessive cerumen
    d. Labyrinthitis

17. Which person has the highest risk for developing hearing problems because of occupation?
    a. Nurse who works night shift in an emergency department
    b. Coach who coaches a high school swim team
    c. Bus driver who picks up elementary school children
    d. Bartender who works in a nightclub with live music

18. Which child is most likely to develop hearing loss in adulthood?
    a. 1-year-old with ear infections related to "night bottles"
    b. 2-year-old who stumbles and bumps his head on a table
    c. 5-year-old who is diagnosed with Down syndrome
    d. 10-year-old with a grandparent who has hearing problems

19. The nurse hears in shift report that a patient suffers from hyperacusis. Which intervention is the nurse most likely to use in the care of this patient?
    a. Supply a writing tablet and pen.
    b. Speak loudly and carefully enunciate.
    c. Ensure that environmental noise is controlled.
    d. Instruct the patient to sit up slowly.

20. The nurse is assisting an inexperienced health care provider who is trying to perform an otoscopic examination on an older patient who is being treated for delirium caused by infection. What should the nurse do?
    a. Quietly talk to the patient to distract him as the provider inserts the speculum.
    b. Gently hold the patient's head to prevent movement during the examination.
    c. Suggest that the otoscopic examination be deferred until the delirium resolves.
    d. Suggest using a Rinne tuning fork test instead of the otoscopic examination.

21. The home health nurse is visiting the patient for the first time. The nurse notices that the patient frequently tilts his head and gives odd answers to simple questions. The nurse has a stethoscope, a digital watch, a pen, and a blood pressure cuff in her supply bag. Which method would the nurse use to test hearing during this visit?
    a. Hold the watch about 5 inches from the each ear and ask the patient what he hears.
    b. Stand 2 feet away and whisper a sentence into the unblocked ear and ask patient to repeat the sentence.
    c. Apply the blood pressure cuff and ask if patient can hear the separation of the Velcro fastener.
    d. Have the patient don the stethoscope and ask the patient to listen to and count his own heartbeat.

22. The nurse reads in the patient's chart that the Weber tuning fork test showed that the patient had lateralization to the right. Based on this information, what would the nurse do while the caring for the patient?
    a. Instruct the patient to turn his head to the right if he is having trouble hearing.
    b. Ask the patient in which ear the sound is louder, because the test is inconclusive.
    c. Position self to the patient's right, so that voice travels directly to the right ear.
    d. Lateralization indicates normal hearing, so the nurse would perform routine care.

23. Which patient is the most likely candidate to benefit from the Rinne tuning fork test?
    a. Patient requires differentiation of hearing by air conduction versus bone conduction.
    b. Patient is a toddler and therefore unable to follow instructions for audiometry or other tests.
    c. Patient has a family history of sensorineural hearing loss and genetic mutation in gene GJB2.
    d. Patient is unable to identify and report which ear has the greater hearing loss.

24. The results of an audiometry test indicate that the patient hears about 50% of the time at 0 decibels. Based on these results, which action is the nurse most likely to perform?
    a. Prepares a brochure about different types of hearing aids
    b. Explains the purpose and procedure of caloric testing
    c. Uses normal conversation speech when speaking to the patient
    d. Asks the patient which ear is better and directs voice towards that side

25. Which patient is most likely to have the lowest threshold for hearing tones and speech?
    a. 25-year-old patient with no previous hearing problems
    b. 76-year-old patient with significant hearing loss
    c. 43-year-old patient who is well-adapted to hearing aid
    d. 60-year-old patient with no known health problems

26. For a person who is just beginning to notice some hearing loss, which sounds would be the most difficult to clearly hear?
    a. A woman singing in the soprano range
    b. Toddler who is angry and screaming
    c. Cell phone ringing with low-frequency tones
    d. Gunfire shots on a television show

27. What is a contraindication for a patient having electronystagmography (ENG)?
    a. Dental problems
    b. Previous ENG
    c. Prostheses
    d. Pacemaker

28. A patient is having problems with speech discrimination. What is the nurse most likely to observe?
    a. Patient speaks very loudly during a conversation.
    b. Patient can hear high tones, but not low tones.
    c. Patient cannot accurately repeat two-syllable words.
    d. Patient repeats back "gay" when the nurse says "gray."

29. Tympanometry is helpful in distinguishing which disorder?
    a. Middle ear infections
    b. External ear infections
    c. Hearing loss for low-pitched tones
    d. Indurated lesions on the pinna

30. What is the normal response to caloric testing?
    a. Vertigo and nystagmus within 20 to 30 seconds
    b. Vertigo and nystagmus immediately
    c. Vertigo and nystagmus within 5 minutes
    d. Nystagmus with no vertigo

31. The examiner is using an otoscope to inspect the external canal. What is the purpose of injecting a gentle puff of air into the canal?
    a. To detect infection
    b. To elicit pain or discomfort
    c. To detect mobility of the eardrum
    d. To verify the patency of the eardrum

32. Which treatments are used for external otitis? *(Select all that apply.)*
    a. Application of heat
    b. Oral analgesics
    c. Topical antibiotics
    d. Myringotomy
    e. Bedrest

33. Which condition caused by trauma results in the calcification and hardening of the pinna?
    a. Squamous cell carcinoma
    b. Furuncle
    c. Tophi
    d. Boxer's ear

34. The nurse uses irrigating fluid that is 98.6° F (37° C) to irrigate a patient's ear to remove cerumen. What is the best rationale for using fluid that is 98.6° F (37° C)?
    a. Evidence-based practice guides the selection of temperature
    b. Reduces the chance of stimulating the vestibular sense
    c. Is less painful than hotter or colder temperatures
    d. Potentiates the melting and mobilization of cerumen

35. An adult patient has external otitis. After the inflammation resolves, which action should the patient avoid?
    a. Using earplugs while swimming
    b. Dropping diluted alcohol in the ear to prevent recurrence
    c. Inserting cotton-tipped applicator into ears after bathing
    d. Using analgesics for pain relief

36. What are potential complications from necrotizing or malignant otitis? *(Select all that apply.)*
    a. Destruction of all cranial nerves
    b. Infection of the ear and skull
    c. Brain abscess
    d. Death
    e. Meningitis

37. An adult patient has otitis media. What does the nurse expect the patient's chief complaint to be?
    a. Ear pain
    b. Rhinitis
    c. Drainage from the ear canal
    d. Swelling of the scalp

38. A patient has been diagnosed with perichondritis. What is the most likely cause of the infection for this patient?
    a. Recent ear piercing
    b. Recent sun exposure
    c. Previous diagnosis of otitis media
    d. Previous treatment of mastoiditis

39. An adult patient with a history of otitis media states that his left ear pain is better. Now the patient has noticed some pus with blood in the affected ear. What does the nurse suspect has happened?
    a. Antibiotics have successfully treated the infection.
    b. The eardrum has perforated.
    c. The condition has worsened.
    d. The ear has been permanently damaged.

40. Which step is a correct part of the procedure for instilling eardrops?
    a. Gently irrigate the ear if the membrane is not intact.
    b. Place the bottle of eardrops in a bowl of hot water for 10 minutes.
    c. Tilt the patient's head in the opposite direction of the affected ear.
    d. Perform hand hygiene and use sterile gloves during the procedure.

41. An adult patient has wax in the left ear. When irrigating his ear, the nurse uses which amount of fluid?
    a. 10 to 30 mL
    b. 50 to 70 mL
    c. 60 to 100 mL
    d. 150 to 200 mL

42. The nurse stops irrigating the ear if the patient reports which symptom?
    a. Persistent pain
    b. Sensation of fullness
    c. Tingling sensation
    d. Fatigue

43. What are the nurse's instructions to a patient after a myringotomy? *(Select all that apply.)*
    a. "Report excessive drainage to your health care provider."
    b. "Restrict hair washing for 1 week."
    c. "Use a straw for drinking liquids."
    d. "Leave the ear dressing in place until the next office visit."
    e. "Blow the nose gently with the mouth open."

44. Lymph node tenderness is most likely to be a symptom of which disorder?
    a. Ménière's disease
    b. Mastoiditis
    c. Otosclerosis
    d. Perichondritis

45. Which patient is most likely to benefit by having music playing during sleeping hours?
    a. Patient has frequent episodes of acute otitis media.
    b. Patient reports an odd sensation of "whirling in space."
    c. Patient has a hearing aid and reports excessive background noise.
    d. Patient reports tinnitus that contributes to emotional disturbance.

46. Tinnitus may be caused by which factors? *(Select all that apply.)*
    a. Tophi of the pinna
    b. Otosclerosis
    c. Continuous exposure to loud noise
    d. Medications
    e. Ménière's disease

47. The patient tells the nurse that he has unpredictable episodes of vertigo. What instructions are the most important to give to the unlicensed assistive personnel (UAP) who is assisting the patient with activities of daily living (ADLs)?
    a. "Face the patient directly whenever speaking to him."
    b. "There is a high risk for falls, so use a gait belt during ambulation."
    c. "Noise from the television or hallway should be minimized."
    d. "Patient is likely to have severe pain, so immediately report pain."

48. Which question will the nurse ask about meclizine (Antivert) to determine if the medication is having the desired therapeutic effect?
    a. "On a scale of 1-10, which number represents your current level of pain?"
    b. "Do you feel the medication helped to relieve the dizziness and nausea?"
    c. "Do you feel the medication decreased the buzzing sound that you reported?"
    d. "Do you think that your hearing has improved after completing the medication?"

49. For a patient with Ménière's disease, what is the purpose of the recommended nutrition therapy?
    a. To ensure an adequate intake of nutrients to slow progression of the disease
    b. To reduce harmful lipid accumulation in the acoustic-vestibular system
    c. To improve general overall health and strengthen the immune system
    d. To stabilize body fluid and prevent excess endolymph accumulation

50. An adult patient has been diagnosed with Ménière's disease. Which points does the nurse include in the teaching plan for this patient? *(Select all that apply.)*
    a. Make slow head movements.
    b. Reduce the intake of salt.
    c. Stop smoking.
    d. Take vitamin supplements
    e. Avoid caffeine.

51. The health care provider tells the nurse that the patient was informed about the diagnosis of acoustic neuroma and was also given information about the prognosis, treatment, and possible complications. Which patient statement indicates that the patient understood the information?
    a. "A tumor that is benign rarely causes a problem."
    b. "Chemotherapy and radiation are recommended."
    c. "The tumor is benign, but can cause neurologic damage."
    d. "Hearing loss is the only expected complication."

52. Which precautions does the nurse instruct a patient to follow after having ear surgery? *(Select all that apply.)*
    a. "Avoid air travel for 5 to 7 days."
    b. "Stay away from people with colds."
    c. "Do not drink through a straw for 2 to 3 weeks."
    d. "Keep your ear dry for 6 weeks."
    e. "Avoid straining when having a bowel movement."

53. Ototoxic drugs are used with caution in patients with which condition?
    a. Heart disease
    b. Liver disease
    c. Renal disease
    d. Lung disease

54. What should the nurse teach a patient who is learning to use a hearing aid?
    a. Soak the hearing aid in a solution of mild soap and water.
    b. Plug the hearing aid into an electrical source when not in use.
    c. Avoid exposing the hearing aid to extreme temperatures.
    d. Adjust volume to the highest setting to maximize hearing.

55. Which action could prevent ear trauma?
    a. Holding the nose when sneezing to reduce pressure
    b. Not using small objects to clean the external ear canal
    c. Occluding one nostril when blowing the nose
    d. Not washing the external ear and canal

56. For which ear condition is a myringotomy performed?
    a. Labyrinthitis
    b. Acoustic neuroma
    c. Otitis media
    d. Perichondrium

57. What should a patient who is having a stapedectomy be told about the procedure? *(Select all that apply.)*
    a. Possible complications include vertigo and infection.
    b. Success rate is high.
    c. There is a risk of total hearing loss on the affected side.
    d. Hearing is immediately improved after surgery.
    e. Facial nerve damage is a possible complication of the surgery.

58. What might the nurse notice if the patient has auditory sensory perception problems?
    a. Patient frequently looks away when being spoken to.
    b. Patient startles very easily at unexpected sounds.
    c. Patient frequently asks speaker to repeat statements.
    d. Patient often seeks out others for assistance.

59. How should the nurse respond to a patient who has auditory sensory perception problems? *(Select all that apply.)*
    a. Reduce the background sound when speaking to the person.
    b. Speak slowly, distinctly, and with a deeper tone.
    c. Initiate fall precautions.
    d. Determine if the patient uses sign language.
    e. Face the patient while speaking.

49 CHAPTER

Assessment of the Musculoskeletal System

1. Which ethnic group has the least risk for developing osteoporosis?
   a. African American
   b. European American
   c. Asian American
   d. Hispanic American

2. The patients with which conditions are most likely to be at risk for osteoporosis related to decreased intake of vitamin D and calcium? *(Select all that apply.)*
   a. Obesity
   b. Bulimia
   c. Anorexia nervosa
   d. Multiple sclerosis
   e. Pancreatitis

3. Which description best defines the Haversian system?
   a. Outer layer of bone tissue
   b. Spongy inner layer of bone
   c. Network connecting bone marrow vessels to outer bone covering
   d. Longitudinal canal network containing microscopic blood vessels

4. Which description best defines the bone diaphysis?
   a. Shaft of a long bone
   b. End of a long bone
   c. Outer layer of bone tissue
   d. Spongy inner layer of bone

5. Which cells are bone-destroyers?
   a. Osteoblasts
   b. Osteoclasts
   c. Osteocytes
   d. Cancellous

6. A patient is at risk for a parathyroid hormone (PTH) imbalance related to a recent surgical procedure. Based on this information, which blood level must the nurse monitor in the patient?
   a. Blood glucose
   b. Serum calcium
   c. Serum potassium
   d. Serum magnesium

7. Which vitamin plays a key role in bone health?
   a. Vitamin A
   b. Vitamin B
   c. Vitamin D
   d. Vitamin E

8. The nurse is caring for an adult patient with a recent increase in growth hormone and acromegaly. In assessing this patient, what does the nurse expect to find?
   a. Bone and soft-tissue deformities
   b. Pain that increases when flexing joints
   c. Unusually tall height for ethnic background
   d. Marked lateral curvature of the spine

9. Pivot joints allow for which type of movement?
   a. Flexion
   b. Rotation
   c. Extension
   d. Hinge

10. Condylar joints provide which types of movement? *(Select all that apply.)*
    a. Extension
    b. Hinge
    c. Slight rotation
    d. Gliding
    e. Flexion

11. The knee provides which type of joint movement?
    a. Condylar
    b. Ball-and-socket
    c. Gliding
    d. Hinge

12. The elbow is considered which type of joint?
    a. Gliding
    b. Ball-and-socket
    c. Flexion and extension
    d. Hinge

13. Biaxial joints provide which type of movement?
    a. Hinge
    b. Gliding
    c. Ball-and-socket
    d. Flexion and extension

14. The patient is an athletic young adult man who broke his leg during a sports accident. The cast, which has been in place for several weeks, is being removed for the first time and the patient is stunned by the appearance of his leg. What is the nurse's best response to this patient's surprise?
    a. "Don't worry; it looks crusty and withered, but the strength and function are normal."
    b. "The cast compresses the tissue, but your leg will look normal in a couple of days."
    c. "Let's just wash off the dead skin and you will see that it is not as bad as it seems."
    d. "Without regular exercise, muscles atrophy; strength can be restored with use."

15. A 55-year-old woman with a small frame is aware of her increased risk for osteoporosis and loss of bone mass, although she currently reports no pain or loss of function. She asks the nurse to recommend a good type of exercise to counteract the risk. What does the nurse suggest?
    a. Swimming
    b. Deep-breathing and isometric exercise
    c. Walking with arm weights
    d. Golfing

16. Which definition best describes the musculoskeletal term *fasciculi*?
    a. Fibrous tissue surrounding muscle
    b. Band of tough, fibrous tissue attaching muscle to bone
    c. Bundles of muscle fibers
    d. Band of tough, fibrous tissue attaching bone to bone

17. Which definition best describes the musculoskeletal term *synovium*?
    a. Collagen fibers at bone ends
    b. Lubricates joints
    c. Small sacs lined with synovial membrane
    d. Membrane that secretes a lubricating fluid

18. Which group has the greatest risk for trauma resulting in injuries to muscles and bones?
    a. Older adult men related to occupational injuries
    b. Young men related to motor vehicle accidents
    c. Young women related to sports injuries
    d. Children who are not supervised during play

19. The nurse is likely to assess which musculoskeletal findings in the average older adult? *(Select all that apply.)*
    a. Increased bone density
    b. Degenerating synovial joint cartilage
    c. Atrophied muscles
    d. Unchanged strength
    e. Slowed movement

20. The patient is a construction worker in his early 30s who was treated with oral antibiotics after stepping on a nail. The wound does not appear to be responding to antibiotic treatment as expected, despite the patient's compliance. The nurse suspects the patient may have a family history of which disorder?
    a. Renal disease
    b. Heart disease
    c. Skin or bone cancer
    d. Diabetes mellitus

21. What concentration level of alkaline phosphatase (ALP) does the nurse expect to monitor for a patient with bone or liver damage?
    a. Increased
    b. Decreased
    c. Normal value
    d. Same as baseline level for the patient

22. A patient has had an arthroscopy in the right leg. In assessing the patient's neurovascular status of the extremity, what does the nurse evaluate? *(Select all that apply.)*
    a. Presence of pain
    b. Hair pattern on skin
    c. Movement
    d. Capillary refill
    e. Sensation

23. Which instrument is used to assess joint range of motion (ROM)?
    a. Odometer
    b. Ergometer
    c. Goniometer
    d. Spectrometer

24. Which assessment finding of the musculoskeletal system indicates an abnormality?
    a. Symmetry in the upper extremities and equal muscle mass
    b. Gait balance and a smooth and regular stride
    c. Flexion, extension, and rotation of the neck
    d. Opposition of three of four fingers to the thumb

25. Which factor is primarily responsible for regulating serum calcium levels?
    a. Calcitonin
    b. Vitamin D
    c. Glucocorticoids
    d. Growth hormone

26. The nurse is reviewing the laboratory results for a patient with severe diarrhea and hypocalcemia. What does the nurse find is present in bone and serum in inverse proportion to calcium?
    a. Estrogen
    b. Phosphorus
    c. Thyroxine
    d. Insulin

27. Which hormones affect bone growth? *(Select all that apply.)*
    a. Glucocorticoids
    b. Renin
    c. Thyroxine
    d. Estrogens
    e. Androgens
    f. Catecholamines

28. Which laboratory result may indicate bone or liver damage, such as metastatic cancer of the bone?
    a. Serum calcium 9.5 mg/dL
    b. Serum calcium 8.2 mg/dL
    c. Lactate dehydrogenase (LDH) 185 units/L
    d. Alkaline phosphatase 140 units/L

29. Which substances affect bone growth and metabolism? *(Select all that apply.)*
    a. Chloride
    b. Calcium
    c. Vitamin C
    d. Phosphorus
    e. Vitamin D

30. A patient reports pain in the left lower ankle. Which questions does the nurse ask to elicit relevant information about this patient's musculoskeletal problem? *(Select all that apply.)*
    a. "Do you have adequate calcium and vitamin D intake?"
    b. "What seems to make the pain worse?"
    c. "What measures seem to help alleviate the symptoms?"
    d. "What did your family doctor tell you?"
    e. "When did your pain start?"
    f. "Do you have a history of diabetes mellitus?"

31. The nurse is assessing a patient's posture and gait, and notes that the patient shifts his shoulders from side to side while walking. How is this finding considered?
    a. Abnormality in the swing phase, called a *lurch*
    b. Abnormality in the stance phase, called an *antalgic gait*
    c. Normal and automatic gait
    d. Limp or other type of asymmetric body movement

32. In assessing a patient's functional ability and ROM, the patient is unable to actively move a joint through the expected ROM. Which technique does the nurse use to assess joint mobility?
    a. The patient relaxes the muscles in the extremity, then moves the joint through the fullest motion possible.
    b. The nurse holds the part with one hand above and one hand below the joint to be evaluated, and allows passive ROM to evaluate joint mobility.
    c. The patient moves the joints while the nurse applies gentle resistance.
    d. The patient moves the joint to the best of ability while the nurse palpates for crepitus.

33. The nurse is assessing a patient who is obese, especially in the abdominal area. What is the most common musculoskeletal assessment finding in this patient?
    a. Scoliosis
    b. Crepitus
    c. Lordosis
    d. Kyphosis

34. What activity does the nurse ask a patient to perform when assessing ROM in the patient's hands?
    a. Wave the hand as though waving good-bye.
    b. Grip the nurse's hand as hard as possible.
    c. Rapidly move the hands into the palm-up and palm-down positions.
    d. Make a fist and then appose each finger to the thumb.

35. A patient has an effusion of the right knee. Which assessment finding does the nurse expect to see in this patient?
    a. Limitations in movement and accompanying pain
    b. Obvious appearance of genu valgum
    c. Crepitus and difficulty bearing weight
    d. Obvious redness and skin breakdown

36. Which of the following must be documented by the nurse with each neurovascular assessment performed? *(Select all that apply.)*
    a. Distal pulses
    b. Capillary refill
    c. Range of motion
    d. Sensation
    e. Pain

37. The nurse is reviewing laboratory results for a patient who was involved in an accident. There is no evidence of fracture or bone damage, but multiple soft tissue injuries were sustained. Which muscle enzymes are expected to be elevated because of the injuries? *(Select all that apply.)*
    a. Creatine kinase (CK)
    b. Aspartate aminotransferase (AST)
    c. ALP
    d. Lactic dehydrogenase (LDH)
    e. Aldolase (ALD)

38. The primary function of which substance is to regulate protein metabolism?
    a. Parathyroid hormone
    b. Growth hormone
    c. Glucocorticoid
    d. Calcitonin

39. How does parathyroid hormone respond when serum calcium levels are lowered in the body? *(Select all that apply.)*
    a. Secretion increases.
    b. It stimulates bone to promote osteoclastic activity.
    c. Secretion decreases.
    d. Secretion raises serum calcium levels back up.
    e. Secretion further decreases serum calcium levels.

40. Which substance promotes absorption of calcium and phosphorus from the small intestine?
    a. Glucocorticoids
    b. Calcitonin
    c. Vitamin D
    d. Parathyroid hormone

41. If serum calcium levels are increased above normal, which substance decreases serum calcium levels by inhibiting bone resorption and increasing renal excretion of calcium and phosphorus?
    a. Glucocorticoids
    b. Calcitonin
    c. Growth hormone
    d. Parathyroid hormone

42. With which radiographic examination is a fiberoptic tube is inserted into a joint (usually the knee or shoulder) for direct visualization.
    a. Myelography
    b. Arthroscopy
    c. Tomography
    d. Xeroradiography

43. Which test uses sound waves to produce an image of the tissue?
    a. Ultrasonography
    b. Electromyography
    c. Computed tomography
    d. Thallium scan

44. Magnetic resonance imaging (MRI) is a diagnostic test used mostly to visualize which of the following? *(Select all that apply.)*
    a. Joints
    b. Fluid accumulation
    c. Soft tissue
    d. Vertebrae
    e. Bony tumors

50 CHAPTER

Care of Patients with Musculoskeletal Problems

1. Which risk factors are associated with osteoporosis?
   a. Male over 50 years of age, European heritage
   b. Female, white, menopausal, thin, lean, immobilized
   c. Older adult, vitamin D deficiency, insufficient exposure to sunlight
   d. Weight-bearing exercise, moderate alcohol intake

2. Which objective patient data are associated with osteomalacia? *(Select all that apply.)*
   a. Unsteady gait
   b. Vertebral fracture
   c. Long bone bowing
   d. Hip flexion contractures
   e. Discomfort on vertebral palpation
   f. Bone tenderness over ribcage

3. The nurse assesses a patient with a musculoskeletal disorder and finds hip flexion contractures, flushed and warm skin, and a soft thick and enlarged skull. Which disorder does the nurse recognize?
   a. Osteoporosis
   b. Osteomalacia
   c. Paget's disease
   d. Osteomyelitis

4. The nurse is conducting an assessment on a patient with osteoporosis. Which factors and/or patient data may be associated with this disorder? *(Select all that apply.)*
   a. Muscle cramps
   b. Sedentary lifestyle
   c. Back pain relieved by rest
   d. Fracture
   e. Urinary or renal stones

5. Which factors and/or patient data may be associated with osteomalacia? *(Select all that apply.)*
   a. Vitamin D deficiency
   b. Drinks 8 cups of coffee per day
   c. Muscle weakness in the pelvic girdle area
   d. Bone pain worsened by walking
   e. Muscle weakness in legs

6. Which factors may be associated with Paget's disease? *(Select all that apply.)*
   a. Loss of height
   b. Apathy or lethargy
   c. Urinary or renal stones
   d. Cigarette smoker
   e. Muscle cramps

7. The nurse is reviewing T-scores for a 68-year-old woman. The patient has a T-score of 2.5. How does the nurse interpret this data?
   a. The patient has osteopenia.
   b. The patient has osteoporosis.
   c. This is a normal score for the patient's age.
   d. There is osteoblastic activity.

8. Which patient is at risk for regional osteoporosis?
   a. Patient who has been in a long leg cast for 10 weeks
   b. Patient on long-term corticosteroid therapy
   c. Patient with a history of hyperparathyroidism
   d. Menopausal patient

9. Which patients are at risk for osteoporosis because of nutritional issues? *(Select all that apply.)*
   a. Older adult female patient who likes to drink a lot of coffee
   b. Patient who has had gastric bypass surgery for obesity
   c. Patient who is on the high-protein Atkins diet
   d. Patient who prefers to drink diluted powdered milk
   e. Patient who drinks two carbonated diet sodas per day
   f. Patient with chronic alcoholism

10. The nurse is assessing an older adult patient at risk for osteoporosis. Which task can be delegated to the unlicensed assistive personnel (UAP)?
    a. Inspect the vertebral column.
    b. Take height and weight measurements.
    c. Compare observations to previous findings.
    d. Ask if the patient is shorter or has gained or lost weight.

11. A patient with osteoporosis moves slowly and carefully with voluntary restriction of movement. The lower thoracic area is tender on palpation. How does the nurse interpret this assessment data?
    a. Vertebral compression fracture
    b. Kyphosis of the dorsal spine
    c. Osteopenia related to immobility
    d. Increased osteoblastic activity

12. The home health nurse is visiting an older adult patient with osteoporosis and severe kyphosis. When the nurse asks about activities she has been doing, the patient replies, "I used to be very active and beautiful when I was younger." What is the nurse's best response?
    a. "You are still very beautiful."
    b. "Activity can help to prevent fractures and complications."
    c. "Tell me what you used to do."
    d. "Do you need information about age-appropriate exercises?"

13. A patient is scheduled to have a dual x-ray absorptiometry (DXA). What information does the nurse give to the patient about preparing for the test?
    a. "Leave metallic objects such as jewelry, coins, and belt buckles at home."
    b. "Have someone come with you to drive you home after the test."
    c. "You will be asked to give a urine specimen prior to the test."
    d. "Bring a comfortable loose nightgown without buttons or snaps."

14. A patient is lactose intolerant and would like suggestions about food sources that supply adequate calcium and vitamin D. In addition to a generally well-balanced diet, what foods does the nurse suggest?
    a. Fresh apples and pears
    b. Whole-wheat bread
    c. Fortified soy or rice products
    d. Prune or cranberry juice

15. A patient has been advised by the health care provider that exercising may help prevent osteoporosis. Which exercise does the nurse recommend to the patient?
    a. Swimming 10 to 15 laps 3 to 5 times a week
    b. Running for 20 minutes 4 times a week
    c. Bowling for 60 minutes 3 times a week
    d. Walking for 30 minutes 3 to 5 times a week

16. Calcitonin (Calcimar) has been prescribed to a patient. What instructions does the nurse provide about this medication? *(Select all that apply.)*
    a. It is a parathyroid hormone that will increase bone density.
    b. It will help prevent bone loss.
    c. It will stimulate the production of bone cells.
    d. Flushing, nausea, and skin rash may be side effects.
    e. Nasal mucosa irritation may occur if taken intranasally.

17. Which osteoporosis drug should not be given to women with a history of venous thromboembolism?
    a. Raloxifene (Evista)
    b. Ibandronate (Boniva)
    c. Risedronate (Actonel)
    d. Alendronate (Fosamax)

18. Which are potential adverse reactions of alendronate (Fosamax)? *(Select all that apply.)*
    a. Difficulty swallowing
    b. Drowsiness
    c. Esophagitis
    d. Constipation
    e. Esophageal ulcers

19. Why do men develop osteoporosis after the age of 50?
    a. Their testosterone levels decrease.
    b. Older men are prescribed more medications.
    c. It is secondary to hyperparathyroidism.
    d. As men age they are less active.

20. The nurse is reviewing the prescriptions for a patient receiving drug therapy for the prevention of osteoporosis. The patient also has hypertension and heart disease. Which prescription order does the nurse question?
    a. Calcium supplements
    b. Hormone replacement therapy
    c. Alendronate (Fosamax)
    d. Raloxifene (Evista)

21. A patient is prescribed calcitonin for treatment of Paget's disease. What does the nurse teach this patient regarding this drug?
    a. Avoid eating salmon because calcitonin is derived from salmon.
    b. Calcitonin is given by subcutaneous injection.
    c. Take a drug holiday after 1 year of therapy.
    d. Store the drug in a cool, dry, dark place.

22. A patient reports pain in the lower legs and pelvis which is aggravated by activity and worse at night. The nurse observes muscle weakness which appears to be causing a waddling and unsteady gait. What additional information supports the likelihood of osteomalacia in this patient?
    a. Recent immigration from a country where famine is common
    b. Taking hormone replacement therapy for a prolonged time
    c. Unable to perform a prescribed exercise regimen
    d. History of recent vertebroplasty for osteoporosis

23. An x-ray shows the presence of radiolucent bands (Looser's lines or zones) in a patient. What is this diagnostic finding specific for?
    a. Osteoporosis
    b. Osteomalacia
    c. Paget's disease
    d. Osteomyelitis

24. The nurse is assessing a patient who reports moderate bone pain in the hip and has a family history of Paget's disease. In performing a musculoskeletal assessment, the nurse pays particular attention to which element?
    a. Size and shape of the skull
    b. Long-bone bowing in the legs
    c. Asymmetrical deformity of the extremities
    d. Loose teeth and difficulty chewing

25. A patient with Paget's disease has complications related to bony enlargements of the skull. Which complication is potentially the most serious and life-threatening?
    a. Basilar complications with compression on the cranial nerves
    b. Platybasia, or basilar invagination with brainstem manifestations
    c. Blockage of cerebrospinal fluid (CSF), resulting in hydrocephalus
    d. Pressure from an enlarged temporal bone leading to deafness and vertigo

26. A patient with Paget's disease comes to the clinic for evaluation. Which symptom reported by the patient alerts the nurse to the possibility of osteogenic sarcoma?
    a. Change in hearing
    b. Warmth and redness of the joints
    c. Changes in balance and gait
    d. Severe bone pain

27. A patient with Paget's disease has a kidney problem associated with increased serum calcium. What is the nursing priority for this patient?
    a. Encourage the patient to increase fluids, unless contraindicated.
    b. Encourage moderate consumption of milk and dairy products.
    c. Assist the patient to problem-solve incontinence issues.
    d. Direct the UAP to measure and record all urine output.

28. A patient is having diagnostic testing to determine the probability of Paget's disease. If the disease is present, which laboratory result does the nurse expect to see?
    a. Slightly decreased serum calcium level
    b. Increased serum alkaline phosphatase (ALP)
    c. Decreased pyridinium (PYD)
    d. Absence of osteocalcin

29. A patient with Paget's disease has been prescribed drug therapy. The nurse prepares patient teaching information for which medication as a first-line therapy?
    a. Calcitonin
    b. Ibuprofen (Motrin)
    c. Plicamycin (Mithracin)
    d. Risedronate (Actonel)

30. A 40-year-old patient is admitted for acute osteomyelitis of the left lower leg. What does the nurse expect to find documented in the patient's admitting assessment?
    a. Temperature greater than 101° F; swelling, tenderness, erythema, and warmth of area
    b. Ulceration resulting with sinus tract formation, localized pain, and drainage
    c. Pain is aching, poorly described, deep, and worsened by pressure and weight bearing
    d. Shortening of the extremity with pain during weight bearing or palpation

31. The nurse is caring for a patient with osteomyelitis. Which laboratory results are of primary concern for this disorder?
    a. Bone-specific alkaline phosphatase and osteocalcin
    b. Serum calcium level and alkaline phosphatase
    c. White blood cell count and erythrocyte sedimentation rate
    d. Thyroid function tests and uric acid levels

32. Which patient is mostly likely to be a candidate for hyperbaric oxygen therapy?
    a. Patient with chronic, unremitting osteomyelitis
    b. Patient with an advanced case of Paget's disease
    c. Patient with osteomalacia related to poverty
    d. Patient with osteoporosis and recurrent fractures

33. A patient comes to the emergency department (ED) after accidentally puncturing his hand with an automatic nail gun. Which disorder is this patient primarily at risk for?
    a. Osteoporosis
    b. Osteomyelitis
    c. Osteomalacia
    d. Dupuytren's contracture

34. The nurse is caring for a patient with acute osteomyelitis. What assessment findings typically accompany this medical diagnosis? *(Select all that apply.)*
    a. Fever; temperature usually above 101° F
    b. Sinus tract formation
    c. Erythema of the affected area
    d. Swelling around the affected area
    e. Decreased peripheral pulses

35. The nurse is teaching a patient about antibiotic therapy for osteomyelitis. What information does the nurse give to the patient?
    a. Single-agent therapy is the most effective treatment for acute infections.
    b. Chronic osteomyelitis may require 1 month of antibiotic therapy.
    c. Patients usually remain hospitalized to complete the full course of antibiotic therapy.
    d. The infected wound may be irrigated with one or more types of antibiotic solutions.

36. A patient is diagnosed with Ewing's sarcoma. Which characteristics are specific to this type of bone cancer? *(Select all that apply.)*
    a. Low-grade fever is present.
    b. Leukocytosis is present.
    c. In 40% of cases, the tumor is found in a distal femur.
    d. Death usually results from metastasis to lungs and other bones.
    e. Ribs and upper extremities are most affected.

37. A patient is being seen in the clinic for dull pain and swelling of the proximal femur over 2-3 months. Which malignant bone tumor might this be?
    a. Ewing's sarcoma
    b. Chondrosarcoma
    c. Fibrosarcoma
    d. Osteosarcoma

38. The nurse is seeing a 49-year-old man in the clinic for left mid-tibia tenderness for the past 3 months. What type of malignant bone tumor might this patient have?
    a. Chondrosarcoma
    b. Ewing's sarcoma
    c. Fibrosarcoma
    d. Osteosarcoma

39. Which radiographic findings are associated with benign bone tumor growth? *(Select all that apply.)*
    a. Intact cortices
    b. Cortical breakthrough
    c. Smooth uniform periosteal bone
    d. Sharp margins
    e. Irregular new periosteal bone

40. What is the most common type of malignant bone tumor?
    a. Ewing's sarcoma
    b. Chondrosarcoma
    c. Fibrosarcoma
    d. Osteosarcoma

41. Which assessment finding in a patient who has undergone a bone graft for a tumor does the nurse report to the health care provider immediately?
    a. Extremity distal to the operative site is warm and pink.
    b. Cast over the operative site is cool to the touch.
    c. Delayed capillary refill presents in digits distal to the site.
    d. Pain is present in the operative extremity.

42. A patient with a bone tumor is grieving and anxious. The nurse includes which psychosocial interventions? *(Select all that apply.)*
    a. Allow the patient to verbalize feelings.
    b. Offer to call the patient's spiritual or religious adviser.
    c. Prepare the patient for death.
    d. Share stories of personal losses.
    e. Redirect the patient to more cheerful topics.
    f. Listen attentively while the patient talks.

43. A patient being evaluated for bone pain has a computed tomography (CT) report that includes a large tumor with a sclerotic center, periphery is soft, and extends through the bone cortex in a sunburst pattern. What do these findings indicate?
    a. Malignant bone tumor such as osteosarcoma
    b. Benign bone tumor such as osteochondroma
    c. Advanced Paget's disease
    d. Osteomalacia with osteoporosis

44. A patient with bone sarcoma had surgery to salvage an upper limb. The nurse has identified the patient has impaired physical mobility related to musculoskeletal impairment. Which intervention does the nurse perform in the early postoperative period?
    a. Encourage the patient to use the opposite hand to achieve forward flexion and abduction of the affected shoulder.
    b. Encourage the patient to emphasize strengthening the quadriceps muscles by using passive and active motion.
    c. Instruct the UAP to completely perform hygiene for the patient until the patient expresses readiness to do self-care.
    d. Evaluate the patient's and family's readiness to use the continuous passive motion machine in the home setting.

45. A patient with bone cancer has had the right lower leg surgically removed. The patient has been brave and uncomplaining, but the nurse recognizes that the patient is likely to experience grieving. What is the nurse's most important role?
    a. Act as a patient advocate to promote the physician-patient relationship.
    b. Encourage the patient to talk to the family and complete an advance directive.
    c. Be an active listener and encourage the patient and family to verbalize feelings.
    d. Help the patient and family cope with and resolve grief and loss issues.

46. Which definition best describes secondary tumors?
    a. Tumors arising from bones
    b. Malignant tumor metastasizing to bone
    c. Malignant tumor arising from underlying tissue
    d. Tumor arising from cartilage

47. Which type of benign tumor is commonly located in the hands and feet?
    a. Chondroma
    b. Giant cell tumor
    c. Osteochondroma
    d. Fibrogenic tumor

48. Which type of malignant bone tumor has manifestations of local tenderness in lower extremity long bones?
    a. Chondrosarcoma
    b. Ewing's sarcoma
    c. Fibrosarcoma
    d. Osteosarcoma

49. A patient who is a long-distance runner reports severe pain in the arch of the foot, especially when getting out of bed and with weight bearing. What does the nurse suspect in this patient?
    a. Morton's neuroma
    b. Plantar fasciitis
    c. Hammertoe
    d. Hallux valgus deformity

50. The nurse is assessing an older Caucasian man and notes there are flexion contractures of the fourth and fifth fingers. The patient reports that he had a similar problem on the other hand and had a fasciectomy which improved the function. What is this condition known as?
    a. Dupuytren's contracture
    b. Ganglion cyst
    c. Bunion
    d. Plantar digital neuritis

51. A patient is diagnosed with plantar fasciitis. What instruction does the nurse give to the patient about self-care for this condition?
    a. Use rest, elevation, and warm packs.
    b. Perform gentle jogging exercises.
    c. Strap the foot to maintain the arch.
    d. Wear loose or open shoes, such as sandals.

52. Which characteristics describe a ganglion hand disorder? *(Select all that apply.)*
    a. Joint discomfort after strain
    b. Progressive palmar flexion deformity
    c. Surgical release is required
    d. Round cyst-like lesion
    e. Painless on palpation
    f. Fourth and fifth digits affected

53. Which characteristics occur with the foot disorder hammertoe? *(Select all that apply.)*
    a. Great toe deviates laterally.
    b. Corns may develop on the dorsal side of the toe.
    c. First metatarsal head becomes enlarged.
    d. Insertion of wires or screws is required for fixation.
    e. Small tumor in a digital nerve of the foot.

54. The nurse is assessing a patient with a spinal deformity. Which technique does the nurse use to accomplish inspection of the spine?
    a. Observe the patient from the front and back while standing and during forward flexion from the hips.
    b. Observe the patient in a sitting and standing position and ask the patient to walk around the room.
    c. Ask the patient to remove the clothes from the waist up and then view the visible curvature of the spine.
    d. Look at the patient's back while the patient moves in different positions: touching toes, lateral bending, twisting.

55. The nurse is caring for a patient with muscular dystrophy. Although all body systems can be affected, the nurse is alert and carefully assesses for which major problem?
    a. Renal failure
    b. Cardiac failure
    c. Muscle weakness
    d. Respiratory failure

56. Which statements about scoliosis are true? *(Select all that apply.)*
    a. Scoliosis screening is best done during middle-school years.
    b. Scoliosis is characterized by a C- or S-shaped lateral curvature of the vertebral spine.
    c. Scoliosis screening is best done during preschool years.
    d. A curvature greater than 50 degrees results in an unstable spine.
    e. The forward-bend test is used to determine scoliosis.

51 Care of Patients with Musculoskeletal Trauma

CHAPTER

1. Which term related to the fracture healing process is the process of bone building and resorption?
   a. Callus
   b. Granulation
   c. Hematoma
   d. Remodeling

2. The nurse is caring for several patients on an orthopedic trauma unit. Which conditions have a high risk for development of acute compartment syndrome? *(Select all that apply.)*
   a. Lower legs caught between the bumpers of two cars
   b. Massive infiltration of IV fluid into forearm
   c. Bivalve cast on the lower leg
   d. Multiple insect bites to lower legs
   e. Daily use of oral contraceptives
   f. Severe burns to the upper extremities

3. A patient has a fracture of the right wrist. What is an early sign that indicates this patient may be having a complication?
   a. Patient loses ability to wiggle fingers without pain.
   b. Fingers are cold and pale; capillary refill is sluggish.
   c. Pain is severe and seems out of proportion to injury.
   d. Patient reports a subjective numbness and tingling.

4. The nurse is assessing a patient for severe pain in the right wrist after falling off a step stool. How does the nurse assess this patient's motor function?
   a. Performing passive range of motion for the wrist
   b. Asking the patient to move the fingers
   c. Having the patient flex and extend the elbow
   d. Instructing the patient to rotate the wrist

5. A patient in traction reports severe pain from a muscle spasm. What is the nurse's priority action?
   a. Assess the patient's body alignment.
   b. Give the patient a prn pain medication.
   c. Notify the health care provider.
   d. Remove some of the weights.

6. The nurse is reviewing the orders for a patient who was admitted for 24-hour observation of a leg fracture. A cast is in place. Which order does the nurse question?
   a. Elevate lower leg above the level of the heart.
   b. Perform neurovascular assessments ("circ checks") every 8 hours.
   c. Apply ice pack for 24 hours.
   d. Provide regular diet as tolerated.

7. A patient with a leg cast denies pain; toes are pink; capillary refill is brisk and toes move freely; the leg is elevated with an ice pack. Six hours later, the patient reports worsening pain unrelieved by medication. The patient's toes are cool and capillary refill is sluggish. What does the nurse suspect is occurring with this patient?
   a. Crush syndrome
   b. Fat embolism syndrome
   c. Acute compartment syndrome
   d. Fasciitis

8. An older adult sustained injury to the lower legs after being trapped underneath a fallen bookcase. Because this patient is at high risk for crush syndrome, which laboratory values will the nurse specifically monitor?
   a. Serum potassium level and myoglobin in urine
   b. White cell count and red cells in the urine
   c. Prothrombin level and serum lipase level
   d. Platelet count and serum calcium level

9. An older adult has been admitted with a hip fracture. Approximately 20 hours postinjury, the patient develops a symptom recognized as an early sign of fat embolism syndrome. Which symptom is the patient displaying?
   a. Severe respiratory distress
   b. Significantly increased pulse rate
   c. Change in mental status
   d. Petechiae rash over the neck

10. The student nurse is assessing a patient with a probable fractured tibia-fibula. What assessment technique used by the student nurse causes the supervising nurse to intervene?
    a. Inspects the fracture site for swelling or deformity
    b. Instructs the patient to wiggle the toes
    c. Assesses the bilateral dorsalis pedis pulse
    d. Pushes on the leg to elicit pain response

11. The nurse is caring for several orthopedic patients who are in different types of traction. What should the nurse do in assessing the traction equipment? *(Select all that apply.)*
    a. Inspect all ropes, knots, and pulleys once every 24 hours.
    b. Inspect ropes and knots for fraying or loosening every 8 to 12 hours.
    c. Check the amount of weight being used against the prescribed weight.
    d. Observe the traction equipment for proper functioning.
    e. Check if the ropes have been changed or cleaned within the past 48 hours.

12. A patient was put into traction at 0800 hours. Hourly neurovascular checks were ordered for the first 24 hours and then every 4 hours thereafter. At what time can the nursing staff start performing the 4-hour checks?
    a. 2000 hours same day
    b. 0000 hours next day
    c. 0800 hours next day
    d. 1200 hours next day

13. The nurse is educating a patient who will have external fixation for treatment of a compound tibial fracture. What information does the nurse include in the teaching session?
    a. "The device allows for early ambulation."
    b. "There is some danger of blood loss, but no danger of infection."
    c. "The device is a substitute therapy for a cast."
    d. "The advantage of the device is rapid bone healing."

14. The nurse is helping to evaluate several patients to determine candidacy for the Ilizaroz external fixation device. Which patient is the best candidate?
    a. Older woman who lives alone with a fracture of nonunion
    b. Child with a congenital bone deformity whose mother is a licensed practical nurse
    c. Teenager with an open fracture and bone loss of the left lower leg
    d. Middle-aged man with a new comminuted fracture of the dominant forearm

15. An older adult patient has a fractured humerus. The physician is considering the use of electrical bone stimulation and asks the nurse to take a medical history on the patient. Which specific condition, which is a contraindication for this therapy, does the nurse ask the patient about?
    a. Seizures
    b. Cardiac pacemaker
    c. Stroke
    d. Peripheral nerve damage

16. A patient is prescribed low-intensity pulsed ultrasound treatments for a very slow-healing fracture of the right lower leg. What instructions does the nurse give this patient related to the treatment?
    a. Test for pregnancy before the therapy and use birth control until treatment is complete.
    b. The treatment is experimental, but there are no known adverse effects.
    c. The device is implanted directly into the fracture site and there is no external apparatus.
    d. Expect to dedicate approximately 20 minutes a day for one treatment.

17. The nursing student is assisting with the care of a patient with musculoskeletal pain related to soft tissue injury and bone disruption. The student sees that the patient has a prn (as needed) order for pain medication. What does the student do first in order to decide when to give the pain medication?
    a. Ask the physician to clarify the order for specific parameters.
    b. Check with the primary nurse or the charge nurse for advice.
    c. Ask the patient about types of activities that increase the pain.
    d. Ask the instructor for help interpreting the order.

18. A patient is receiving scheduled and prn narcotics for severe pain related to a musculoskeletal injury. The nurse finds that the patient's abdomen is distended and bowel sounds are hypoactive. Because the nurse suspects that the patient is having a medication side effect, which question does the nurse ask the patient?
    a. "Are you having nausea and vomiting?"
    b. "When was your last bowel movement?"
    c. "Does your abdomen hurt?"
    d. "Are you having diarrhea or loose stool?"

19. A patient comes into the ED after falling off his four-wheeler. His lower leg is obviously broken; it is bleeding and bone fragments are protruding from the skin. What type of fracture does this patient likely have?
    a. Impacted
    b. Open (compound)
    c. Comminuted (fragmented)
    d. Displaced

20. A patient comes to the ED after slipping on some chalk in her classroom. She did not fall far and was able to walk with the assistance of one of her students. What type of fracture does this patient likely have?
    a. Closed, nondisplaced
    b. Oblique
    c. Impacted
    d. Incomplete

21. A female patient with osteoporosis comes to the ED after falling suddenly while opening her car door. She said it felt as though her "leg gave way" and caused her to fall. What type of fracture does this patient likely have?
    a. Pathologic (spontaneous)
    b. Spiral
    c. Impacted
    d. Incomplete

22. The nurse is caring for a patient with an open fracture. Which intervention does the nurse perform to prevent infection of the fracture?
    a. Use clean or aseptic technique for dressing changes and wound irrigations.
    b. Use clean technique for dressing changes and wound irrigations.
    c. Place the patient in contact isolation and wear sterile gloves.
    d. Place the patient in reverse isolation and perform scrupulous hand hygiene.

23. The nurse must adjust a pair of crutches to properly fit a patient. Which description illustrates correct crutch adjustment?
    a. Axilla rests lightly on the top of the crutch when the crutch is moved forward.
    b. Patient can easily use the crutch without subjective complaints.
    c. Elbow is flexed no more than 30 degrees when the palm is on the handle.
    d. Adult patient is of average height and the crutches are medium-sized.

24. An older patient's family is trying to find an appropriate cane for the patient to use because of chronic pain in the right ankle. The nurse instructs the family to purchase which type of cane?
    a. One with the top being parallel to the greater trochanter of the femur
    b. One that creates about 45 degrees of flexion of the elbow
    c. One that is based on the patient's weight to provide adequate support
    d. One that has padding on the handle grip to ensure safety

25. What members of the health care team will be consulted to teach a patient about proper use of the cane? *(Select all that apply.)*
    a. Occupational therapist
    b. Physical therapist
    c. Registered nurse
    d. Unlicensed assistive personnel
    e. Medical social worker

26. The nurse is caring for a patient with an external fixation of a bone fracture. What are the advantages of this type of treatment? *(Select all that apply.)*
    a. It is less painful than other treatments.
    b. It allows for earlier ambulation.
    c. It decreases the risk for infection.
    d. It maintains bone alignment.
    e. It stabilizes commuted fractures that require bone grafting.

27. An older patient with a lower leg fracture is having difficulty performing the weight-bearing exercises. Based on fracture pathophysiology and the patient's abilities, which condition could the patient develop?
    a. Osteomyelitis
    b. Internal derangement
    c. Neuroma
    d. Pulmonary embolism

28. The nurse case manager is making a home visit to assist an older patient with a hip fracture. During the home visit, the nurse reviews home environment safety. Which observation indicates a need for additional teaching?
    a. Patient's bed has been moved to the ground floor level.
    b. There are handle bars around the toilet and tub.
    c. Floors are clean and shiny and covered with throw rugs.
    d. Patient's walker is close to the patient's bedside.

29. Which is a potentially fatal complication of acute compartment syndrome?
    a. Myoglobinuric renal failure
    b. Ischemic heart failure
    c. Acute liver failure
    d. Hypovolemic shock

30. A patient comes to the ED with crush syndrome from a crush injury to his right upper extremity and right lower extremity when heavy equipment fell on him at a construction site. The patient has signs and symptoms of hypovolemia, hyperkalemia, and compartment syndrome. Management of care for this patient will focus on preventing which complications? *(Select all that apply.)*
    a. Sepsis
    b. Cardiac dysrhythmias
    c. Respiratory failure
    d. Acute kidney failure
    e. Fluid overload

31. A chronic complication of bone healing is called *avascular necrosis*. Which statements about this complication are true? *(Select all that apply.)*
    a. It involves disrupting the blood supply to the bone.
    b. It occurs when fat globules disrupt the blood supply to the bone.
    c. It involves disrupting the nerve supply to the bone.
    d. It results in the death of bone tissue.
    e. It is most often a complication of hip fractures.

32. A 30-year-old patient who is hospitalized for repair of a fractured tibia and fibula reports shortness of breath. Which complication related to the injury might the patient be experiencing?
    a. Hypovolemic shock
    b. Fat embolism
    c. Acute compartment syndrome
    d. Pneumonia

33. The older patient has a fracture that has failed to heal. Which fracture complication best describes this situation?
    a. Malunion
    b. Avascular necrosis
    c. Nonunion
    d. Crush syndrome

34. A patient who tripped and fell down several stairs reports having heard a popping sound and fears that she has broken her ankle. How does the nurse initially assess for fracture in this patient?
    a. Measuring the circumference of the distal leg
    b. Gently moving the ankle through the full range of motion
    c. Inspecting for crepitus and skin color
    d. Observing for deformity or misalignment

35. The nurse is assessing a patient with an injury to the shoulder and upper arm after being thrown from a horse. What is the best position for this patient's assessment?
    a. Supine so that the extremity can be elevated
    b. Low Fowler's on an exam table for patient comfort
    c. Sitting to observe for shoulder droop
    d. Slow ambulation to observe for natural arm movement

36. The nurse is caring for a patient with skeletal pins that have been placed for traction. What does the nurse expect to see in the first 48 hours?
    a. Clear fluid drainage weeping from the pin insertion site
    b. Some bloody drainage, but very minimal
    c. Swelling at the site with tenderness to gentle touch
    d. Dressings around the pin sites to be dry and intact

37. What potential adverse effect prevents meperidine (Demerol) from being used in older adults?
    a. Hypertension
    b. Angina
    c. Kidney failure
    d. Seizures

38. The unlicensed assistive personnel (UAP) is assisting the orthopedic physician to cut a window in a patient's cast. What does the nurse instruct the UAP to do?
    a. Check the pulse that is accessed after the window is cut.
    b. Clean up and dispose of all casting debris.
    c. Inform the patient that the procedure is painless.
    d. Save the plaster piece that was cut so it can be taped in place.

39. The nurse is caring for a patient in Buck's (skin) traction. Which task is best to delegate to the UAP (with supervision)?
    a. Turning and repositioning
    b. Inspecting heels and sacral area
    c. Asking the patient about muscle spasms
    d. Adjusting the weights on the apparatus

40. The nurse is instructing a teenage patient with a tibia-fibula fracture that was treated with internal fixation and a long leg cast. He is anxious to know when the cast will be removed so that he can resume football practice. Which statement by the patient indicates a need for additional teaching?
    a. "There's a possibility that the cast could be removed in 4 weeks."
    b. "The plates and screws reduce the length of time I'll be in the cast."
    c. "The cast could remain in place as long as 6 weeks."
    d. "I'll use crutches for 2 weeks and then the cast will be removed."

41. In the emergency care of a patient with a fracture, which action does the nurse implement first?
    a. Check the neurovascular status of the area distal to the extremity: temperature, color, sensation, movement, and capillary refill. Compare affected and unaffected limbs.
    b. Remove the patient's clothing (cut if necessary) to inspect the affected area while supporting the injured area above and below the injury. Do not remove shoes because this can cause increased trauma.
    c. Apply direct pressure on the area if there is bleeding and pressure over the proximal artery nearest the fracture.
    d. Immobilize the extremity by splinting; include joints above and below the fracture site. Recheck circulation after splinting.

42. According to the patient's chart, there is a family history of osteoporosis. In order to plan interventions related to this finding, what action does the nurse take?
    a. Ask the patient's age and assess for weight loss.
    b. Review the patient's dietary intake of calcium.
    c. Assess the patient for kyphoscoliosis or other deformities.
    d. Assess the patient for occult fractures of the long bones.

43. The nurse's neighbor comes running over because her husband "cut his finger off with a power saw." After calling for help, what is the first priority action when the nurse gets to the neighbor's house?
    a. Examine the amputation site.
    b. Assess for airway or breathing problems.
    c. Elevate the hand above the heart.
    d. Assess the severed finger.

44. An excited group of teenagers brings a friend to the ED who severed a finger while playing sports. The bleeding from the site is well-controlled and the patient is alert and stable. What does the nurse do with the severed finger?
    a. Place it directly into a bag of ice and then put the bag into a refrigerator.
    b. Wrap it in moist sterile gauze and ensure that it stays with the patient.
    c. Wrap it in dry gauze, place it in a water-proof bag, and put the bag in ice water.
    d. Carefully clean it with sterile saline, and then place it in a sterile container.

45. Which nursing intervention is best to prevent increased pain in a patient experiencing phantom limb pain?
    a. Handle the residual limb carefully when assessing the site or changing the dressing.
    b. Advise the patient that the sensation is temporary and will diminish over time.
    c. Remind the patient that the part is not really there, so the pain is not real.
    d. Encourage the patient to mourn the loss of the body part and express grief.

46. A young patient had a great toe amputated because of severe injury. The patient is depressed and withdrawn after the physician tells him that the amputation will affect balance and gait. What is the nurse's best response?
    a. "The physical therapy department can help you with exercises for balance and gait."
    b. "Let me get your parents and we can talk about rehabilitation programs."
    c. "When the doctor was explaining things to you, what were you thinking about?"
    d. "How have you usually handled stressful situations in the past?"

47. The patient is a middle-aged man with a history of uncontrolled diabetes. His right foot is a dark brownish-purple color and there is no palpable dorsalis pedis or posterior tibial pulse. The nurse prepares the patient for which diagnostic test?
    a. X-ray of the foot and ankle
    b. Doppler ultrasound
    c. Electromyelogram
    d. Arthrogram

48. The pain a patient experiences from a bone fracture results from which processes? *(Select all that apply.)*
    a. Loss of muscle tone
    b. Edema
    c. Neuropathy
    d. Bone healing
    e. Muscle spasms

49. A patient injured a lower extremity and has been placed in a running traction. What instructions does the nurse give to the UAP?
    a. Support the weights when turning the patient every 2 hours.
    b. Apply countertraction before moving the patient.
    c. Defer hygienic care and moving the patient until traction is removed.
    d. Moving the patient or the bed during care can alter the countertraction.

50. The nurse is caring for a patient with an above-the-knee amputation (AKA). In order to prevent hip flexion contractures, how does the nurse position the patient?
    a. Supine position with the residual limb elevated on a pillow
    b. Prone position every 3 to 4 hours for 20- to 30-minute periods
    c. Supine position with an abduction pillow placed between the legs
    d. Head of the bed elevated 30 degrees with assurance that the bandage is wrapped around the limb

51. The nurse applies bandages to a patient's residual limb in order to help shape and shrink the limb for a prosthesis. What is the proper technique for the nurse to use?
    a. Reapply the bandages every 8 hours or more often if they become loose.
    b. Use a proximal-to-distal direction when wrapping.
    c. Use soft, flexible bandage material and pad the area with gauze.
    d. Use a figure-eight wrapping method to prevent restriction of blood flow.

52. An older patient is discharged to home following an orthopedic injury. Which mobilization device is usually preferred for older patients who need additional support for balance?
    a. Crutches
    b. Cane
    c. Walker
    d. Wheelchair

53. The nurse is interviewing an older adult with a history of osteoporosis who reports falling and catching her weight on her outstretched dominant hand. This patient is most likely to have sustained what type of fracture?
    a. Carpal scaphoid bone
    b. Phalanges fracture
    c. Humeral fracture
    d. Colles' wrist fracture

54. Which factor carries the greatest risk for hip fracture?
    a. Decreased visual acuity
    b. Joint stiffness
    c. Osteoporosis
    d. Cardiac drug regimen

55. An older adult patient has skin traction in place for a hip fracture. What is the main purpose of this type of traction?
    a. It decreases painful muscle spasms.
    b. It helps heal the fracture.
    c. It prevents extension of the fracture.
    d. It prevents compression syndrome.

56. The nurse is caring for a patient with open reduction and internal fixation (ORIF) for a hip fracture. Because the patient is at risk for hip dislocation, the nurse ensures that the hip is maintained in which position?
    a. Adduction
    b. Anatomically neutral
    c. Abduction
    d. Extended

57. A patient reports dramatic changes in color and temperature of the skin over the left foot with intense burning pain, sensitive skin, excessive sweating, and edema. The physician makes a preliminary medical diagnosis of complex regional pain syndrome. What is the priority for nursing care?
    a. Patient education
    b. Care of the skin to prevent skin breakdown
    c. Management of pain
    d. Assessment of circulation

58. A patient is admitted to the same-day surgery unit following a meniscectomy. What does postoperative care for this patient include? *(Select all that apply.)*
    a. Perform neurovascular checks every hour for the first few hours and then every 4 hours.
    b. Check the surgical dressing for bleeding.
    c. Monitor vital signs.
    d. Strict intake and output (I&O).
    e. Teach about signs and symptoms of infection.
    f. Keep patient NPO until fully awake.

59. Following a meniscectomy, the nurse assists a patient to immediately start performing which exercises?
    a. Range-of-motion exercises to both legs
    b. Straight leg raises on both legs
    c. Flexion and extension of knees
    d. Flexion and extension of ankles

60. A patient arrives in the emergency department (ED) reporting pain and immobility of the right shoulder. The patient reports a history of recurrent dislocations of the same shoulder. The nurse observes for which other signs and symptoms that are associated with a dislocation injury? *(Select all that apply.)*
    a. Alteration in contour of the joint
    b. Deviation in length of the extremity
    c. Muscle atrophy
    d. Mottled skin discoloration
    e. Rotation of the extremity

61. Which descriptions are true about sprains? *(Select all that apply.)*
    a. They involve an injury to a ligament.
    b. Second- and third-degree sprains require immobilization.
    c. Sprains are usually precipitated by twisting motions from a sports injury.
    d. They are caused by excessive stretching of a muscle or tendon.
    e. Surgical repair is required for second- and third-degree sprains.

62. Which statements are true about dislocations? *(Select all that apply.)*
    a. Surgical repair is usually performed to re-align a dislocated joint.
    b. Dislocation of a joint occurs when two bones are moved away from each other.
    c. Partial dislocation of a joint is referred to as "subluxation."
    d. A health care provider performs closed reductions on dislocated joints.
    e. Joint dislocation is most common in the hip, spine, and fingers.

63. The health care provider tells a patient that she has a mild first-degree sprain to the ankle. What instructions does the nurse give to the patient about the treatment for the injury? *(Select all that apply.)*
    a. Rest.
    b. Apply ice for the first 4 to 6 hours.
    c. Apply a compression bandage for a few days to reduce swelling and provide joint support.
    d. Elevate the foot.
    e. Perform range-of-motion exercises every 4 hours.

64. A patient is informed by the physician that he must have a fiberglass cast applied to the lower extremity. What does the nurse teach the patient about the procedure before the cast is applied?
    a. "The cast will be applied after a stockinette if fitted to your skin."
    b. "The cast material will dry and become rigid in a few minutes."
    c. "The cast will increase your risk for skin breakdown."
    d. "The plaster is not a waterproof material."

65. The nurse is caring for a patient with a plaster splint applied to the ankle. The patient received oral pain medication at 0900. At 1100, the patient reports that the pain is getting worse, not better. What is the nurse's priority action?
    a. Give the patient IV pain medication.
    b. Reposition the extremity on a pillow and place an ice pack.
    c. Assess the pulses and skin temperature distal to the splint.
    d. Call the physician to report the patient's increasing pain.

66. Which factors affect bone healing after a fracture has occurred? *(Select all that apply.)*
    a. Patient's age
    b. Patient's occupation
    c. Type of bone injured
    d. How the fracture is managed
    e. Presence of infection at the fracture site

67. The nurse is providing teaching for a patient with a forearm cast. What information does the nurse give to the patient?
    a. "The hand should be elevated above the shoulder when resting."
    b. "Use an ice pack for the first 6 to 8 hours, and cover the pack with a towel to absorb condensation."
    c. "The sling should distribute the weight over a large area of the shoulders and trunk."
    d. "Limit movement of the fingers or wrist joints to prevent pain."

68. The patient has a musculoskeletal injury that resulted from excessive stretching of a muscle or tendon. Which type best describes this patient's injury?
    a. Dislocation
    b. Sprain
    c. Strain
    d. Subluxation

69. A patient with a lower extremity injury is being treated by external fixation. What nursing assessment is of particular concern in the care of this patient with this type of system?
   a. Maintaining a 30-degree flexed position of the knee
   b. Measuring the weights used for counter-traction
   c. Observing the patient's ability to adjust the clickers
   d. Observing the points of entry of the pins and wires

70. The nurse is caring for a patient who had a kyphoplasty. What does postoperative care for this patient include? *(Select all that apply.)*
   a. Monitor and record vital signs.
   b. Perform frequent neurologic assessments.
   c. Apply a warm pack to the puncture site if needed to relieve pain.
   d. Assess the patient's pain level and compare it to the preoperative level.
   e. Give opioid analgesics as needed.
   f. Monitor for bleeding at the puncture site.

71. A patient in a body cast reports nausea, vomiting, and epigastric pain. The nurse notifies the physician for orders. Which intervention is the most conservative, and therefore the first thing to try, to address this patient's symptoms?
   a. Insert a nasogastric tube and attach to low wall suction.
   b. Cut a window over the abdominal area of the cast.
   c. Obtain an order for an x-ray to diagnose a paralytic ileus.
   d. Administer prn antiemetic and prn pain medication.

72. A patient with a long leg cast that was applied in the ED is being admitted to the orthopedic unit. Which task is best for the nurse to delegate to the UAP?
   a. Obtain a fracture pan and use caution to prevent spillage on the cast.
   b. Obtain several plastic-covered pillows for elevation of the leg.
   c. Check flexion/extension and color of the toes.
   d. Turn the patient every 4 to 6 hours to allow the cast to dry.

73. A patient who has sustained a traumatic amputation of the left leg expresses concern about working and taking care of his family after his injury. What resources does the nurse recommend to help the patient adjust to his lost limb? *(Select all that apply.)*
   a. Chaplain
   b. Medical social worker
   c. Physical therapist
   d. Physician
   e. National Amputation Foundation

52
CHAPTER

Assessment of the Gastrointestinal System

1. What is the name of the first 12 inches of the small intestine?
   a. Jejunum
   b. Ileum
   c. Duodenum
   d. Esophagus

2. Which structure is involved in the protective function of the liver?
   a. Sphincter of Oddi
   b. Gallbladder
   c. Pancreas
   d. Kupffer cells

3. The pancreas performs which functions? (Select all that apply.)
   a. Breaks down amino acids
   b. Secretes enzymes for digestion from the exocrine part of the organ
   c. Breaks down fatty acids and triglycerides
   d. Produces glucagon from the endocrine part of the organ
   e. Produces enzymes that digest carbohydrates, fats, and proteins

4. Which statements about intrinsic factor are correct? (Select all that apply.)
   a. It is produced by the parietal cells.
   b. It is essential to fat emulsification.
   c. It aids in the absorption of vitamin B_{12}.
   d. It forms and secretes bile.
   e. Its absence causes pernicious anemia.

5. Which statements about Kupffer cells are true? (Select all that apply.)
   a. They are located in the epithelial cell layer lining in the GI tract.
   b. They are cells found in the liver.
   c. They phagocytize harmful bacteria.
   d. They are part of the substance that aids in the absorption of vitamin B_{12}.
   e. They are part of the body's reticuloendothelial system.

6. Which drugs predispose a patient to peptic ulcer disease and gastrointestinal (GI) bleeding? (Select all that apply.)
   a. Nonsteroidal antiinflammatory drugs
   b. Anticoagulants
   c. Aspirin
   d. Lasix
   e. Digitalis

7. Which gastrointestinal problem is related to anorexia?
   a. Heartburn
   b. Constipation
   c. Steatorrhea
   d. Loss of appetite

8. Dyspepsia is characterized by which factors? (Select all that apply.)
   a. Indigestion associated with eating
   b. Loss of appetite for food
   c. Heartburn associated with eating
   d. Vomiting that occurs after eating
   e. Malabsorption

9. The nurse is caring for a patient with abdominal pain. While assessing the patient, which questions will the nurse ask the patient? *(Select all that apply.)*
   a. "Is the pain burning, gnawing, or stabbing?"
   b. "Can you point to where you feel the pain?"
   c. "Do you have a family history of cancer?"
   d. "When did you first notice the pain?"
   e. "Does the pain spread anywhere?"

10. In which quadrant does the abdominal examination usually begin?
    a. Right lower quadrant (RLQ)
    b. Left lower quadrant (LLQ)
    c. Left upper quadrant (LUQ)
    d. Right upper quadrant (RUQ)

11. When examining the abdomen, which technique for abdominal assessment is used second?
    a. Inspection
    b. Percussion
    c. Palpation
    d. Auscultation

12. The nurse is performing an abdominal assessment on a patient. For which finding does the nurse alert the physician immediately?
    a. Borborygmus
    b. Blumberg's sign
    c. Bulging, pulsating mass
    d. Cullen's sign

13. On assessment, the patient has areas of the abdomen with pain that also show rebound tenderness. What is the correct term for this finding?
    a. Blumberg's sign
    b. Bruits
    c. Tympanic
    d. Cullen's sign

14. The nurse ascultates a patient's abdomen and hears high-pitched, loud, musical sounds in an air-filled abdomen. How does the nurse best describe this finding?
    a. Bruits
    b. Tympanic
    c. Dull
    d. Medium-pitched

15. What will laboratory values for a patient with liver disease most likely show? *(Select all that apply.)*
    a. Increased prothrombin time
    b. Increased aspartate transaminase (AST) and alanine aminotransferase (ALT)
    c. Increased albumin levels
    d. Decreased ammonia levels
    e. Increased unconjugated bilirubin

16. Laboratory values for a patient with acute pancreatitis may show which abnormal findings? *(Select all that apply.)*
    a. Increased hemoglobin
    b. Decreased serum amylase
    c. Increased serum lipase
    d. Decreased urine nitrates
    e. Increased serum amylase

17. A patient being seen the emergency department (ED) has been vomiting blood for the past 12 hours. What test will likely be ordered for the patient?
    a. Endoscopic retrograde cholangiopancreatography (ERCP)
    b. Upper GI radiographic series
    c. Esophagogastroduodenoscopy (EGD)
    d. Barium enema

18. The nurse is providing care for a patient after an EGD. What is the first priority action after this diagnostic study?
    a. Monitor vital signs.
    b. Auscultate breath sounds.
    c. Keep patient NPO until gag reflex returns.
    d. Keep accurate intake and output.

19. The nurse is caring for a patient who received a barium swallow with a small bowel follow-through. What key points must the nurse include in teaching this patient after the procedure? *(Select all that apply.)*
    a. "Drink lots of fluids."
    b. "Depending on the results, you may need a colonoscopy."
    c. "You will be on bedrest for about 6 to 8 hours."
    d. "A laxative will be provided to help remove the barium."
    e. "Your stools will be chalky white for 1 to 3 days."

20. Which diagnostic test does the nurse expect the health care provider to order to visually examine a patient's liver, gallbladder, bile ducts, and pancreas to identify the cause and location of an obstruction?
    a. EGD
    b. Upper GI radiographic series
    c. Percutaneous transhepatic cholangiography (PTC)
    d. ERCP

21. The nurse is caring for a patient scheduled for a colonoscopy in three days after discharge. What does the nurse teach the patient about preparations for this diagnostic test? *(Select all that apply.)*
    a. "Take only clear liquids the day before your colonoscopy."
    b. "Drink lots of red, orange, or purple (grape) beverages the day before the test."
    c. "You should take nothing by mouth for 4 to 6 hours before the test."
    d. "Do not take aspirin, NSAIDs, or anticoagulants for several days before the test."
    e. "After you drink the bowel-cleansing solution, you will have watery diarrhea in about an hour."
    f. "You will have an IV placed to receive medication to help you relax during the procedure."

22. The nurse is monitoring a patient after endoscopy. Vital signs are stable and side rails are raised but the patient tells the nurse that he is very thirsty. What is the nurse's best action?
    a. Administer a small amount of ice chips only.
    b. Give the patient small sips of water through a straw.
    c. Check to see if the patient's gag reflex has returned.
    d. Keep the patient NPO for at least 4 hours.

23. Which diagnostic test is a noninvasive imaging procedure that can get multidimensional views of the entire colon?
    a. Abdominal ultrasound
    b. Computed tomography colonography
    c. Colonoscopy
    d. Sigmoidoscopy

24. Mild gas pain and flatulence may be experienced as a result of air instilled into the rectum during the examination, and if a biopsy specimen is obtained, a small amount of bleeding may be observed. For which endoscopic procedure is this follow-up care describing?
    a. Colonoscopy
    b. Proctosigmoidoscopy
    c. Enteroscopy
    d. ERCP

25. A feeling of fullness, cramping, and passage of flatus can be expected for several hours after the test, and a small amount of blood may be in the first stool after the test if a biopsy specimen is taken or a polypectomy is performed. Vital signs should be checked every 15 minutes, the patient should be monitored for signs of perforation or hemorrhage, and excessive bleeding should be reported immediately. For which procedure is this follow-up care describing?
    a. EGD
    b. Enteroscopy
    c. Small bowel series
    d. Colonoscopy

26. The patient should be observed for cholangitis, perforation, sepsis, and pancreatitis, and the patient should report abdominal pain, fever, nausea, or vomiting that fails to resolve. The patient is on NPO status until the gag reflex returns. For which procedure is this follow-up care describing?
    a. Enteroscopy
    b. EGD
    c. ERCP
    d. PTC

27. The patient should be monitored for signs of perforation such as pain, bleeding, or fever, and the patient is instructed not to drive for 12 hours after the test. A hoarse voice and sore throat may persist for several days; throat lozenges may be used to relieve the discomfort. For which procedure is this follow-up care describing?
    a. EGD
    b. ERCP
    c. Enteroscopy
    d. Small bowel series

28. Which body structures are located in the RUQ of the abdomen? *(Select all that apply.)*
    a. Duodenum
    b. Liver
    c. Stomach
    d. Spleen
    e. Gallbladder
    f. Pancreas head

29. Which gastrointestinal changes occur in older adults? *(Select all that apply.)*
    a. Increased hydrochloric acid secretion
    b. Decreased absorption of iron and vitamin B_{12}
    c. Decreased peristalsis may cause constipation
    d. Increased cholesterol synthesis
    e. Decreased lipase with decreased fat digestion

30. The nurse is taking a GI health history from a newly admitted patient. Which questions would the nurse be sure to ask? *(Select all that apply.)*
    a. "Have you lost or gained weight recently?"
    b. "Have you had any recent cardiac or respiratory surgeries?"
    c. "Do you wear dentures and if so, how do they fit you?"
    d. "Do you have difficulty chewing or swallowing?"
    e. "Have you traveled in the USA recently and where?"
    f. "What is your usual bowel elimination pattern?"

31. The patient's potassium level is 3.1 mEq/L. Which condition would cause this value?
    a. Malabsorption
    b. Gastric suctioning
    c. Acute pancreatitis
    d. Kidney failure

32. The patient tells the nurse that she is experiencing emotional stress related to concerns about her children and husband and whether she will be able to return to her job. Which GI condition is she at increased risk for?
    a. Exacerbation of irritable bowel syndrome
    b. Nausea accompanied with vomiting
    c. Stomach or duodenal ulcers
    d. Esophagitis

33. During abdominal assessment, the nurse detects a loud bruit near midline. What must the nurse do?
    a. Measure the patient's abdomen just under the diaphragm.
    b. Check the patient's record for a history of stomach ulcers.
    c. Avoid palpation or percussion of the abdomen.
    d. Ask the patient about nausea and gastric reflux.

34. Which findings does the nurse document after inspecting a patient's abdomen? *(Select all that apply.)*
    a. Symmetry of the abdomen
    b. Presence of borborygmus
    c. Distention of the abdomen
    d. Taut, glistening skin
    e. Discoloration or scars

53 CHAPTER

Care of Patients with Oral Cavity Problems

1. What statement is true about the *Candida albicans* form of stomatitis?
   a. It is a common type of primary stomatitis.
   b. *Candida albicans* is a bacterial infection.
   c. This infection is uncommon in patients who are immunocompromised.
   d. Patients on steroid therapy often experience this infection.

2. The nurse has provided teaching to a patient on ways to prevent the recurrence of aphthous ulcers. Which statement by the patient indicates teaching has been effective?
   a. "I will rinse with the tetracycline syrup for 2 minutes then swallow the syrup."
   b. "Potatoes have nothing to do with the development of the ulcers."
   c. "I will continue to eat peanut butter and jelly sandwiches."
   d. "It doesn't matter what types of foods I eat as long as I brush my teeth after every meal."

3. When caring for a patient with stomatitis, what is most important for the nurse to assess?
   a. Nutritional status
   b. Level of pain
   c. Self-care abilities
   d. Airway status

4. The nurse is performing an oral assessment on a patient and notes white plaque-like lesions on the tongue, palate, pharynx, and buccal mucosa. When the patches are wiped away, the underlying surface is red and sore. What disorder does the nurse suspect the patient has?
   a. Leukoplakia
   b. Candida albicans
   c. Erythroplakia
   d. Kaposi's sarcoma

5. The unlicensed assistive personnel (UAP) is providing care to a patient with stomatitis. Which intervention by the UAP illustrates correct care for this patient?
   a. Using a hard-bristled toothbrush to thoroughly clean the oral cavity
   b. Rinsing the mouth with a commercial mouthwash
   c. Using a warm saline, hydrogen peroxide, or sodium bicarbonate solution to rinse the mouth
   d. Rinsing the mouth frequently with cold tap water and vinegar solution

6. What is the drug of choice for the treatment of a fungal mouth infection?
   a. Nystatin (Mycostatin)
   b. Acyclovir (Zovirax)
   c. Minocycline
   d. Benzocaine (Kenalog in Orabase)

7. Which statement by the student nurse indicates the need for a better understanding of the care of patients with oral cavity problems?
   a. "I will use lemon-glycerin swabs to clean the patient's mouth."
   b. "The patient should eat a soft, bland diet."
   c. "Dentures should be removed."
   d. "Gauze may be used for oral care."

8. A patient is in the clinic for a nonhealing sore on the lower left corner of her bottom lip and right side of her tongue. The lesions are red, raised, and have erosions. After taking a history, the nurse suspects the patient may have which type of oral cancer?
   a. Basal cell carcinoma
   b. Kaposi's sarcoma
   c. Squamous cell carcinoma
   d. Erythroplakia

9. A patient has a Kaposi's sarcoma lesion on his hard palate. How is this lesion described? *(Select all that apply.)*
   a. Small raised lesion
   b. Dark-yellow nodule
   c. Lesions are painful
   d. Purplish-brown nodule
   e. Usually not painful

10. Which type of oral cavity tumor appears as a red, velvety lesion on the tongue, palate, floor of the mouth or mandibular mucosa?
    a. Leukoplakia
    b. Erythroplakia
    c. Basal cell carcinoma
    d. Kaposi's sarcoma

11. Which oral cavity tumor appears as a raised scab, primarily on the lips and evolves to an ulcer with a raised pearly border?
    a. Leukoplakia
    b. Erythroplakia
    c. Basal cell carcinoma
    d. Kaposi's sarcoma

12. A patient is scheduled for multiple tests to evaluate an oral tumor. The patient asks the nurse which of the tests is the best to determine if the tumor is cancerous. How does the nurse respond?
    a. "All of the tests need to be looked at together because no single test can tell if you have cancer."
    b. "Magnetic resonance imaging is the only diagnostic test that will need to be done."
    c. "Biopsy is the definitive method for diagnosing oral cancer."
    d. "An aqueous solution of toluidine blue 1% can be applied to the oral lesion. If the lesion is malignant it will not absorb the solution; however, the preparation stains the normal tissue."

13. During an assessment of a patient with an oral tumor, the nurse notes that the patient develops stridor. What functional assessment is the least important for the nurse to complete?
    a. Ability to speak
    b. Gag reflex
    c. Quality of respirations
    d. Pain rating

14. Which operative procedure includes excision of a segment of the mandible with the oral lesion, and radical neck dissection?
    a. Oropharyngeal resection
    b. Glossectomy
    c. Mandibulectomy
    d. Commando procedure

15. The nurse is teaching a patient who will have a radical neck dissection. What must the nurse teach the patient will be removed during this procedure? *(Select all that apply.)*
    a. Sternocleidomastoid muscle
    b. Removal of the jaw
    c. Excision of cervical lymph nodes on the affected side
    d. Cranial nerve XI
    e. Excision of the tongue
    f. Internal jugular vein

16. After a patient has undergone a radical neck dissection, what is the priority nursing intervention?
    a. Manage the patient's pain.
    b. Maintain fluid and electrolyte balance.
    c. Maintain the patient's airway.
    d. Enhance the patient's ability to communicate.

17. Which interventions prevent or minimize the risk factors in patients at risk for aspiration? *(Select all that apply.)*
    a. Requesting medications in pill form
    b. Providing liquids with a thickening agent
    c. Positioning the patient upright at 90 degrees
    d. Keeping the head of bed elevated for five minutes after eating
    e. Keeping suction equipment nearby
    f. Feeding the patient small bites

18. How is xerostomia characterized?
    a. Reduction of taste sensation
    b. Inflammation of a salivary gland
    c. Excessive mouth dryness
    d. Inflammation of the mouth

19. Which are considered acute effects of radiation therapy? *(Select all that apply.)*
    a. Excessive drooling
    b. Stomatitis
    c. Herpes simplex
    d. Treatment-related mucositis
    e. Alteration in taste

20. The UAP is caring for a patient undergoing radiation therapy to the neck. Which action by the UAP requires intervention by the supervising nurse?
    a. Using powder on the patient's neck
    b. Shaving the patient with an electric razor
    c. Avoiding use of alcohol-based aftershave lotion
    d. Using gentle nondeodorant soap to wash the patient

21. Which patient is at lowest risk for development of acute sialadentitis?
    a. Patient with Sjögren's syndrome
    b. Patient with HIV infection
    c. Patient with anemia
    d. Patient prescribed phenothiazine drugs

22. When assessing a patient with a salivary gland tumor, the nurse pays particular attention to the facial nerve. Which requests by the nurse are likely to determine if the tumor has affected the facial nerve? *(Select all that apply.)*
    a. "Puff out your cheeks."
    b. "Wrinkle your nose."
    c. "Cough."
    d. "Raise your eyebrows."
    e. "Turn your head back and forth."
    f. "Pucker your lips."

23. The nurse has taught a patient with acute sialadenitis to use sialagogues to stimulate saliva. The patient demonstrates teaching has been effective when the patient states he will eat which food?
    a. Lemon slices
    b. Apple slices
    c. Bananas
    d. Bread

24. Which patients are at risk for development of oral cavity disorders? *(Select all that apply.)*
    a. Homeless veteran
    b. Overweight adult with type 2 diabetes
    c. Older adult living in a long-term care facility
    d. Middle-aged smoker who is alcoholic
    e. Underweight teen with anorexia

25. The nurse is assessing a patient's mouth for lesions. Which actions will the nurse implement? *(Select all that apply.)*
    a. Wear clean gloves.
    b. Assure adequate lighting with a penlight.
    c. Ask the patient to say "ahh."
    d. Use a tongue blade.
    e. Instruct the patient to perform the Valsalva maneuver.

54 CHAPTER

Care of Patients with Esophageal Problems

1. Which physiologic factor contributes to gastroesophageal reflux disease (GERD)?
   a. Accelerated gastric emptying
   b. Irritation from reflux of stomach contents
   c. Competent lower esophageal sphincter
   d. Increased esophageal clearance

2. Which statement is true about Barrett's epithelium in the patient with GERD?
   a. While the body heals, a different type of cell forms on the lower part of the esophagus.
   b. This new tissue is less resistant to acid so it must be taken care of.
   c. Barrett's epithelium is resistant to the development of cancer.
   d. Esophageal strictures are less likely to occur with this type of epithelium.

3. Which statements about GERD are correct? *(Select all that apply.)*
   a. Overweight and obese patients are at an increased risk.
   b. Thin and underweight patients are at an increased risk.
   c. It is a common disorder in the Asian and Hispanic populations.
   d. There is a high incidence in patients who eat mostly hot and spicy foods.
   e. It is a common upper gastrointestinal disorder in the United States.

4. Which are the two most common manifestations of GERD? *(Select all that apply.)*
   a. Dyspepsia
   b. Eructation
   c. Water brash
   d. Regurgitation
   e. Odynophagia
   f. Flatulence

5. The patient with GERD describes painful swallowing. Which symptom does the nurse recognize?
   a. Dyspepsia
   b. Regurgitation
   c. Odynophagia
   d. Dysphagia

6. A patient is scheduled to have several diagnostic tests to verify the medical diagnosis of GERD. Which diagnostic test is the most accurate method of diagnosing this disorder?
   a. Esophagogastroduodenoscopy (EGD)
   b. 24-hour ambulatory pH monitoring
   c. Esophageal manometry
   d. Motility testing

7. The nurse has provided teaching to a patient with GERD. Which statement by the patient indicates the teaching has been effective?
   a. "I will eat three meals a day."
   b. "I won't snack for 1 hour before I go to bed."
   c. "I won't nap for 30 minutes after eating dinner."
   d. "I won't lift heavy objects."

8. A patient with GERD is on a medication that raises the pH of gastric contents. Which drug does the nurse expect to administer?
   a. Ranitidine
   b. Mylanta
   c. Gaviscon
   d. Omeprazole

9. A patient who has been prescribed famotidine (Pepcid) is being discharged home. Which statement by the patient indicates a need for further discharge teaching by the nurse?
   a. "This drug will increase acid secretion to break down food faster."
   b. "Famotidine will facilitate healing of my esophagus."
   c. "I will call the health care provider if I continue to have heartburn."
   d. "This drug is available over the counter."

10. Which statement is true about the drug rabeprazole (Aciphex) for treatment of GERD?
    a. It is rapidly released into the body after it is administered.
    b. The tablets are large and may be crushed if the patient has difficulty swallowing them.
    c. It is a histamine receptor antagonist.
    d. If once-a-day dosing does not control symptoms, it may be taken twice a day.

11. A patient has returned to the unit after a Stretta procedure for GERD. Which action by the student nurse requires the supervising nurse to intervene?
    a. The patient is offered clear liquids in the early postprocedure period.
    b. The patient's routine 81 mg of aspirin is held.
    c. A proton pump inhibitor is administered.
    d. A nasogastric tube is prepared for insertion.

12. Which lifestyle adjustment may a patient have to make to best control GERD?
    a. Sleep in the Trendelenburg position.
    b. Attain and maintain ideal body weight.
    c. Wear snug-fitting belts and waistbands.
    d. Engage in strenuous exercise such as weightlifting.

13. Which statements will the nurse include when providing health teaching for a patient with hiatal hernia? *(Select all that apply.)*
    a. "Elevate the head of your bed at least 6 inches for sleeping at night."
    b. "Remain in the upright position for several hours after eating."
    c. "Avoid straining or excessive vigorous exercise."
    d. "After surgery, you will have no dietary restriction."
    e. "Avoid wearing clothing that is tight around the abdomen."
    f. "Avoid eating in the late evening."

14. What diagnostic test best identifies a hiatal hernia?
    a. EGD
    b. 24-hour ambulatory pH monitoring
    c. Esophageal manometry
    d. Barium swallow study with fluoroscopy

15. Which statements about Barrett's esophagus are accurate? *(Select all that apply.)*
    a. It is considered to be a premalignant condition.
    b. It is associated with excessive intake of fresh fruits and vegetables.
    c. It results from exposure to acid and pepsin.
    d. It is associated with pickled and fermented foods.
    e. Normal cells undergo dysplasia to become cancerous.

16. The nurse has provided postoperative teaching for a patient who underwent a laparoscopic Nissen fundoplication (LNF). Which statement by the patient indicates a need for additional teaching?
    a. "I will walk every day."
    b. "I will no longer need the antireflux drugs after the surgery."
    c. "I will report a fever above 101° F."
    d. "I'll remove the gauze dressing 2 days after surgery and shower."

17. What is the primary focus of care after conventional surgery for hiatal hernia?
    a. Prevention of respiratory complications
    b. Pain management
    c. Management of fluid balance
    d. Teaching the patient self-care activities

18. Uncontrolled GERD can be a cause of which adult-onset disorders? *(Select all that apply.)*
    a. Dental caries
    b. Aspiration pneumonia
    c. Laryngitis
    d. Diverticulitis
    e. Asthma

19. The nurse is assessing a patient's nasogastric drainage following a conventional fundoplication procedure. How does the nurse expect the drainage to appear the first 8 hours after surgery?
    a. Dark brown
    b. Bright red mixed with brown
    c. Yellowish to green
    d. Green to clear

20. The nurse is giving discharge instructions to a patient after a fundoplication procedure. The patient is instructed to avoid which activities? *(Select all that apply.)*
    a. Drinking more than 8 oz of carbonated beverage at one time
    b. Chewing gum
    c. Drinking with a straw
    d. Eating gas-producing foods
    e. Drinking noncarbonated beverages

21. A patient is prescribed pantoprazole (Protonix). What does the nurse tell the patient is the major action of this medication?
    a. It produces a coating on the stomach lining.
    b. It neutralizes gastric acid.
    c. It heals esophageal irritation.
    d. It inhibits gastric acid secretion.

22. A patient is undergoing a workup for carcinoma of the esophagus. What are the two primary risk factors associated with the development of this carcinoma?
    a. High-fat, low-fiber diet and tobacco use
    b. Tobacco use and obesity
    c. Sedentary lifestyle and family history of squamous cell carcinoma
    d. Heavy alcohol intake and high-fat, low-fiber diet

23. The definitive diagnosis for esophageal cancer is made with which procedure?
    a. Barium swallow
    b. Esophageal manometry
    c. Esophageal ultrasound with fine needle aspiration
    d. EGD

24. Nonsurgical treatment options for cancer of the esophagus can include which therapies? *(Select all that apply.)*
    a. Swallowing therapy
    b. Chemoradiation
    c. Targeted therapies
    d. Smoking cessation programs
    e. Photodynamic therapy
    f. Endoscopic therapies

25. Which procedure would the health care provider recommend for immediate relief of dysphagia?
    a. Photodynamic therapy
    b. Esophageal dilation
    c. Targeted therapy
    d. Chemoradiation therapy

26. The nurse is caring for a patient with esophageal cancer who is scheduled to undergo an esophagogastrostomy with a section of the jejunum to replace the esophagus. Which procedure does the nurse expect to perform preoperatively?
    a. Complete bowel preparation
    b. Chest tube placement
    c. Urinary catheter placement
    d. Nasogastric tube placement for feeding

27. After an esophagectomy, what is the nurse's priority for patient care?
    a. Wound care
    b. Nutrition care
    c. Respiratory care
    d. Hydration care

28. The nurse is caring for a postoperative patient after esophageal surgery. On assessment, the nurse discovers that the patient's temperature is 101° F, heart rate is 120/minute, and respiratory rate is 32/minute. Lung sounds include bilateral crackles. What is the nurse's priority first action?
    a. Raise the head of the patient's bed.
    b. Call the Rapid Response Team.
    c. Apply oxygen at 2 L per nasal cannula.
    d. Administer IV normal saline at 75 mL/hour.

29. The nurse is supervising a senior nursing student in the care of a patient after esophageal surgery. For which action by the student must the nurse intervene?
    a. Student secures the NG tube to prevent dislodgment.
    b. Student prepares to irrigate NG tube.
    c. Student provides mouth care every 2 to 4 hours.
    d. Student elevates the head of the patient's bed.

30. What manifestations are expected when a patient has esophageal diverticula? *(Select all that apply.)*
    a. Halitosis
    b. Dysphagia
    c. Swelling with difficulty breathing
    d. Nocturnal cough
    e. Regurgitation

Care of Patients with Stomach Disorders

1. Which are pathologic changes associated with acute gastritis? *(Select all that apply.)*
   a. Vascular congestion
   b. Severe mucosal damage and ruptured vessels
   c. Edema
   d. Acute inflammatory cell infiltration
   e. Increased cell production in the superficial epithelium of the stomach lining

2. Which are possible complications of chronic gastritis? *(Select all that apply.)*
   a. Pernicious anemia
   b. Thickening of the stomach lining
   c. Gastric cancer
   d. Decreased gastric acid secretion
   e. Peptic ulcer disease

3. Which statements about gastritis are accurate? *(Select all that apply.)*
   a. The diagnosis of gastritis is made solely on clinical symptoms.
   b. The onset of infection with *Helicobacter pylori* can result in acute gastritis.
   c. Long-term use of acetaminophen (Tylenol) is a high risk factor for acute gastritis.
   d. Atrophic gastritis is a form of chronic gastritis that is seen most in older adults.
   e. Type B chronic gastritis affects the glands in the antrum, but may affect all of the stomach.

4. The nurse is teaching a patient about health promotion and maintenance to prevent gastritis. Which information does the nurse include? *(Select all that apply.)*
   a. "A balanced diet can help prevent gastritis."
   b. "To prevent gastritis, you should limit your intake of salt."
   c. "If you stop smoking, there is less of a chance that you will develop gastritis."
   d. "Yoga has been found to be effective in preventing gastritis."
   e. "Although regular exercise is good for you, it has not been found to have an effect on the prevention of gastritis."

5. A patient with chronic gastritis is being admitted. Which sign/symptom does the nurse identify as being associated with this patient's condition?
   a. Pernicious anemia
   b. Gastric hemorrhage
   c. Hematemesis
   d. Dyspepsia

6. When teaching a patient about pernicious anemia, which statement does the nurse include?
   a. "Patients with pernicious anemia are not able to digest fats."
   b. "Pernicious anemia results in a deficiency of vitamin B_{12}."
   c. "All patients with gastrointestinal bleeding will eventually develop pernicious anemia."
   d. "Oral iron supplements are an effective treatment for pernicious anemia."

7. A patient comes to the emergency department (ED) reporting rapid onset of epigastric pain with nausea and vomiting. The patient says the pain is worse than any heartburn he has had, and that he has not had an appetite for the past day. What does the nurse suspect this patient has?
   a. Peritonitis
   b. *H. pylori* infection
   c. Duodenal ulcer
   d. Acute gastritis

8. Which diagnostic test is the gold standard for diagnosing gastritis?
   a. Esophagogastroduodenoscopy (EGD)
   b. Computed tomography (CT) scan
   c. Upper gastrointestinal (GI) series
   d. Cholangiogram

9. The nurse is teaching a patient about ranitidine (Zantac) prescribed for gastritis. Which statement by the patient indicates effective teaching by the nurse?
   a. "The drug will heal the areas of my stomach that are sore."
   b. "This drug will block the secretions of my stomach."
   c. "Zantac will coat the inside of my stomach to protect it from acid."
   d. "This pill kills the bacterial infection I have in my stomach."

10. A patient with acute gastritis is receiving treatment to block and buffer gastric acid secretions to relieve pain. Which drug does the nurse identify as an antisecretory agent (proton-pump inhibitor)?
    a. Sucralfate (Carafate)
    b. Ranitidine (Zantac)
    c. Mylanta
    d. Omeprazole (Prilosec)

11. The nursing student caring for a patient with a duodenal ulcer is about to administer a proton pump inhibitor (PPI). Which statement about this medication is true?
    a. These drugs should not be used for a prolonged period of time because they may contribute to osteoporotic-related fractures.
    b. PPIs may not be given via feeding tube.
    c. These drugs help prevent stress-induced ulcers.
    d. PPIs work by coating the stomach with a protective barrier.

12. The nurse is teaching a patient being discharged home about taking prescribed medications that include sucralfate (Carafate). Which statement by the patient indicates teaching has been effective?
    a. "The main side effect of sucralfate is diarrhea."
    b. "I will take sucralfate with meals."
    c. "I will take sucralfate along with the antacid medication I take."
    d. "Sucralfate works to heal my ulcer."

13. Which types of ulcers are included in peptic ulcer disease? *(Select all that apply.)*
    a. Esophageal ulcers
    b. Gastric ulcers
    c. Pressure ulcers
    d. Duodenal ulcers
    e. Stress ulcers

14. Which type of gastric ulcer does the nurse expect may occur when caring for a patient with extensive burns?
    a. Curling's ulcer
    b. Cushing's ulcer
    c. Stress ulcer
    d. Ischemic ulcer

15. Which type of nonsteroidal antiinflammatory (NSAID) drug is less likely to cause mucosal damage to the stomach?
    a. Ibuprofen
    b. Aspirin
    c. Acetaminophen
    d. Celecoxib

16. The nurse is caring for a patient who vomited coffee-ground blood. Where does the nurse suspect the patient is bleeding?
    a. Colon
    b. Rectum
    c. Small intestine
    d. Upper GI system

17. The patient with a gastric ulcer suddenly develops sharp epigastric pain that spreads over the entire abdomen. What complication has the patient most likely developed?
    a. Hemorrhage
    b. Gastric erosion
    c. Perforation
    d. Gastric cancer

18. The gastric ulcer patient's abdomen is rigid, tender, and painful. He prefers lying in a knee-chest (fetal) position. What is the nurse's priority action at this time?
    a. Notify the health care provider.
    b. Administer opioid pain medication.
    c. Reposition the patient supine.
    d. Measure the abdominal circumference.

19. Drug therapy for peptic ulcer disease is implemented for which purposes? *(Select all that apply.)*
    a. Pain relief
    b. Rebuild the mucosal lining of the stomach
    c. Eliminate *H. pylori* infection
    d. Heal ulcerations
    e. Prevent recurrence

20. Which peptic ulcer disease drug is useful to protect patients against NSAID-induced ulcers?
    a. Magnesium hydroxide (Maalox)
    b. Omeprazole (Prilosec)
    c. Esomeprazole (Nexium)
    d. Misoprostol (Cytotec)

21. Which statement about the use of antacids in the treatment of gastric ulcers is true?
    a. Antacids should be administered with meals.
    b. Patients should take calcium carbonate (Tums) if they still have pain after taking their usual antacid.
    c. The patient should take antacid on an empty stomach.
    d. Avoid using antacids with phenytoin (Dilantin).

22. A patient with peptic ulcer disease is receiving Maalox. Which actions does the nurse take when administering this medication? *(Select all that apply.)*
    a. Give the medication 2 hours after the patient's meal.
    b. Do not give other drugs within 1 to 2 hours of antacids.
    c. Assess the patient for a history of renal disease before giving Maalox.
    d. Assess the patient for a history of heart failure before giving Maalox.
    e. Observe the patient for the side effect of constipation.

23. The nurse has provided instruction for a patient prescribed sucralfate (Carafate) to treat a gastric ulcer. Which statement by the patient indicates that teaching has been effective?
    a. "This drug will stop the secretion of acid in my stomach."
    b. "I will take this drug on an empty stomach."
    c. "I will not be able to take ranitidine (Zantac) with this drug."
    d. "The main side effect of this drug that I can expect is diarrhea."

24. An older adult patient is admitted with an upper GI bleed. Which finding does the nurse expect to assess in the patient?
    a. Decreased pulse
    b. Increased hemoglobin and hematocrit
    c. Acute confusion
    d. Increased blood pressure

25. A patient develops an active upper GI bleed. Which are the priority actions the nurse takes in caring for this patient? *(Select all that apply.)*
    a. Provide oxygen.
    b. Start 1 or 2 large-bore IV lines.
    c. Prepare to infuse 0.9% normal saline solution or lactated Ringer's solution.
    d. Monitor serum electrolytes.
    e. Prepare for nasogastric (NG) tube insertion.

26. When performing an assessment on a patient with an active upper GI bleed, which conditions does the nurse identify as common causes of upper GI bleeding? *(Select all that apply.)*
    a. Esophageal cancer
    b. Esophageal varices
    c. Gastroesophageal reflux disease
    d. Duodenal ulcer
    e. Gastritis
    f. Gastric cancer

27. The student nurse is performing a gastric lavage on a patient with an active upper GI bleed. Which action by the student requires intervention by the supervising nurse?
    a. Using an ice-cold solution to perform lavage of the stomach
    b. Instilling the lavage solution in volumes of 200 to 300 mL
    c. Continuing the lavage until the solution returned is clear or light pink without clots
    d. Positioning the patient on his left side during the procedure

28. Which drug would the health care provider prescribe to treat *H. pylori* infection?
    a. Ranitidine (Zantac)
    b. Omeprazole (Prilosec)
    c. Clarithromycin (Biaxin)
    d. Pantoprazole (Protonix)

29. The nurse is caring for several patients with gastric and duodenal ulcers. Which differential features of gastric ulcers compared to duodenal ulcers does the nurse identify? *(Select all that apply.)*
    a. Normal secretion or hyposecretion
    b. Relieved by ingestion of food
    c. Hematemesis more common than melena
    d. No gastritis present
    e. Most often, the patient has type O blood

30. The nurse is assessing a patient who has had a total gastrectomy today and notes bright-red blood in the NG and abdominal distention. What does the nurse do next?
    a. Irrigate the NG tube.
    b. Reposition the NG tube.
    c. Inform the surgeon of these findings.
    d. Remove the NG tube.

31. Which are symptoms of early dumping syndrome? *(Select all that apply.)*
    a. Tachycardia
    b. Confusion
    c. Desire to lie down
    d. Syncope
    e. Occurs 30 minutes after eating

32. What is the cause of late dumping syndrome?
    a. Rapid emptying of food into the small intestine
    b. Shift of fluids into the gut leading to abdominal distention
    c. Release of an excessive amount of insulin
    d. Rapid entry of high-protein foods into the jejunum

33. Which strategies does the nurse expect to implement in the management of dumping syndrome? *(Select all that apply.)*
    a. Provide more frequent smaller meals.
    b. Provide a high-carbohydrate diet.
    c. Eliminate liquids ingested with meals.
    d. Increase protein and fat in the diet.
    e. Administer acarbose to decrease carbohydrate absorption.

34. The nurse is caring for a patient who underwent gastric resection. On assessment, the nurse notes that the patient's tongue is smooth, shiny, and appears "beefy." What does the nurse suspect has occurred?
    a. Vitamin B_{12} deficiency
    b. Anemia
    c. Hypovolemia
    d. Inadequate nutrition

35. The nurse is teaching a patient with dumping syndrome about diet. Which statement by the patient indicates that teaching has been effective?
    a. "I will use sugar-free gelatin with caution."
    b. "I will avoid rice in my diet."
    c. "Meat in my diet will consist of a total of 8 ounces a day."
    d. "I will limit fluids with my meals to 8 ounces."

36. Which statement about general principles of diet therapy for patients with dumping syndrome is true?
    a. Patients with dumping syndrome should have liquids between meals only.
    b. Patients with dumping syndrome should be encouraged to eat a diet high in roughage.
    c. Patients with dumping syndrome should eat a high-carbohydrate diet.
    d. The diet for a patient with dumping syndrome must be low in fat and protein.

37. The nurse is providing discharge teaching for a patient after gastrectomy. Which teaching points will the nurse include to help the patient minimize dumping syndrome? *(Select all that apply.)*
    a. "Eat small frequent meals."
    b. "Drink an 8-ounce glass of water with each meal."
    c. "Eliminate alcohol and caffeine from your diet."
    d. "Lie flat for a short time after eating."
    e. "Take B_{12} injections as prescribed by your health care provider."

56

CHAPTER

Care of Patients with Noninflammatory Intestinal Disorders

1. The patient has a diagnosis of irritable bowel syndrome (IBS). Which forms can IBS take? *(Select all that apply.)*
   a. Diarrhea (IBS-D)
   b. Constipation (IBS-C)
   c. Bloating (IBS-B)
   d. Alternating diarrhea and constipation (IBS-A)
   e. Mix of constipation and diarrhea (IBS-M)

2. Which test may be used in diagnosing IBS?
   a. Erythrocyte sedimentation rate
   b. Stool sample for ova and parasites
   c. Hydrogen breath test
   d. Blood cultures for infection

3. The patient with IBS reports abdominal distention and feeling bloated to the nurse. The patient states she had a bowel movement that morning. What drug treatment does the nurse expect the health care provider to order?
   a. Loperamide (Imodium)
   b. Psyllium hydrophilic mucilloid (Metamucil)
   c. Lubiprostone (Amitiza)
   d. Rifaximin (Xifaxan)

4. Darifenacin (Enablex) is an example of a new group of drugs that may be used to manage IBS. What action of this drug would make it suitable for treatment of IBS?
   a. Inhibits intestinal motility
   b. Decreases abdominal distention
   c. Eliminates constipation
   d. Increases fluid in the intestines

5. Which drug is the drug of choice for the treatment of IBS when pain is the predominant symptom?
   a. Amitriptyline (Elavil)
   b. Fesoterodine (Toviaz)
   c. Loperamide (Imodium)
   d. Psyllium hydrophilic mucilloid (Metamucil)

6. The nurse is teaching a patient with IBS about complementary and alternative therapies for the disease. Which patient statements indicate that teaching has been effective? *(Select all that apply.)*
   a. "Hydrotherapy may help decrease symptoms."
   b. "Probiotics can help decrease bacteria and decrease my IBS symptoms."
   c. "Peppermint oil has been used to expel gas and relax spastic intestinal muscles."
   d. "Fish oil can be used to ease constipation."
   e. "Ginkgo can be used for abdominal discomfort and to expel gas."

7. The patient has an abdominal hernia with a sac that can be replaced into the abdominal cavity by gentle pressure. Which type of hernia does the nurse recognize?
   a. Incisional
   b. Irreducible
   c. Indirect inguinal
   d. Reducible

8. The nurse assesses a patient with a hernia and finds that the patient's symptoms include abdominal distention, nausea, vomiting, and pain. The patient's heart rate is 118/minute and temperature is 101° F. Which type of hernia does the nurse suspect?
   a. Incisional
   b. Incarcerated
   c. Strangulated
   d. Umbilical

9. The nurse is performing an abdominal assessment on a patient suspected of having an abdominal hernia. The nurse auscultates the abdomen and determines the absence of bowel sounds. What does the nurse suspect in this patient?
   a. Peritonitis
   b. IBS
   c. Obstruction and strangulation
   d. Low intraabdominal pressure

10. Which are true statements about caring for a patient with a truss? *(Select all that apply.)*
   a. A surgical binder holds the truss in place.
   b. The truss is removed only for bathing.
   c. The truss is only used after the hernia has been reduced by the physician.
   d. The truss is applied before the hernia is reduced to decrease pain.
   e. Powder should be applied to the skin under the truss daily.

11. Which activity does the nurse tell the patient to *avoid* after surgery for a hernia repair?
   a. Ambulating
   b. Turning
   c. Coughing
   d. Deep-breathing

12. What do postoperative measures for a male patient who has had an inguinal herniorrhaphy include?
   a. Applying a warm pack to the scrotum
   b. Elevating the scrotum on a pillow
   c. Encouraging use of a bedpan to void
   d. Decreasing fluid intake to decrease bladder emptying

13. The nurse is providing teaching about ways to reduce the risk for colorectal cancer. Which dietary suggestions will the nurse be sure to include? *(Select all that apply.)*
   a. Low fat
   b. Low protein
   c. High fiber
   d. High in red meat
   e. Low in refined carbohydrates

14. Which are the most common signs of colorectal cancer (CRC)? *(Select all that apply.)*
   a. Change in stool consistency
   b. Absent bowel sounds
   c. Abdominal cramping
   d. Anemia
   e. Rectal bleeding

15. Which test is definitive for the diagnosis of CRC?
   a. Carcinoembryonic antigen (CEA)
   b. Barium swallow
   c. Colonoscopy with biopsy
   d. Fecal occult blood test (FOBT)

16. After colostomy surgery, which intervention does the nurse employ?
   a. Cover the stoma with a dry, sterile dressing.
   b. Apply a pouch system as soon as possible.
   c. Make a hole in the pouch for gas to escape.
   d. Watch for the colostomy to start functioning on day 1.

17. Which discharge instruction does the nurse include for a patient after abdominoperitoneal (AP) resection?
   a. "Use a soft pillow to sit on whenever you sit down."
   b. "Lie on your back when you are resting in bed."
   c. "Use a rubber doughnut device for sitting on when in the car."
   d. "Sit in a chair for at least 4 consecutive hours a day."

18. Which findings does the nurse expect for a postoperative colostomy patient? *(Select all that apply.)*
    a. Reddish-pink, moist stoma
    b. Small amount of bleeding
    c. Large amount of stoma swelling
    d. Mucocutaneous separation
    e. Smooth, intact peristomal skin

19. Which findings for a patient with a new colostomy will the nurse report to the surgeon? *(Select all that apply.)*
    a. A dark-red, dry stoma
    b. Stoma protruding about 2 cm from the abdominal wall
    c. Mucocutaneous separation
    d. A slight amount of edema in the initial postoperative period
    e. Large amount of bleeding

20. The nurse is teaching a patient about what to expect after a descending colon colostomy. The nurse tells the patient to expect the stool to have what kind of form?
    a. Similar to that of stool expelled from the rectum
    b. Thick and paste-like
    c. Thin and gelatin-like
    d. Watery

21. Which sign/symptom is a patient who had an AP resection instructed to report to the health care provider immediately?
    a. Serosanguineous drainage from the wound
    b. Sensations of having a bowel movement
    c. Constant perineal odor and pain
    d. Occasional perineal pain and itching

22. The nurse is teaching a patient about colostomy care. Which information does the nurse include in the teaching plan?
    a. The stoma will enlarge within 6 to 8 weeks of surgery.
    b. Use a moisturizing soap to cleanse the area around the stoma.
    c. Place the colostomy bag on the skin when the skin sealant is still damp.
    d. An antifungal cream or powder can be used if a fungal rash develops.

23. A patient with a colostomy may safely include which food item in the diet?
    a. Burritos
    b. Yogurt
    c. Cabbage
    d. Carbonated beverages

24. The nurse is teaching a patient about how to control gas and odor from a colostomy. Which information does the nurse include?
    a. Do not chew gum.
    b. Place an aspirin in the colostomy.
    c. Do not consume buttermilk.
    d. Do not eat parsley.

25. Which are examples of mechanical bowel obstructions? *(Select all that apply.)*
    a. Paralytic ileus
    b. Adhesions
    c. Tumors
    d. Absent peristalsis
    e. Fecal impaction

26. Which acid-base abnormality results from a bowel obstruction high in the small intestine?
    a. Respiratory acidosis
    b. Respiratory alkalosis
    c. Metabolic acidosis
    d. Metabolic alkalosis

27. Which description best defines intussusception of the intestine?
    a. Twisting of the intestine
    b. Fecal constipation or impaction
    c. Telescoping of a segment of the intestine within itself
    d. Adhesions forming scar tissue

28. The nurse is assessing a patient newly admitted with obstipation and failure to pass flatus. Which condition is the most likely cause of this patient's symptoms?
    a. Complete obstruction
    b. Partial obstruction
    c. Colorectal cancer
    d. Crohn's disease

29. Which key feature does the nurse most likely find when performing a physical assessment on a patient with a small-bowel obstruction?
    a. Visible peristaltic waves in the upper and middle abdomen
    b. Minimal or no vomiting
    c. No major fluid and electrolyte imbalances
    d. Metabolic acidosis

30. What nursing care does a patient with a nasogastric (NG) tube require? *(Select all that apply.)*
    a. Assessment of proper placement at least every 12 hours
    b. Keep patient in a semi-Fowler's position
    c. Confirmation of NG tube placement by x-ray if it is repositioned
    d. Monitor contents of the NG tube
    e. Irrigation of the tube with 30 mL of normal saline as ordered
    f. Questioning the patient about the passage of flatus

31. Which NG tubes can be connected to low continuous suction?
    a. Salem sump
    b. Levin
    c. Anderson
    d. Carney

32. The nurse providing care for a patient with a bowel obstruction notes that the patient has started passing flatus and had a small bowel movement. What has occurred with this patient?
    a. Blockage is complete.
    b. Peristalsis has returned.
    c. Peritonitis has occurred.
    d. The patient is rehydrated.

33. Which intervention applies to the nursing care of an older patient with heart failure and hypovolemia related to an intestinal obstruction?
    a. Provide frequent mouth care with lemon-glycerin swabs.
    b. Offer ice chips to suck on before surgery.
    c. Offer a small glass of water.
    d. Assess for crackles in the lungs.

34. The nurse is to administer alvimopan (Entereg) to a patient with postoperative ileus (POI). What is the action of this drug?
    a. Increases gastrointestinal (GI) motility
    b. Laxative for bowel movement
    c. Antibiotic to prevent infection
    d. Prevents nausea and vomiting

35. Which observation of a patient with an intestinal obstruction does the nurse report immediately?
    a. Urinary output of 1000 mL in an 8-hour period
    b. The patient's request for something to drink
    c. Abdominal pain changing from colicky to constant discomfort
    d. The patient is changing positions frequently

36. Which discharge information does the nurse include for the patient who has had an intestinal obstruction caused by fecal impaction?
    a. Encourage the patient to report abdominal distention, nausea or vomiting, and constipation.
    b. Provide the patient a written description of a low-fiber diet.
    c. Remind the patient to limit activity.
    d. Remind the patient to decrease fluid intake.

37. Which nursing care actions should the nurse delegate to the unlicensed assistive personnel (UAP) for an older patient with a bowel obstruction? *(Select all that apply.)*
    a. Administer analgesics as needed.
    b. Provide mouth care every 2 hours.
    c. Assess abdomen for distention.
    d. Teach the patient about surgical procedures.
    e. Provide the patient with a few ice chips.

38. Why does the nurse place a patient with a bowel obstruction in semi-Fowler's position? *(Select all that apply.)*
    a. To promote increased peristalsis
    b. To alleviate the pressure of abdominal distention on the chest
    c. To decrease the likelihood of nausea and vomiting
    d. To facilitate breathing
    e. To prevent aspiration

39. Emergency care of a patient with abdominal trauma includes which interventions? *(Select all that apply.)*
    a. Insertion of at least two large-bore IV catheters in the lower extremities
    b. Type and cross-matching of 4 to 8 units of blood
    c. Measurement of arterial blood gases
    d. Continuous hemodynamic monitoring
    e. Insertion of a Foley catheter

40. The emergency department (ED) nurse is assessing a patient with abdominal trauma after a motor vehicle accident. The patient has become somewhat confused, his skin is pale, cool, and moist and he has had only 20 mL of urine output during the past hour. What does the nurse suspect?
    a. Hypovolemic shock
    b. Head injury
    c. Liver laceration
    d. Large bowel injury

41. The trauma patient has ecchymosis (bruising) in the shape and distribution of a seat belt. What is the nurse's best first action?
    a. Start a third large-bore IV.
    b. Notify the health care provider.
    c. Insert a urinary catheter.
    d. Get a 12-lead electrocardiogram.

42. Which statement about intraabdominal pressure (IAP) monitoring is correct?
    a. The normal IAP for adults is 15 to 20 mm Hg.
    b. Patients with high IAP have bradycardia.
    c. High IAP leads to increased afterload and decreased preload.
    d. Patients with high IAP are hypertensive.

43. Which are potential complications of polyps? *(Select all that apply.)*
    a. Gross rectal bleeding
    b. Colorectal cancer
    c. Intestinal obstruction
    d. Septic shock
    e. Intussusception

44. Which information does the nurse include when teaching a patient with new-onset hemorrhoids about prevention of hemorrhoid flare-up? *(Select all that apply.)*
    a. "Increase the fiber in your diet to prevent constipation."
    b. "Do not participate in any physical exercise."
    c. "Maintain a healthy weight."
    d. "Increase your amount of fluid intake."
    e. "Prolonged sitting or standing will not affect the development of hemorrhoids."

45. Which intervention is contraindicated in the nonsurgical management of hemorrhoids?
    a. Diets low in fiber and fluids
    b. Dibucaine (Nupercainal) ointment
    c. Warm sitz baths three or four times a day
    d. Cleansing the anal area with moistened cleaning tissues

46. Which statement by a patient indicates an understanding of surgical management of hemorrhoids?
    a. "It will take 10 to 14 days for the rubber band used on the hemorrhoid to fall off."
    b. "My first bowel movement after the surgery may be very painful."
    c. "After surgery, I will need to eat a low-fiber, low-fluid diet."
    d. "Stool softeners and laxatives are avoided after hemorrhoid surgery."

47. What is the classic symptom of malabsorption syndrome?
    a. Unintentional weight loss
    b. Decreased libido
    c. Bloating with flatus
    d. Chronic diarrhea

48. Which laboratory results are expected with malabsorption syndrome resulting in hypochromic microcytic anemia? *(Select all that apply.)*
    a. Low mean corpuscular hemoglobin (MCH)
    b. High serum vitamin A level
    c. Elevated fecal fat content
    d. Increased mean corpuscular volume (MCV)
    e. Decreased serum cholesterol level
    f. Low mean corpuscular hemoglobin concentration (MCHC)

49. Which diagnostic test measures urinary excretion of vitamin B_{12} for diagnosis of pernicious anemia and other malabsorption syndromes?
    a. Bile acid breath test
    b. Schilling test
    c. Hydrogen breath test
    d. D-xylose absorption test

50. What are the major focus areas for interventions aimed at treating malabsorption syndromes? *(Select all that apply.)*
    a. Avoiding substances that aggravate malabsorption
    b. Use of complementary and alternative therapies
    c. Supplementation of nutrients
    d. Assessment and supplementation of coping strategies
    e. Curative radiation therapy

57

CHAPTER

Care of Patients with Inflammatory Intestinal Disorders

1. The patient comes to the emergency department (ED) with right lower quadrant pain. What does the ED nurse suspect?
   a. Gastroenteritis
   b. Ulcerative colitis
   c. Appendicitis
   d. Crohn's disease

2. The nurse is caring for the patient with acute appendicitis. Which interventions will the nurse perform? *(Select all that apply.)*
   a. Maintain the patient on NPO status.
   b. Administer IV fluids as prescribed.
   c. Apply warm compresses to the right lower abdominal quadrant.
   d. Maintain the patient in the supine position.
   e. Administer laxatives.

3. The patient has been diagnosed with acute appendicitis. Based on this diagnosis, which intervention does the nurse perform?
   a. Start a bowel cleansing program.
   b. Prepare the patient for surgery.
   c. Apply a heating pad to the lower abdomen.
   d. Assess the patient's knowledge about dietary modifications.

4. The nurse on the surgical unit is expecting to admit the patient who has had an appendectomy with abscess. What does the nurse anticipate care for this patient will include? *(Select all that apply.)*
   a. Clear liquids
   b. Wound drains
   c. IV antibiotics
   d. Nonsteroidal antiinflammatory drugs (NSAIDs) for pain control
   e. Nasogastric (NG) tube care

5. Which laboratory finding does the nurse expect may occur with a diagnosis of appendicitis?
   a. Decreased hematocrit and hemoglobin
   b. Increased coagulation time
   c. Decreased potassium
   d. Increased WBC count

6. Which statements about peritonitis are true? *(Select all that apply.)*
   a. Peritonitis is caused by contamination of the peritoneal cavity by bacteria or chemicals.
   b. Continuous ambulatory peritoneal dialysis (CAPD) can cause peritonitis.
   c. White blood cell counts are often decreased with peritonitis.
   d. Abdominal wall rigidity is a classic finding in patients with peritonitis.
   e. Chemical peritonitis is caused by leakage of pancreatic enzymes or gastric acids.

7. The fluid shift that occurs in peritonitis may result in which of the following?
   a. Intracellular fluid moving into the peritoneal cavity
   b. Significant increase in circulatory volume
   c. Decreased circulatory volume and hypovolemic shock
   d. Increased bowel motility caused by increased fluid volume

8. The respiratory problems that may accompany peritonitis are a result of which factor?
   a. Associated pain interfering with ventilation
   b. Decreased pressure against the diaphragm
   c. Fluid shifts to the thoracic cavity
   d. Decreased oxygen demands related to the infectious process

9. Which nursing intervention is part of nonsurgical management for a patient with peritonitis?
   a. Monitor weekly weight and intake and output.
   b. Insert a nasogastric tube to decompress the stomach.
   c. Order a breakfast tray when the patient is hungry.
   d. Administer NSAIDs for pain.

10. What are the cardinal signs of peritonitis?
    a. Fever and headache
    b. Dizziness with nausea and vomiting
    c. Abdominal pain, distention, and tenderness
    d. Nausea and loss of appetite

11. Which intervention does the nurse delegate to the unlicensed assistive personnel (UAP) when caring for a postoperative patient with peritonitis?
    a. Measure intake and output.
    b. Assess wound drainage.
    c. Administer IV antibiotics.
    d. Teach patient about wound care.

12. The nurse is instructing a patient about home care after an exploratory laparotomy for peritonitis. Which statement by the patient indicates that teaching has been effective?
    a. "It is normal for the incision site to be warm."
    b. "I will stop taking the antibiotics if diarrhea develops."
    c. "I will call the health care provider for a temperature greater than 101° F."
    d. "I will resume activity with my bowling league this week for exercise."

13. The patient with gastroenteritis due to infection with the norovirus asks the nurse how this illness occurred. Which statement by the patient indicates correct understanding of the nurse's teaching?
    a. "I got this infection from being around my grandchildren when they had respiratory illnesses."
    b. "It is likely that I got this illness from either contaminated water or food."
    c. "I may have gotten sick when I was travelling last month."
    d. "It's really important that everything I eat is cooked until it is well done."

14. Which interventions are useful in preventing spread of gastroenteritis? *(Select all that apply.)*
    a. Careful handwashing
    b. Sanitize all surfaces that may be contaminated
    c. Prophylactic use of antibiotics
    d. Easily accessible hand sanitizers
    e. Test all food preparation employees

15. The nurse is assessing a patient with viral gastroenteritis. Which symptom is the nurse most concerned about?
    a. Orthostatic blood pressure changes
    b. Poor skin turgor
    c. Dry mucous membranes
    d. Rebound tenderness

16. What is the priority nursing concern for a patient with gastroenteritis?
    a. Nutrition therapy
    b. Fluid replacement
    c. Skin care
    d. Drug therapy

17. Which are common manifestations in a 28-year-old patient with dehydration secondary to gastroenteritis? *(Select all that apply.)*
    a. Peripheral edema
    b. Elevated temperature
    c. Dry mucous membranes
    d. Hypertension
    e. Oliguria

18. As part of the routine treatment plan for a patient with bacterial gastroenteritis, which drugs does the nurse anticipate the patient will most likely be prescribed?
    a. Anticholinergics
    b. Antiemetics
    c. Antiperistaltic drugs
    d. Antibiotics

19. The nurse is caring for a patient with gastroenteritis who has frequent stools. Which task is best to delegate to the UAP?
    a. Teach the patient to avoid toilet paper and harsh soaps.
    b. Instruct the patient on how to take a sitz bath.
    c. Use a warm washcloth to remove stool from the skin.
    d. Dry the skin with absorbent cotton.

20. Which characteristics pertain to Crohn's disease (CD)? *(Select all that apply.)*
    a. Begins in the rectum and proceeds in a continuous manner toward the cecum
    b. Fistulas commonly develop
    c. Five to six soft, loose stools per day that are nonbloody
    d. Increased risk of colon cancer
    e. Some patients experience extraintestinal manifestations such as migratory polyarthritis, ankylosing spondylitis, and erythema nodosum
    f. Cobblestone appearance of the internal intestine

21. A patient is suspected to have ulcerative colitis (UC). Which definitive diagnostic test does the nurse expect the patient to undergo in order to confirm the diagnosis?
    a. Colonoscopy
    b. C-reactive protein
    c. Albumin levels
    d. Erythrocyte sedimentation rate

22. A patient is prescribed sulfasalazine (Azulfidine) for the treatment of UC. Which patient statement indicates the patient is experiencing a side effect of this drug?
    a. "My skin is covered with a rash."
    b. "My knees hurt."
    c. "My appetite has increased."
    d. "I wake up at night sweating sometimes."

23. Which statement is true about the medical treatment of UC?
    a. Infliximab (Remicade) is approved as a first-line therapy.
    b. Immunomodulators are not thought to be effective; however, in combination with steroids, they may offer a synergistic effect.
    c. When a therapeutic level of glucocorticoids is reached, the dosage of the drug stays the same to maintain the therapeutic effect.
    d. The method of action for the aminosalicylates is interruption of the pain pathway.

24. A patient with UC who has had an ileostomy is being discharged home. The nurse has provided discharge teaching. Which statements by the patient indicate the teaching has been effective? *(Select all that apply.)*
    a. "I will avoid foods that cause gas."
    b. "I will call the health care provider if I have a fever over 101° F."
    c. "I will change the adhesive for the appliance daily."
    d. "I know the pouch needs emptying when I feel pain in that area."
    e. "I will call the health care provider if I feel like my heart is beating fast."

25. Which statement is true about drug therapy for CD?
    a. Budesonide (Entocort EC) is a rapid-release compound that delivers low local glucocorticoid concentrations to the terminal ileum for patients with CD.
    b. Methotrexate (Rheumatrex) is contraindicated in the treatment of CD.
    c. Metronidazole (Flagyl) has been helpful in patients with fistulas and CD.
    d. Adalimumab (Humira) is a glucocorticoid approved for the treatment of CD.

26. A patient with CD has a fistula. Which assessment finding indicates possible dehydration?
    a. Weight gain of 2 pounds in one day
    b. Abdominal pain
    c. Foul-smelling urine
    d. Decreased urinary output

27. In caring for a patient with CD, the nurse observes for which complications? *(Select all that apply.)*
    a. Peritonitis
    b. Small bowel obstruction
    c. Nutritional and fluid imbalances
    d. Presence of fistulas
    e. Appendicitis
    f. Severe nausea and vomiting

28. Which surgical procedure involves removal of the colon, rectum, and anus with surgical closure of the anus?
    a. Restorative proctolectomy with ileo pouch-anal anastomosis (RPC-IPAA)
    b. Natural orifice transluminal endoscopic surgery (NOTES)
    c. Sigmoid colostomy
    d. Total proctocolectomy with a permanent ileostomy

29. Which type of diet has been implicated in the formation of diverticula?
    a. High-fat diet
    b. Low-protein diet
    c. High-cholesterol diet
    d. Low-fiber diet

30. What is the nature of pain associated with diverticulitis?
    a. Intermittent becoming progressively steady
    b. Sharp and continuous
    c. Localized to the right upper quadrant
    d. Severe and incapacitating

31. The nurse is assessing an older adult patient with abdominal pain. Assessment findings include generalized abdominal pain with rigidity, nausea and vomiting, elevated temperature (101.2°F), increased heart rate (122/minute) and chills. The patient is also somewhat confused and does not know where he is. What does the nurse suspect with this patient?
    a. Crohn's disease
    b. Ulcerative colitis
    c. Diverticulitis
    d. Peritonitis

32. Which drug is often used in older patients for pain management of moderate to severe diverticulitis?
    a. Ibuprofen (Motrin)
    b. Acetaminophen (Tylenol)
    c. Aspirin (Anacin)
    d. Morphine sulfate (Duramorph)

33. Which statement about diverticular disease is true?
    a. Most diverticula occur in the sigmoid colon.
    b. Diverticula are uncomfortable even when not inflamed.
    c. High-fiber diets contribute to diverticula occurrence.
    d. Diverticula form where intestinal wall muscles are weak.

34. Which is a preventive measure for diverticular disease?
    a. Excluding whole-grain breads from the diet
    b. Avoiding fresh apples, broccoli, and lettuce
    c. Taking bulk agents such as psyllium hydrophilic mucilloid (Metamucil)
    d. Taking routine anticholinergics to reduce bowel spasms

35. Which type of stoma will a patient with diverticulitis most likely have postoperatively?
    a. Ileostomy
    b. Jejunostomy
    c. Colostomy
    d. Cecostomy

36. Which interventions does the nurse expect to implement when caring for a patient with diverticulitis? *(Select all that apply.)*
    a. Laxative and enemas as ordered
    b. IV fluids to prevent dehydration
    c. Broad-spectrum antibiotics
    d. Teach the patient to refrain from lifting or straining
    e. Keep the patient NPO if symptoms are severe

37. Which description best defines an anal fissure?
    a. Perianal tear that can be very painful
    b. Duct obstruction and infection
    c. Communicating tract
    d. Localized area of induration with pus

38. The nurse is providing teaching for a patient with an anal fissure as a complication of CD. Which statement by the patient indicates the need for further teaching?
    a. "I will use warm sitz baths."
    b. "A diet that is low in bulk-producing agents is best for me."
    c. "Hydrocortisone cream may be helpful to decrease discomfort."
    d. "Topical antiinflammatory agents will help if I am uncomfortable."

39. Which parasitic infection is manifested by diarrhea and occurs most commonly in immunosuppressed patients, especially those with human immunodeficiency virus (HIV)?
    a. *Entamoeba histolytica*
    b. *Cryptosporidium*
    c. *Giardia lamblia*
    d. *Escherichia coli*

40. Which statements does the nurse include while providing discharge instructions for a patient with giardiasis? *(Select all that apply.)*
    a. "Avoid contact with stool from dogs and beavers."
    b. "All household and sexual partners should have stool examinations for parasites."
    c. "Treatment will most likely consist of metronidazole (Flagyl)."
    d. "The infection can be transmitted to others until the amebicides kill the parasites."
    e. "Stools are examined 6 days after treatment to assess for eradication."

41. The ED nurse is assessing a patient admitted with frequent, liquid, foul-smelling stools containing mucus and blood. Assessment findings include temperature 103.8° F, tenesmus, abdominal tenderness, and vomiting. Which additional laboratory tests does the nurse expect to collect?
    a. Serial stool samples
    b. Urine culture
    c. Throat culture
    d. Sputum culture

1. A patient with decompensated cirrhosis is at risk for which complications? *(Select all that apply.)*
   a. Jaundice
   b. Esophageal varices
   c. Coagulation defects
   d. Hepatitis A virus (HAV)
   e. Spontaneous bacterial peritonitis
   f. Ascites

2. What is the most common cause for Laennec's cirrhosis?
   a. Hepatitis C virus (HPC)
   b. Chronic biliary obstruction
   c. Autoimmune disorders
   d. Chronic alcoholism

3. The nurse is assessing a patient with massive ascites. What related complication must the nurse monitor for with this patient?
   a. Bleeding due to fragile, thin-walled veins
   b. Hematemesis due to absence of clotting factors
   c. Increased ascites due to sodium and water retention
   d. Bruising due to low platelet count

4. When admitting the patient with cirrhosis, the nurse assesses for which conditions related to splenomegaly as possible complications of the disease? *(Select all that apply.)*
   a. Thrombocytopenia
   b. Bleeding esophageal varices
   c. Hepatorenal syndrome
   d. Portal hypertensive gastropathy

5. Patients with cirrhosis are susceptible to bleeding and easy bruising because there is a decrease in the production of bile in the liver preventing the absorption of which vitamin?
   a. Vitamin A
   b. Vitamin D
   c. Vitamin E
   d. Vitamin K

6. Which key points does the nurse include when teaching the patient with cirrhosis and his family about drug therapy before discharge? *(Select all that apply.)*
   a. "Do not take over-the-counter medications unless approved by your health care provider."
   b. "The beta blocker called propranolol (Inderal) will cause your heart rate to increase."
   c. "The lactulose syrup should cause you to have two to three bowel movements every day."
   d. "Take your furosemide (Lasix) early in the day so that it does not keep you up at night."
   e. "Report any muscle weakness or lightheadedness to your health care provider right away."

7. The nurse identifies which laboratory value as the usual indication of hepatic encephalopathy?
   a. Elevated sodium level
   b. Elevated ammonia level
   c. Increased blood urea nitrogen (BUN)
   d. Increased clotting time

8. The nurse is assessing a male patient with cirrhosis. Which male-specific characteristics does the nurse expect to find? *(Select all that apply.)*
   a. Gynecomastia
   b. Testicular atrophy
   c. Ascites
   d. Impotence
   e. Spider angiomas

9. Which assessment finding indicates neurologic function deterioration in a patient with stage II cirrhosis?
   a. Fetor hepaticus
   b. Asterixis
   c. Palmar erythema
   d. Icterus

10. Which intervention should the nurse delegate to the unlicensed assistive personnel (UAP) when caring for a patient with cirrhosis experiencing pruritus?
    a. Apply lotion to soothe the patient's skin
    b. Use lots of soap and hot water to cleanse the skin
    c. Assess the patient for signs of skin infection
    d. Encourage the patient to use distraction to avoid scratching

11. Which elevated laboratory test results indicate hepatic cell destruction? *(Select all that apply.)*
    a. Elevated serum aspartate aminotransferase (AST)
    b. Elevated serum alanine aminotransferase (ALT)
    c. Elevated lactate dehydrogenase (LDH)
    d. Decreased serum total bilirubin
    e. Increased fecal urobilinogen
    f. Increased International Normalized Ratio (INR)

12. A patient is scheduled for a procedure to place a stent in the biliary tract. For which procedure does the nurse provide patient teaching?
    a. Esophagogastroduodenoscopy (EGD)
    b. Endoscopic retrograde cholangiopancreatography (ERCP)
    c. Upper gastrointestinal (GI) series
    d. Cholangiogram

13. The nurse is teaching a patient with cirrhosis about nutrition therapy. Which statement by the patient indicates teaching has been effective?
    a. "I will only use table salt with my dinner meal."
    b. "I will read the sodium content labels on all food and beverages."
    c. "I will avoid the use of vinegar."
    d. "I will not take vitamin supplements."

14. When preparing a patient for paracentesis, what does the nurse do? *(Select all that apply.)*
    a. Ask the patient to void before the procedure.
    b. Place the patient in the supine position.
    c. Weigh the patient before the procedure.
    d. Obtain the patient's heart rate.
    e. Assess the patient's respiratory rate.
    f. Obtain the patient's blood pressure.

15. A patient will undergo an abdominal paracentesis. Which factor provides an additional safety measure?
    a. The procedure is performed using ultrasound.
    b. The procedure is performed at the bedside.
    c. A trocar is inserted into the peritoneal cavity.
    d. General anesthesia is administered.

16. The student nurse is caring for a patient with cirrhosis. Which action by the student nurse causes the supervising nurse to intervene?
    a. Uses a straight-edge razor to shave the patient
    b. Monitors for orthostatic changes of blood pressure
    c. Avoids intramuscular injections
    d. Uses a toothette for oral care

17. The nurse who is assessing a patient with portal-systemic encephalopathy finds that the patient has fetor hepaticus, a positive Babinski's sign, and seizures, but no asterixis. The nurse identifies the patient as being in which stage of portal-systemic encephalopathy?
    a. Stage I prodromal
    b. Stage II impending
    c. Stage III stuporous
    d. Stage IV comatose

18. Which statements about a patient with cirrhosis and esophageal varices are accurate? (*Select all that apply.*)
    a. All patients with cirrhosis should be screened for esophageal varices to detect them before they bleed.
    b. Bleeding esophageal varices are a medical emergency.
    c. Esophageal balloon tamponade is often used to control bleeding esophageal varices.
    d. A nonselective beta blocker such as propranolol (Inderal) is prescribed to prevent varices from bleeding.
    e. Bleeding esophageal varices can be managed by use of endoscopic variceal ligation.

19. The nurse is teaching a patient with cirrhosis about lactulose therapy. Which statement by the patient indicates the teaching has been effective?
    a. "This therapy will promote the removal of ammonia in my stool."
    b. "Constipation is a frequent side effect of this therapy."
    c. "I will know the therapy is working when I am less itchy."
    d. "The drug tastes bitter and is watery."

20. How is neomycin sulfate (Mycifradin) used to treat patients with cirrhosis?
    a. It treats the current infection the patient has.
    b. It prevents future infections of the liver.
    c. It restores normal function to the liver cells.
    d. It decreases the rate of ammonia production.

21. The patient with liver cancer will be discharged with a tunneled ascites drain. What statements by the patient indicate an understanding of the purpose of this device? (*Select all that apply.*)
    a. "I will have this drain until I am able to get the tumor removed."
    b. "I will not remove more than 2000 mL of fluid at a time."
    c. "The drain will make breathing more comfortable for me after some fluid is removed."
    d. "After I drain off the extra fluid, I can remove the drain."
    e. "This drain will be useful to remove fluid from my belly when there is too much."

22. Which statements about hepatitis are accurate? (*Select all that apply.*)
    a. Hepatitis D is the leading cause of cirrhosis and liver failure in the U.S.
    b. Hepatitis A is spread through the fecal-oral route.
    c. Hepatitis B can be transmitted through unprotected sexual intercourse.
    d. Hepatitis carriers have chronic obvious signs of hepatitis B.
    e. Hepatitis C is transmitted by casual contact or intimate household contact.
    f. Hepatitis D only occurs with hepatitis B to cause viral replication.

23. When teaching a group of adult patients measures for preventing hepatitis A (HAV), which information does the nurse include? (*Select all that apply.*)
    a. Perform proper handwashing, especially after handling shellfish.
    b. Receive immune globulin within 14 days if exposed to the virus.
    c. Receive the HAV vaccine before traveling to Mexico or the Caribbean.
    d. After exposure, HAV symptoms always let the patient know something is wrong.
    e. Receive the vaccine if working in a long-term care facility.

24. Which people are in need of immunization against hepatitis B (HBV)? *(Select all that apply.)*
    a. People who have unprotected sex with more than one partner
    b. Men who have sex with men
    c. Any patient scheduled for a surgical procedure
    d. Firefighters
    e. Health care providers

25. What is the major source of hepatitis B transmission to health care workers?
    a. Improper handwashing
    b. Needlesticks
    c. Touching contaminated surfaces
    d. Contact with infected stool

26. How many injections does a health care worker usually need to be protected with the hepatitis B vaccine?
    a. 1
    b. 2
    c. 3
    d. 4

27. Which actions will help prevent viral hepatitis in health care workers? *(Select all that apply.)*
    a. Wash hands before and after each patient
    b. Needleless systems
    c. Use contact and respiratory precautions
    d. After exposure to hepatitis A, get immunoglobulin (Ig)
    e. Report all cases of hepatitis to the health department.

28. Which laboratory test result indicates permanent immunity to hepatitis A?
    a. Immunoglobulin G (IgG) antibodies
    b. Immunoglobulin M (IgM) antibodies
    c. A positive enzyme-linked immunosorbent assay (ELISA)
    d. The presence of anti-HAV antibodies

29. Which antiviral drugs are given to patients with chronic hepatitis B virus? *(Select all that apply.)*
    a. Lamivudine (Epivir-HBV)
    b. Entecavir (Baraclude)
    c. Tenofovir (Viread)
    d. Oral ribavirin (Rebetol)
    e. Adefovir (Hepsera)

30. Which conditions place a patient at high risk for the development of fatty liver (steatosis)? *(Select all that apply.)*
    a. Hypertension
    b. Diabetes mellitus
    c. Obesity
    d. Elevated lipid profile
    e. Alcohol abuse

31. In performing an assessment on a patient with liver trauma, what does the nurse expect to find? *(Select all that apply.)*
    a. Right upper quadrant pain
    b. Increased blood pressure
    c. Guarding of the abdomen
    d. Bradypnea
    e. Kehr's sign

32. The nurse is assessing a patient with liver trauma and finds that the patient is confused with a blood pressure of 86/50 mm Hg; heart rate of 128/minute; and cool, clammy skin. What does the nurse suspect?
    a. Septic shock
    b. Liver hemorrhage
    c. Liver cancer
    d. GI bleeding

33. What is the tumor marker for cancers of the liver?
    a. Decreased alkaline phosphatase
    b. Increased serum ammonia
    c. Decreased serum total bilirubin
    d. Increased alpha-fetoprotein (AFP)

34. Which treatment offers the patient with liver cancer the possibility of long-term survival?
    a. Chemotherapy
    b. Selective internal radiation therapy
    c. Liver transplantation
    d. Hepatic arterial embolization

35. What is the priority focus in caring for a patient with advanced liver cancer?
    a. Hospice and end-of life care
    b. Getting placed on the liver transplant list
    c. Hepatic arterial infusion of chemotherapy
    d. Cryotherapy to freeze and destroy liver tumors

36. Administration of which drug has greatly improved the success of organ transplants?
    a. Telaprevir (Incivek)
    b. Entecavir (Baraclude)
    c. Tenofovir (Viread)
    d. Cyclosporine (Cyclosporin A)

37. The patient who had a liver transplant develops a heart rate of 134/minute, temperature of 102° F, jaundiced skin, and right upper quadrant pain. What does the nurse suspect?
    a. Liver infection
    b. Hypovolemic shock
    c. Liver transplant rejection
    d. Liver trauma from the transplant surgery

38. Which procedure uses energy waves to heat cancer cells and kill them?
    a. Cryotherapy
    b. Selective internal radiation therapy (SIRT)
    c. Hepatic artery embolization
    d. Radiofrequency ablation (RFA)

39. Which patients would not be considered candidates for a liver transplant? *(Select all that apply.)*
    a. Patient with metastatic tumors
    b. Patient with type 2 diabetes
    c. Patient with severe respiratory disease
    d. Patient with chronic liver disease
    e. Patient with advanced cardiac disease

40. The nurse is teaching a patient with cirrhosis about nutrition therapy. Which key points must the nurse include? *(Select all that apply.)*
    a. Do not use table salt.
    b. Adding salt when cooking is acceptable.
    c. Eat small frequent meals.
    d. Drink supplemental liquids such as Ensure.
    e. Be sure to take a multivitamin every day.

59 CHAPTER

Care of Patients with Problems of the Biliary System and Pancreas

1. A patient is admitted to the patient care unit with obstructive jaundice. Which sign/symptom does the nurse expect to find upon assessment of the patient?
   a. Pruritus
   b. Pale urine in increased amounts
   c. Pink discoloration of sclera
   d. Dark, tarry stools

2. The daughter of a patient with cholelithiasis has heard that there is a genetic disposition for cholelithiasis. The daughter asks the nurse about the risk factors. How does the nurse respond?
   a. "There is no evidence that first-degree relatives have an increased risk for this disease."
   b. "Cholecystitis is seen more frequently in patients who are underweight."
   c. "Hormone replacement therapy has been associated with increased risk for cholecystitis."
   d. "Patients with diabetes mellitus are at increased risk for cholecystitis."

3. Which patient is at low risk for the development of gallbladder disorders?
   a. Patient with sickle cell anemia
   b. Patient who is Mexican American
   c. Patient who is 20 years old and male
   d. Patient with a history of prolonged parenteral nutrition

4. The nurse on a medical-surgical unit is caring for several patients with acute cholecystitis. Which task is best to delegate to the unlicensed assistive personnel (UAP)?
   a. Obtain the patients' vital signs.
   b. Determine if any foods are not tolerated.
   c. Assess what measures relieve the abdominal pain.
   d. Ask the patients to describe their daily activity or exercise routines.

5. Which are common manifestations of acute cholecystitis? (Select all that apply.)
   a. Anorexia
   b. Ascites
   c. Eructation
   d. Steatorrhea
   e. Jaundice
   f. Rebound tenderness

6. The nurse is assessing a patient with acute cholecystitis whose abdominal pain is severe. The patient has a heart rate of 118/minute, is pale, diaphoretic, and describes extreme fatigue. What is the nurse's priority action at this time?
   a. Instruct the UAP to check a complete set of vital signs.
   b. Auscultate the patient's abdomen in all four quadrants.
   c. Notify the patient's health care provider.
   d. Administer the ordered opioid analgesic.

7. The health care provider has assessed a patient's abdomen and found rebound tenderness on deep palpation. What does the nurse recognize?
   a. Steatorrhea
   b. Eructation
   c. Biliary colic
   d. Blumberg's sign

8. A patient is scheduled for tests to verify the medical diagnosis of cholecystitis. For which diagnostic test does the nurse provide patient teaching?
   a. Extracorporeal shock wave lithotripsy (ESWL)
   b. Ultrasonography of the right upper quadrant
   c. Endoscopic retrograde cholangiopancreatography (ERCP)
   d. Serum level of aspartate aminotransferase (AST)

9. Which type of drug is used to treat acute severe biliary pain?
   a. Acetaminophen (Tylenol)
   b. Nonsteroidal antiinflammatory drugs (NSAIDs) (Ibuprofen)
   c. Antiemetics (Compazine)
   d. Opioids (Morphine)

10. The nurse is administering ketorolac (Toradol) to a 78-year-old patient for mild to moderate pain management. Which assessment finding indicates the patient is experiencing a side effect of this drug?
    a. Abdominal bloating and cramping
    b. Ventricular cardiac dysrhythmias
    c. Decreased urinary output
    d. Jaundice

11. The nurse is caring for an older adult patient with acute biliary pain. Which drug order does the nurse question?
    a. Ketorolac (Toradol, Acular)
    b. Meperidine (Demerol)
    c. Morphine
    d. Hydromorphone (Dilaudid)

12. Which factor renders a patient the least likely to benefit from ESWL for the treatment of gallstones?
    a. Height 5 feet 10 inches, 325 lbs.
    b. Cholesterol-based stones
    c. Height 5 feet 7 inches, 138 lbs.
    d. Small gallstones

13. Which statements are true regarding laparoscopic cholecystectomy? *(Select all that apply.)*
    a. Laparoscopic cholecystectomy is considered the "gold standard" and is performed far more often than the traditional open approach.
    b. Patients with chronic lung disease or heart failure who are unable to tolerate the oxygen used in the laparoscopic procedure are examples of patients who have the open surgical approach (abdominal laparotomy).
    c. Removing the gallbladder with the laparoscopic technique reduces the risk of wound complications.
    d. Patients who have their gallbladders removed by the laparoscopic technique should be taught the importance of early ambulation to promote absorption of carbon dioxide.
    e. Use of laparoscopic cholecystectomy puts the patient at increased risk for bile duct injuries.

14. Which statement about the care of a patient with a Jackson-Pratt (JP) drain after a traditional cholecystectomy is true?
    a. The patient is maintained in the prone position.
    b. When the patient is allowed to eat, the JP drain is clamped continuously.
    c. The JP drain is irrigated every hour for the first 24 hours.
    d. Serosanguineous drainage stained with bile is expected for 24 hours.

15. The female patient is to have her gallbladder removed by natural orifice transluminal endoscopic surgery. What does the nurse teach about this surgery?
    a. The surgeon will use powerful shock waves to break up the gallstones.
    b. The surgeon will insert a transhepatic biliary catheter to open blocked bile ducts.
    c. The surgeon will use a vaginal approach to remove your gallbladder.
    d. The surgeon will inject ursodeoxycholic acid to dissolve any remaining gallstone fragments.

16. After removal of the gallbladder, a patient experiences abdominal pain with vomiting for several weeks. What does the nurse recognize?
    a. Chronic cholecystitis
    b. Recurrence of acute cholecystitis
    c. Unremoved gallstones
    d. Postcholecystectomy syndrome

17. The patient with acute cholecystitis had a pacemaker. Which diagnostic test is contraindicated?
    a. ERCP
    b. Magnetic resonance cholangiopancreatography (MRCP)
    c. Ultrasonography of the right upper quadrant
    d. Hepatobiliary (HIDA) scan

18. The nurse is evaluating electrolyte values for a patient with acute pancreatitis and notes that the serum calcium is 6.8 mEq/L. How does the nurse interpret this finding?
    a. Within normal limits considering the diagnosis of acute pancreatitis
    b. A result of the body not being able to use bound calcium
    c. A protective measure that will reduce the risk of complications
    d. Full compensation of the parathyroid gland

19. Disseminated intravascular coagulation (DIC) is a complication of pancreatitis. What pathophysiology leads to this complication?
    a. Hypovolemia
    b. Peritoneal irritation and seepage of pancreatic enzymes
    c. Disruption of alveolar-capillary membrane
    d. Consumption of clotting factors and microthrombi formation

20. The patient with acute pancreatitis experiences abdominal pain. What is the best intervention to begin management of this pain?
    a. IV opioids by means of patient-controlled analgesia (PCA)
    b. Oral opioids such as morphine sulfate given as needed
    c. Intramuscular opioids given every 6 hours
    d. Oral hydromorphone (Dilaudid) given twice a day

21. The patient comes to the emergency department (ED) with severe abdominal pain in the midepigastric area. The patient states that the pain began suddenly, is continuous, radiates to his back, and is worst when he lies flat on his back. What condition does the nurse suspect?
    a. Acute cholecystitis
    b. Pancreatic cancer
    c. Acute pancreatitis
    d. Pancreatic pseudocyst

22. Which diagnostic test is the most accurate in verifying a diagnosis of acute pancreatitis?
    a. Trypsin
    b. Lipase
    c. Alkaline phosphatase
    d. Alanine aminotransferase

23. A patient with acute pancreatitis is at risk for the development of paralytic (adynamic) ileus. Which action provides the nurse with the best indication of bowel function?
    a. Observing contents of the nasogastric drainage
    b. Weighing the patient every day at the same time
    c. Asking the patient if he or she has passed flatus or had a stool
    d. Obtaining a computed tomography (CT) scan of the abdomen with contrast medium

24. Which condition is most likely to be treated with antibiotics?
    a. Cancer of the gallbladder
    b. Acute cholelithiasis
    c. Chronic pancreatitis
    d. Acute necrotizing pancreatitis

25. The nurse has instructed a patient in the recovery phase of acute pancreatitis about diet therapy. Which statement by the patient indicates that teaching has been successful?
    a. "I will eat the usual three meals a day that I am used to."
    b. "I am eating tacos for my first meal back home."
    c. "I will avoid eating chocolate and drinking coffee."
    d. "I will limit the amount of protein in my diet."

26. The nursing student is caring for a patient with chronic pancreatitis who is receiving pancreatic enzyme replacement therapy. Which statement by the student indicates the need for further study concerning this therapy?
    a. "The enzymes will be administered with meals."
    b. "The patient will take the drugs with a glass of water."
    c. "If the patient has difficulty swallowing the enzyme preparation, I will crush it and mix it with foods."
    d. "The effectiveness of pancreatic enzyme treatment is monitored by the frequency and fat content of stools."

27. Which statements about pancreatic cancer are accurate? *(Select all that apply.)*
    a. Venous thromboembolism (VTE) is a common complication of pancreatic cancer.
    b. Pancreatic cancer often presents in a slow and vague manner.
    c. The most common concern of the patient with pancreatic cancer is pain.
    d. There are no specific blood tests to diagnose pancreatic cancer.
    e. Chemotherapy is the treatment of choice for pancreatic cancer.
    f. Chronic pancreatitis predisposes a patient to pancreatic cancer.

28. The nurse detects an epigastric mass while assessing a patient with acute pancreatitis. The patient describes epigastric pain that radiates to his back. What does the nurse suspect?
    a. Liver cirrhosis
    b. Pancreatic pseudocyst
    c. Gallstones
    d. Chronic pancreatitis

29. The nurse is caring for a patient with pancreatic cancer who had a Whipple procedure. Which interventions and assessments does the nurse implement? *(Select all that apply.)*
    a. Place the patient in semi-Fowler's position.
    b. Place the NG tube on intermittent suction.
    c. Monitor NG drainage, which should be bile-tinged and contain blood.
    d. Keep the patient NPO.
    e. Check blood glucose often.

30. What is the most common and serious complication after a Whipple procedure?
    a. Diabetes mellitus
    b. Wound infection
    c. Fistula development
    d. Bowel obstruction

31. Which are manifestations of pancreatic cancer? *(Select all that apply.)*
    a. Light-colored urine and dark-colored stools
    b. Anorexia and weight loss
    c. Splenomegaly
    d. Ascites
    e. Leg or calf pain
    f. Weakness and fatigue

32. The nurse is teaching a patient and family how to prevent exacerbations of chronic pancreatitis. Which teaching point does the nurse include?
    a. Moderation in the use of caffeinated beverages
    b. Avoidance of alcohol and nicotine
    c. Consume a bland, high-fat, low-protein diet
    d. Regular exercise, stressing aerobic activities

33. The patient is to continue pancreatic enzyme replacement therapy (PERT) after discharge. Which statement indicates that the patient understands teaching about this therapy?
    a. "I will take the enzymes before meals with a full glass of water."
    b. "I will take the enzymes after I take my ranitidine (Zantac)."
    c. "I will mix the enzymes with chopped meat."
    d. "I will chew the capsules before swallowing the enzymes."

34. Which are potential cardiovascular complications for a patient after surgery for a Whipple procedure? *(Select all that apply.)*
    a. Thrombophlebitis
    b. Pulmonary embolism
    c. Myocardial infarction
    d. Heart failure
    e. Renal failure

35. Which abnormal laboratory findings are cardinal findings in acute pancreatitis? *(Select all that apply.)*
    a. Elevated serum lipase
    b. Increased serum amylase
    c. Decreased serum trypsin
    d. Elevated serum elastase
    e. Elevated serum glucose

60 CHAPTER

Care of Patients with Malnutrition and Obesity

1. The nurse is assisting a patient who follows a lacto-vegetarian diet to fill out a menu. Based on this diet, which foods could the patient select for breakfast? *(Select all that apply.)*
   a. Milk
   b. Scrambled eggs
   c. Toast
   d. Sausage
   e. Cereal

2. The nurse is assisting a patient who follows a lacto-ovo-vegetarian diet to fill out a menu. Based on this diet, which foods could the patient select for breakfast? *(Select all that apply.)*
   a. Milk
   b. Scrambled eggs
   c. Toast
   d. Sausage
   e. Cereal

3. When caloric energy is inadequate, what does the body use for energy?
   a. Carbohydrates
   b. Proteins
   c. Glucose
   d. Fats

4. Which statement by the new graduate nurse about nutritional assessment requires clarification by the student's mentor?
   a. "A complete nutritional assessment must be completed on every patient admitted to the hospital."
   b. "A nutritional screening must be completed on every patient admitted to the hospital."
   c. "An unintentional weight loss of 10% within a 6-month period should be evaluated."
   d. "Measurement of height and weight are part of the nutritional assessment."

5. Which activity of a nutritional assessment can be delegated to the unlicensed assistive personnel (UAP)?
   a. Review of the patient's nutritional history
   b. Review of the patient's laboratory data
   c. Obtaining the patient's height and weight
   d. Psychosocial assessment of the patient

6. Which signs/symptoms in an older adult can be an indication of "failure to thrive?" *(Select all that apply.)*
   a. Weakness
   b. Slow walking speed
   c. Decreased meal enjoyment
   d. Low physical activity
   e. Unintentional weight loss
   f. Exhaustion

7. The nurse is providing teaching about the risk factors for malnutrition for a group of older adults. What factors does the nurse emphasize in the teaching plan? *(Select all that apply.)*
   a. Poor dental health
   b. Hypersecretion of saliva
   c. Depression
   d. Fatigue
   e. Lack of transportation

8. A patient is malnourished. What is the priority nursing intervention?
   a. Determine the patient's food preferences.
   b. Provide the patient with high-calorie, high-protein food.
   c. Weigh the patient.
   d. Offer the patient snacks.

9. The nurse is caring for three patients who have undergone bariatric surgery. Which activity is most appropriate for the nurse to delegate to the UAP?
   a. Give analgesics about 1 hour before mealtimes.
   b. Document the percentage of food eaten at mealtimes.
   c. Assess the patient's food preferences.
   d. Teach the patient about portion control.

10. After the UAP tells the nurse that an older patient will not eat her dinner, the nurse enters the patient's room to assess the situation. Which factors likely contribute to the patient's lack of desire to eat? *(Select all that apply.)*
    a. An emesis basin is on the bedside table.
    b. The volume of the television is loud.
    c. The food is cold.
    d. The cleaning lady is in the room disinfecting the bathroom.
    e. Cartons and packages are opened and food has been cut into bite-sized pieces.
    f. The patient's roommate has two adults and three children visiting.

11. The nurse is teaching a male patient about the 2010 Dietary Guidelines for Americans. Which statement by the patient indicates a need for additional teaching?
    a. "I'll limit consumption of alcohol to two drinks a day."
    b. "I'll consume at least 6 cups of whole milk products a day."
    c. "I'll increase my intake of fruits and vegetables."
    d. "I'll limit added sugar and salt in my diet."

12. Which manifestation(s) would the nurse expect to see in a patient with a vitamin D deficit?
    a. Swollen, bleeding gums
    b. Hepatomegaly
    c. Osteomalacia, bone pain, rickets
    d. Xerosis of conjunctiva

13. The patient has alopecia. Which nutritional deficiency is the likely cause?
    a. Zinc
    b. Vitamin A
    c. Riboflavin
    d. Vitamin C

14. What is the most reliable indicator of fluid status?
    a. Intake and output
    b. Trends in weight
    c. Skin turgor
    d. Edema

15. The nurse hears the UAP instructing a new UAP about obtaining patients' weights. Which statements by the UAP indicate a need for clarification? *(Select all that apply.)*
    a. "It is best to weigh the patients before breakfast."
    b. "Just ask the patients how much they weigh."
    c. "You can weigh the patients whenever you have time during your shift."
    d. "Weigh the patients while they are in minimal clothing and no shoes."
    e. "Ambulatory patients can be weighed on the upright scales."

16. Which is the most accurate way to obtain a height measurement for a patient who cannot stand?
    a. Review the patient's old chart.
    b. Ask the patient's family member.
    c. Estimate height based on the patient's position in bed.
    d. Use a sliding blade knee height caliper.

17. Which statements about body mass index (BMI) measurements are accurate? *(Select all that apply.)*
    a. It is a measure of nutritional status that varies according to frame size.
    b. It is based on a formula using height and weight.
    c. Health risks are associated with BMIs >25.
    d. It indirectly estimates total fat scores.
    e. There are no health risks associated with a low BMI.

18. The nurse is providing discharge instructions to the family of an older female patient who was admitted for failure to thrive. The patient has a history of osteoarthritis, stroke, and dementia. What information does the nurse include to promote nutritional intake? *(Select all that apply.)*
    a. Do not allow her to get out of bed while eating.
    b. Withhold analgesics prior to meals.
    c. Be sure she has her glasses and hearing aid on.
    d. Encourage self-feeding as much as possible.
    e. Keep environmental noise to a minimum.

19. The nurse is assessing a patient with acquired immune deficiency syndrome (AIDS) who has muscle wasting related to poor nutrition. How does the nurse interpret this finding?
    a. Cachexia
    b. Candidiasis
    c. Protein catabolism
    d. Positive nitrogen balance

20. Which characteristics are consistent with bulimia nervosa? *(Select all that apply.)*
    a. It is self-induced starvation.
    b. There are episodes of binge eating.
    c. Binge eating is followed by purging.
    d. It is most often seen in older adults.
    e. It is most often seen in teens and young adults.

21. The nurse assesses for which potential complications in a patient who is malnourished? *(Select all that apply.)*
    a. Poor wound healing
    b. Intolerance to heat
    c. Infection
    d. Lethargy
    e. Edema

22. Which intervention does the nurse delegate to the UAP to promote nutritional intake for an older patient?
    a. Feed the patient even if he/she is able to self-feed.
    b. Assess which foods the patient likes to eat.
    c. Administer analgesic medication before meals.
    d. Assist the patient to sit up in a chair for meals.

23. Which laboratory test is a sensitive indicator of protein deficiency in a malnourished patient?
    a. Cholesterol
    b. Total lymphocyte count (TLC)
    c. Serum albumin
    d. Prealbumin

24. Which lab value is usually low in patients with malabsorption, liver disease, pernicious anemia, terminal cancer, and sepsis?
    a. Cholesterol
    b. Hematocrit
    c. Hemoglobin
    d. Albumin

25. The nurse is providing discharge instructions to a patient who is malnourished and will be taking iron supplements at home. Which statement by the patient indicates a correct understanding of the instructions?
    a. "These supplements may cause me to have diarrhea."
    b. "I will take these supplements with my meals."
    c. "I will limit my fiber intake from now on."
    d. "I will limit my fluid intake from now on."

26. Total enteral nutrition (TEN) is contraindicated for which patient?
    a. Older adult receiving chemotherapy
    b. Patient who has had a stroke and has dysphagia
    c. Patient who has had extensive jaw and mouth surgery
    d. Patient with intestinal obstruction that has progressed to diffuse peritonitis

27. The patient is receiving intermittent feedings of a specified amount at specified times through a feeding tube. Which type of feeding is the patient receiving?
    a. Bolus feeding tube
    b. Continuous feeding tube
    c. Cycle feeding tube
    d. Gravity tube feeding

28. What is the most reliable method to confirm initial placement of nasoduodenal or nasogastric (NG) tube placement?
    a. Auscultation
    b. X-ray
    c. Capnometry
    d. Testing pH of gastric contents

29. After initial placement of nasoduodenal and NG tubes is confirmed, how often must the placement be checked? (Select all that apply.)
    a. Before intermittent feeding
    b. Before medication administration
    c. Every 4 to 8 hours during feeding
    d. It is not necessary to recheck placement
    e. According to facility policy

30. The nurse is using capnometry testing to check NG tube placement prior to medication administration and the capnometry test is positive for carbon dioxide. What action does the nurse take?
    a. Administer the medication orally.
    b. Remove the NG tube.
    c. Administer the medication through the NG tube.
    d. Verify placement by auscultation.

31. The nurse is caring for a patient receiving a continuous feeding through an NG tube. Which position is best to prevent aspiration?
    a. Semi-Fowler's
    b. Trendelenburg
    c. Supine
    d. Sims'

32. Which interventions are necessary to provide safe, quality care to a patient receiving enteral tube feeding? (Select all that apply.)
    a. Check the residual volume every 4 to 6 hours.
    b. Change the feeding bag and tubing every 12 hours.
    c. Keep the head of the bed elevated at least 30 degrees.
    d. Use clean technique when changing the feeding system.
    e. Allow closed system containers to hang for 24 hours.

33. A patient is receiving a tube feeding. Which action by the student nurse requires intervention by the supervising nurse?
    a. Weighing the patient
    b. Placing food coloring in the tube feeding to assess for aspiration
    c. Discarding any unused open cans of feeding solution after 24 hours
    d. Monitoring the patient for the development of diarrhea

34. Which statement about a patient with a tube feeding indicates best practice for patient safety and quality care?
    a. If the tube becomes clogged, use 30 mL of water for flushing, while applying gentle pressure with a 50-mL piston syringe.
    b. Use cranberry juice to flush the tube if it is clogged.
    c. When administering medications, use cold water to dissolve the drug before administering it.
    d. Administer drugs down the feeding tube without flushing first, but flush the feeding tube after the drug is given.

35. A patient in a starvation state has been started on enteral feedings. The nurse assesses the patient and finds shallow respirations, weakness, acute confusion, and oozing from the IV site. What does the nurse suspect is happening in this patient?
    a. Septicemia
    b. Hypoglycemia
    c. Aspiration
    d. Refeeding syndrome

36. Which statement describes the correct method of testing the pH of gastrointestinal (GI) contents at the bedside?
    a. The tube is in the stomach if the pH reading is 8.0.
    b. Before aspirating the GI contents, flush the tube with 10 mL of air.
    c. If the patient takes certain medications such as H_2 blockers, the pH of the stomach is usually 2.0.
    d. Wait at least 1 hour after drug administration before assessing the pH of GI contents.

37. A patient receiving intravenous fat emulsions should be monitored closely for which manifestations of fat overload syndrome? *(Select all that apply.)*
    a. Increased triglycerides
    b. Clotting problems
    c. Fever
    d. Multisystem organ failure
    e. Excessive weight gain
    f. Infection

38. The nurse is assessing a patient receiving total parenteral nutrition (TPN) at 100 mL/hour. The TPN solution has 50 mL left in the bag. The nurse looks for the next bag of TPN, but it is not on the unit. When the pharmacy is called, the nurse is told it will take at least 1 hour for the next bag of TPN solution to be delivered. What does the nurse do?
    a. Call the health care provider.
    b. Administer 10% dextrose/water (D/W) until the TPN is available.
    c. Prepare to treat the patient for hyperglycemia.
    d. Cap the TPN line until the next TPN solution is available.

39. Which definition best describes morbid obesity?
    a. Weight that has a severely negative effect on health
    b. Excessive amount of body fat when compared to lean body mass
    c. Increase in body weight for height as compared to a standard
    d. Excessive amount of body weight requiring surgical intervention

40. Which statements about obesity are accurate? *(Select all that apply.)*
    a. Waist-to-hip ratio (WHR) is a strong predictor of colon cancer.
    b. Obesity is the second-leading cause of preventable deaths in the United States.
    c. Genetics have been found to have no role in obesity.
    d. Drug therapy is the first-line treatment for obesity.
    e. Waist circumference is a stronger predictor of coronary artery disease than is BMI.

41. The nurse is performing an admission assessment on a morbidly obese patient. Which common complications of obesity does the nurse assess for? *(Select all that apply.)*
    a. Type 1 diabetes mellitus
    b. Metabolic syndrome
    c. Urinary incontinence
    d. Gout
    e. Early osteoarthritis

42. Which prescribed drugs can contribute to weight gain when they are taken on a long-term basis? *(Select all that apply.)*
    a. Estrogens
    b. Acetaminophen
    c. Corticosteroids
    d. Nonsteroidal antiinflammatory drugs (NSAIDs)
    e. Antiepileptics

43. Which drugs are available for long-term treatment of obesity? *(Select all that apply.)*
    a. Phentermine-topiramate (Qsymia)
    b. Lorcaserin (Belviq)
    c. Sibutramine (Meridia)
    d. Orlistat (Xenical)
    e. Diethylpropion (Tenuate)

44. The nurse is caring for a patient after bariatric surgery. What is the nursing priority for this patient?
    a. Nutritional intake
    b. Pain management
    c. Prevention of infection
    d. Airway management

45. Which criteria make a patient a candidate for surgical treatment of obesity? *(Select all that apply.)*
    a. Repeated failure with nonsurgical interventions
    b. Waist circumference greater than 40 inches
    c. A BMI greater than or equal to 40
    d. Waist-to-hip ratio of greater than 0.95
    e. Weight more than 100% above ideal body weight

46. A patient comes to the clinic after having bariatric surgery and says, "After I eat, I feel really funny. My heart races, I feel nauseated, and my abdomen cramps up. I even have diarrhea." What does the nurse suspect is happening with this patient?
    a. Hyperglycemia
    b. Intestinal obstruction
    c. Peritonitis
    d. Dumping syndrome

47. The nurse is assessing a patient after bariatric surgery. The patient has increased back pain, is restless, has a heart rate of 126/minute and has only 15 mL of urine output for the past hour. What does the nurse suspect?
    a. Anastomotic leak
    b. Hypovolemic shock
    c. Bowel obstruction
    d. Hemorrhage

48. After bariatric surgery, which interventions does the nurse implement to prevent complications? *(Select all that apply.)*
    a. Apply an abdominal binder.
    b. Place the patient in semi-Fowler's position.
    c. Keep the patient on bedrest for 24 hours.
    d. Monitor oxygen saturation.
    e. Apply sequential compression stockings.
    f. Observe skin folds for redness and excoriation.

49. The nurse is preparing discharge teaching for a patient after bariatric surgery. Which key teaching points will the nurse be sure to include? *(Select all that apply.)*
    a. Diet progression, importance of vitamin supplements and hydration
    b. Take analgesics every 4 hours whether there is pain or not
    c. Restrictions on activities such as heavy lifting
    d. Follow the health care provider's instructions for progression of activity
    e. Cover wound during bath or shower

50. The patient who had bariatric surgery and is to be discharged asks the nurse when to expect the panniculectomy surgery. What is the nurse's best response?
    a. Usually in 6 to 8 months
    b. Usually in 12 to 18 months
    c. Usually in 18 to 24 months
    d. When your weight stabilizes

61 CHAPTER

Assessment of the Endocrine System

1. Which glands are parts of the endocrine system? *(Select all that apply.)*
   a. Thyroid
   b. Occipital
   c. Parathyroid
   d. Adrenal
   e. Pituitary

2. What is the name of the substance secreted by the endocrine glands?
   a. Vasoactive amines
   b. Chemotaxins
   c. Hormones
   d. Cytotoxins

3. Which mechanism is used to transport the substance produced by the endocrine glands to their target tissue?
   a. Lymph system
   b. Bloodstream
   c. Direct seeding
   d. Gastrointestinal system

4. Which hormones are secreted by the posterior pituitary gland? *(Select all that apply.)*
   a. Testosterone
   b. Oxytocin
   c. Growth hormone (GH)
   d. Antidiuretic hormone (ADH)
   e. Cortisol

5. Which hormones are secreted by the thyroid gland? *(Select all that apply.)*
   a. Calcitonin
   b. Somatostatin
   c. Glucagon
   d. Thyroxine (T_4)
   e. Aldosterone
   f. Triiodothyronine (T_3)

6. A patient has a low serum cortisol level. Which hormone would the nurse expect to be secreted to correct this?
   a. Thyroid-stimulating hormone (TSH)
   b. Adrenocorticotropic hormone
   c. Parathyroid hormone
   d. Antidiuretic hormone

7. The target tissue for ADH is which organ?
   a. Hypothalamus
   b. Thyroid
   c. Ovary
   d. Kidney

8. Which statements about hormones and the endocrine system are accurate? *(Select all that apply.)*
   a. There are specific normal blood levels of each hormone.
   b. Hormones exert their effects on specific target tissues.
   c. Each hormone can bind with multiple receptor sites.
   d. The endocrine system works independently to regulate homeostasis.
   e. More than one hormone can be stimulated before the target tissue is affected.

9. The binding of a hormone to a specific receptor site is an example of which endocrine process?
   a. "Lock and key" manner
   b. Negative feedback mechanism
   c. Neuroendocrine regulation
   d. "Fight-or-flight" response

10. What are tropic hormones?
    a. Hormones that trigger female and male sex characteristics.
    b. Hormones that have a direct effect on final target tissues.
    c. Hormones produced by the anterior pituitary gland that stimulate other endocrine glands.
    d. Hormones that are synthesized in the hypothalamus and stored in the posterior pituitary gland.

11. Which hormone is directly suppressed when circulating levels of cortisol are above normal?
    a. Corticotropin-releasing hormone (CRH)
    b. ADH
    c. Adrenocorticotropic hormone (ACTH)
    d. Growth hormone–releasing hormone (GH-RH)

12. The maintenance of internal body temperature at approximately 98.6° F (37° C) is an example of which endocrine process?
    a. "Lock and key" manner
    b. Neuroendocrine regulation
    c. Positive feedback mechanism
    d. Stimulus-response theory

13. Which statements about the pituitary glands are correct? *(Select all that apply.)*
    a. The main role of the anterior pituitary is to secrete tropic hormones.
    b. The posterior pituitary gland stores hormones produced by the hypothalamus.
    c. The anterior pituitary is connected to the thalamus gland.
    d. The anterior pituitary releases stored hormones produced by the hypothalamus.
    e. The anterior pituitary gland secretes gonadotropins.

14. The anterior pituitary gland secretes tropic hormones in response to which hormones from the hypothalamus?
    a. Releasing hormones
    b. Target tissue hormones
    c. Growth hormones
    d. Demand hormones

15. Which statement about pituitary hormones is correct?
    a. ACTH acts on the adrenal medulla.
    b. Follicle-stimulating hormone (FSH) stimulates sperm production in men.
    c. Growth hormone promotes protein catabolism.
    d. Vasopressin decreases systolic blood pressure.

16. Which statement about the gonads is correct?
    a. Gonads are reproductive glands found in males only.
    b. The function of the hormones begins at birth in low, undetectable levels.
    c. The placenta secretes testosterone for the development of male external genitalia.
    d. External genitalia maturation is stimulated by gonadotropins during puberty.

17. Which statements about the adrenal glands are correct? *(Select all that apply.)*
    a. The cortex secretes androgens in men and women.
    b. Catecholamines are secreted from the cortex.
    c. Glucocorticoids are secreted by the medulla.
    d. The medulla secretes hormones essential for life.
    e. The cortex secretes aldosterone that maintains extracellular fluid volume.

18. Which is the major function of the hormones produced by the adrenal cortex?
    a. "Fight-or-flight" response
    b. Control of potassium, sodium, and water
    c. Regulation of cell growth
    d. Calcium and stress regulation

19. Which statements about the hormone cortisol being secreted by the adrenal cortex are accurate? *(Select all that apply.)*
    a. Cortisol peaks occur late in the day, with lowest points 12 hours after each peak.
    b. Cortisol has an effect on the body's immune function.
    c. Stress causes an increase in the production of cortisol.
    d. Blood levels of cortisol have no effect on its secretion.
    e. Cortisol affects carbohydrate, protein, and fat metabolism.

20. Which assessment findings does the nurse monitor in response to catecholamines released by the adrenal medulla? *(Select all that apply.)*
    a. Increased heart rate related to vasoconstriction
    b. Increased blood pressure related to vasoconstriction
    c. Increased perspiration
    d. Constriction of pupils
    e. Increased blood glucose in response to glycogenolysis

21. Which statements about the thyroid gland and its hormones are correct? *(Select all that apply.)*
    a. The gland is located in the posterior neck below the cricoid cartilage.
    b. The gland has two lobes joined by a thin tissue called the *isthmus*.
    c. T_4 and T_3 are two thyroid hormones.
    d. Thyroid hormones increase red blood cell production.
    e. Thyroid hormone production depends on dietary intake of iodine and potassium.

22. Which hormone responds to a low serum calcium blood level by increasing bone resorption?
    a. Parathyroid hormone (PTH)
    b. T_4
    c. T_3
    d. Calcitonin

23. Which hormone responds to elevated serum calcium blood level by decreasing bone resorption?
    a. PTH
    b. T_4
    c. T_3
    d. Calcitonin

24. Which statements about T_3 and T_4 hormones are correct? *(Select all that apply.)*
    a. The basal metabolic rate is affected.
    b. Hypothalamus is stimulated by cold and stress to secrete thyrotropin-releasing hormone (TRH).
    c. These hormones need intake of protein and iodine for production.
    d. Circulating hormone in the blood directly affects the production of TSH.
    e. T_3 and T_4 increase oxygen use in tissues.

25. Which are the target organs of PTH in the regulation of calcium and phosphorus? *(Select all that apply.)*
    a. Stomach
    b. Kidney
    c. Bone
    d. Gastrointestinal tract
    e. Thyroid gland

26. Which statement about the pancreas is correct?
    a. Endocrine functions of the pancreas include secretion of digestive enzymes.
    b. Exocrine functions of the pancreas include secretion of glucagon and insulin.
    c. The islets of Langerhans are the only source of somatostatin secretion.
    d. Somatostatin inhibits pancreatic secretion of glucagon and insulin.

27. Which statement about glucagon secretion is correct?
    a. It is stimulated by an increase in blood glucose levels.
    b. It is stimulated by a decrease in amino acid levels.
    c. It exerts its primary effect on the pancreas.
    d. It acts to increase blood glucose levels.

28. Which statements about insulin secretion are correct? *(Select all that apply.)*
    a. Insulin levels increase following the ingestion of a meal.
    b. Insulin is stimulated primarily by fat ingestion.
    c. Basal levels are secreted continuously.
    d. Insulin promotes glycogenolysis and gluconeogenesis.
    e. Carbohydrate intake is the main trigger for insulin secretion.

29. In addition to the pancreas that secretes insulin, which gland secretes hormones that affect protein, carbohydrate, and fat metabolism?
    a. Posterior pituitary
    b. Thyroid
    c. Ovaries
    d. Parathyroid

30. The bloodstream delivers glucose to the cells for energy production. Which hormone controls the cells' use of glucose?
    a. T_4
    b. Growth hormone
    c. Adrenal steroids
    d. Insulin

31. Which disease involves a disorder of the islets of Langerhans?
    a. Diabetes insipidus
    b. Diabetes mellitus
    c. Addison's disease
    d. Cushing's disease

32. Which endocrine tissues are most commonly found to have reduced function as a result of aging? *(Select all that apply.)*
    a. Hypothalamus
    b. Ovaries
    c. Testes
    d. Pancreas
    e. Thyroid gland

33. Which statement about age-related changes in older adults and the endocrine system is true?
    a. All hormone levels are elevated.
    b. Thyroid hormone levels decrease.
    c. Adrenal glands enlarge.
    d. The thyroid gland enlarges.

34. In the older adult female, which physiologic changes occur as a result of decreased function of the ovaries?
    a. Decreased bone density, decreased production of estrogen
    b. Decreased sensitivity of peripheral tissues to the effects of insulin
    c. Decreased urine-concentrating ability of the kidneys
    d. Decreased metabolic rate

35. An older adult reports a lack of energy and not being able to do the usual daily activities without several naps during the day. Which problem may these symptoms indicate that is often seen in the older adult?
    a. Hypothyroidism
    b. Hyperparathyroidism
    c. Overproduction of cortisol
    d. Underproduction of glucagon

36. The nurse is performing a physical assessment of a patient's endocrine system. Which gland can be palpated?
    a. Pancreas
    b. Thyroid
    c. Adrenal glands
    d. Parathyroids

37. Which statement about performing a physical assessment of the thyroid gland is correct?
    a. The thyroid gland is easily palpated in all patients.
    b. The patient is instructed to swallow sips of water to aid palpation.
    c. The anterior approach is preferred for thyroid palpation.
    d. The thumbs are used to palpate the thyroid lobes.

38. Which are diagnostic methods to measure patient hormone levels? *(Select all that apply.)*
    a. Stimulation testing
    b. Suppression testing
    c. 24-hour urine testing
    d. Chromatographic assay
    e. Needle biopsy

39. What is the correct nursing action before beginning a 24-hour urine collection for endocrine studies?
    a. Place each voided specimen in a separate collection container.
    b. Check whether any preservatives are needed in the collection container.
    c. Start the collection with the first voided urine.
    d. Weigh the patient before beginning the collection.

40. Which instructions are included when teaching a patient about urine collection for endocrine studies? *(Select all that apply.)*
    a. Fast before starting the urine collection.
    b. Measure the urine in mL rather than ounces.
    c. Empty the bladder completely, and then start timing.
    d. Time the test for exactly the instructed number of hours.
    e. Avoid taking any unnecessary drugs during endocrine testing.
    f. Empty the bladder at the end of the time period and keep that specimen.

41. Which are the types of radiographic tests that may be used for an endocrine assessment? *(Select all that apply.)*
    a. Ultrasonography
    b. Skull x-ray
    c. Chest x-ray
    d. Magnetic resonance imaging (MRI)
    e. Computed tomography (CT)

42. A patient is suspected of having a pituitary tumor. Which radiographic test aids in determining this diagnosis?
    a. Skull x-rays
    b. MRI/CT
    c. Angiography
    d. Ultrasound

43. After an ultrasound of the thyroid gland, which diagnostic test determines the need for surgical intervention for thyroid nodules?
    a. CT scan
    b. MRI
    c. Angiography
    d. Needle biopsy

44. A patient is at risk for falling related to the effect of pathologic fractures as a result of bone demineralization. Which endocrine problem is this pertinent to?
    a. Underproduction of PTH
    b. Overproduction of PTH
    c. Underproduction of thyroid hormone
    d. Overproduction of thyroid hormone

62
CHAPTER

Care of Patients with Pituitary and Adrenal Gland Problems

1. Problems in the hypothalamus that change the function of the anterior pituitary gland result in which condition?
   a. Adenohypophysis
   b. Panhypopituitarism
   c. Primary pituitary dysfunction
   d. Secondary pituitary dysfunction

2. A malfunctioning posterior pituitary gland can result in which disorders? *(Select all that apply.)*
   a. Hypothyroidism
   b. Altered sexual function
   c. Diabetes insipidus (DI)
   d. Growth retardation
   e. Syndrome of inappropriate antidiuretic hormone (SIADH)

3. A malfunctioning anterior pituitary gland can result in which disorders? *(Select all that apply.)*
   a. Pituitary hypofunction
   b. Pituitary hyperfunction
   c. DI
   d. Hypothyroidism
   e. Osteoporosis

4. The assessment findings of a male patient with anterior pituitary tumor include reports of changes in secondary sex characteristics, such as episodes of impotence and decreased libido. The nurse explains to the patient that these findings are a result of overproduction of which hormone?
   a. Gonadotropins inhibiting prolactin (PRL)
   b. Thyroid hormone inhibiting PRL
   c. PRL inhibiting secretion of gonadotropins
   d. Steroids inhibiting production of sex hormones

5. A patient with a PRL-secreting tumor is likely to be treated with which medication?
   a. Dopamine agonists
   b. Vasopressin
   c. Steroids
   d. Growth hormone (GH)

6. A patient is prescribed bromocriptine mesylate (Parlodel). Which information does the nurse teach the patient? *(Select all that apply.)*
   a. Get up slowly from a lying position.
   b. Take medication on an empty stomach.
   c. Take daily for purposes of raising GH levels to reduce symptom of acromegaly.
   d. Begin therapy with a maintenance level dose.
   e. Report watery nasal discharge to the health care provider immediately.

7. Patients diagnosed with an anterior pituitary tumor can have symptoms of acromegaly or gigantism. These symptoms are a result of overproduction of which hormone?
   a. ACTH
   b. PRL
   c. Gonadotropins
   d. GH

8. The nurse is performing an assessment of an adult patient with new-onset acromegaly. What does the nurse expect to find?
   a. Extremely long arms and legs
   b. Thickened lips
   c. Changes in menses with infertility
   d. Rough, extremely dry skin

9. When analyzing laboratory values, the nurse expects to find which value as a direct result of overproduction of GH?
   a. Hyperglycemia
   b. Hyperphosphatemia
   c. Hypocalcemia
   d. Hypercalcemia

10. In caring for a patient with hyperpituitarism, which symptoms does the nurse expect the patient to report? *(Select all that apply.)*
    a. Joint pain
    b. Visual disturbances
    c. Changes in menstruation
    d. Increased libido
    e. Headache
    f. Fatigue

11. A deficiency of which anterior pituitary hormones is considered life-threatening? *(Select all that apply.)*
    a. GH
    b. Melanocyte-stimulating hormone (MSH)
    c. PRL
    d. Thyroid-stimulating hormone (TSH)
    e. ACTH

12. Which statements about the etiology of hypopituitarism are correct? *(Select all that apply.)*
    a. Dysfunction can result from radiation treatment to the head or brain.
    b. Dysfunction can result from infection or a brain tumor.
    c. Infarction following systemic shock can result in hypopituitarism.
    d. Severe malnutrition and body fat depletion can depress pituitary gland function.
    e. There is always an underlying cause of hypopituitarism.

13. Which statement about hormone replacement therapy for hypopituitarism is correct?
    a. Once manifestations of hypofunction are corrected, treatment is no longer needed.
    b. The most effective route of androgen replacement is the oral route.
    c. Testosterone replacement therapy is contraindicated in men with prostate cancer.
    d. Clomiphene citrate (Clomid) is used to suppress ovulation in women.

14. A female patient has been prescribed hormone replacement therapy. What does the nurse instruct the patient to do regarding this therapy?
    a. Report any recurrence of symptoms, such as decreased libido, between injections.
    b. Monitor blood pressure at least weekly for potential hypotension.
    c. Treat leg pain, especially in the calves, with gentle muscle stretching.
    d. Take measures to reduce risk for hypertension and thrombosis.

15. A patient requires 100 g of oral glucose for suppression testing and GH levels are measured serially for 120 minutes. The results of the suppression testing are abnormal. The nurse assesses for the signs and symptoms of which endocrine disorder?
    a. Adrenal insufficiency
    b. DI
    c. Hyperpituitarism
    d. Hypothyroidism

16. A patient is recovering from a transsphenoidal hypophysectomy. What postoperative nursing interventions apply to this patient? *(Select all that apply.)*
    a. Encouraging the patient to perform deep-breathing exercises
    b. Vigorous coughing and deep-breathing exercises
    c. Instructing on the use of a soft-bristled toothbrush for brushing the teeth
    d. Strict monitoring of fluid balance
    e. Hourly neurologic checks for first 24 hours
    f. Instructing the patient to alert the nurse regarding postnasal drip

17. Following a hypophysectomy, the patient requires instruction on hormone replacement for which hormones? *(Select all that apply.)*
    a. Cortisol
    b. Thyroid
    c. Gonadal
    d. Vasopressin
    e. PRL

18. After a hypophysectomy, home care monitoring by the nurse includes assessing which factors? *(Select all that apply.)*
    a. Hypoglycemia
    b. Bowel habits
    c. Possible leakage of cerebrospinal fluid (CSF)
    d. 24-hour intake of fluids and urine output
    e. 24-hour diet recall
    f. Activity level

19. Postoperative care for a patient who has had a transsphenoidal hypophysectomy includes which intervention?
    a. Encouraging coughing and deep-breathing to decrease pulmonary complications
    b. Testing nasal drainage for glucose to determine whether it contains CSF
    c. Keeping the bed flat to decrease central CSF leakage
    d. Assisting the patient with brushing the teeth to reduce risk of infection

20. While caring for a postoperative patient following a transsphenoidal hypophysectomy, the nurse observes nasal drainage that is clear with yellow color at the edge. This "halo sign" is indicative of which condition?
    a. Worsening neurologic status of the patient
    b. Drainage of CSF from the patient's nose
    c. Onset of postoperative infection
    d. An expected finding following this surgery

21. A patient with a hypophysectomy can postoperatively experience transient DI. Which manifestation alerts the nurse to this problem?
    a. Output much greater than intake
    b. Change in mental status indicating confusion
    c. Laboratory results indicating hyponatremia
    d. Nonpitting edema

22. The action of antidiuretic hormone (ADH) influences normal kidney function by stimulating which mechanism?
    a. Glomerulus to control the filtration rate
    b. Proximal nephron tubules to reabsorb water
    c. Distal nephron tubules and collecting ducts to reabsorb water
    d. Constriction of glomerular capillaries to prevent loss of protein in urine

23. What is the disorder that results from a deficiency of vasopressin (ADH) from the posterior pituitary gland called?
    a. SIADH
    b. DI
    c. Cushing's syndrome
    d. Addison's disease

24. Which statements about DI are accurate? *(Select all that apply.)*
    a. It is caused by ADH deficiency.
    b. It is characterized by a decrease in urination.
    c. Urine output of greater than 4 L/24 hours is the first diagnostic indication.
    d. The water loss increases plasma osmolarity.
    e. Nephrogenic DI can be caused by lithium (Eskalith).

25. What does the nurse instruct patients with permanent DI to do? *(Select all that apply.)*
    a. Continue vasopressin therapy until symptoms disappear.
    b. Monitor for recurrence of polydipsia and polyuria.
    c. Monitor and record weight daily.
    d. Check urine specific gravity three times a week.
    e. Wear a medical alert bracelet.

26. A hospitalized patient is prescribed desmopressin acetate metered dose spray as a replacement hormone for ADH. Which is an indication for another dose? *(Select all that apply.)*
    a. Excessive urination
    b. Specific gravity of 1.003
    c. Dark, concentrated urine
    d. Edema in the legs
    e. Decreased urination

27. The nurse is caring for a patient with DI. What is the priority goal of collaborative care?
    a. Correct the water metabolism problem.
    b. Control blood sugar and blood pH.
    c. Measure urine output, specific gravity, and osmolality hourly.
    d. Monitor closely for respiratory distress.

28. Which medication is used to treat DI?
    a. Desmopressin acetate (DDAVP)
    b. Lithium (Eskalith)
    c. Vasopressin (Pitressin)
    d. Demeclocycline (Declomycin)

29. Which patient's history puts him or her at risk for developing SIADH?
    a. 27-year-old patient on high-dose steroids
    b. 47-year-old hospitalized adult patient with acute renal failure
    c. 58-year-old with metastatic lung or breast cancer
    d. Older adult with history of a stroke within the last year

30. Which statement about the pathophysiology of SIADH is correct?
    a. ADH secretion is inhibited in the presence of low plasma osmolality.
    b. Water retention results in dilutional hyponatremia and expanded extracellular fluid (ECF) volume.
    c. The glomerulus is unable to increase its filtration rate to reduce the excess plasma volume.
    d. Renin and aldosterone are released and help decrease the loss of urinary sodium.

31. The effect of increased ADH in the blood results in which effect on the kidney?
    a. Urine concentration tends to decrease.
    b. Glomerular filtration tends to decrease.
    c. Tubular reabsorption of water increases.
    d. Tubular reabsorption of sodium increases.

32. In SIADH, as a result of water retention from excess ADH, which laboratory value does the nurse expect to find? *(Select all that apply.)*
    a. Increased sodium in urine
    b. Elevated serum sodium level
    c. Increased specific gravity (concentrated urine)
    d. Decreased serum osmolarity
    e. Decreased urine specific gravity

33. Which nursing intervention is the priority for a patient with SIADH?
    a. Restrict fluid intake.
    b. Monitor neurologic status at least every 2 hours.
    c. Offer ice chips frequently to ease discomfort of dry mouth.
    d. Monitor urine tests for decreased sodium levels and low specific gravity.

34. Which type of IV fluid does the nurse use to treat a patient with SIADH when the serum sodium level is very low?
    a. $D_5$1/2 normal saline
    b. D_5W
    c. 3% normal saline
    d. Normal saline

35. In addition to IV fluids, a patient with SIADH is on a fluid restriction as low as 500 to 600 mL/24 hours. Which serum and urine results demonstrate effectiveness of this treatment? *(Select all that apply.)*
    a. Decreased urine specific gravity
    b. Decreased serum sodium
    c. Increased urine output
    d. Increased urine specific gravity
    e. Increased serum sodium
    f. Decreased urine output

36. Which medications are used in SIADH to promote water excretion without causing sodium loss? *(Select all that apply.)*
    a. Tolvaptan (Samsca)
    b. Demeclocycline (Declomycin)
    c. Furosemide (Lasix)
    d. Conivaptan (Vaprisol)
    e. Spironolactone (Aldactone)

37. Which statement about pheochromocytoma is correct?
    a. It is most often malignant.
    b. It is a catecholamine-producing tumor.
    c. It is found only in the adrenal medulla.
    d. It is manifested by hypotension.

38. A patient in the emergency department is diagnosed with possible pheochromocytoma. What is the priority nursing intervention for this patient?
    a. Monitor the patient's intake and output and urine specific gravity.
    b. Monitor blood pressure for severe hypertension.
    c. Monitor blood pressure for severe hypotension.
    d. Administer medication to increase cardiac output.

39. The nurse expects to perform which diagnostic test for pheochromocytoma?
    a. 24-hour urine collection for sodium, potassium, and glucose
    b. Catecholamine-stimulation test
    c. Administration of beta-adrenergic blocking agent and monitor results
    d. 24-hour urine collection for fractionated metanephrine and catecholamine levels

40. Which intervention applies to a patient with pheochromocytoma?
    a. Assist to sit in a chair for blood pressure monitoring.
    b. Instruct not to smoke, drink coffee, or change positions suddenly.
    c. Encourage to maintain an active exercise schedule including activity such as running.
    d. Encourage one glass of red wine nightly to promote rest.

41. Which intervention is contraindicated for a patient with pheochromocytoma?
    a. Monitoring blood pressure
    b. Palpating the abdomen
    c. Collecting 24-hour urine specimens
    d. Instructing the patient to limit activity

42. Which diuretic is ordered by the health care provider to treat hyperaldosteronism?
    a. Furosemide (Lasix)
    b. Ethacrynic acid (Edecrin)
    c. Bumetanide (Bumex)
    d. Spironolactone (Aldactone)

43. Which statement about hyperaldosteronism is correct?
    a. Painful "charley horses" are common from hyperkalemia.
    b. It occurs more often in men than in women.
    c. It is a common cause of hypertension in the population.
    d. Hypokalemia and hypertension are the main issues.

44. When diagnosed with Cushing's syndrome, the manifestations are most likely related to an excess production of which hormone?
    a. Insulin from the pancreas
    b. ADH from posterior pituitary gland
    c. PRL from anterior pituitary gland
    d. Cortisol from the adrenal cortex

45. What is the most common cause of endogenous hypercortisolism, or Cushing's disease?
    a. Pituitary hypoplasia
    b. Insufficient ACTH production
    c. Adrenocortical hormone deficiency
    d. Hyperplasia of the adrenal cortex

46. Which are physical findings of Cushing's disease? *(Select all that apply.)*
    a. "Moon-faced" appearance
    b. Decreased amount of body hair
    c. Truncal obesity
    d. Coarse facial features
    e. Thin, easily damaged skin
    f. Extremity muscle wasting

47. Which laboratory findings does the nurse expect to find with Cushing's syndrome? *(Select all that apply.)*
    a. Decreased serum sodium
    b. Increased serum glucose
    c. Increased serum sodium
    d. Increased serum potassium
    e. Decreased serum calcium

48. The nurse determines a priority patient problem of altered self-concept in a female patient with Cushing's syndrome who expresses concern about the changes in her general appearance. What is the expected outcome for this patient?
    a. To verbalize an understanding that treatment will reverse many of the problems
    b. To ventilate about the frustration of these lifelong physical changes
    c. To verbalize ways to cope with the changes such as joining a support group or changing style of dress
    d. To achieve a personal desired level of sexual functioning

49. Which drug is an adrenal cytotoxic agent used for inoperable adrenal tumors?
    a. Mitotane (Lysodren)
    b. Aminoglutethimide (Cytadren)
    c. Cyproheptadine (Periactin)
    d. Fludrocortisone (Florinef)

50. Which drug decreases cortisol production?
    a. Mitotane (Lysodren)
    b. Aminoglutethimide (Cytadren)
    c. Cyproheptadine (Periactin)
    d. Hydrocortisone (Cortef)

51. A patient is scheduled for bilateral adrenalectomy. Before surgery, steroids are to be given. Which is the reasoning behind the administration of this drug?
    a. To promote glycogen storage by the liver for body energy reserves
    b. To compensate for sudden lack of adrenal hormones following surgery
    c. To increase the body's inflammatory response to promote scar formation
    d. To enhance urinary excretion of salt and water following surgery

52. The nurse is teaching a patient being discharged after bilateral adrenalectomy. What medication information does the nurse emphasize in the teaching plan?
    a. The dosage of steroid replacement drugs will be consistent throughout the patient's lifetime.
    b. The steroid drugs should be taken in the evening so as not to interfere with sleep.
    c. The patient should take the drugs on an empty stomach.
    d. The patient should learn how to give himself an intramuscular injection of hydrocortisone.

53. Which statement about a patient with hyperaldosteronism after a successful unilateral adrenalectomy is correct?
    a. The low-sodium diet must be continued postoperatively.
    b. Glucocorticoid replacement therapy is temporary.
    c. Spironolactone (Aldactone) must be taken for life.
    d. Additional measures are needed to control hypertension.

54. Which patient is at risk for developing secondary adrenal insufficiency?
    a. Patient who suddenly stops taking high-dose steroid therapy
    b. Patient who tapers the dosages of steroid therapy
    c. Patient deficient in ADH
    d. Patient with an adrenal tumor causing excessive secretion of ACTH

55. An ACTH stimulation test is the most definitive test for which disorder?
    a. Adrenal insufficiency
    b. Cushing's syndrome
    c. Pheochromocytoma
    d. Acromegaly

56. Which interventions are necessary for a patient with acute adrenal insufficiency (Addisonian crisis)? *(Select all that apply.)*
    a. IV infusion of normal saline
    b. IV infusion of 3% saline
    c. Hourly glucose monitoring
    d. Insulin administration
    e. IV potassium therapy

57. A patient in the emergency department who reports lethargy, muscle weakness, nausea, vomiting, and weight loss over the past weeks is diagnosed with Addisonian crisis (acute adrenal insufficiency). Which drug(s) does the nurse expect to administer to this patient?
    a. Beta blocker to control the hypertension and dysrhythmias
    b. Solu-Cortef IV along with IM injections of hydrocortisone
    c. IV fluids of D_5 NS with KCl added for dehydration
    d. Spironolactone (Aldactone) to promote diuresis

58. The nurse determines that the administration of hydrocortisone for Addisonian crisis is effective when which assessment is made?
    a. Increased urine output
    b. No signs of pitting edema
    c. Weight gain
    d. Lethargy improving; patient alert and oriented

59. Which nursing intervention is a preventive measure for adrenocortical insufficiency?
    a. Maintaining diuretic therapy
    b. Instructing the patient on salt restriction
    c. Reducing high-dose glucocorticoid therapy quickly
    d. Reducing high-dose glucocorticoid doses gradually

60. The nurse should instruct a patient who is taking hydrocortisone to report which symptoms to the health care provider for possible dose adjustment? *(Select all that apply.)*
    a. Rapid weight gain
    b. Round face
    c. Fluid retention
    d. Gastrointestinal irritation
    e. Urinary incontinence

63 CHAPTER

Care of Patients with Problems of the Thyroid and Parathyroid Glands

1. The nurse is performing a physical examination of a patient's thyroid gland. Precautions are taken in performing the correct technique because palpation can result in which occurrence?
   a. Damage to the esophagus causing gastric reflux
   b. Obstruction of the carotid arteries causing a stroke
   c. Pressure on the trachea and laryngeal nerve causing hoarseness
   d. Exacerbation of symptoms by releasing additional thyroid hormone

2. Which assessment findings indicate hyperthyroidism? *(Select all that apply.)*
   a. Weight loss with increased appetite
   b. Constipation
   c. Increased heart rate
   d. Insomnia
   e. Decreased libido
   f. Heat intolerance

3. The nurse assesses a patient in the emergency department (ED) and finds the following: constipation, fatigue with increased sleeping time, impaired memory, facial puffiness, and weight gain. Which deficiency does the nurse recognize?
   a. Hyperthyroidism
   b. Hypothyroidism
   c. Hyperparathyroidism
   d. Hypoparathyroidism

4. Which factor is a hallmark assessment finding that signifies hyperthyroidism?
   a. Weight loss
   b. Increased libido
   c. Heat intolerance
   d. Diarrhea

5. Which factor is a main assessment finding that signifies hypothyroidism?
   a. Irritability
   b. Cold intolerance
   c. Diarrhea
   d. Fatigue

6. Which sign/symptom is one of the first indicators of hyperthyroidism that is often noticed by the patient?
   a. Eyelid or globe lag
   b. Vision changes or tiring of the eyes
   c. Protruding eyes
   d. Photophobia

7. Which laboratory result is consistent with a diagnosis of hyperthyroidism?
   a. Decreased serum triiodothyronine (T_3) and thyroxine (T_4) levels
   b. Elevated serum thyrotropin-releasing hormone (TRH) level
   c. Decreased radioactive iodine uptake
   d. Increased serum T_3 and T_4

8. The laboratory results for a 53-year-old patient indicate a low T_3 level and elevated thyroid-stimulating hormone (TSH). What do these results indicate?
   a. Hyperthyroidism
   b. Hypothyroidism
   c. Malfunctioning pituitary gland
   d. Normal laboratory values for this age

9. The clinical manifestations of hyperthyroidism are known as which condition?
   a. Thyrotoxicosis
   b. Euthyroid function
   c. Graves' disease
   d. Hypermetabolism

10. What is the most common cause of hyperthyroidism?
    a. Radiation to thyroid
    b. Graves' disease
    c. Thyroid cancer
    d. Thyroiditis

11. The nurse assessing a patient palpates enlargement of the thyroid gland, along with noticeable swelling of the neck. How does the nurse interpret this finding?
    a. Globe lag
    b. Myxedema
    c. Exophthalmos
    d. Goiter

12. The nurse is assessing a patient diagnosed with hyperthyroidism and observes dry, waxy swelling of the front surfaces of the lower legs. How does the nurse interpret this finding?
    a. Globe lag
    b. Pretibial myxedema
    c. Exophthalmos
    d. Goiter

13. Which statement best describes globe lag in a patient with hyperthyroidism?
    a. Abnormal protrusion of the eyes
    b. Upper eyelid fails to descend when the patient gazes downward
    c. Upper eyelid pulls back faster than the eyeball when the patient gazes upward
    d. Inability of both eyes to focus on an object simultaneously

14. The nurse is assessing a patient with Graves' disease and observes an abnormal protrusion of both eyeballs. How does the nurse document this assessment finding?
    a. Globe lag
    b. Pretibial myxedema
    c. Exophthalmos
    d. Goiter

15. Which statements about hyperthyroidism are accurate? *(Select all that apply.)*
    a. It is most commonly caused by Graves' disease.
    b. It can be caused by overuse of thyroid replacement medication.
    c. It occurs more often in men between the ages of 20-40.
    d. Weight gain is a common manifestation.
    e. Serum T_3 and T_4 results will be elevated.

16. The nurse is providing instructions to a patient taking levothyroxine (Synthroid). When does the nurse tell the patient to take this medication?
    a. With breakfast in the morning
    b. At lunchtime immediately after eating
    c. In the morning on an empty stomach
    d. At dinnertime within 15 minutes after eating

17. The nurse is providing instructions to a patient who is taking the antithyroid medication propylthiouracil (PTU). The nurse instructs the patient to notify the health care provider immediately if which sign/symptom occurs?
    a. Weight gain
    b. Dark-colored urine
    c. Cold intolerance
    d. Headache

18. The patient who is prescribed methimazole (Tapazole) 4 mg orally every 8 hours tells the nurse that his heart rate is slow (60/minute), he has gained 7 pounds, and he wears a sweater even on warm days. What does the nurse suspect?
    a. Indications of hypothyroidism will require a lower dosage.
    b. Indications of hypothyroidism will require a higher dosage.
    c. Indications of hyperthyroidism will require a lower dosage.
    d. Indications of hyperthyroidism will require a higher dosage.

19. A patient who has been diagnosed with Graves' disease is going to receive radioactive iodine (RAI) in the oral form of ^{131}I. What does the nurse teach the patient about how this drug works?
    a. It destroys the hormones T_3 and T_4.
    b. It destroys the tissue that produces thyroid hormones.
    c. It blocks thyroid hormone production.
    d. It prevents T_4 from being converted to T_3.

20. A patient who has been diagnosed with Graves' disease is to receive RAI in the oral form of ^{131}I as a treatment. What instructions does the nurse include in the teaching plan about preventing radiation exposure to others? *(Select all that apply.)*
    a. Do not share a toilet with others for 2 weeks after treatment.
    b. Flush the toilet three times after each use.
    c. Wash clothing separately from others in the household.
    d. Limit contact with pregnant women, infants, and children.
    e. Do not use a laxative within 2 weeks of having the treatment.

21. Which statements about hypothyroidism are accurate? *(Select all that apply.)*
    a. It occurs more often in women.
    b. It can be caused by iodine deficiency.
    c. Weight loss is a common manifestation.
    d. It can be caused by autoimmune thyroid destruction.
    e. Myxedema coma is a rare but serious complication.

22. The nurse is assessing a patient with a diagnosis of Hashimoto's disease. What are the primary manifestations of this disease? *(Select all that apply.)*
    a. Dysphagia
    b. Painless enlargement of the thyroid gland
    c. Painful enlargement of the thyroid gland
    d. Weight loss
    e. Intolerance to heat

23. Laboratory findings of elevated T_3 and T_4, decreased TSH, and high thyrotropin receptor antibody titer indicate which condition?
    a. Multinodular goiter
    b. Hyperthyroidism related to overmedication
    c. Pituitary tumor suppressing TSH
    d. Graves' disease

24. The patient has multiple thyroid nodules resulting in thyroid hyperfunction. What is the most likely cause of this hyperthyroidism?
    a. Thyroid carcinoma
    b. Graves' disease
    c. Toxic multinodular goiter
    d. Pituitary hyperthyroidism

25. After a visit to the health care provider's office, a patient is diagnosed with general thyroid enlargement and elevated thyroid hormone level. Which condition do these findings indicate?
    a. Hyperthyroidism and goiter
    b. Hypothyroidism and goiter
    c. Nodules on the parathyroid gland
    d. Thyroid or parathyroid cancer

26. Which condition is a life-threatening emergency and serious complication of untreated or poorly treated hypothyroidism?
    a. Endemic goiter
    b. Myxedema coma
    c. Toxic multinodular goiter
    d. Thyroiditis

27. A patient with exophthalmos from hyperthyroidism reports dry eyes, especially in the morning. The nurse teaches the patient to perform which intervention to help correct this problem?
    a. Wear sunglasses at all times when outside in the bright sun.
    b. Use cool compresses to the eye four times a day.
    c. Tape the eyes closed with nonallergenic tape.
    d. There is nothing that can be done to relieve this problem.

28. Which factors are considered to be triggers for thyroid storm? *(Select all that apply.)*
    a. Infection
    b. Cold temperatures
    c. Vigorous palpation of a goiter
    d. Diabetic ketoacidosis
    e. Extremely warm temperatures

29. A patient has the following assessment findings: elevated TSH level, low T_3 and T_4 levels, difficulty with memory, lethargy, and muscle stiffness. These are clinical manifestations of which disorder?
    a. Hypothyroidism
    b. Hyperthyroidism
    c. Hypoparathyroidism
    d. Hyperparathyroidism

30. A patient has been prescribed thyroid hormone for treatment of hypothyroidism. Within what time frame does the patient expect improvement in mental awareness with this treatment?
    a. A few days
    b. 2 weeks
    c. 1 month
    d. 3 months

31. Which signs and symptoms are assessment findings indicative of thyroid storm? *(Select all that apply.)*
    a. Abdominal pain and nausea
    b. Hypothermia
    c. Elevated temperature
    d. Tachycardia
    e. Elevated systolic blood pressure
    f. Bradycardia

32. Management of the patient with hyperthyroidism focuses on which goals? *(Select all that apply.)*
    a. Blocking the effects of excessive thyroid secretion
    b. Treating the signs and symptoms the patient experiences
    c. Establishing euthyroid function
    d. Preventing spread of the disease
    e. Maintaining an environment of reduced stimulation

33. Which are preoperative instructions for a patient having thyroid surgery? *(Select all that apply.)*
    a. Teach postoperative restrictions such as no coughing and deep-breathing exercises to prevent strain on the suture line.
    b. Teach the moving and turning technique of manually supporting the head and avoiding neck extension to minimize strain on the suture line.
    c. Inform the patient that hoarseness for a few days after surgery is usually the result of a breathing tube (endotracheal tube) used during surgery.
    d. Humidification of air may be helpful to promote expectoration of secretions. Suctioning may also be used.
    e. Clarify any questions regarding placement of incision, complications, and postoperative care.
    f. A supine position and lying flat will be maintained postoperatively to avoid strain on suture line.

34. The nurse is preparing for a patient to return from thyroid surgery. What priority equipment does the nurse ensure is immediately available? *(Select all that apply.)*
    a. Tracheostomy equipment
    b. Calcium gluconate or calcium chloride for IV administration
    c. Mechanical ventilator
    d. Humidified oxygen
    e. Suction equipment
    f. Pillows

35. After a thyroidectomy, a patient reports tingling around the mouth and muscle twitching. Which complication do these assessment findings indicate to the nurse?
    a. Hemorrhage
    b. Respiratory distress
    c. Thyroid storm
    d. Hypocalcemia

36. The nurse assesses a patient postthyroidectomy for laryngeal nerve damage. Which findings indicate this complication? *(Select all that apply.)*
    a. Dyspnea
    b. Sore throat
    c. Hoarseness
    d. Weak voice
    e. Dry cough

37. The nurse is assessing a patient after thyroid surgery and discovers harsh, high-pitched respiratory sounds. What is the nurse's best first action?
    a. Administer oxygen at 5 L via nasal cannula.
    b. Administer IV calcium chloride.
    c. Notify the Rapid Response Team.
    d. Suction the patient for oral secretions.

38. After hospitalization for myxedema, a patient is prescribed thyroid replacement medication. Which statement by the patient demonstrates a correct understanding of this therapy?
    a. "I'll be taking this medication until my symptoms are completely resolved."
    b. "I'll be taking thyroid medication for the rest of my life."
    c. "Now that I'm feeling better, no changes in my medication will be necessary."
    d. "I'm taking this medication to prevent symptoms of an overactive thyroid gland."

39. Which statements about thyroiditis are accurate? *(Select all that apply.)*
    a. It is an inflammation of the thyroid gland.
    b. Hashimoto's disease is the most common type.
    c. It always resolves with antibiotic therapy.
    d. There are three types: acute, subacute, and chronic.
    e. The patient must take thyroid hormones.

40. Which statements about acute thyroiditis are accurate? *(Select all that apply.)*
    a. It is caused by a bacterial infection of the thyroid gland.
    b. It is treated with antibiotic therapy.
    c. It results from a viral infection of the thyroid gland.
    d. Subtotal thyroidectomy is a form of treatment.
    e. Manifestations include neck tenderness, fever, and dysphagia.

41. What is the hallmark of thyroid cancer?
    a. Aggressive tumors
    b. Elevated serum thyroglobulin level
    c. Metastasis to other organs
    d. Invasion of blood vessels

42. Serum calcium levels are maintained by which hormone?
    a. Cortisol
    b. Luteinizing hormone
    c. Antidiuretic hormone (ADH)
    d. Parathyroid hormone (PTH)

43. Production of which hormone causes lower levels of calcium?
    a. Calcitonin
    b. PTH
    c. T_4
    d. TSH

44. Bone changes in the older adult are often seen with endocrine dysfunction and increased secretion of which substance?
    a. PTH
    b. Calcitonin
    c. Insulin
    d. Testosterone

45. In addition to regulation of calcium levels, PTH and calcitonin regulate the circulating blood levels of which substance?
    a. Potassium
    b. Sodium
    c. Phosphate
    d. Chloride

46. A patient has positive Trousseau's and Chvostek's signs resulting from hypoparathyroidism. What condition does this assessment finding indicate?
    a. Hypercalcemia
    b. Hypocalcemia
    c. Hyperphosphatemia
    d. Hypophosphatemia

47. Which foods will the nurse instruct a patient with hypoparathyroidism to avoid? *(Select all that apply.)*
    a. Canned vegetables
    b. Yogurt
    c. Fresh fruit
    d. Red meat
    e. Milk
    f. Processed cheese

48. A patient with continuous spasms of the muscles is diagnosed with hypoparathyroidism. The muscle spasms are a clinical manifestation of which condition?
    a. Nerve damage
    b. Seizures
    c. Tetany
    d. Decreased potassium

49. Which disorders/conditions can cause hyperparathyroidism? *(Select all that apply.)*
    a. Chronic kidney disease
    b. Neck trauma
    c. Thyroidectomy
    d. Vitamin D deficiency
    e. Parathyroidectomy

50. A patient has hyperparathyroidism and high levels of serum calcium. Which initial treatment does the nurse prepare to administer to the patient?
    a. Furosemide (Lasix) with IV saline
    b. Calcitonin
    c. Oral phosphates
    d. Mithramycin

51. Which are assessment findings of hypocalcemia? *(Select all that apply.)*
    a. Numbness and tingling around the mouth
    b. Muscle cramping
    c. Bone fractures
    d. Fever
    e. Tachycardia

52. Which medication therapies does the nurse expect patients with hypoparathyroidism to receive? *(Select all that apply.)*
    a. Calcium chloride
    b. Calcium gluconate
    c. Calcitrol (Rocaltrol)
    d. Propranolol (Inderal)
    e. Ergocalciferol

53. Discharge planning for a patient with chronic hypoparathyroidism includes which instructions? *(Select all that apply.)*
    a. Prescribed medications must be taken for the patient's entire life.
    b. Eat foods low in vitamin D and high in phosphorus.
    c. Eat foods high in calcium, but low in phosphorus.
    d. After several weeks, medications can be discontinued.
    e. Kidney stones are no longer a risk to the patient.

54. In older adults, assessment findings of fatigue, altered thought processes, dry skin, and constipation are often mistaken for signs of aging rather than assessment findings for which endocrine disorder?
    a. Hyperthyroidism
    b. Hypothyroidism
    c. Hyperparathyroidism
    d. Hypoparathyroidism

55. What is the most common cause of death from myxedema coma?
    a. Myocardial infarction
    b. Acute kidney failure
    c. High serum level of iodide
    d. Respiratory failure

56. Which conditions may precipitate myxedema coma? *(Select all that apply.)*
    a. Rapid withdrawal of thyroid medication
    b. Vitamin D deficiency
    c. Untreated hypothyroidism
    d. Surgery
    e. Excessive exposure to iodine

Care of Patients with Diabetes Mellitus

1. Which descriptors are typical of type 2 diabetes mellitus (DM)? *(Select all that apply.)*
   a. Autoimmune process causes beta cell destruction.
   b. Cells have decreased ability to respond to insulin.
   c. Diagnosis is based on results of 100-g glucose tolerance test.
   d. Most patients diagnosed are obese adults.
   e. Usually has abrupt onset of thirst and weight loss.

2. Which statement is true about insulin?
   a. It is secreted by alpha cells in the islets of Langerhans.
   b. It is a catabolic hormone that builds up glucagon reserves.
   c. It is necessary for glucose transport across cell membranes.
   d. It is stored in muscles and converted to fat for storage.

3. Why is glucose vital to the body's cells?
   a. It is used to build cell membranes.
   b. It is used by cells to produce energy.
   c. It affects the process of protein metabolism.
   d. It provides nutrients for genetic material.

4. A patient with diabetes presents to the emergency department (ED) with a blood sugar of 640 mg/dL and reports being constantly thirsty and having to urinate "all of the time." How does the nurse document this subjective finding?
   a. Polydipsia and polyphagia
   b. Polydipsia and polyuria
   c. Polycoria and polyuria
   d. Polyphagia and polyesthesia

5. Which cultures tend to have a higher incidence of DM? *(Select all that apply.)*
   a. Mexican American
   b. African American
   c. Caucasian
   d. American Indian
   e. Eastern European

6. Which individual is at greatest risk for developing type 2 DM?
   a. 25-year-old African-American woman
   b. 36-year-old African-American man
   c. 56-year-old Hispanic woman
   d. 40-year-old Hispanic man

7. According to the American Diabetes Association (ADA), which laboratory finding is most indicative of DM?
   a. Fasting blood glucose = 80 mg/dL
   b. 2-hour postprandial blood glucose = 110 mg/dL
   c. 1-hour glucose tolerance blood glucose = 110 mg/dL
   d. 2-hour glucose tolerance blood glucose = 210 mg/dL

8. Untreated hyperglycemia results in which condition?
   a. Respiratory acidosis
   b. Metabolic alkalosis
   c. Respiratory alkalosis
   d. Metabolic acidosis

9. In a patient with hyperglycemia, the respiratory center is triggered in an attempt to excrete more carbon dioxide and acid, thus causing a rapid and deep respiratory pattern. What is the term for this respiratory pattern?
   a. Tachypnea
   b. Cheyne-Stokes respiration
   c. Kussmaul respiration
   d. Biot respiration

10. Which electrolyte is most affected by hyperglycemia?
    a. Sodium
    b. Chloride
    c. Potassium
    d. Magnesium

11. Which complications of DM are considered emergencies? *(Select all that apply.)*
    a. Diabetic ketoacidosis (DKA)
    b. Hypoglycemia
    c. Diabetic retinopathy
    d. Hyperglycemic-hyperosmolar state (HHS)
    e. Diabetic neuropathy

12. In determining if a patient is hypoglycemic, the nurse looks for which characteristics in addition to checking the patient's blood glucose? *(Select all that apply.)*
    a. Nausea
    b. Hunger
    c. Irritability
    d. Palpitations
    e. Profuse perspiration
    f. Rapid, deep respirations

13. Which factors differentiate DKA from HHS? *(Select all that apply.)*
    a. Level of hyperglycemia
    b. Amount of ketones produced
    c. Serum bicarbonate levels
    d. Amount of volume depletion
    e. Dosage of insulin needed

14. A patient is admitted with a blood glucose level of 900 mg/dL. IV fluids and insulin are administered. Two hours after treatment is initiated, the blood glucose level is 400 mg/dL. Which complication is the patient most at risk for developing?
    a. Hypoglycemia
    b. Pulmonary embolus
    c. Renal shutdown
    d. Pulmonary edema

15. What type of insulin is used in the emergency treatment of DKA and hyperglycemic-hyperosmolar nonketotic syndrome (HHNS)?
    a. NPH
    b. Lente
    c. Regular
    d. Protamine zinc

16. Early treatment of DKA and HHNS includes IV administration of which fluid?
    a. Glucagon
    b. Potassium
    c. Bicarbonate
    d. Normal saline

17. Glucagon is used primarily to treat the patient with which disorder?
    a. DKA
    b. Idiosyncratic reaction to insulin
    c. Severe hypoglycemia
    d. HHNS

18. In which situations does the nurse teach a patient to perform urine ketone testing? *(Select all that apply.)*
    a. Acute illness or stress
    b. When blood glucose levels are above 240 mg/dL
    c. When symptoms of DKA are present
    d. To evaluate the effectiveness of DKA treatment
    e. When a diabetic patient is in a weight-loss program

19. When glucagon is administered, what does it do?
    a. Competes for insulin at the receptor sites
    b. Frees glucose from hepatic stores of glycogen
    c. Supplies glycogen directly to the vital tissues
    d. Provides a glucose substitute for rapid replacement

20. Which statements about type 1 DM are accurate? *(Select all that apply.)*
    a. It is an autoimmune disorder.
    b. Most people with type 1 DM are obese.
    c. Age of onset is typically younger than 30.
    d. Etiology can be attributed to viral infections.
    e. It can be treated with oral antidiabetic medications and insulin.

21. Which statements about type 2 DM are accurate? *(Select all that apply.)*
    a. It peaks at about the age of 50.
    b. Most people with type 2 DM are obese.
    c. It typically has an abrupt onset.
    d. People with type 2 DM have insulin resistance.
    e. It can be treated with oral antidiabetic medications and insulin.

22. Which are modifiable risk factors for type 2 DM? *(Select all that apply.)*
    a. Age
    b. Family history
    c. Working in a low-stress environment
    d. Maintaining ideal body weight
    e. Maintaining adequate physical activity

23. A diabetic patient is scheduled to have a blood glucose test the next morning. What does the nurse tell the patient to do before coming in for the test?
    a. Eat the usual diet but have nothing after midnight.
    b. Take the usual oral hypoglycemic tablet in the morning.
    c. Eat a clear liquid breakfast in the morning.
    d. Follow the usual diet and medication regimen.

24. The nurse is providing discharge teaching to a patient about self-monitoring of blood glucose (SMBG). What information does the nurse include? *(Select all that apply.)*
    a. Only perform SMBG before breakfast.
    b. Wash hands before using the meter.
    c. Do a retest if the results seem unusual.
    d. It is okay to reuse lancets in the home setting.
    e. Do not share the meter.

25. Which are considered the early signs of diabetic nephropathy? *(Select all that apply.)*
    a. Positive urine red blood cells
    b. Microalbuminuria
    c. Positive urine glucose
    d. Positive urine white blood cells
    e. Elevated serum uric acid

26. Which class of antidiabetic medication should be taken with the first bite of a meal to be fully effective?
    a. Alpha-glucosidase inhibitors, which include miglitol (Glyset)
    b. Biguanides, which include metformin (Glucophage)
    c. Meglitinides, which include nateglinide (Starlix)
    d. Second-generation sulfonylureas, which include glipizide (Glucotrol)

27. Which class of antidiabetic medication must be held after using contrast media until adequate kidney function is established?
    a. Alpha-glucosidase inhibitors, which include miglitol (Glyset)
    b. Biguanides, which include metformin (Glucophage)
    c. Meglitinides, which include nateglinide (Starlix)
    d. Second-generation sulfonylureas, which include glipizide (Glucotrol)

28. Which class of antidiabetic medication is most likely to cause a hypoglycemic episode because of the long duration of action?
    a. Alpha-glucosidase inhibitors, which include miglitol (Glyset)
    b. Biguanides, which include metformin (Glucophage)
    c. Meglitinides, which include nateglinide (Starlix)
    d. Second-generation sulfonylureas, which include glipizide (Glucotrol)

29. Which class of antidiabetic medication should be given 1-30 minutes before meals?
    a. Alpha-glucosidase inhibitors, which include miglitol (Glyset)
    b. Biguanides, which include metformin (Glucophage)
    c. Meglitinides, which include nateglinide (Starlix)
    d. Sulfonylureas, which include chlorpromadine (Diabinese)

30. Which oral agent may cause lactic acidosis?
    a. Nateglinide
    b. Repaglinide
    c. Metformin
    d. Miglitol

31. For which patient should the health care provider avoid prescribing rosiglitazone (Avandia)?
    a. Patient with symptomatic heart failure
    b. Patient with new-onset asthma
    c. Patient with kidney disease
    d. Patient with hyperthyroidism

32. The patient with type 2 diabetes is prescribed sitagliptin (Januvia) for glucose regulation. Which key changes does the nurse teach a patient to report to the health care provider immediately? *(Select all that apply.)*
    a. Report any signs of jaundice.
    b. Report any signs of bleeding.
    c. Report any blue-grey discoloration of the abdomen.
    d. Report any cough or flu symptoms.
    e. Report any sudden onset of abdominal pain.

33. Which statement about insulin is true?
    a. Exogenous insulin is necessary for management of all cases of type 2 DM.
    b. Insulin's effectiveness depends on the individual patient's absorption of the drug.
    c. Insulin doses should be regulated according to self-monitoring urine glucose levels.
    d. Insulin administered in multiple doses per day decreases the flexibility of a patient's lifestyle.

34. Which statement about insulin administration is correct?
    a. Insulin may be given orally, intravenously, or subcutaneously.
    b. Insulin injections should be spaced no closer than one-half inch apart.
    c. Rotating injection sites improves absorption and prevents lipohypertrophy.
    d. Shake the bottle of intermediate-acting insulin, and then draw it into the syringe.

35. A diabetic patient is on a mixed-dose insulin protocol of 8 units regular insulin and 12 units NPH insulin at 7 AM. At 10:30 AM, the patient reports feeling uneasy, shaky, and has a headache. Which is the probable explanation for this?
    a. The NPH insulin's action is peaking, and there is an insufficient blood glucose level.
    b. The regular insulin's action is peaking, and there is an insufficient blood glucose level.
    c. The patient consumed too many calories at breakfast and now has an elevated blood glucose level.
    d. The symptoms are unrelated to the insulin administered in the early morning or food taken in at lunchtime.

36. A patient asks the nurse how insulin injection site rotation should be accomplished. What is the nurse's best response?
    a. "Rotation within one site is preferred to avoid changes in insulin absorption."
    b. "Change rotation sites after a week or two to avoid lipohypertrophy."
    c. "Rotation from site to site each day is best for the best insulin absorption."
    d. "Always rotate insulin injection sites within 4 to 5 inches from the umbilicus."

37. A patient will be using an external insulin pump. What does the nurse tell the patient about the pump?
    a. SMBG levels should be done three or more times a day.
    b. The insulin supply must be replaced every 2 to 4 weeks.
    c. The pump's battery should be checked on a regular weekly schedule.
    d. The needle site must be changed every day.

38. A 47-year-old patient with a history of type 2 DM and emphysema who reports smoking three packs of cigarettes per day is admitted to the hospital with a diagnosis of acute pneumonia. The patient is placed on the regular oral antidiabetic agents, sliding-scale insulin, and antibiotic medications. On day 2 of hospitalization, the health care provider orders prednisone therapy. What does the nurse expect the blood glucose to do?
    a. Decrease
    b. Stay the same
    c. Increase
    d. Return to normal

39. Which laboratory test is the best indicator of a patient's average blood glucose level and/or compliance with the DM regimen over the last 3 months?
    a. Postprandial blood glucose test
    b. Oral glucose tolerance test (OGTT)
    c. Casual blood glucose test
    d. Glycosylated hemoglobin (HbA$_{1c}$)

40. A patient with diabetic ketoacidosis is on an insulin drip of 50 units of regular insulin in 250 mL of normal saline. The current blood glucose level is 549 mg/dL. According to insulin protocol, the insulin drip needs to be changed to 8 units per hour. At what rate does the nurse set the pump?
    a. 40 mL/hr
    b. 50 mL/hr
    c. 60 mL/hr
    d. 75 mL/hr

41. Which insulins are considered to have a rapid onset of action? *(Select all that apply.)*
    a. Novolin 70/30
    b. Glulisine
    c. Humulin N
    d. Aspart
    e. Lispro

42. A patient with type 2 DM, usually controlled with a second-generation sulfonylurea, develops a urinary tract infection. Due to the stress of the infection, the patient must be treated with insulin. What additional information about this treatment does the nurse relay to the patient?
    a. The sulfonylurea must be discontinued and insulin taken until the infection clears.
    b. Insulin will now be necessary to control the patient's diabetes for life.
    c. The sulfonylurea dose must be reduced until the infection clears.
    d. The insulin is necessary to supplement the second-generation sulfonylurea until the infection clears.

43. The diabetic patient experiences early morning hyperglycemia (Somogyi effect) as a result of the counterregulatory response to hypoglycemia. What treatment does the nurse expect for this condition? *(Select all that apply.)*
    a. Administer a 10 PM dose of intermediate-acting insulin.
    b. Provide an evening snack to ensure adequate dietary intake.
    c. Evaluate insulin dosage and exercise program.
    d. Add an oral antidiabetic drug to patient's regimen.
    e. Increase blood glucose checks to every 2 hours around the clock.

44. Which diabetic complication is associated with neuropathy?
    a. End-stage kidney disease
    b. Muscle weakness
    c. Permanent blindness
    d. Eye hemorrhage

45. A patient will be using an external insulin pump. What does the nurse tell the patient about the pump?
    a. SMBG levels can be done only twice a day.
    b. The insulin supply must be replaced every 2 to 4 weeks.
    c. The pump's battery should be checked on a regular weekly schedule.
    d. The needle must be changed every two to three days.

46. The patient's urinalysis shows proteinuria. Which pathophysiology does the nurse suspect?
    a. Nephropathy
    b. Neuropathy
    c. Retinopathy
    d. Gastroparesis

47. Which infection control measures must the nurse teach a patient who will be performing SMBG? *(Select all that apply.)*
    a. Always wash hands before monitoring glucose.
    b. Regular cleaning of the meter is critical.
    c. Do not reuse lancets.
    d. Do not share blood glucose monitoring equipment.
    e. Sterilize blood glucose monitor before each use.

48. Which statements about sensory alteration in patients with diabetes are accurate? *(Select all that apply.)*
    a. Healing of foot wounds is reduced because of impaired sensation.
    b. Very few patients with diabetic foot ulcers have peripheral sensory neuropathy.
    c. Loss of pain, pressure, and temperature sensation in the foot increases the risk for injury.
    d. Sensory neuropathy causes loss of normal sweating and skin temperature regulation.
    e. It can be delayed by keeping the blood glucose level as close to normal as possible.

49. Intensive therapy with good glucose control results in delays in which diabetic complications? *(Select all that apply.)*
    a. Macrovascular disease
    b. Cardiovascular disease
    c. Stroke
    d. Retinopathy
    e. Nephropathy
    f. Neuropathy

50. The patient with diabetes has a foot that is warm, swollen, and painful. Walking causes the arch of the foot to collapse and gives the food a "rocker bottom" shape. Which foot deformity does the nurse recognize?
    a. Hallux valgus
    b. Claw-toe deformity
    c. Charcot foot
    d. Diabetic foot ulcer

51. In developing an individualized meal plan for a patient with diabetes, which goals will be focal points of the plan? *(Select all that apply.)*
    a. Maintaining blood glucose levels at or as close to the normal range as possible
    b. Patient food preferences
    c. Allowing patients to eat as much as they desire
    d. Patient cultural preferences
    e. Limiting food choices only when guided by scientific evidence

52. What is the basic principle of meal planning for a patient with type 1 DM?
    a. Five small meals per day plus a bedtime snack
    b. Taking extra insulin when planning to eat sweet foods
    c. High-protein, low-carbohydrate, and low-fiber foods
    d. Considering the effects and peak action times of the patient's insulin

53. Which statement about dietary concepts for a patient with diabetes is true?
    a. Alcoholic beverage consumption is unrestricted.
    b. Carbohydrate counting is emphasized when adjusting dietary intake of nutrients.
    c. Sweeteners should be avoided because of the side effects.
    d. Both soluble and insoluble fiber foods should be limited.

54. What is the recommended protocol for patients with type 2 DM who must lose weight?
    a. Participate in an aerobic program twice a week for 20 minutes each session.
    b. Slowly increase insulin dosage until mild hypoglycemia occurs.
    c. Reduce calorie intake moderately and increase exercise.
    d. Reduce daily calorie intake to 1000 calories and monitor urine for ketones.

55. Along with exercise, what is the recommended calorie reduction for a patient with diabetes who must lose weight?
    a. 100-200 calories/day
    b. 250-500 calories/day
    c. 501-600 calories/day
    d. 601-750 calories/day

56. What type of exercise does the nurse recommend for the patient with diabetic retinopathy?
    a. Non–weight-bearing activities such as swimming
    b. Weight-bearing activities such as jogging
    c. Vigorous aerobic and resistance exercises
    d. Weight training and heavy lifting

57. The nurse is teaching a patient with diabetes about proper foot care. Which instructions does the nurse include? *(Select all that apply.)*
    a. Use rubbing alcohol to toughen the skin on the soles of the feet.
    b. Wear open-toed shoes or sandals in warm weather to prevent perspiration.
    c. Apply moisturizing cream to the feet after bathing, but not between the toes.
    d. Use cold water for bathing the feet to prevent inadvertent thermal injury.
    e. Do not go barefoot.
    f. Inspect the feet daily.

58. A 25-year-old female patient with type 1 DM tells the nurse, "I have two kidneys and I'm still young. I expect to be around for a long time, so why should I worry about my blood sugar?" What is the nurse's best response?
    a. "You have little to worry about as long as your kidneys keep making urine."
    b. "You should discuss this with your physician because you are being unrealistic."
    c. "You would be right if your diabetes was managed with insulin."
    d. "Keeping your blood sugar under control now can help to prevent damage to both kidneys."

59. SMBG levels is most important in which patients? *(Select all that apply.)*
    a. Patients taking multiple daily insulin injections
    b. Patients with mild type 2 diabetes
    c. Patients with hypoglycemic unawareness
    d. Patients using a portable infusion device for insulin administration
    e. Patients with acute illnesses
    f. Pregnant patients

60. Which statement about sexual intercourse for patients with diabetes is true?
    a. The incidence of sexual dysfunction is lower in men than women.
    b. Retrograde ejaculation does not interfere with male fertility.
    c. Impotence is associated with DM in male patients.
    d. Sexual dysfunction in female patients includes inability to achieve pregnancy.

61. A patient with type 1 DM is planning to travel by air and asks the nurse about preparations for the trip. What does the nurse tell the patient to do?
    a. Pack insulin and syringes in a labeled, crushproof kit in the checked luggage.
    b. Carry all necessary diabetes supplies in a clearly identified pack aboard the plane.
    c. Ask the flight attendant to put the insulin in the galley refrigerator once on the plane.
    d. Take only minimal supplies and get the prescription filled at his or her destination.

62. Which statement by a patient with DM indicates an understanding of the principles of self-care?
    a. "I don't like the idea of sticking myself so often to measure my sugar."
    b. "I plan to measure the sugar in my urine at least four times a day."
    c. "I plan to get my spouse to exercise with me to keep me company."
    d. "If I get a cold, I can take my regular cough medication until I feel better."

63. After a 2-hour glucose challenge, which result demonstrates impaired glucose tolerance?
    a. Less than 100 mg/dL
    b. Less than 140 mg/dL
    c. Greater than 140 mg/dL
    d. Greater than 250 mg/dL

64. The nurse is caring for a patient with DM. The patient's urine is positive for ketones. What does the nurse instruct the patient with regard to exercise?
    a. "When urine ketones are present, you should not exercise."
    b. "You may exercise as long as serum ketones are negative."
    c. "If you exercise now, be sure to perform aerobic exercises."
    d. "Exercise is always a good option because it helps with glucose utilization."

65. A patient with type 2 DM often has which laboratory value?
    a. Elevated thyroid studies
    b. Elevated triglycerides
    c. Ketones in the urine
    d. Low hemoglobin

66. A patient has been diagnosed with DM. Which aspects does the nurse consider in formulating the teaching plan for this patient? *(Select all that apply.)*
    a. Covering all needed information in one teaching session
    b. Assessing visual impairment regarding insulin labels and markings on syringes
    c. Assessing manual dexterity to determine if the patient is able to draw insulin into a syringe
    d. Assessing patient motivation to learn and comprehend instructions
    e. Assessing the patient's ability to read printed material

67. Which are signs and symptoms of *mild* hypoglycemia? *(Select all that apply.)*
    a. Headache
    b. Weakness
    c. Cold, clammy skin
    d. Irritability
    e. Pallor
    f. Tachycardia

68. The older adult with DM asks the nurse for advice about beginning an exercise program. What is the nurse's best response? *(Select all that apply.)*
    a. Begin with high-intensity activities.
    b. Start low-intensity activities in short sessions.
    c. Be sure to include warm-up and cool-down periods.
    d. Start with periods of 20 minutes or less.
    e. Changes in activity should be gradual.

69. A patient with type 1 DM is taking a mixture of NPH and regular insulin at home. The patient has been NPO for surgery since midnight. What action does the nurse take regarding the patient's morning dose of insulin?
    a. Administer the dose that is routinely prescribed at home because the patient has type 1 DM and needs the insulin.
    b. Administer half the dose because the patient is NPO.
    c. Hold the insulin with all the other medications because the patient is NPO and there is no need for insulin.
    d. Contact the health care provider for an order regarding the insulin.

70. What glucose level range does the American Association of Clinical Endocrinologists recommend for a critically ill patient?
    a. Between 100 and 130 mg/dL
    b. Between 140 and 180 mg/dL
    c. Between 180 and 200 mg/dL
    d. Between 200 and 240 mg/dL

71. The patient with DM had a pancreas transplant and takes daily doses of cyclosporine (Neoral). For which key lab assessment does the nurse monitor?
    a. Serum electrolytes
    b. CBC with differential count
    c. Serum creatinine
    d. Clotting studies

72. Which diabetic patient is at greatest risk for diabetic foot ulcer formation?
    a. 75-year-old African-American male with history of cardiovascular disease
    b. 53-year-old Caucasian female with history of renal insufficiency
    c. 38-year-old American Indian with history of gastric ulcers
    d. 28-year-old Caucasian male with history of chronic kidney disease

73. A patient with DM has signs and symptoms of hypoglycemia. The patient is alert and oriented with a blood glucose of 56 mg/dL. What does the nurse do next?
    a. Give a glass of orange juice with two packets of sugar and continue to monitor the patient.
    b. Give 8 oz of skim milk and then a carbohydrate and protein snack.
    c. Give a complex carbohydrate and continue to monitor the patient.
    d. Administer D50 IV push and give the patient something to eat.

74. A patient with diabetes has signs and symptoms of hypoglycemia. The patient has a blood glucose of 56 mg/dL, is not alert but responds to voice, and is confused and is unable to swallow fluids. What does the nurse do next?
    a. Give a glass of orange juice with two packets of sugar and continue to monitor the patient.
    b. Give a glass of orange or other type of juice and continue to monitor the patient.
    c. Give a complex carbohydrate and continue to monitor the patient.
    d. Administer D50 IV push.

75. A patient has been receiving insulin in the abdomen for 3 days. On day 4, where does the nurse give the insulin injection?
    a. Deltoid
    b. Thigh
    c. Abdomen, but in an area different from the previous day's injection
    d. Abdomen, in the same area as the previous day's injection

76. From which injection site is insulin absorbed most rapidly?
    a. Buttocks
    b. Abdomen
    c. Deltoid
    d. Thigh

77. Which are characteristics of regular insulin? *(Select all that apply.)*
    a. This insulin does not have a peak time.
    b. When mixing types of insulin, this insulin is always drawn up first.
    c. This insulin is given once daily for basal insulin coverage.
    d. This insulin should be given 30 minutes before meals.
    e. This insulin should not be diluted or mixed with any other insulin.

78. The nurse is preparing to teach a diabetic patient how to select appropriate shoes. Which points must be included in the teaching plan? *(Select all that apply.)*
    a. "It is best to have the shoes fitted by an experienced shoe fitter such as a podiatrist."
    b. "The shoes should be 1 to 1.5 inches longer than your longest toe."
    c. "The heels of the shoes should be less than 2 inches high."
    d. "Avoid tight-fitting shoes, which can cause tissue damage to your feet."
    e. "You should get at least two pairs of shoes so you can change them at midday and in the evening."

79. The male diabetic patient asks the nurse for advice about alcohol consumption. What is the nurse's best response?
    a. "It is best to have alcohol near bedtime."
    b. "As long as your diabetes is under control you can drink as much as you like."
    c. "You should drink only one alcoholic beverage with each meal."
    d. "Avoid more than two drinks a day and have them with or shortly after meals."

80. The nurse is caring for a diabetic patient in the ED. The patient's lab values include serum glucose 353 mg/dL, positive serum ketones, and positive urine ketones. What complication does the nurse suspect?
    a. DKA
    b. HHS
    c. Hyperglycemia
    d. Hypoglycemia

81. The critical care nurse is caring for an older patient admitted with HHS. What is the first priority in caring for this patient?
    a. Slowly decreasing blood glucose
    b. Fluid replacement to increase blood volume
    c. Potassium replacement to prevent hypokalemia
    d. Diuretic therapy to maintain kidney function

65
CHAPTER

Assessment of the Renal/Urinary System

1. A patient has sustained a minor kidney injury. Which structure must remain functional in order to form urine from blood?
   a. Medulla
   b. Nephron
   c. Calyx
   d. Capsule

2. Which event is most likely to trigger renin production?
   a. Patient participates in strenuous exercise.
   b. Patient becomes anxious and nervous.
   c. Patient has urge to urinate during the night.
   d. Patient sustains significant blood loss.

3. In which circumstance is the regulatory role of aldosterone most important in order for the person to maintain homeostasis?
   a. Person is having pain related to a kidney stone.
   b. Person has been hiking in the desert for several hours.
   c. Person experiences stress incontinence when coughing.
   d. Person experiences a burning sensation during urination.

4. Which hormone is released from the posterior pituitary and makes the distal convoluted tubule and the collecting duct permeable to water to maximize reabsorption and produce concentrated urine?
   a. Aldosterone
   b. Vasopressin
   c. Bradykinins
   d. Natriuretic

5. Based on the nurse's knowledge of the normal function of the kidney, which large particles are not found in the urine because they are too large to filter through the glomerular capillary walls? *(Select all that apply.)*
   a. Blood cells
   b. Albumin
   c. Other proteins
   d. Electrolytes
   e. Water

6. What is the average urine output of a healthy adult for a 24-hour period?
   a. 500 mL to 1000 mL per day
   b. 1500 mL to 2000 mL per day
   c. 3000 mL to 5000 mL per day
   d. 5000 mL to 7000 mL per day

7. The nurse is caring for a patient who sustained major injuries in an automobile accident. Which blood pressure will result in compromised kidney function, in particular the glomerular filtration rate (GFR)?
   a. 150/70 mm Hg
   b. 70/40 mm Hg
   c. 80/60 mm Hg
   d. 140/80 mm Hg

8. Damage to which renal structure or tissues can change the actual production of urine?
   a. Kidney parenchyma
   b. Convoluted tubules
   c. Calyces
   d. Ureters

9. Which hematologic disorder is most likely to occur if the hormonal function of the kidneys is not working properly?
    a. Leukemia
    b. Thrombocyopenia
    c. Neutropenia
    d. Anemia

10. Which patient is most likely to exceed the renal threshold if there is noncompliance with the prescribed therapeutic regimen?
    a. Has recurrent kidney stone formation
    b. Has type 2 diabetes mellitus
    c. Has functional urinary incontinence
    d. Has biliary obstruction

11. Which personal action is most likely to cause the kidneys to produce and release erythropoietin?
    a. Person moves to a low desert area where the humidity is very low.
    b. Person moves to a high-altitude area where atmospheric oxygen is low.
    c. Person drinks an excessive amount of fluid that results in fluid overload.
    d. Person eats a large high-protein meal after a rigorous exercise workout.

12. Vitamin D is converted to its active form in the kidney. If this function fails, which electrolyte imbalance will occur?
    a. Hyperkalemia
    b. Hypocalcemia
    c. Hypernatremia
    d. Hypoglycemia

13. Mastering voluntary micturition is a normal developmental task for which person?
    a. A healthy 20-month-old toddler
    b. A 56-year-old woman with stress incontinence
    c. A healthy 8-year-old child
    d. A 25-year-old with a spinal cord injury

14. An elderly patient has been in bed for several days after a fall. The nurse encourages ambulation to stimulate the movement of urine through the ureter by what phenomenon?
    a. Peristalsis
    b. Gravity
    c. Pelvic pressure
    d. Backflow

15. Which renal change associated with aging does the nurse expect an older adult patient to report?
    a. Nocturnal polyuria
    b. Micturition
    c. Hematuria
    d. Dysuria

16. An older adult male patient has a history of an enlarged prostate. The patient is most likely to report which symptom associated with this condition?
    a. Inability to sense the urge to void
    b. Difficulty starting the urine stream
    c. Excreting large amounts of very dilute urine
    d. Burning sensation when urinating

17. Impairment in the thirst mechanism associated with aging makes an older adult patient more vulnerable to which disorder?
    a. Hypernatremia
    b. Hypocalcemia
    c. Hyperkalemia
    d. Hypoglycemia

18. The nurse is talking to a group of older women about changes in the urinary system related to aging. What symptom is likely to be the common concern for this group?
    a. Incontinence
    b. Hematuria
    c. Retention
    d. Dysuria

19. Which ethnic group has the highest risk for kidney failure and needs special attention for patient teaching related to hypertension and sodium intake?
    a. Caucasian Americans
    b. African Americans
    c. Asian Americans
    d. Native Americans

20. The nurse is taking a history on a patient with a change in urinary patterns. In addition to the medical and surgical history, what does the nurse ask the patient about to complete the assessment? *(Select all that apply.)*
    a. Occupational exposure to toxins
    b. Use of illicit substances, such as cocaine
    c. Financial resources for payment of treatments
    d. Likelihood of complying with treatment recommendations
    e. Recent travel to geographic regions that pose infectious disease risks

21. Which patient narrative describes the symptom of dysuria?
    a. "I have to pee all the time."
    b. "I have to wait before the pee starts."
    c. "It burns when I pee."
    d. "It feels like I am going to pee in my pants."

22. The nurse is interviewing a 35-year-old woman who needs evaluation for a potential kidney problem. The woman reports she has been pregnant twice and has two healthy children. What would the nurse ask about health problems that occurred during pregnancy?
    a. "How much weight did you gain during the pregnancy?"
    b. "Were you treated for gestational diabetes?"
    c. "Did both of your pregnancies go to full-term?"
    d. "Did you have a urinary catheter inserted during labor?"

23. The nurse tells the patient that the health care provider recommends a fluid intake of at least 2 liters per day. The nurse then asks the patient to report on fluid intake over the past 24 hours to assess typical intake. The patient reports 15 ounces of coffee and 10 ounces of juice for breakfast; 10 ounces of skim milk for a mid-morning snack, 12 ounces of protein shake for lunch, ½ liter of sports drink in the afternoon and 3 ounces of wine for dinner. After calculating the 24-hour fluid intake, what does the nurse tell the patient?
    a. Fluid consumption should be increased by at least 2 more servings.
    b. Fluid consumption is meeting the 2 liter/day recommendation.
    c. Fluid consumption exceeds recommendation, therefore eliminate the wine.
    d. Fluid consumption only includes liquids such as water, juice, or milk.

24. The nurse is taking a history on a 55-year-old patient who denies any serious chronic health problems. Which sudden onset sign/symptom suggests possible kidney disease in this patient?
    a. Weakness
    b. Hypertension
    c. Confusion
    d. Dysrhythmia

25. The nurse is determining whether a patient has a history of hypertension because of the potential for kidney problems. Which question is best to elicit this information?
    a. "Do you have high blood pressure?"
    b. "Do you take any blood pressure medications?"
    c. "Have you ever been told that your blood pressure was high?"
    d. "When was the last time you had your blood pressure checked?"

26.   A patient appears very uncomfortable with the nurse's questions about urinary functions and patterns. What is the best technique for the nurse to use to elicit relevant information and decrease the patient's discomfort?
a.   Defer the questions until a later time.
b.   Direct the questions toward a family member.
c.   Use anatomic or medical terminology.
d.   Use the patient's own terminology.

27.   The nurse is taking a nutritional history on a patient. The patient states, "I really don't drink as much water as I should." What is the nurse's best response?
a.   "We should probably all drink more water than we do."
b.   "It's an easy thing to forget; just try to remember to drink more."
c.   "What would encourage you to drink the recommended 2 liters per day?"
d.   "I'd like you to read this brochure about kidney health and fluids."

28.   When patients have problems with the kidneys or urinary tract, what is the most common symptom that prompts them to seek medical attention?
a.   Change in the frequency or amount of urination
b.   Pain in flank or abdomen or pain when urinating
c.   Noticing a change in the color or odor of the urine
d.   Exposure to a nephrotoxic substance

29.   Which over-the-counter product used by a patient does the nurse further explore for potential impact on kidney function?
a.   Mouthwash with alcohol
b.   Fiber supplement
c.   Vitamin C
d.   Acetaminophen

30.   The nurse is performing an assessment of the renal system. What is the first step in the assessment process?
a.   Percuss the lower abdomen; continue toward the umbilicus.
b.   Observe the flank region for asymmetry or discoloration.
c.   Listen for a bruit over each renal artery.
d.   Lightly palpate the abdomen in all quadrants.

31.   A patient with chronic kidney disease (CKD) develops anorexia, nausea and vomiting, muscle cramping, and pruritus. How does the nurse interpret these findings?
a.   Oliguria
b.   Azotemia
c.   Anuria
d.   Uremia

32.   The nurse hears in report that the patient is having renal colic pain. When performing the physical assessment of this patient during a severe pain episode, what additional sign/symptom may the nurse expect to observe?
a.   Diaphoresis
b.   Redness over the flank
c.   Jaundice
d.   Bruit in the renal artery

33.   The nurse is assessing a patient with a chronic kidney problem. The nurse notes that the patient has pedal edema and periorbital edema. What additional assessments will the nurse make to assess for fluid overload? *(Select all that apply.)*
a.   Obtain a urine specimen.
b.   Compare current blood pressure to baseline.
c.   Measure the residual urine with a bladder scanner.
d.   Weigh the patient and compare to baseline.
e.   Auscultate lung fields to determine if fluid is present.

34. A patient is diagnosed with renal artery stenosis. Which sound does the nurse expect to hear by auscultation when a bruit is present in a renal artery?
    a. Quiet, pulsating sound
    b. Swishing sound
    c. Faint wheezing
    d. No sound at all

35. The nurse is assisting an inexperienced health care provider to assess a patient who has an aneurysm. The nurse would intervene if the provider performed which action?
    a. Inspected the flank for bruising or redness
    b. Listened for a bruit over the renal artery
    c. Auscultated the abdomen for bowel sounds
    d. Palpated deeply to locate masses or tenderness

36. The nurse reads in the assessment note made by the advanced-practice nurse that the "left kidney cannot be palpated." How does the nurse interpret this notation?
    a. The left kidney is smaller than normal, which indicates CKD.
    b. The left kidney is normally deeper and often cannot be palpated.
    c. The palpation of kidneys should be repeated by another provider.
    d. The patient is too obese for this type of examination.

37. The nurse is assessing a patient for bladder distention. What technique does the nurse use?
    a. Gently palpate for the outline of the bladder, percuss the lower abdomen, continue toward the umbilicus until dull sounds are no longer produced.
    b. Gently palpate for the outline of the bladder, auscultate for sounds in the lower abdomen.
    c. Place one hand under the back and palpate with the other hand over the bladder, percuss the lower abdomen until tympanic sounds are no longer produced.
    d. Use the hand to depress the bladder as the patient takes a deep breath, then percuss.

38. A patient reports flank pain and tenderness. What technique does the nurse use to assess for costovertebral angle (CVA) tenderness?
    a. Percuss the nontender flank and assess for rebound.
    b. Thump the CVA area with the flat surface of the hand.
    c. Thump the CVA area with a clenched fist.
    d. Place one palm over the CVA area, thump with other fist.

39. The nurse is preparing to assess a female patient's urethra prior to the insertion of a Foley catheter. In addition to gloves, which equipment does the nurse obtain to perform the initial assessment?
    a. Glass slide
    b. Good light source
    c. Speculum
    d. Cotton ball

40. A healthy female patient has no physical symptoms, but urinalysis results reveal a protein level of >0.8 mg/dL and a white blood cell count of 4 per high-powered field. What question would the nurse ask the patient in order to assist the health care provider to correctly interpret the urinalysis results?
    a. "Have you ever been treated for a urinary tract infection?"
    b. "Do you have a family history of cardiac or biliary disease?"
    c. "Are you sexually active and if so, do you use condoms?"
    d. "Have you recently performed any strenuous exercise?"

41. Ketones in the urine may indicate which occurrence or process?
    a. Increased glomerular membrane permeability
    b. Chronic kidney infection
    c. Body's use of fat for cellular energy
    d. Urinary tract infection

42. The nurse and nutritionist are evaluating the diet and nutritional therapies for a patient with kidney problems. Blood urea nitrogen (BUN) levels for this patient are tracked because of the direct relationship to the intake and metabolism of which substance?
    a. Lipids
    b. Carbohydrates
    c. Protein
    d. Fluids

43. The nurse is caring for a patient with dehydration. Which laboratory test results does the nurse anticipate to see for this patient?
    a. BUN and creatinine ratio stay the same.
    b. BUN rises faster than creatinine level.
    c. Creatinine rises faster than BUN.
    d. BUN and creatinine have a direct relationship.

44. What does the BUN test measure?
    a. Kidney excretion of urea nitrogen
    b. Urine osmolality
    c. Creatinine clearance
    d. Urine output

45. A healthy 34-year-old male with no physical complaints has a BUN of 26 mg/dL. Which questions would the nurse ask to identify non-renal factors that could be contributing to this laboratory result? *(Select all that apply.)*
    a. "Did you drink a lot of extra fluid before the blood sample was drawn?"
    b. "Have you been on a severe protein- or calorie-restricted diet?"
    c. "Are you taking or have you recently taken any steroid medications?"
    d. "Have you recently experienced any physical or emotional stress?"
    e. "Have you noticed any blood in the stool or have you vomited any blood?"

46. The nurse sees that an older patient has a blood osmolarity of 303 mOsm/L. Which additional assessment will the nurse make before notifying the health care provider about the laboratory results?
    a. Patient's mental status
    b. Signs of dehydration
    c. Patient's temperature
    d. Odor of the urine

47. Which patient is most likely to have a decreased calcium level?
    a. Patient with kidney disease
    b. Patient with cystitis
    c. Patient with a Foley catheter
    d. Patient with urinary retention

48. The nurse performs a dipstick urine test for a patient being evaluated for kidney problems. Glucose is present in the urine. How does the nurse interpret this result?
    a. Blood glucose level is greater than 220 mg/dL.
    b. The kidneys are failing to filter any glucose.
    c. The patient is at risk for hypoglycemia.
    d. The renal threshold has not been exceeded.

49. In addition to kidney disease, which patient condition causes the BUN to rise above the normal range?
    a. Anemia
    b. Asthma
    c. Infection
    d. Malnutrition

50. The community health nurse is talking to a group of African-American adults about renal health. The nurse encourages the participants to have which type of yearly examination to screen for kidney problems?
    a. Kidney ultrasound
    b. Serum creatinine and blood urea nitrogen
    c. Urinalysis and microalbuminuria
    d. 24-hour urine collection

51. Which test is the best indicator of kidney function?
    a. Urine osmolarity
    b. Serum creatinine
    c. Urine pH
    d. BUN

52. Which patient is most likely to produce urine with a specific gravity of less than 1.005?
    a. Takes diuretic medication everyday
    b. Has dehydration secondary to vomiting
    c. Is hypovolemic due to blood loss
    d. Has syndrome of inappropriate antidiuretic hormone

53. What does an increase in the ratio of BUN to serum creatinine indicate?
    a. Highly suggestive of kidney dysfunction
    b. Definitive for kidney infection
    c. Suggests nonkidney factors causing an elevation in BUN
    d. Suggests nonkidney factors causing an elevation in serum creatinine

54. Which urine characteristic listed on a urinalysis report arouses the nurse's suspicion of a problem in the urinary tract?
    a. Cloudiness
    b. Straw color
    c. Ammonia odor
    d. One cast per high-powered field

55. A patient has a urinalysis ordered. When is the best time for the nurse to collect the specimen?
    a. In the evening
    b. After a meal
    c. In the morning
    d. After a fluid bolus

56. During the day, the nursing student is measuring urine output and observing for urine characteristics in a patient. Which abnormal finding is the most urgent, which must be reported to the supervising nurse?
    a. Specific gravity is decreased.
    b. Output is decreased.
    c. pH is decreased.
    d. Color has changed.

57. A 24-hour urine specimen is required from a patient. Which strategy is best to ensure that all the urine is collected for the full 24-hour period?
    a. Instruct the unlicensed assistive personnel (UAP) to collect all the urine.
    b. Put a bedpan or commode next to the bed as a reminder.
    c. Place a sign in the bathroom reminding everyone to save the urine.
    d. Verbally remind the patient about the test.

58. Place the steps of using a bedside bladder scanner in the correct order using the numbers 1 through 6.
    _____ a. Select the male or female icon on the bladder scanner.
    _____ b. Aim the scan head towards the expected location of the bladder.
    _____ c. Place the probe midline about 1.5 inches (4 cm) above the pubic bone.
    _____ d. Explain the purpose and what sensations to expect.
    _____ e. Place the ultrasound probe with gel right above the symphysis pubis.
    _____ f. Press and release the scan button.

59. A patient is scheduled for a computed tomography (CT) with iodinated contrast medium. Which medication is discontinued 24 hours before the procedure and for at least 48 hours until kidney function has been reevaluated?
    a. Glucophage (Metformin)
    b. Morphine (MS Contin)
    c. Furosemide (Lasix)
    d. Oral acetylcysteine (Mucomyst)

60. Several patients are scheduled for testing to diagnose potential kidney problems. Which test requires a patient to have a urinary catheter inserted before the test?
    a. Urine stream testing
    b. Computed tomography
    c. Cystography
    d. Renal scan

61. A patient had a renal scan. What is included in the postprocedural care for this patient?
    a. Administer laxatives to cleanse the bowel.
    b. Encourage oral fluids to assist excretion of isotope.
    c. Administer captopril (Capoten) to increase blood flow.
    d. Insert a urinary catheter to measure urine output.

62. Which diagnostic test incorporates contrast dye, but does not place a patient at risk for nephrotoxicity?
    a. Renal scan
    b. Renal angiography
    c. Voiding cystourethrogram
    d. Computed tomography

63. The nurse is reviewing the results of a patient's ultrasound of the kidney. The report reveals an enlarged kidney which suggests which possible problem?
    a. Polycystic kidney
    b. Kidney infection
    c. Renal carcinoma
    d. Chronic kidney disease

64. A patient returns to the unit after a renal scan. Which instruction about the patient's urine does the nurse give to the UAP caring for the patient?
    a. It is radioactive, so it should be handled with special biohazard precautions.
    b. It does not place anyone at risk because of the small amount of radioactive material.
    c. Its radioactivity is dangerous only to those who are pregnant.
    d. It is potentially dangerous if allowed to sit for prolonged periods in the commode.

65. What is an advantage of a renal scan compared to a CT scan for diagnosing the perfusion, function, and structure of the kidneys?
    a. Renal scan is more readily tolerated by elderly patients and small children.
    b. Renal scan is preferred if the patient is allergic to iodine or has impaired kidney function.
    c. Renal scans are more likely to detect pathologic changes that CT scans do not detect.
    d. Renal scan requires less pre- and postprocedural care than CT scan.

66. The nurse is teaching a patient scheduled for an ultrasonography. What preprocedural instruction does the nurse give the patient?
    a. Void just before the test begins.
    b. Drink water to fill the bladder.
    c. Stop routine medications.
    d. Have nothing to eat or drink after midnight.

67. A patient had a cystoscopy. After the procedure, what does the nurse expect to see in this patient?
    a. Pink-tinged urine
    b. Bloody urine
    c. Very dilute urine
    d. Decreased urine output

68. A patient is scheduled for retrograde urethrography. Postprocedural care is similar to postprocedural care given for which test?
    a. Ultrasonography
    b. Computed tomography
    c. Renal angiogram
    d. Cystoscopy

69. A patient has undergone a kidney biopsy. What does the nurse monitor for in the patient related to this procedure?
    a. Nephrotoxicity
    b. Hemorrhage
    c. Urinary retention
    d. Hypertension

70. The health care provider informs the nurse that there is a change in orders because the patient has a decrease in creatinine clearance rate. What change does the nurse anticipate?
    a. Fluid restriction
    b. Reduction of drug dosage
    c. Limitations on activity level
    d. Modification of diet

71. The nurse is planning the care for several patients who are undergoing diagnostic testing. Which patient is likely to need the most time for postprocedural care?
    a. Will have a kidney, ureter, and bladder x-ray
    b. Needs a kidney ultrasound
    c. Will have a cystoscopy
    d. Needs urine for culture and sensitivity

72. A patient has undergone a kidney biopsy. In the immediate postprocedural period, the nurse notifies the health care provider about which findings? *(Select all that apply.)*
    a. Hematuria with blood clots
    b. Localized pain at the site
    c. "Tamponade effect"
    d. Decreasing urine output
    e. Flank pain
    f. Decreasing blood pressure

73. Limiting fluid intake would have what effect on urine?
    a. Increases the concentration of urine
    b. Makes the urine less irritating
    c. Decreases the risk for urine infection
    d. Decreases the pH of urine

74. Which abnormal finding would be associated with chronic kidney disease?
    a. Hematuria
    b. Pus in the urine
    c. Blood at the urethral meatus
    d. Decreased urine specific gravity

66 CHAPTER

Care of Patients with Urinary Problems

1. The home health nurse reads in the patient's chart that the patient has asymptomatic bacterial urinary tract infection (ABUTI). Which intervention will the nurse perform?
   a. Obtain an order for urinalysis and urine culture and sensitivity.
   b. Check the patient's medication list for appropriate antibiotic order.
   c. Closely monitor for conditions that cause progression to acute infection.
   d. Ask the patient when the ABUTI first started and when it was diagnosed.

2. Which group has the highest prevalence of urinary tract infections (UTIs)?
   a. Young men
   b. Older women
   c. Older men
   d. School-aged girls

3. Which patient has the highest risk for developing a complicated UTI?
   a. 26-year-old woman who is sexually active, but not currently pregnant
   b. 22-year-old man who has a neurogenic bladder due to spinal cord injury
   c. 35-year-old woman who had three full-term pregnancies and a miscarriage
   d. 53-year-old woman who is having some menstrual irregularities

4. The nurse is working in a long-term care facility. Which circumstance is cause for greatest concern, because the facility has a large number of residents who are developing UTIs?
   a. Residents are not drinking enough fluids with meals.
   b. Unlicensed personnel are not assisting with toileting in a timely fashion.
   c. A large percentage of residents have indwelling urinary catheters.
   d. Many residents have severe dementia and functional incontinence.

5. The nurse is caring for a patient with an indwelling catheter. What intervention does the nurse use to minimize catheter-related infections?
   a. Assess the patient daily to determine need for catheter.
   b. Irrigate the catheter daily with sterile solution to remove debris.
   c. Use sterile technique when opening system to obtain urine samples.
   d. Apply antiseptic solutions or antibiotic ointments to the perineal area.

6. Which task related to care of patients who have indwelling catheters can be delegated to unlicensed assistive personnel (UAP)?
   a. Perform daily catheter care by washing the perineum and proximal portion of the catheter with soap and water.
   b. Use sterile technique when inserting the urinary catheter or when opening the system to obtain urine samples.
   c. Determine whether use of condom catheters is appropriate for male patients and apply the devices accordingly.
   d. Keep urine collection bag in a place that is readily visible to the patient, so that the patient is reassured of kidney function.

7. In which patient circumstance would the nurse question the order for the insertion of an indwelling catheter?
   a. Patient is critically ill and at risk for hypovolemic shock.
   b. Patient has urinary retention with beginnings of hydronephrosis.
   c. Patient was in a car accident and has a possible spinal cord injury.
   d. Patient has functional incontinence related to Alzheimer's disease.

8. For a patient who needs an indwelling catheter for at least 2 weeks, which intervention would help reduce the bacterial colonization along the catheter?
   a. Secure the catheter to the female patient's thigh.
   b. Consider the use of a coated catheter.
   c. Wash the urine bag and outflow tube every day.
   d. Apply antiseptic ointment to the catheter tubing.

9. The nurse hears in report that the patient is being treated for a fungal UTI. In addition to performing routine care and assessments, the nurse is extra-vigilant for signs/symptoms of which systemic disorder that may underlie the fungal UTI?
   a. Chronic cardiac disease
   b. Immune system compromise
   c. Respiratory system dysfunction
   d. Connective tissue disorder

10. The nurse is caring for a patient who has an indwelling catheter and subsequently developed a UTI. The patient has been receiving antibiotics for several days, but develops hypotension, a rapid pulse, and confusion. The nurse suspects urosepsis and alerts the health care provider. Which diagnostic test is the provider most likely to order to confirm urosepsis?
    a. Culture of the drainage bag
    b. Culture of the catheter tip
    c. Blood culture
    d. Repeat urinalysis

11. The nurse is teaching a woman how to prevent UTIs. What information does the nurse include?
    a. Clean the perineal area from front to back.
    b. Always use a condom if spermicides are used for contraception.
    c. Obtain prescription for oral estrogen for vaginal dryness.
    d. Avoid urinary stasis by urinating every 6 to 8 hours.

12. The nurse is teaching a man about how to prevent UTIs. What information does the nurse include?
    a. "Have a minimal fluid intake of 5 L daily, unless contraindicated."
    b. "Empty your bladder before and after sexual intercourse."
    c. "Make sure that spermicides are used with condoms."
    d. "Gently wash the genital area before intercourse."

13. Patients who have central nervous system lesions from stroke, multiple sclerosis, or parasacral spinal cord lesions may have which type of urinary incontinence?
    a. Detrusor hyperreflexia
    b. Mixed
    c. Stress
    d. Functional

14. A patient reports intense urgency, frequency, and bladder pain. Urinalysis results show white blood cells (WBCs) and red blood cells (RBCs) and urine culture results are negative for infection. How does the nurse interpret these findings?
    a. Interstitial cystitis
    b. Urethritis
    c. Bacteriuria
    d. Infectious cystitis

15. A patient has been started on oxybutynin (Ditropan) for urinary incontinence. What is the major action of this medication?
    a. Increases blood flow to the urethra
    b. Blocks acetylcholine receptors
    c. Causes slight numbing of the bladder
    d. Relaxes bladder muscles

16. A young female patient reports experiencing burning with urination. What question does the nurse ask to differentiate between a vaginal infection and a urinary infection?
    a. "Have you noticed any blood in the urine?"
    b. "Have you had recent sexual intercourse?"
    c. "Have you noticed any vaginal discharge?"
    d. "Have you had fever or chills?"

17. A patient reports symptoms indicating a UTI. Results from which diagnostic test will verify a UTI?
    a. Urinalysis to test for leukocyte esterase and nitrate
    b. Urinalysis for glucose and red blood cells
    c. Urinalysis to test for ketones and protein
    d. Urinalysis for pH and specific gravity

18. A patient is diagnosed with a fungal UTI. Which drug does the nurse anticipate the patient will be treated with?
    a. Trimethoprim/sulfamethoxazole (Bactrim)
    b. Ciprofloxacin (Cipro)
    c. Fluconazole (Diflucan)
    d. Amoxicillin (Amoxil)

19. The nurse is teaching a patient about self-care measures to prevent UTIs. Which daily fluid intake does the nurse recommend to the patient to prevent a bladder infection?
    a. 2 to 3 L of water
    b. 3 to 6 glasses of iced tea
    c. 4 to 6 cups of electrolyte fluid
    d. 3 to 4 glasses of juice

20. The nursing student sees an order for a urinalysis for a patient with frequency, urgency, and dysuria. In order to collect the specimen, what does the student do?
    a. Use sterile technique to insert a small-diameter (6 Fr) catheter.
    b. Instruct the patient on how to collect a clean-catch specimen.
    c. Tell the patient to urinate approximately 10 mL into a specimen cup.
    d. Take the urine from a bedpan and transfer it into a specimen cup.

21. The nurse is reviewing the laboratory results for an older adult patient with an indwelling catheter. The urine culture is pending, but the urinalysis shows greater than 10^5 colony-forming units, and the differential WBC count shows a "left shift." How does the nurse interpret these findings?
    a. Interstitial cystitis
    b. Urosepsis
    c. Complicated cystitis
    d. Radiation-induced cystitis

22. A patient has UTI symptoms but there are no bacteria in the urine. The health care provider suspects interstitial cystitis. The nurse prepares patient teaching material for which diagnostic test?
    a. Urography
    b. Abdominal sonography
    c. Computed tomography (CT)
    d. Cystoscopy

23. Several patients at the clinic have just been diagnosed with UTIs. Which patients may need longer antibiotic treatment (7 to 21 days) or different agents than the typical first-line medications? *(Select all that apply.)*
    a. Postmenopausal patient
    b. Patient with urethritis
    c. Diabetic patient
    d. Immunosuppressed patient
    e. Pregnant patient

24. The nurse is counseling a patient with recurrent symptomatic UTIs about dietary therapy. What information does the nurse give to the patient?
    a. Drink 50 mL of concentrated cranberry juice every day.
    b. Low consumption of protein may prevent recurrent UTIs.
    c. Caffeine, carbonated beverages, and tomato products cause UTI.
    d. Cranberry tablets are more effective than juice or fluids.

25. A patient received an antibiotic prescription several hours ago and has started the medication, but requests "some relief from the burning." What comfort measures does the nurse suggest to the patient?
    a. Take over-the-counter acetaminophen.
    b. Sit in a sitz bath and urinate into the warm water.
    c. Place a cold pack over the perineal area.
    d. Rest in a recumbent position with legs elevated.

26. A patient's recurrent cystitis appears to be related to sexual intercourse. The patient seems uncomfortable talking about the situation. What communication technique does the nurse use to assist the patient?
    a. Have a frank and sensitive discussion with the patient.
    b. Give the patient reading material with instructions to call with any questions.
    c. Call the patient's partner and invite the partner to discuss the problem.
    d. Talk about other topics until the patient feels more comfortable disclosing.

27. The cystoscopy results for a patient include a small-capacity bladder, the presence of Hunner's ulcers, and small hemorrhages after bladder distention. How does the nurse interpret this report?
    a. Urosepsis
    b. Complicated cystitis
    c. Interstitial cystitis
    d. Urethritis

28. A male college student comes to the clinic reporting burning or difficulty with urination and a discharge from the urethral meatus. Based on the patient's chief complaint, what is the most logical question for the nurse to ask about the patient's past medical history?
    a. "Do you have a history of a narrow urethra or a stricture?"
    b. "Could you have been exposed to a sexually transmitted disease (STD)?"
    c. "Do you have a history of kidney stones?"
    d. "Have you been drinking an adequate amount of fluids?"

29. The health care provider verbally informs the nurse that the patient needs a fluoroquinolone antibiotic to treat a UTI. The pharmacy delivers gabapentin (Neurontin). What should the nurse do first?
    a. Administer the medication as ordered.
    b. Call the pharmacist and ask for a read back of the order.
    c. Call the health care provider for clarification of the order.
    d. Look at the written order to clarify the name of the medication.

30. Which patient should not be advised to take cranberry juice?
    a. 26-year-old pregnant woman with a history of uncomplicated UTI
    b. 23-year-old man with history of recurrent kidney stones
    c. 65-year-old man with urinary retention secondary to enlarged prostate
    d. 33-year-old woman with dysuria associated with interstitial cystitis

31. Which urine characteristic suggests that the patient is drinking a sufficient amount of fluid?
    a. Urine pH is between 6 to 6.5.
    b. Urine has a high specific gravity.
    c. Urine has a faint ammonia odor.
    d. Urine is a pale yellow color.

32. A young woman tells the nurse that she gets frequent UTIs that seem to follow sexual intercourse. Which questions would the nurse ask? *(Select all that apply.)*
    a. "Do you use a diaphragm or spermicides for contraception?"
    b. "Do you feel guilty or embarrassed about your sexual activities?"
    c. "Have you considered abstaining from intercourse?"
    d. "Do you and your partner(s) wash the perineal area before intercourse?"
    e. "Some positions cause more irritation during sex. Have you noticed this?"

33. A patient is diagnosed with urethral stricture. What findings does the nurse expect to see documented in the patient's chart for this condition?
    a. Pain on urination
    b. Pain on ejaculation
    c. Overflow incontinence
    d. Hematuria and pyuria

34. A patient is diagnosed with a urethral stricture. The nurse prepares the patient for which temporary treatment?
    a. Dilation of the urethra
    b. Antibiotic therapy
    c. Fluid restriction
    d. Urinary diversion

35. A patient reports the loss of small amounts of urine during coughing, sneezing, jogging, or lifting. Which type of incontinence do these symptoms describe?
    a. Urge
    b. Overflow
    c. Functional
    d. Stress

36. The nurse is caring for an obese older adult patient with dementia. The patient is alert and ambulatory, but has functional incontinence. Which nursing intervention is best for this patient?
    a. Help the patient to lose weight.
    b. Help the patient apply an estrogen cream.
    c. Offer assistance with toileting every 2 hours.
    d. Intermittently catheterize the patient.

37. Which patient is mostly likely to have mixed incontinence?
    a. 54-year-old woman who had four full-term pregnancies
    b. 52-year-old man who had a stroke with neurologic deficits
    c. 76-year-old man with benign prostatic hyperplasia
    d. 25-year-old woman who has a pelvic fracture

38. The nurse is caring for an older adult patient with urinary incontinence. The patient is alert and oriented, but refuses to use the call bell and has fallen several times while trying to get to the bathroom. What is the nurse's priority concern for this patient?
    a. Managing noncompliance
    b. Accurately measuring urinary output
    c. Providing fall prevention measures
    d. Managing urinary incontinence

39. The nurse is performing an assessment on a patient with probable stress incontinence. Which assessment technique does the nurse use to validate stress incontinence?
    a. Assess the abdomen to estimate bladder fullness.
    b. Check for residual urine using a portable ultrasound.
    c. Catheterize the patient immediately after voiding.
    d. Ask the patient to cough while wearing a perineal pad.

40. The advanced-practice nurse is performing a digital rectal examination (DRE) and notes that the rectal sphincter contracts on digital insertion. How does the nurse interpret this finding?
    a. Nerve supply to the bladder is most likely intact.
    b. There is adequate strength in the pelvic floor.
    c. A rectocele is placing pressure on the bladder.
    d. Abnormal function for the bladder is unlikely.

41. A middle-aged woman has urinary stress incontinence related to weak pelvic muscles. The patient is highly motivated to participate in self-care. Which interventions does the nurse include in the treatment plan? *(Select all that apply.)*
    a. Suggest keeping a detailed diary of urine leakage, activities, and foods eaten.
    b. Suggest wearing absorbent undergarments during the assessment process.
    c. Teach pelvic floor (Kegel) exercise therapy.
    d. Teach about vaginal cone therapy.
    e. Encourage drinking orange juice every day for 4 to 6 weeks.
    f. Refer to a nutritionist for diet therapy for weight reduction.

42. A patient has been performing Kegel exercises for 2 months. How does the nurse know whether the exercises are working?
    a. Incontinence is still present, but the patient states that it is less.
    b. The patient is able to stop the urinary stream.
    c. There are no complaints of urgency from the patient.
    d. The patient is using absorbent undergarments for protection.

43. The home health nurse is assessing an older adult patient who refuses to leave the house to see friends or participate in usual activities. She reports taking a bath several times a day and becomes very upset when she has an incontinent episode. What is the priority problem for this patient?
    a. Negative self-image
    b. Stress urinary incontinence
    c. Social isolation
    d. Potential for skin breakdown

44. The nurse is evaluating outcome criteria for a patient being treated for urge incontinence. Which statement indicates the treatment has been successful?
    a. "I'm following the prescribed therapy, but I think surgery is my best choice."
    b. "I still lose a little urine when I sneeze, but I have been wearing a thin pad."
    c. "I had trouble at first, but now I go to the toilet every 3 hours."
    d. "I have been using the bladder compression technique and it works."

45. The nurse is teaching a patient with urge incontinence about dietary modifications. What is the best information the nurse gives to the patient about fluid intake?
    a. Drink at least 2000 mL per day unless contraindicated.
    b. Drink 120 mL every hour or 240 mL every 2 hours and limit fluids after dinner.
    c. Drink fluid freely in the morning hours, but limit intake before going to bed.
    d. Drinking water is especially good for bladder health.

46. A patient has agreed to try a bladder training program. What is the priority nursing intervention in starting this therapy?
    a. Start a schedule for voiding (e.g., every 2-3 hours).
    b. Teach the patient how to be alert, aware, and able to resist the urge to urinate.
    c. Convince the patient that the bladder issues are controlling his/her lifestyle.
    d. Give a thorough explanation of the problem of stress incontinence.

47. An older adult patient with a cognitive impairment is living in an extended-care facility. The patient is incontinent, but as the family points out, "he will urinate in the toilet if somebody helps him." Which type of incontinence does the nurse suspect in this patient?
    a. Urge
    b. Overflow
    c. Functional
    d. Stress

48. The nurse is designing a habit training bladder program for an older adult patient who is alert but mildly confused. What task associated with the training program is delegated to the UAP?
    a. Tell the patient it is time to go to the toilet and assist him to go on a regular schedule.
    b. Help the patient record the incidents of incontinence in a bladder diary.
    c. Change the patient's incontinence pants (or pad) every 4 hours.
    d. Gradually encourage independence and increase the intervals between voidings.

49. Which patient with incontinence is most likely to benefit from a surgical intervention?
    a. Patient with vaginal atrophy and altered urethral competency
    b. Patient with reflex (overflow) incontinence caused by obstruction
    c. Patient with functional incontinence related to musculoskeletal weakness
    d. Patient with urge incontinence or overactive bladder

50. The nurse is teaching a patient a behavioral intervention for bladder compression. In order to correctly perform the Credé method, what does the nurse teach the patient to do?
    a. Insert the fingers into the vagina and gently push against the vaginal wall.
    b. Breathe in deeply and direct the pressure towards the bladder during exhalation.
    c. Empty the bladder, wait a few minutes, and attempt a second bladder emptying.
    d. Apply firm and steady pressure over the bladder area with the palm of the hand.

51. The health care provider has recommended intermittent self-catheterization for a patient with long-term problems of incomplete bladder emptying. Which information does the nurse give the patient about the procedure?
    a. Perform proper handwashing and cleaning of the catheter to reduce the risk for infection.
    b. Use a large-lumen catheter and good lubrication for rapid emptying of the bladder.
    c. Catheterize yourself whenever the bladder gets distended.
    d. Use sterile technique, especially if catheterization is done by a family member.

52. The nurse is reviewing a care plan for a patient who has functional incontinence. There is a note that containment is recommended, especially at night. What is the major concern with this approach?
    a. Skin integrity
    b. Cost of care and materials
    c. Self-esteem of the patient
    d. Fall risk

53. The nurse is caring for a patient with functional incontinence. The UAP reports that "the linens have been changed four times within the past 6 hours, but the patient refuses to wear a diaper." What does the nurse do next?
    a. Thank the UAP for the hard work and advise to continue to change the linens.
    b. Call the health care provider to obtain an order for an indwelling catheter.
    c. Instruct the UAP to stop using the word "diaper" and instead use "incontinence pants."
    d. Assess the patient for any new urinary problems and ask about toileting preferences.

54. Which dietary changes does the nurse suggest to a patient with urge incontinence?
    a. Limit fluid intake to no more than 2 L/day.
    b. Peel all fruit before consuming.
    c. Avoid alcohol and caffeine.
    d. Avoid smoked or salted foods.

55. A patient is considering vaginal cone therapy, but is a little hesitant because she does not understand how it works. What does the nurse tell her about how vaginal cone therapy improves incontinence?
    a. It mechanically obstructs urine loss from the urethra.
    b. It repositions the bladder to reduce compression.
    c. It increases the normal flora of the perineum.
    d. It strengthens pelvic floor muscles.

56. A patient with urinary incontinence is prescribed oxybutynin (Ditropan). What precautions or instructions does the nurse provide related to this therapy?
    a. Avoid aspirin or aspirin-containing products.
    b. Increase fluids and dietary fiber intake.
    c. Report any unusual vaginal bleeding.
    d. Change positions slowly, especially in the morning.

57. Teaching intermittent self-catheterization for incontinence is appropriate for which patient?
    a. 25-year-old male patient with paraplegia
    b. 35-year-old female patient with stress incontinence
    c. 70-year-old patient who wears absorbent briefs
    d. 18-year-old patient with a severe head injury

58. What role does drug therapy have as an intervention for reflex (overflow) urinary incontinence?
    a. Captopril (Capoten) is given to lower urine cystine levels.
    b. Levofloxacin (Levaquin) is given to prevent UTIs with this type of incontinence.
    c. Midorine (ProAmatine) is given to increase the contractile force of the bladder.
    d. Bethanechol chloride (Urecholine) may be used short-term after surgery.

59. A patient is admitted for an elective orthopedic surgical procedure. The patient also has a personal and family history for urolithiasis. Which circumstance creates the greatest risk for recurrent urolithiasis?
    a. Giving the patient milk with every meal tray
    b. Keeping the patient NPO for extended periods
    c. Giving the patient an opioid narcotic for pain
    d. Inserting an indwelling catheter for the procedure

60. A patient reports severe flank pain. The report indicates that urine is turbid, malodorous, and rust-colored; RBCs, WBCs, and bacteria are present; and microscopic analysis shows crystals. What does this data suggest?
    a. Pyuria and cystitis
    b. Staghorn calculus with infection
    c. Urolithiasis and infection
    d. Dysuria and urinary retention

61. A patient comes to the clinic and reports severe flank pain, bladder distention, and nausea and vomiting with increasingly smaller amounts of urine with frank blood. The patient states, "I have kidney stones and I just need a prescription for pain medication." What is the nurse's priority concern?
    a. Controlling the patient's pain
    b. Checking the quantity of blood in the urine
    c. Flushing the kidneys with oral fluids
    d. Determining if there is an obstruction

62. The nurse is caring for a patient with urolithiasis. Which medication is likely to be given in the acute phase to relieve the patient's severe pain?
    a. Ketorolac (Toradol)
    b. Oxybutynin chloride (Ditropan)
    c. Propantheline bromide (Pro-Banthine)
    d. Morphine sulfate (Astramorph)

63. A patient returns to the medical-surgical unit after having shock wave lithotripsy (SWL). What is an appropriate nursing intervention for the postprocedural care of this patient?
    a. Strain the urine to monitor the passage of stone fragments.
    b. Report bruising that occurs on the flank of the affected side.
    c. Continuously monitor electrocardiogram (ECG) for dysrhythmias.
    d. Apply a local anesthetic cream to the skin of the affected side.

64. The nurse is teaching self-care measures to a patient who had lithotripsy for kidney stones. What information does the nurse include? *(Select all that apply.)*
    a. Finish the entire prescription of antibiotics to prevent UTIs.
    b. Balance regular exercise with sleep and rest.
    c. Drink at least 3 L of fluid a day.
    d. Watch for and immediately report bruising after lithotripsy.
    e. Urine may be bloody for several days.
    f. Pain in the region of the kidneys or bladder is expected.

65. A patient with a history of kidney stones presents with severe flank pain, nausea, vomiting, pallor, and diaphoresis. He reports freely passing urine, but it is bloody. The priority for nursing care is to monitor for which patient problem?
    a. Possible dehydration
    b. Impaired tissue perfusion
    c. Impaired urinary elimination
    d. Severe pain

66. Which clinical manifestation indicates to the nurse that interventions for the patient's renal colic are effective?
    a. Urine is pink-tinged.
    b. Patient reports that pain is relieved.
    c. Urine output is 50 mL/min.
    d. Bladder scan shows no residual urine.

67. The urine output of a patient with a kidney stone has decreased from 40 mL/hr to 5 mL/hr. What is the nurse's priority action?
    a. Ensure IV access and notify the health care provider.
    b. Perform the Credé maneuver on the patient's bladder.
    c. Test the urine for ketone bodies.
    d. Document the finding and continue monitoring.

68. What does the nurse include in the care plan for a patient who had pyelolithotomy? *(Select all that apply.)*
    a. Monitor the amount of bleeding from incisions.
    b. Restrict fluids to prevent edema and fluid overload.
    c. Strain the urine to monitor the passage of stone fragments.
    d. Encourage fluids to avoid dehydration and supersaturation.
    e. Monitor changes in urine output.
    f. Administer antibiotics to eliminate or prevent infections.

69. Which patient has the highest risk for bladder cancer?
    a. 60-year-old male patient with malnutrition secondary to chronic alcoholism and self-neglect
    b. 25-year-old male patient with type 1 diabetes mellitus, who is noncompliant with therapeutic regimen
    c. 60-year-old female patient who smokes two packs of cigarettes per day and works in a chemical factory
    d. 25-year-old female patient who has had three episodes of bacterial *(Escherichia coli)* cystitis in the past year

70. The nurse is talking to a 68-year-old male patient who has lifestyle choices and occupational exposure that put him at high risk for bladder cancer. The nurse is most concerned about which urinary characteristic?
    a. Frequency
    b. Nocturia
    c. Painless hematuria
    d. Incontinence

71. A patient has had surgery for bladder cancer. To prevent recurrence of superficial bladder cancer, the nurse anticipates that the health care provider is likely to recommend which treatment?
    a. No treatment is needed for this benign condition.
    b. Intravesical instillation of single-agent chemotherapy.
    c. Radiation therapy to the bladder, ureters, and urethra.
    d. Intravesical instillation of bacille Calmette-Guérin.

72. Which statement by a patient indicates effective coping with a Kock's pouch?
    a. "I don't have any discomfort, but the pouch frequently overflows."
    b. "My wife has been irrigating the pouch daily. She likes to do it."
    c. "I check the pouch every 2 to 3 hours depending on my fluid and diet."
    d. "I never undress in front of anyone anymore, but I guess that is okay."

73. A patient has had a bladder suspension and a suprapubic catheter is in place. The patient wants to know how long the catheter will remain in place. What is the nurse's best response?
    a. "Typically it remains for 24 hours postoperatively."
    b. "It will be removed at your first clinic visit."
    c. "When you can void on your own, it will be removed."
    d. "It will be removed when you can void and residual urine is less than 50 mL."

74. The employee health nurse is conducting a presentation for employees who work in a paint manufacturing plant. In order to protect against bladder cancer, the nurse advises that everyone who works with chemicals should do what?
    a. Shower with mild soap and rinse well before they come to work.
    b. Use personal protective equipment such as gloves and masks.
    c. Limit their exposure to chemicals and fumes at all times.
    d. Avoid hobbies such as furniture refinishing that further expose to chemicals.

75. A patient is returning from the postanesthesia care unit after surgery for bladder cancer resulting in a cutaneous ureterostomy. Where does the nurse expect the stoma to be located?
    a. On the perineum
    b. At the beltline
    c. On the posterior flank
    d. In the midabdominal area

67

CHAPTER

Care of Patients with Kidney Disorders

1. A 22-year-old patient comes to the clinic for a wellness check-up. History reveals that the patient's parent has the autosomal-dominant form of polycystic kidney disease (PKD). Which vital sign suggests that the patient should be evaluated for PKD?
   a. Pulse of 90 beats/min
   b. Temperature of 99.6° F
   c. Blood pressure of 136/88 mm Hg
   d. Respiratory rate of 22/min

2. Which description of the recessive form of PKD is correct?
   a. Prognosis is better for the recessive form compared to the dominant form.
   b. 100% of people with this form of PKD develop kidney failure around age 50.
   c. Most people with this form of PKD die in early childhood.
   d. The recessive form only manifests if other kidney problems occur.

3. Which description of the autosomal-dominant form of PKD is correct?
   a. 25% of patients with this form of PKD develop acute kidney failure by age 30.
   b. The dominant form is responsive to newer gene therapy treatments.
   c. 50% of people with this form of PKD develop kidney disease by age 50.
   d. Most people with this form of PKD die in young adulthood.

4. The nurse is interviewing a patient with suspected PKD. What questions does the nurse ask the patient? *(Select all that apply.)*
   a. "Is there any family history of PKD or kidney disease?"
   b. "Do you have a history of sexually transmitted disease?"
   c. "Have you had any constipation or abdominal discomfort?"
   d. "Have you noticed a change in urine color or frequency?"
   e. "Have you had any problems with headaches?"
   f. "Is there a family history of sudden death from a myocardial infarction?"

5. A patient has a family history of the autosomal-dominant form of PKD and has therefore been advised to monitor for and report symptoms. What is an early symptom of PKD?
   a. Headache
   b. Pruritus
   c. Edema
   d. Nocturia

6. A patient with a history of PKD reports dull, aching flank pain and the urinalysis is negative for infection. The health care provider tells the nurse that the pain is chronic and related to enlarging kidneys compressing abdominal contents. What nursing intervention is best for this patient?
   a. Administer trimethoprim/sulfamethoxazole (Bactrim).
   b. Apply cool compresses to the abdomen or flank.
   c. Teach methods of relaxation such as deep-breathing.
   d. Administer around-the-clock nonsteroidal antiinflammatory drugs (NSAIDs).

7. Why may a patient with PKD experience constipation?
   a. Polycystic kidneys enlarge and put pressure on the large intestine.
   b. Patient becomes dehydrated because the kidneys are dysfunctional.
   c. Constipation is a side effect from the medications given to treat PKD.
   d. Patients with PKD have special dietary restrictions that cause constipation.

8. The nurse is developing a teaching plan for a patient with PKD. Which topics does the nurse include? *(Select all that apply.)*
   a. Teach how to measure and record blood pressure.
   b. Assist to develop a schedule for self-administering drugs.
   c. Instruct to take and record weight twice a month.
   d. Explain the potential side effects of the drugs.
   e. Review high-protein, low-fat diet plan.

9. A patient with PKD reports sharp flank pain followed by blood in the urine. How does the nurse interpret these signs/symptoms?
   a. Infection
   b. Ruptured cyst
   c. Increased kidney size
   d. Ruptured renal artery aneurysm

10. A patient with PKD reports a severe headache and is at risk for a berry aneurysm. What is the nurse's priority action?
    a. Assess the pain and give a prn pain medication.
    b. Reassure the patient that this is an expected aspect of the disease.
    c. Assess for neurologic changes and check vital signs.
    d. Monitor for hematuria and decreased urinary output.

11. A patient with PKD reports nocturia. What is the nocturia caused by?
    a. Increased fluid intake in the evening
    b. Increased hypertension
    c. Decreased urine-concentrating ability
    d. Detrusor irritability

12. The nurse is reviewing laboratory results for a patient with PKD. Which laboratory abnormality indicates glomeruli involvement?
    a. Low specific gravity of urine
    b. Bacteria in urine
    c. Proteinuria
    d. Hematuria

13. A patient is suspected of having PKD. Which diagnostic study has minimal risks and can reveal PKD?
    a. Kidneys-ureters-bladder (KUB) x-ray
    b. Urography
    c. Renal sonography
    d. Renal angiography

14. Which pain management strategy does the nurse teach a patient who has pain from infected kidney cysts of PKD?
    a. Take nothing by mouth.
    b. Increase the dose of NSAIDs.
    c. Assume a high-Fowler's position.
    d. Apply dry heat to the abdomen or flank.

15. A patient with PKD usually experiences constipation. What does the nurse recommend?
    a. Increased dietary fiber and increased fluids
    b. Decreased dietary fiber and laxatives
    c. Daily laxatives and increased exercise
    d. Tap-water enemas and fiber supplements

16. A patient with PKD has nocturia. What does the nurse encourage the patient to do?
    a. Drink at least 2 liters of fluid daily.
    b. Restrict fluid in the evening.
    c. Drink 1000 mL early in the morning
    d. Add a pinch of salt to water in the evenings.

17. For the patient with PKD, which antihypertensive medication may be used because it helps control the cell growth aspects of PKD and reduce microalbuminuria?
    a. Angiotensin-converting enzyme inhibitors
    b. Beta blockers
    c. Calcium channel blockers
    d. Vasodilators

18. After the nurse instructs a patient with PKD on home care, the patient knows to contact the health care provider immediately when what sign/symptom occurs?
    a. Urine is a clear, pale yellow color.
    b. Weight has increased by 3 pounds in 2 days.
    c. Two days have passed since the last bowel movement.
    d. Morning systolic blood pressure has decreased by 5 mm Hg.

19. The health care provider tells the nurse that the patient with PKD has salt wasting. Which intervention is the nurse likely to use related to nutrition therapy?
    a. Talk to the patient about seasonings that are alternatives for salt.
    b. Help the patient select a lunch tray with low-sodium items.
    c. Obtain an order for fluid restriction to prevent loss of sodium during urination.
    d. Advise that a low-sodium diet is not currently necessary.

20. The health care team is using a collaborative and interdisciplinary approach to design a treatment plan for a patient with PKD. What is the top priority?
    a. Controlling hypertension
    b. Preventing rupture of cysts
    c. Providing genetic counseling
    d. Identifying community resources

21. A patient with PKD would exhibit which signs/symptoms? *(Select all that apply.)*
    a. Frequent urination
    b. Increased abdominal girth
    c. Hypertension
    d. Kidney stones
    e. Diarrhea

22. In PKD, the effect on the renin-angiotensin system in the kidney has which result?
    a. Adrenal insufficiency
    b. Increased blood pressure
    c. Increased urine output
    d. Oliguria

23. What is the common problem of hydronephrosis, hydroureter, and urethral stricture in kidney function?
    a. Dilute urine
    b. Tubular cell damage
    c. Dehydration
    d. Obstruction

24. An older adult male patient calls the clinic because he has "not passed any urine all day long." What is the nurse's best response?
    a. "Try drinking several large glasses of water and waiting a few more hours."
    b. "If you develop flank pain or fever, then you should probably come in."
    c. "You could have an obstruction, so you should come in to be checked."
    d. "I am sorry, but I really can't comment about your problem over the phone."

25. A patient reports straining to pass very small amounts of urine today, despite a normal fluid intake, and reports having the urge to urinate. The nurse palpates the bladder and finds that it is distended. Which condition is most likely to be associated with these findings?
    a. Urethral stricture
    b. Hydroureter
    c. Hydronephrosis
    d. PKD

26. A patient is diagnosed with hydronephrosis. What is a complication that could result from this condition?
    a. Damage to the nephrons
    b. Kidney cancer
    c. Kidney stone
    d. Structural defects

27. Which clinical manifestation in a patient with an obstruction in the urinary system is associated specifically with a hydronephrosis?
    a. Flank asymmetry
    b. Chills and fever
    c. Urge incontinence
    d. Decreased urine volume

28. An older adult male patient reports an acute problem with urine retention. The nurse advises the patient to seek medical attention because permanent kidney damage can occur in what time frame?
   a. In less than 6 hours
   b. In less than 48 hours
   c. Within several weeks
   d. Within several years

29. The nurse is reviewing the laboratory results for a patient being evaluated for trouble with passing urine. The urinalysis shows tubular epithelial cells on microscopic examination. How does the nurse interpret this finding?
   a. The obstruction is resolving.
   b. The obstruction is prolonged.
   c. Glomerular filtration rate is reduced.
   d. Glomerular filtration rate is adequate.

30. A patient had a nephrostomy and a nephrostomy tube is in place. What is included in the postoperative care of this patient?
   a. Assess the amount of drainage in the collection bag.
   b. Irrigate the tube to ensure patency.
   c. Keep the patient NPO for 6 to 8 hours.
   d. Review the results of the clotting studies.

31. The nurse is caring for a patient with a nephrostomy. The nurse notifies the health care provider about which assessment finding?
   a. Urine drainage is red-tinged 4 hours postsurgery.
   b. Amount of drainage decreases and the patient has back pain.
   c. There is a small steady drainage for the first 4 hours postsurgery.
   d. The nephrostomy site looks dry and intact.

32. The off-going nurse is giving shift report to the oncoming nurse about the care of a patient who had a nephrostomy tube placed 3 days ago and it is to remain in place until the urinary obstruction is resolved. What is the most important point to clearly communicate about the urine drainage?
   a. "Urine is draining only into the collection bag, not the bladder; therefore the minimum expected drainage is 30 mL/hour."
   b. "For the first 24 hours postoperatively, the amount of urinary drainage was assessed every hour."
   c. "The surgeon placed ureteral tubes so all the urine may pass through the bladder or all of the urine might go directly into the collection bag."
   d. "The nephrostomy site has not been leaking any blood or urine and you should continue to monitor the site for leakage."

33. What are the key features associated with chronic pyelonephritis? *(Select all that apply.)*
   a. Abscess formation
   b. Hypertension
   c. Inability to conserve sodium
   d. Decreased urine-concentrating ability, resulting in nocturia
   e. Tendency to develop hyperkalemia and acidosis

34. Which factor/manifestation is primarily associated with acute pyelonephritis?
   a. Obstruction caused by hydroureter
   b. Active bacterial infection
   c. Decreased urine specific gravity
   d. Alcohol abuse

35. The nurse is assessing a patient who reports chills, high fever, and flank pain with urinary urgency and frequency. On physical examination, the patient has costovertebral angle (CVA) tenderness, pulse is 110 beats/min, and respirations are 28/min. How does the nurse interpret these findings?
   a. Complicated cystitis
   b. Acute pyelonephritis
   c. Chronic pyelonephritis
   d. Acute glomerulonephritis

36. The health care provider advises the patient that diagnostic testing is needed to identify the possible presence of a renal abscess. Which test does the nurse prepare the patient for?
    a. Renal arteriography
    b. Cystourethrogram
    c. Radionuclide renal scan
    d. Urodynamic flow studies

37. A patient with chronic pyelonephritis returns to the clinic for follow-up. Which behavior indicates the patient is meeting the expected outcomes to conserve existing kidney function?
    a. Drinks a liter of fluid every day
    b. Considers buying a home blood pressure cuff
    c. Reports taking antibiotics as prescribed
    d. Takes pain medication on a regular basis

38. Which patient has the greatest risk for developing chronic pyelonephritis?
    a. 80-year-old woman who takes diuretics for mild heart failure
    b. 80-year-old man who drinks four cans of beer per day
    c. 36-year-old woman with diabetes mellitus who is pregnant
    d. 36-year-old man with diabetes insipidus

39. A patient is diagnosed with acute pyelonephritis. What is the priority for nursing care for this patient?
    a. Providing information about the disease process
    b. Controlling hypertension
    c. Managing pain
    d. Preventing constipation

40. A patient has come to the clinic for follow-up of acute pyelonephritis. Which action does the nurse reinforce to the patient?
    a. Complete all antibiotic regimens.
    b. Report episodes of nocturia.
    c. Stop taking the antibiotic when pain is relieved.
    d. Avoid taking any over-the-counter drugs.

41. A patient is admitted for acute glomerulonephritis. In reviewing the patient's past medical history, which systemic conditions does the nurse suspect may have caused acute glomerulonephritis and will include in the overall plan of care?
    a. Systemic lupus erythematosus and diabetic nephropathy
    b. Myocardial infarction and atrial fibrillation
    c. Ischemic stroke and hemiparesis
    d. Blunt trauma to the kidney with hematuria

42. The nurse is assessing a patient with possible acute glomerulonephritis. During the inspection of the hands, face, and eyelids, what is the nurse primarily observing for?
    a. Redness
    b. Edema
    c. Rashes
    d. Dryness

43. The nurse is assessing a patient with glomerulonephritis and notes crackles in the lung fields and neck vein distention. The patient reports mild shortness of breath. Based on these findings, what does the nurse do next?
    a. Check for CVA tenderness or flank pain.
    b. Obtain a urine sample to check for proteinuria.
    c. Assess for additional signs of fluid overload.
    d. Alert the health care provider about the respiratory symptoms.

44. For a patient with acute glomerulonephritis, a 24-hour urine test was initiated and the glomerular filtration rate (GFR) results are pending. What are the clinical implications of the test results?
    a. GFR is normal; the therapy can be discontinued.
    b. GFR is high; the patient is at risk for dehydration.
    c. GFR is low; the patient is at risk for infection.
    d. GFR is low; the patient is at risk for fluid overload.

45. A patient is very ill and is admitted to the intensive care unit with rapidly progressing glomerulonephritis. The nurse monitors the patient for manifestations of which organ system failure?
    a. Immune system
    b. Cardiovascular system
    c. Neurologic system
    d. Renal system

46. Kidney tissue changes in chronic glomerulonephritis are caused by which factors? *(Select all that apply.)*
    a. Ischemia
    b. Fluid overload
    c. Hypertension
    d. Obstruction
    e. Infection

47. A patient is diagnosed with chronic glomerulonephritis. The patient's spouse reports that the patient is irritable, forgetful, and has trouble concentrating. Which assessment finding does the nurse expect on further examination?
    a. Increased respiratory rate
    b. Elevated blood urea nitrogen
    c. High white count with a left shift
    d. Low blood pressure and bradycardia

48. The nurse is reviewing the laboratory results for a patient with chronic glomerulonephritis. The serum albumin level is low. What else does the nurse expect to see?
    a. Proteinuria
    b. Elevated hematocrit
    c. High specific gravity
    d. Low white blood cell count

49. A patient has chronic glomerulonephritis. In order to assess for uremic symptoms, what does the nurse do?
    a. Evaluate the blood urea nitrogen (BUN).
    b. Ask the patient to extend the arms and hyperextend the wrists.
    c. Gently palpate the flank for asymmetry and tenderness.
    d. Auscultate for the presence of an S_3 heart sound.

50. The nurse is reviewing the laboratory results of a patient with chronic glomerulonephritis. The phosphorus level is 5.3 mg/dL. What else does the nurse expect to see?
    a. Serum calcium level below the normal range
    b. Serum potassium level below the normal range
    c. Falsely elevated serum sodium level
    d. Elevated serum levels for all other electrolytes

51. The nurse is reviewing arterial blood gas results of a patient with acute glomerulonephritis. The pH of the sample is 7.35. As acidosis is likely to be present because of hydrogen ion retention and loss of bicarbonate, how does the nurse interpret this data?
    a. Normal pH with respiratory compensation
    b. Acidosis with failure of respiratory compensation
    c. Alkalosis with failure of metabolic compensation
    d. Normal pH with metabolic compensation

52. The nurse is taking a history on a patient with chronic glomerulonephritis. What is the patient most likely to report?
    a. History of antibiotic allergy
    b. Intense flank pain
    c. Poor appetite and weight loss
    d. Occasional edema and fatigue

53. Which patient history factor is considered causative for acute glomerulonephritis?
    a. Urinary incontinence 6 months ago
    b. Strep throat 3 weeks ago
    c. Kidney stones 2 years ago
    d. Mild hypertension diagnosed 1 year ago

54. A patient with acute glomerulonephritis has edema of the face. The blood pressure is moderately elevated and the patient has gained 2 pounds within the past 24 hours. The patient reports fatigue and refuses to eat. What is the priority for nursing care?
    a. Cluster care to allow rest periods for the patient.
    b. Obtain a dietary consult to plan an adequate nutritional diet.
    c. Monitor urine output with accurate intake and output amounts.
    d. Assess for signs and symptoms of fluid volume overload.

55. A patient with acute glomerulonephritis is required to provide a 24-hour urine specimen. What does the nurse expect to see when looking at the specimen?
    a. Smoky or cola-colored urine
    b. Clear and very dilute urine
    c. Urine that is full of pus and very thick
    d. Bright orange-colored urine

56. Which nursing intervention is applicable for a patient with acute glomerulonephritis?
    a. Restricting visitors who have infections
    b. Assessing the incision site
    c. Inspecting the vascular access
    d. Measuring weight daily

57. Which diagnostic tests and results does the nurse expect to see with acute glomerulonephritis? (Select all that apply.)
    a. Urinalysis revealing hematuria
    b. Urinalysis revealing proteinuria
    c. Microscopic red blood cell casts
    d. Serum albumin levels increased
    e. Serum potassium decreased

58. A patient has late-stage chronic glomerulonephritis. Which educational brochure would be the most appropriate to prepare for the patient?
    a. "How to Take Your Antiinfective Medications"
    b. "Important Points to Know about Dialysis"
    c. "What Are the Side Effects of Radiation Therapy?"
    d. "Precautions to Take During Immunosuppressive Therapy"

59. The nurse is caring for a patient with nephrotic syndrome. What interventions are included in the plan of care for this patient? (Select all that apply.)
    a. Fluids should be restricted.
    b. Administer mild diuretics.
    c. Assess for edema.
    d. Administer antihypertensive medications.
    e. Frequently assess the patient's mental status.

60. The nurse is reviewing the patient's history, assessment findings, and laboratory results for a patient with suspected kidney problems. Which manifestation is the main feature of nephrotic syndrome?
    a. Flank asymmetry
    b. Proteinuria greater than 3.5 g of protein in 24 hours
    c. Serum sodium 148 mmol/L
    d. Serum cholesterol (total) 190 mg/dL

61. A patient is newly admitted with nephrotic syndrome and has proteinuria, edema, hyperlipidemia, and hypertension. What is the priority for nursing care?
    a. Consult the dietitian to provide adequate nutritional intake.
    b. Prevent urinary tract infection.
    c. Monitor fluid volume and the patient's hydration status.
    d. Prepare the patient for a renal biopsy.

62. A patient is diagnosed with interstitial nephritis. Which nursing action is relevant and specific for this patient's medical condition?
    a. Avoid analgesic use.
    b. Use disposable gloves.
    c. Monitor for fever.
    d. Place the patient in isolation.

63. Which ethnic groups are mostly likely to develop end-stage kidney disease related to hypertension? (Select all that apply.)
    a. Caucasian Americans
    b. Asian Americans
    c. American Indians
    d. African Americans
    e. Hispanic Americans

64. A patient with diabetic nephropathy reports having frequent hypoglycemic episodes "so my doctor reduced my insulin, which means my diabetes is improving." What is the nurse's best response?
    a. "Congratulations! You must be following the diet and lifestyle instructions very carefully."
    b. "When kidney function is reduced, the insulin is available for a longer time and thus less of it is needed."
    c. "You should probably talk to your doctor again. You have been diagnosed with nephropathy and that changes the situation."
    d. "Let me get you a brochure about the relationship of diabetes and kidney disease. It is a complex topic and hard to understand."

65. The student nurse is assisting in the postoperative care of a patient who had a recent nephrectomy. The student demonstrates a reluctance to move the patient to change the linens because "the patient seems so tired." The nurse reminds the student that a priority assessment for this patient is to assess for which factor?
    a. Skin breakdown on the patient's back
    b. Blood on the linens beneath the patient
    c. Urinary incontinence and moisture
    d. The patient's ability to move self in bed

66. After a nephrectomy, a patient has a large urine output because of adrenal insufficiency. What does the nurse anticipate the priority intervention for this patient will be?
    a. ACE inhibitor to control the hypertension and decrease protein loss in urine
    b. Straight catheterization or bedside bladder scan to measure residual urine
    c. IV fluid replacement because of subsequent hypotension and oliguria
    d. IV infusion of temsirolimus (Torisel), to inhibit cell division

67. Which patient has the greatest risk of developing a kidney abscess?
    a. Patient is diagnosed with acute pyelonephritis
    b. Patient has flank asymmetry related to hydronephrosis
    c. Patient developed a urinary tract infection secondary to a urinary catheter
    d. Patient is diagnosed with hypertension and nephrosclerosis

68. A 53-year-old patient is newly diagnosed with renal artery stenosis. What clinical manifestation is the nurse most likely to observe when the patient first seeks health care?
    a. Sudden onset of hypertension
    b. Urinary frequency and dysuria
    c. Nausea and vomiting
    d. Flank pain and hematuria

69. A patient has been informed by the health care provider that treatment will be needed for renal artery stenosis. The nurse prepares to teach about a variety of treatment options. What treatments will the nurse include in the teaching plan? (Select all that apply.)
    a. Kidney transplant
    b. Hypertension control
    c. Balloon angioplasty
    d. Renal artery bypass surgery
    e. Synthetic blood vessel graft
    f. Percutaneous ultrasonic pyelolithotomy

70. What change in diabetic therapy may be needed for a patient who has diabetic nephropathy?
    a. Fluid restriction
    b. Decreased activity level
    c. Decreased insulin dosages
    d. Increased caloric intake

71. A patient is newly diagnosed with type 2 diabetes mellitus. Which screening recommendation does the nurse give to the patient regarding the early detection of diabetic kidney disease?
    a. Urine should be tested annually for protein and microalbuminuria.
    b. Blood urea nitrogen and serum creatinine should tested within 5 years.
    c. Urine should be tested within 5 years for protein and microalbuminuria.
    d. Urine should be tested annually for protein, glucose, and blood.

72. Which data set indicates that the patient with diabetes is achieving the goals of care to prevent the development of microalbuminuria and delay the progression to end-stage kidney disease?
    a. A_{1C} <7%, BP is 125/75 mm Hg, LDL cholesterol is 90 mg/dL
    b. A_{1C} >7%, BP is 140/80 mm Hg, LDL cholesterol is 200 mg/dL
    c. A_{1C} <7%, BP is 130/80 mm Hg with proteinuria 2.0 g/24 hours
    d. A_{1C} >7%, BP is 120/70 mm Hg, LDL cholesterol is 300 mg/dL

73. A patient diagnosed with renal cell carcinoma that has metastasized to the lungs is considered to be in which stage of cancer?
    a. I
    b. II
    c. III
    d. IV

74. A patient has had one kidney removed as a treatment for kidney cancer. The patient's spouse asks, "Does the good kidney take over immediately? I know a person can live with just one kidney." What is the nurse's best response?
    a. "The other kidney will provide adequate function, but this may take days or weeks."
    b. "The other kidney alone isn't able to provide adequate function, so supplemental therapies will be needed."
    c. "That's a good question. Remember to ask your doctor next time he or she comes in."
    d. "It varies a lot, but within a few days we expect everything to normalize."

75. After a nephrectomy, one adrenal gland remains. Based on this knowledge, which type of medication replacement therapy does the nurse expect if the remaining adrenal gland function is insufficient?
    a. Potassium
    b. Steroid
    c. Calcium
    d. Estrogen

76. The nurse is caring for a patient with kidney cell carcinoma who manifests paraneoplastic syndromes. What findings does the nurse expect to see in this patient? *(Select all that apply.)*
    a. Urinary tract infection
    b. Erythrocytosis
    c. Hypercalcemia
    d. Liver dysfunction
    e. Decreased sedimentation rate
    f. Hypertension

77. The nurse is caring for a patient with kidney cell carcinoma. What does the nurse expect to find documented about the patient's initial assessment?
    a. Flank pain, gross hematuria, palpable kidney mass, and renal bruit
    b. Gross hematuria, hypertension, diabetes, and oliguria
    c. Dysuria, polyuria, dehydration, and palpable kidney mass
    d. Nocturia and urinary retention with difficulty starting stream

78. A patient is diagnosed with kidney cancer and the health care provider recommends the best therapy. Which treatment does the nurse anticipate teaching the patient about?
    a. Chemotherapy
    b. Surgical removal
    c. Hormonal therapy
    d. Radiation therapy

79. A patient returning to the unit after a left radical nephrectomy for kidney cell carcinoma reports having some soreness on the right side. What does the nurse tell the patient?
    a. "The right kidney was repositioned to take over the function of both kidneys."
    b. "I'll call your doctor for an order to increase your pain medication."
    c. "The soreness is likely to be from being positioned on your right side during surgery."
    d. "Would you like to talk with someone who had this surgery last year and now is fully recovered?"

80. The nurse is caring for a postoperative nephrectomy patient. The nurse notes during the first several hours of the shift a marked and steady downward trend in blood pressure. How does the nurse interpret this finding?
    a. Hypertension has been corrected.
    b. Internal hemorrhage is possible.
    c. The other kidney is failing.
    d. This is an expected response to medication.

81. The nurse is caring for a patient after a nephrectomy. The nurse notes that the urine flow was 50 mL/hr at the beginning of the shift, but several hours later has dropped to 30 mL. What would the nurse do first?
    a. Notify the health care provider for an order for an IV fluid bolus.
    b. Document the finding and continue to monitor for downward trend.
    c. Check the drainage system for kinks or obstructions to flow.
    d. Obtain the patient's weight and compare it to baseline.

82. The nurse is caring for a patient who had a nephrectomy yesterday. To manage the patient's pain, what is the best plan for analgesia therapy?
    a. Limit narcotics because of respiratory depression.
    b. Give an oral analgesic when the patient can eat.
    c. Alternate parenteral and oral medications.
    d. Give parenteral medications on a schedule.

83. A patient is brought to the emergency department (ED) after being involved in a fight in which the patient was kicked and punched repeatedly in the back. What does the nurse include in the initial physical assessment? *(Select all that apply.)*
    a. Take complete vital signs.
    b. Check apical and peripheral pulses.
    c. Inspect both flanks for asymmetry or penetrating injuries of the lower chest or back.
    d. Inspect the abdomen for bruising or penetrating wounds.
    e. Deeply palpate the abdomen for signs of rigidity.
    f. Inspect the urethra for gross bleeding.

84. The ED nurse is preparing a patient with kidney trauma for emergency surgery. What is the best task to delegate to the unlicensed assistive personnel (UAP)?
    a. Set the automated blood pressure machine to cycle every 2 hours.
    b. Inform the family about surgery and assist them to the surgery waiting area.
    c. Go to the blood bank and pick up the units of packed red cells.
    d. Insert a urinary catheter if there is no gross bleeding at the urethra.

85. A patient has sustained a kidney injury. In order to assist the patient to undergo the best diagnostic test to determine the extent of injury, what does the nurse do?
    a. Obtain a clean-catch urine specimen for urinalysis.
    b. Give an IV fluid bolus before renal arteriography.
    c. Give an explanation of computed tomography.
    d. Obtain a blood sample for hemoglobin and hematocrit.

86. What might the nurse notice if the patient is experiencing problems with urinary elimination as a result of acute pyelonephritis? *(Select all that apply.)*
    a. Patient urinates large amounts of dilute urine.
    b. Patient reports pain and burning on urination.
    c. Patient reports back or flank pain.
    d. Urine is cloudy and foul-smelling.
    e. Urine may be darker or smoky or have obvious blood in it.

87. What laboratory values would the nurse interpret for a patient experiencing problems with urinary elimination as a result of acute pyelonephritis? *(Select all that apply.)*
    a. Observe complete blood count for elevation of differentials.
    b. Observe for elevation of BUN and serum creatinine levels.
    c. Observe for electrolyte imbalances, such as hypokalemia.
    d. Observe arterial blood gases for alkalosis and respiratory compensation.
    e. Observe urinalysis for bacteria, leukocyte esterase, nitrate, or red blood cells.

68 CHAPTER

Care of Patients with Acute Kidney Injury and Chronic Kidney Disease

1. Which problems occur with acute kidney injury (AKI)? *(Select all that apply.)*
   a. Decreased peristalsis
   b. Anemia
   c. Metabolic acidosis
   d. Hypokalemia
   e. Peripheral edema

2. The community health nurse is designing programs to reduce kidney problems and kidney injury among the general public. In order to do so, the nurse targets health promotion and compliance with therapy for people with which conditions?
   a. Diabetes mellitus and hypertension
   b. Frequent episodes of sexually transmitted disease
   c. Osteoporosis and other bone diseases
   d. Gastroenteritis and poor eating habits

3. What are common causes of prerenal kidney injury? *(Select all that apply.)*
   a. Urethral cancer
   b. Hypovolemic shock
   c. Enlarged prostate gland
   d. Sepsis
   e. Severe burns

4. A patient can develop intrarenal kidney injury from which causes? *(Select all that apply.)*
   a. Vasculitis
   b. Pyelonephritis
   c. Strenuous exercise
   d. Exposure to nephrotoxins
   e. Bladder cancer

5. Postrenal kidney injury can result from which conditions? *(Select all that apply.)*
   a. Septic shock
   b. Cervical cancer
   c. Nephrolithiasis or ureterolithiasis
   d. Heart failure
   e. Neurogenic bladder
   f. Prostate cancer

6. When shock or other problems cause an acute reduction in blood flow to the kidneys, how do the kidneys compensate? *(Select all that apply.)*
   a. Constrict blood vessels in the kidneys.
   b. Activate the renin-angiotensin-aldosterone pathway.
   c. Release beta blockers.
   d. Dilate blood vessels throughout the body.
   e. Release antidiuretic hormones.

7. The nurse reads in the patient's chart that he has *acute-on-chronic* kidney disease. How does the nurse interpret this information?
   a. Kidney disease has progressed to the need for dialysis or transplant.
   b. Patient has chronic kidney disease and has sustained an acute kidney injury.
   c. Acute kidney injury requires aggressive management to prevent chronic disease.
   d. The condition could by acute or chronic; further diagnostic testing is needed.

8. The nurse is talking to a group of healthy young college students about maintaining good kidney health and preventing AKI. Which health promotion point is the nurse most likely to emphasize with this group?
   a. "Have your blood pressure checked regularly."
   b. "Find out if you have a family history of diabetes."
   c. "Avoid dehydration by drinking at least 2 to 3 L of water daily."
   d. "Have annual testing for microalbuminuria and urine protein."

9. The nurse is caring for a patient who had hypovolemic shock secondary to trauma in the emergency department (ED) 2 days ago. Based on the pathophysiology of hypovolemia and prerenal azotemia, what does the nurse assess at least every hour?
   a. Urinary output
   b. Presence of edema
   c. Urine color
   d. Presence of pain

10. The nurse is talking to an older adult male patient who is reasonably healthy for his age, but has benign prostatic hyperplasia (BPH). Which condition does the BPH potentially place him at risk for?
    a. Prerenal acute kidney injury
    b. Postrenal acute kidney injury
    c. Polycystic kidney disease
    d. Acute glomerulonephritis

11. Which combination of drugs is the most nephrotoxic?
    a. Angiotensin-converting enzyme (ACE) inhibitors and aspirin
    b. Angiotensin II receptor blockers and antacids
    c. Aminoglycoside antibiotics and nonsteroidal antiinflammatory drugs (NSAIDs)
    d. Calcium channel blockers and antihistamines

12. The nurse is caring for several patients on a medical-surgical unit. None of the patients currently has any acute or chronic kidney problems. Which patient has the greatest risk to develop AKI?
    a. 73-year-old male who has hypertension and peripheral vascular disease
    b. 32-year-old female who is pregnant and has gestational diabetes
    c. 49-year-old male who is obese and has a history of skin cancer
    d. 23-year-old female who has been treated for a urinary tract infection

13. For a patient with AKI, the nurse would consider questioning the order for which diagnostic test?
    a. Kidney biopsy
    b. Ultrasonography
    c. Computed tomography with contrast dye
    d. Kidney, ureter, bladder (KUB) x-ray

14. The nurse is caring for a postoperative patient and is evaluating the patient's intake and output as a measure to prevent AKI. The patient weighs 60 kilograms and has produced 180 mL of urine in the past 4 hours. What should the nurse do?
    a. Perform other assessments related to fluid status and record the output.
    b. Call the health care provider and obtain an order for a fluid bolus.
    c. Encourage the patient to drink more fluid, so that the output is increased.
    d. Compare the patient's weight to baseline to determine fluid retention.

15. The nurse is caring for a patient receiving gentamicin. Because this drug has potential for nephrotoxicity, which laboratory results does the nurse monitor? *(Select all that apply.)*
    a. Blood urea nitrogen (BUN)
    b. Creatinine
    c. Drug peak and trough levels
    d. Prothrombin time (PT)
    e. Platelet count
    f. Hemoglobin and hematocrit

16. According to the RIFLE classification *(Risk, Injury, Failure, Loss, End-stage kidney failure).* How would the nurse interpret the following data? Serum creatinine increased × 1.5 or glomerular filtration rate (GFR) decrease >25%; Urine output is <0.5 mL/kg/hr for ≥ 6 hours.
    a. Risk stage
    b. Injury stage
    c. Failure stage
    d. End-stage kidney disease (ESKD)

17. A patient has been diagnosed with AKI, but the cause is uncertain. The nurse prepares patient educational material about which diagnostic test?
    a. Flat plate of the abdomen
    b. Renal ultrasonography
    c. Computed tomography
    d. Kidney biopsy

18. A patient is in the diuretic phase of AKI. During this phase, what is the nurse mainly concerned about?
    a. Assessing for hypertension and fluid overload
    b. Monitoring for hypovolemia and electrolyte loss
    c. Adjusting the dosage of diuretic medications
    d. Balancing diuretic therapy with intake

19. A patient with prerenal azotemia is administered a fluid challenge. In evaluating response to the therapy, which outcome indicates that the goal was met?
    a. Patient reports feeling better and indicates an eagerness to go home.
    b. Patient produces urine soon after the initial bolus.
    c. The therapy is completed without adverse effects.
    d. The health care provider orders a diuretic when the challenge is completed.

20. The nurse is caring for a patient with AKI and notes a trend of increasingly elevated BUN levels. How does the nurse interpret this information?
    a. Breakdown of muscle for protein which leads to an increase in azotemia
    b. Sign of urinary retention and decreased urinary output
    c. Expected trend that can be reversed by increasing dietary protein
    d. Ominous sign of impending irreversible kidney failure

21. The nurse is caring for a patient with AKI that developed after a severe anaphylactic reaction. What is a primary treatment goal of the initial phase that will help to prevent permanent kidney damage for this patient?
    a. Correct fluid volume by administering IV normal saline.
    b. Maintain a mean arterial pressure (MAP) of 65 mm Hg.
    c. Prevent kidney infections by administering antibiotics.
    d. Give antihistamines to prevent allergic response.

22. A patient sustained extensive burns and depletion of vascular volume. The nurse expects which changes in vital signs and urinary function?
    a. Decreased urine output, hypotension, tachycardia
    b. Increased urine output, hypertension, tachycardia
    c. Bradycardia, hypotension, polyuria
    d. Dysrhythmias, hypertension, oliguria

23. The nurse is taking a history of a patient at risk for kidney failure. What does the nurse ask the patient about during the interview? *(Select all that apply.)*
    a. Exposure to nephrotoxic chemicals
    b. Increased appetite
    c. History of diabetes mellitus, hypertension, systemic lupus erythematosus
    d. Recent surgery, trauma, or transfusions
    e. Leakage of urine when coughing or laughing
    f. Recent or prolonged use of antibiotics and NSAIDs

24. Which disorder could be a complication from AKI?
    a. Heart failure
    b. Diabetes mellitus
    c. Kidney cancer
    d. Compartment syndrome

25. A patient with AKI is ill and has a poor appetite. What would the health care team try first?
    a. IV normal saline to prevent dehydration
    b. Familiar foods brought by the family
    c. Nasogastric tube for enteral feedings
    d. Oral supplements designed for kidney patients

26. The nurse is caring for a patient with AKI who does not have signs or symptoms of fluid overload. A fluid challenge is performed to promote kidney perfusion by doing what?
    a. Administering normal saline 500 to 1000 mL infused over 1 hour
    b. Administering drugs to suppress aldosterone release
    c. Instilling warm, sterile normal saline into the bladder
    d. Having the patient drink several large glasses of water

27. Which signs/symptoms does the nurse expect to see in the patient with AKI that has progressed in severity? *(Select all that apply.)*
    a. Oliguria
    b. Hypotension
    c. Shortness of breath
    d. Pulmonary crackles
    e. Weight loss

28. A patient has AKI related to nephrotoxins. In order to maintain cell integrity, improve GFR, and improve blood flow to the kidneys, which type of medication does the nurse anticipate the health care provider will prescribe?
    a. Loop diuretics
    b. Alpha-adrenergic blockers
    c. Beta blockers
    d. Calcium channel blockers

29. A patient with AKI has a high rate of catabolism. What is this related to?
    a. Increased levels of catecholamines, cortisol, and glucagon
    b. Inability to excrete excess electrolytes
    c. Conversion of body fat into glucose
    d. Presence of retained nitrogenous wastes

30. The nurse requests a dietary consult to address the patient's high rate of catabolism. Which nutritional element is directly related to this metabolic process?
    a. Carbohydrates
    b. Proteins
    c. Liquids
    d. Fats

31. The nurse is caring for a patient in the intensive care unit who sustained blood loss during a traumatic accident. For early identification of signs and symptoms that would suggest the development of kidney dysfunction, what does the nurse observe for? *(Select all that apply.)*
    a. Hypotension
    b. Bradycardia
    c. Decreased urine output
    d. Decreased cardiac output
    e. Increased central venous pressure

32. A patient with AKI is receiving total parenteral nutrition (TPN). What is the therapeutic goal of using TPN?
    a. Preserve lean body mass
    b. Promote tubular reabsorption
    c. Create a negative nitrogen balance
    d. Prevent infection

33. The nurse and the dietitian are planning dietary intake for a patient with AKI who is currently not on dialysis therapy. The dietitian informs the nurse that 0.6 g/kg of body weight of protein are needed. The patient weighs 130 pounds. How many grams of protein should the patient receive? (Round grams to the nearest whole number.) _____ grams

34. What are the characteristics of continuous venovenous hemofiltration (CVVH)? *(Select all that apply.)*
    a. Requires placement of arterial and venous access
    b. Uses a pump to drive blood from the patient catheter into the dialyzer
    c. Risk of air embolus
    d. More commonly used for patients who are critically ill
    e. Most convenient method for home care patients

35. Which characteristics are associated with ESKD? *(Select all that apply.)*
    a. Severe fluid overload
    b. Renal osteodystrophy
    c. Nephrons compensate
    d. Dialysis or transplant needed to maintain homeostasis
    e. Excessive waste products

36. The nurse is taking a history on a patient with diabetes and hypertension. Because of the patient's high risk for developing kidney problems, which early sign of chronic kidney disease (CKD) does the nurse assess for?
    a. Decreased output with subjective thirst
    b. Urinary frequency of very small amounts
    c. Pink or blood-tinged urine
    d. Increased output of very dilute urine

37. Increased BUN and creatinine, hyperkalemia, and hypernatremia are all characteristics of which stage of kidney disease?
    a. Stage 1 CKD
    b. Mild CKD
    c. Moderate CKD
    d. ESKD

38. A patient's laboratory results show an elevated creatinine level. The patient's history reveals no risk factors for kidney disease. Which question does the nurse ask the patient to shed further light on the laboratory result?
    a. "How many hours of sleep did you get the night before the test?"
    b. "How much fluid did you drink before the test?"
    c. "Did you take any type of antibiotics before taking the test?"
    d. "When and how much did you last urinate before having the test?"

39. The nurse is reviewing a patient's laboratory results. In the early phase of CKD, the patient is at risk for which electrolyte abnormality?
    a. Hyperkalemia
    b. Hyponatremia
    c. Hypercalcemia
    d. Hypokalemia

40. A patient with CKD has a potassium level of 8 mEq/L. The nurse notifies the health care provider after assessing for which sign/symptom?
    a. Cardiac dysrhythmias
    b. Respiratory depression
    c. Tremors or seizures
    d. Decreased urine output

41. The nurse is assessing a patient with kidney injury and notes a marked increase in the rate and depth of breathing. The nurse recognizes this as Kussmaul respiration, which is the body's attempt to compensate for which condition?
    a. Hypoxia
    b. Alkalosis
    c. Acidosis
    d. Hypoxemia

42. A patient is diagnosed with renal osteodystrophy. What does the nurse instruct the unlicensed assistive personnel (UAP) to do in relation to this patient's diagnosis?
    a. Assist the patient with toileting every 2 hours.
    b. Gently wash the patient's skin with a mild soap and rinse well.
    c. Handle the patient gently because of risk for fractures.
    d. Assist the patient with eating because of loss of coordination.

43. A patient with CKD develops severe chest pain, an increased pulse, low-grade fever, and a pericardial friction rub with a cardiac dysrhythmia and muffled heart tones. The nurse immediately alerts the health care provider and prepares for which emergency procedure?
    a. Pericardiocentesis
    b. CVVH
    c. Kidney dialysis
    d. Endotracheal intubation

44. All patients with hypertension or diabetes should have yearly screenings for which factor?
    a. Creatinine
    b. BUN
    c. Glycosuria
    d. Microalbuminuria

45. The nurse is reviewing urinalysis results for a patient who is in the early stages of CKD, What results might the nurse expect to see?
    a. Excessive protein, glucose, red blood cells, and white blood cells
    b. Increased specific gravity with a dark amber discoloration
    c. Dramatically increased urine osmolarity
    d. Pink-tinged urine with obvious small blood clots

46. The night shift nurse sees a patient with kidney failure sitting up in bed. The patient states, "I feel a little short of breath at night or when I get up to walk to the bathroom." What assessment does the nurse do?
    a. Check for orthostatic hypotension because of potential volume depletion.
    b. Auscultate the lungs for crackles, which indicate fluid overload.
    c. Check the pulse and blood pressure for possible decreased cardiac output.
    d. Assess for normal sleep pattern and need for a prn sedative.

47. What type of breath odor is most likely to be noted in a patient with CKD?
    a. Fruity smell
    b. Fecal smell
    c. Smells like urine
    d. Smells like blood

48. The patient with CKD reports chronic fatigue and lethargy with weakness and mild shortness of breath with dizziness when rising to a standing position. In addition, the nurse notes pale mucous membranes. Based on the patient's illness and the presenting symptoms, which laboratory result does the nurse expect to see?
    a. Low hemoglobin and hematocrit
    b. Low white cell count
    c. Low blood glucose
    d. Low oxygen saturation

49. The nurse is assessing the skin of a patient with ESKD. Which clinical manifestation is considered a sign of very late, premorbid, advanced uremic syndrome?
    a. Ecchymoses
    b. Sallowness
    c. Pallor
    d. Uremic frost

50. The nurse notes an abnormal laboratory test finding for a patient with CKD and alerts the health care provider. The nurse also consults with the registered dietitian because an excessive dietary protein intake is directly related to which factor?
    a. Elevated serum creatinine level
    b. Protein presence in the urine
    c. Elevated BUN level
    d. Elevated serum potassium level

51. In collaboration with the registered dietitian, the nurse teaches the patient about which diet recommendations for management of CKD? *(Select all that apply.)*
    a. Controlling protein intake
    b. Limiting fluid intake
    c. Restricting potassium
    d. Increasing sodium
    e. Restricting phosphorus
    f. Reducing calories

52. A patient receives dialysis therapy and the health care provider has ordered sodium restriction to 3 g daily. What does the nurse teach the patient?
    a. Add smaller amounts of salt at the table or during cooking.
    b. Identify foods that are high in sodium (e.g., bacon, potato chips, fast foods).
    c. Avoid foods that have a metallic, salty, or bitter taste.
    d. Eat larger amounts of bland foods with very minimal amounts of spicing.

53. In order to assist a patient in the prevention of osteodystrophy, which intervention does the nurse perform?
    a. Administer phosphate binders with meals.
    b. Encourage high-quality protein foods.
    c. Administer iron supplements.
    d. Encourage extra milk at mealtimes.

54. The home health nurse is reviewing the medication list of a patient with CKD. The nurse calls the health care provider as a reminder that the patient might need which nutritional supplements? *(Select all that apply.)*
    a. Iron
    b. Magnesium
    c. Phosphorus
    d. Calcium
    e. Vitamin D
    f. Water-soluble vitamins

55. The nurse is caring for a patient with ESKD and dialysis has been initiated. Which drug order does the nurse question?
    a. Erythropoietin
    b. Diuretic
    c. ACE inhibitor
    d. Calcium channel blocker

56. The nurse monitors a CKD patient's daily weights because of the risk for fluid retention. What instructions does the nurse give to the UAP?
    a. Weigh the patient daily at the same time each day, same scale, with the same amount of clothing.
    b. Weigh the patient daily and add 1 kilogram of weight for the intake of each liter of fluid.
    c. Weigh the patient in the morning before breakfast and weigh the patient at night just before bedtime.
    d. Ask the patient what his or her normal weight is and then weigh the patient before and after each voiding.

57. A patient with CKD is taking digoxin (Lanoxin). Which signs of digoxin toxicity does the nurse vigilantly monitor for? *(Select all that apply.)*
    a. Nausea and vomiting
    b. Visual changes
    c. Respiratory depression
    d. Restlessness or confusion
    e. Headache or fatigue
    f. Tachycardia

58. The nurse is reviewing the medication list and appropriate dose adjustments made for a patient with CKD. The nurse would question the use and/or dosage adjustment of which type of medication?
    a. Antibiotics
    b. Magnesium antacids
    c. Oral antidiabetics
    d. Opioids

59. The nurse is evaluating a patient's treatment response to erythropoietin (Epogen). Which hemoglobin reading indicates that the goal is being met?
    a. Around 10 g/dL
    b. Greater than 20 g/dL
    c. Upward trend
    d. At baseline for gender

60. A patient has been receiving erythropoietin (Epogen). Which statement by the patient indicates that the therapy is producing the desired effect?
    a. "I can do my housework with less fatigue."
    b. "I have been passing more urine than I was before."
    c. "I have less pain and discomfort now."
    d. "I can swallow and eat much better than before."

61. Which behavior is the strongest indicator that a patient with ESKD is not coping well with the illness and may need a referral for psychological counseling?
    a. Displays irritability when the meal tray arrives
    b. Refuses to take one of the drugs because it causes nausea
    c. Repeatedly misses dialysis appointments
    d. Seems distracted when the health care provider talks about the prognosis

62. A patient with CKD is restless, anxious, and short of breath. The nurse hears crackles that begin at the base of the lungs. The pulse rate is increased and the patient has frothy, blood-tinged sputum. What does the nurse do first?
    a. Facilitate transfer to the ICU for aggressive treatment.
    b. Place the patient in a high-Fowler's position.
    c. Continue to monitor vital signs and assess breath sounds.
    d. Administer a loop diuretic such as furosemide (Lasix).

63. Which patient is the most likely candidate for CVVH?
    a. Patient with fluid volume overload
    b. Patient who needs long-term management
    c. Patient who is critically ill
    d. Patient who is ready for discharge to home

64. As a patient with ESKD experiences isosthenuria, what must the nurse be alert for?
    a. The diuretic stage
    b. Fluid volume overload
    c. Dehydration
    d. Alkalosis

65. The nurse is caring for a patient with CKD. The family asks about when renal replacement therapy will begin. What is the nurse's best response?
    a. "As early as possible to prevent further damage in stage I."
    b. "When there is reduced kidney function and metabolic wastes accumulate."
    c. "When the kidneys are unable to maintain a balance in body functions."
    d. "It will be started with diuretic therapy to enhance the remaining function."

66. Which are the most accurate ways to monitor kidney function in the patient with CKD? *(Select all that apply.)*
    a. Monitoring intake and output
    b. Checking urine specific gravity
    c. Reviewing BUN and serum creatinine levels
    d. Reviewing x-ray reports
    e. Consulting the dietitian's notes

67. As a result of kidney failure, excessive hydrogen ions cannot be excreted. With acid retention, the nurse is most likely to observe what type of respiratory compensation?
    a. Cheyne-Stokes respiratory pattern
    b. Increased depth of breathing
    c. Decreased respiratory rate and depth
    d. Increased arterial carbon dioxide levels

68. The nurse is assessing a patient with uremia. Which gastrointestinal changes does the nurse expect to find? *(Select all that apply.)*
    a. Halitosis
    b. Hiccups
    c. Anorexia
    d. Nausea
    e. Vomiting
    f. Salivation

69. Which patients with CKD are candidates for intermittent hemodialysis? *(Select all that apply.)*
    a. Patient with fluid overload who does not respond to diuretics
    b. Patient with injury stage according to the RIFLE classification
    c. Patient with symptomatic toxin ingestion
    d. Patient with uremic manifestations, such as decreased cognition
    e. Patient with symptomatic hyperkalemia and calciphylaxis

70. The home health nurse is evaluating the home setting for a patient who wishes to have in-home hemodialysis. What is important to have in the home setting to support this therapy?
    a. Specialized water treatment system to provide a safe, purified water supply
    b. Large dust-free space to accommodate and store the dialysis equipment
    c. Modified electrical system to provide high voltage to power the equipment
    d. Specialized cooling system to maintain strict temperature control

71. The nursing student is explaining principles of hemodialysis to the nursing instructor. Which statement by the student indicates a need for additional study and research on the topic?
    a. "Dialysis works as molecules from an area of higher concentration move to an area of lower concentration."
    b. "Blood and dialyzing solution flow in opposite directions across an enclosed semipermeable membrane."
    c. "Excess water, waste products, and excess electrolytes are removed from the blood."
    d. "Bacteria and other organisms can also pass through the membrane, so the dialysate must be kept sterile."

72. A patient and family are trying to plan a schedule that coordinates with the patient's dialysis regimen. The patient asks, "How often will I have to go and how long does it take?" What is the nurse's best response?
    a. "If you are compliant with the diet and fluid restrictions, you spend less time in dialysis; about 12 hours a week."
    b. "Most patients require about 12 hours per week; this is usually divided into three 4-hour treatments."
    c. "It varies from patient to patient. You will have to call your health care provider for specific instructions."
    d. "If you gain a large amount of fluid weight, a longer treatment time may be needed to prevent severe side effects."

73. A patient is undergoing a dialysis treatment and exhibits a progression of symptoms which include headache, nausea, and vomiting; and fatigue. How does the nurse interpret these symptoms?
    a. Mild dialysis disequilibrium syndrome
    b. Expected manifestations in ESKD
    c. Transient symptoms in a new dialysis patient
    d. Adverse reaction to the dialysate

74. The nurse is caring for a patient with an arteriovenous fistula. What instructions are given to the UAP regarding the care of this patient?
    a. Palpate for thrills and auscultate for bruits every 4 hours.
    b. Check for bleeding at needle insertion sites.
    c. Assess the patient's distal pulses and circulation.
    d. Do not take blood pressure readings in the arm with the fistula.

75. The nurse is assessing a patient's extremity with an arteriovenous graft. The nurse notes a thrill and a bruit, and the patient reports numbness and a cool feeling in the fingers. How does the nurse interpret this information in regard to the graft?
    a. The graft is functional and these symptoms are expected.
    b. The patient has "steal syndrome" and may need surgical intervention.
    c. The graft is patent, but the blood is flowing in the wrong direction.
    d. The patient needs to increase active use of hands and fingers.

76. The nurse is providing postdialysis care for a patient. In comparing vital signs and weight measurements to the predialysis data, what does the nurse expect to find?
    a. Blood pressure and weight are reduced.
    b. Blood pressure is increased and weight is reduced.
    c. Blood pressure and weight are slightly increased.
    d. Blood pressure is low and weight is the same.

77. The nurse is assessing a patient who has just returned from hemodialysis. Which assessment finding is cause for greatest concern?
    a. Feeling of malaise
    b. Headache
    c. Muscle cramps in the legs
    d. Bleeding at the access site

78. The nurse is caring for a patient with an arteriovenous fistula. What is included in the nursing care for this patient? *(Select all that apply.)*
    a. Keep small clamps handy by the bedside.
    b. Encourage routine range-of-motion exercises.
    c. Avoid venipuncture or IV administration on the arm with the access device.
    d. Instruct the patient to carry heavy objects to build muscular strength.
    e. Assess for manifestations of infection of the fistula.
    f. Instruct the patient to sleep on the side with the affected arm in the dependent position.

79. A patient has returned to the medical-surgical unit after having a dialysis treatment. The nurse notes that the patient is also scheduled for an invasive procedure on the same day. What is the primary rationale for delaying the procedure for 4 to 6 hours?
    a. The patient was heparinized during dialysis.
    b. The patient will have cardiac dysrhythmias after dialysis.
    c. The patient will be incoherent and unable to give consent.
    d. The patient needs routine medications that were delayed.

80. The nurse is talking to a patient with ESKD. The patient frequently displays weight gain and increased blood pressure beyond the baseline measurements. Which question is the nurse most likely to ask to determine if the patient is doing something that is contributing to these assessment findings?
    a. "Are you controlling your salt intake?"
    b. "Are you following the protein restrictions?"
    c. "Have you been eating a lot of sweets?"
    d. "Have you been exercising regularly?"

81. Which patient with kidney problems is the best candidate for peritoneal dialysis (PD)?
    a. Patient with peritoneal adhesions
    b. Patient with a history of extensive abdominal surgery
    c. Patient with peritoneal membrane fibrosis
    d. Patient with a history of difficulty with anticoagulants

82. Place the sequence of steps of continuous ambulatory peritoneal dialysis (CAPD) in the correct order using the numbers 1 through 4.
    _____ a. Fluid stays in the cavity for a specified time prescribed by the health care provider.
    _____ b. 1 to 2 L of dialysate is infused by gravity over a 10- to 20-minute period.
    _____ c. Fluid flows out of the body by gravity into a drainage bag.
    _____ d. Warm the dialysate bags before instillation by using a heating pad to wrap the bag.

83. The health care provider has ordered intra-peritoneal heparin for a patient with a new PD catheter to prevent clotting of the catheter by blood and fibrin formation. How does the nurse advise the patient?
    a. Watch for bruising or bleeding from the gums.
    b. Make a follow-up appointment for coagulation studies.
    c. Intraperitoneal heparin does not affect clotting times.
    d. Heparin will be given with a small subcutaneous needle.

84. What is the best description of CAPD?
    a. Daily infusion of four 2 L exchanges of dialysate every 4 to 6 hours while awake.
    b. Is a form of automated dialysis that uses an automated cycling machine.
    c. Functions of the cycling machine are programmed to the patient's needs.
    d. This form decreases the risk of peritonitis and poor dialysate flow.

85. The home health nurse is visiting a patient who independently performs PD. Which question does the nurse ask the patient to assess for the major complication associated with PD?
    a. "Have you noticed any signs or symptoms of infection?"
    b. "Are you having any pain during the dialysis treatments?"
    c. "Is the dialysate fluid slow or sluggish?"
    d. "Have you noticed any leakage around the catheter?"

86. The nurse is teaching a patient about performing PD at home. In order to identify the earliest manifestation of peritonitis, what does the nurse instruct the patient to do?
    a. Monitor temperature before starting PD.
    b. Check the effluent for cloudiness.
    c. Be aware of feelings of malaise.
    d. Monitor for abdominal pain.

87. During PD, the nurse notes slowed dialysate outflow. What does the nurse do to trouble-shoot the system? *(Select all that apply.)*
    a. Ensure that the drainage bag is elevated.
    b. Inspect the tubing for kinking or twisting.
    c. Ensure that clamps are open.
    d. Turn the patient to the other side.
    e. Make sure the patient is in good body alignment.
    f. Instruct the patient to stand or cough.

88. A patient has recently started PD therapy and reports some mild pain when the dialysate is flowing in. What does the nurse do next?
    a. Immediately report the pain to the health care provider.
    b. Try warming the dialysate in the microwave oven.
    c. Reassure that pain should subside after the first week or two.
    d. Assess the connection tubing for kinking or twisting.

89. The nurse is caring for a patient requiring PD. In order to monitor the patient's weight, what does the nurse do?
    a. Check the weight after a drain and before the next fill to monitor the patient's "dry weight."
    b. Calculate the "dry weight" by weighing the patient every day and comparing the measurements to baseline.
    c. Determine "dry weight" by comparing the patient's weight to a standard weight chart based on height and age.
    d. Weigh the patient each day and count fluid intake and dialysate volume to determine the patient's "dry weight."

90. The nurse is monitoring a patient's PD treatment. The total outflow is slightly less than the inflow. What does the nurse do next?
    a. Instruct the patient to ambulate.
    b. Notify the health care provider.
    c. Record the difference as intake.
    d. Put the patient on fluid restriction.

91. Which patients are likely to be excluded from receiving a transplant? *(Select all that apply.)*
    a. Patient who had breast cancer 6 years ago
    b. Patient with advanced and uncorrectable heart disease
    c. Patient with a chemical dependency
    d. Patient who is 70 years old and has a living related donor
    e. Patient with diabetes mellitus

92. A daughter is considering donating a kidney to her mother for organ transplant. What information does the nurse give to the daughter about the criteria for donation? *(Select all that apply.)*
    a. Age limit is at least 21 years old.
    b. Systemic disease and infection must be absent.
    c. There must be no history of cancer.
    d. Hypertension or kidney disease must be absent.
    e. There must be adequate kidney function as determined by diagnostic studies.
    f. The donor must understand the surgery and be willing to give up the organ.

93. The nurse is caring for the kidney transplant patient in the immediate postoperative period. During this initial period, the nurse will assess the urine output at least every hour for how many hours?
    a. First 8 hours
    b. First 12 hours
    c. First 24 hours
    d. First 48 hours

94. The intensive care nurse is caring for the kidney transplant patient who was just transferred from the recovery unit. Which finding is the most serious within the first 12 hours after surgery and warrants immediate notification of the transplant surgeon?
    a. Diuresis with increased output
    b. Pink and bloody urine
    c. Abrupt decrease in urine
    d. Small clots in bladder irrigation fluid

95. The nurse is caring for the kidney transplant patient who is 3 days postsurgery. The nurse notes a sudden and abrupt decrease in urine. The nurse alerts the health care provider because this is a sign of which anomaly?
    a. Rejection
    b. Thrombosis
    c. Stenosis
    d. Infection

96. What might the nurse notice if the patient is experiencing reduced perfusion and altered urinary elimination related to AKI? *(Select all that apply.)*
    a. Hemodynamic instability, especially persistent hypotension and tachycardia
    b. Urine output of less than 0.5 mL/kg/hour for 6 or more hours
    c. Serum creatinine below baseline or admission values
    d. Urine may be clear or have a pale yellow color
    e. Abnormal serum and urine potassium and sodium values

69 CHAPTER

Assessment of the Reproductive System

1. What is the site for a Papanicolaou (Pap) test?
   a. Cervix
   b. Vaginal wall
   c. Uterus
   d. Fallopian tubes

2. The nurse is interviewing a 52-year-old woman who reports irregular and decreased flow of menses for several months. Which question does the nurse ask the patient?
   a. "Is there any chance you could be pregnant?"
   b. "Are you having any discomfort during intercourse?"
   c. "Do your breasts feel tender or swollen?"
   d. "Are you having any problems with urination?"

3. The nurse is assisting a patient to assume the correct position for a hysteroscopy procedure. Which position is correct?
   a. Lithotomy position
   b. Side-lying position
   c. Slight Trendelenburg position
   d. Low-Fowler's position

4. An insufficient estrogen level is related to what condition?
   a. Osteoporosis
   b. Diabetes mellitus
   c. Endometriosis
   d. Decreased immune function

5. A male patient had mumps as a child which caused orchitis. Which potential complication could result?
   a. Decreased libido
   b. Chronic urinary infection
   c. Enlarged prostate gland
   d. Testicular atrophy

6. A male patient reports that he has a decreased libido. The nurse assesses for which factors related to this condition? (Select all that apply.)
   a. Tobacco use
   b. Type of exercise
   c. Alcohol consumption
   d. Occupation
   e. Illicit drug use

7. Most diseases that alter a woman's metabolism or nutrition can result in which condition?
   a. Excessive bleeding
   b. Endometriosis
   c. Amenorrhea
   d. Pelvic inflammatory disease

8. A 60-year-old female patient informs the nurse that she has experienced some vaginal changes since menopause. What gynecologic change is the patient most likely to report?
   a. Thin, white vaginal drainage
   b. Vaginal odor
   c. Excessive vaginal bleeding
   d. Vaginal dryness

9. The mother of a 17-year-old adolescent girl tells the nurse that her daughter has been purging, showing anorexic behavior, and continuously exercising. Based on the mother's report, which question related to the reproductive system would the nurse ask the girl?
   a. "When was your last normal menstrual period?"
   b. "Are you sexually active?"
   c. "Are you having any unusual vaginal discharge?"
   d. "Have you had any problems with urination?"

10. A 29-year-old patient has strictures and adhesions in her fallopian tubes. This may be the result of which condition?
    a. Pelvic inflammatory disease
    b. Frequent bouts of colitis
    c. Gallbladder disease
    d. Frequent urinary tract infections

11. In a patient with a reproductive health problem, what health and lifestyle habits would the nurse assess? *(Select all that apply.)*
    a. Diet
    b. Socioeconomic status
    c. Exercise pattern
    d. Occupation
    e. Sleep pattern

12. A patient is diagnosed with a chlamydial infection, but is reluctant to spend the money for treatment because she is asymptomatic and does not have a job or health insurance. The nurse advises her that chlamydial infections can result in which condition?
    a. Female infertility
    b. Male partner infertility
    c. Amenorrhea
    d. Teratogenic effects

13. A 40-year-old woman has heavy vaginal bleeding. Which question is the priority in evaluating the patient's chief complaint?
    a. "Is the bleeding related to the menstrual cycle or intercourse?"
    b. "Are you having any sensations of pain or cramping?"
    c. "Are you sexually active and do you use oral contraceptives?"
    d. "Are you feeling weak, dizzy, or lightheaded?"

14. A 37-year-old patient reports abnormal vaginal bleeding not related to her menstrual cycle. The nurse would ask the patient about which associated symptoms? *(Select all that apply.)*
    a. Pain
    b. Change in bowel habits
    c. Breast mass
    d. Abdominal fullness
    e. Urinary difficulties

15. According to the American Cancer Society (ACS) recommendations, which healthy woman with no previous history of an abnormal Pap test should be advised to have a Pap test every 3 years?
    a. 18-year-old
    b. 21-year-old
    c. 35-year-old
    d. 70-year-old

16. The health care provider has just informed the patient about the diagnosis and complications of salpingitis. Which intervention is the nurse most likely to use with this patient?
    a. Review nonpharmacologic methods to control chronic pain.
    b. Use empathetic listening for feelings related to possible infertility.
    c. Inform that annual Pap smears are recommended for salpingitis.
    d. Review expected changes that will occur with menstrual flow.

17. For a patient with a low testosterone level, which symptom is the patient most likely to report?
    a. Increased muscle mass
    b. Problems passing urine
    c. Change in sexual performance
    d. Testicular pain with nausea

18. What features would be considered normal findings for the scrotum of a young white male? *(Select all that apply.)*
    a. Suspended below the pubic bone
    b. Tenderness with gentle palpation
    c. Contracts with exposure to cold
    d. Sparse hair follicles
    e. Dark cherry-red coloration

19. What is the function of the prostate gland?
    a. Production and storage of testosterone
    b. Secretes fluid to enhance sperm movement
    c. Secretes hormone to increase libido
    d. Production of androgen and relaxin

20. A 72-year-old patient admitted to the medical-surgical unit tells the nurse that he has benign prostatic hyperplasia. Which question will the nurse ask?
    a. "Have you had chemotherapy or radiation treatments?"
    b. "Were you recently diagnosed with benign prostatic hyperplasia?"
    c. "Would you like to review information about nutrition therapy?"
    d. "Are you having urinary incontinence or frequency at night?"

21. A young woman reports that she has a genital discharge causing irritation and odor. She feels embarrassed, but insists that she has not had recent sexual relations. Which question is the nurse most likely to ask?
    a. "Have you recently taken any antibiotic medications?"
    b. "Do you have a family history for cervical cancer?"
    c. "How old were you when you first had sexual intercourse?"
    d. "Have you had a change of diet or noticed weight loss?"

22. The nurse is interviewing a patient who reports a discharge from his penis that started 3 days ago. What does the nurse ask the patient regarding this problem? *(Select all that apply.)*
    a. "Has your sexual partner(s) noticed a discharge?"
    b. "Does the discharge have an odor?"
    c. "Have you noticed a mass or lump in the scrotum?"
    d. "Have you noticed a change in bowel habits?"
    e. "What is the consistency of the discharge?"

23. A nurse is working at an ambulatory clinic. Which patient is most likely to need to be prepared for a pelvic examination?
    a. 12-year-old whose mother desires a "virgin check"
    b. 25-year-old with a possible urinary tract infection
    c. 62-year-old who reports resumption of menses
    d. 53-year-old who reports decreased libido

24. A 31-year-old woman is diagnosed with salpingitis. On the figure below, indicate which area of the reproductive system is most affected by this condition.

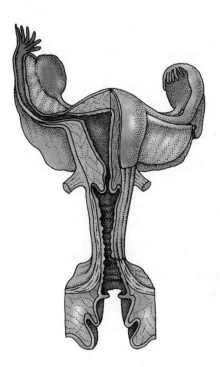

25. Which diagnostic test is used to differentiate solid tissue masses from cystic or hemorrhagic structures in the abdomen and pelvis?
    a. Hysterosalpingography
    b. Computed tomography
    c. Hysteroscopy
    d. Colposcopy

26. Which test detects cancerous and precancerous cells of the cervix?
    a. Serologic studies
    b. Vaginal culture
    c. Pap smear
    d. Human papilloma virus (HPV) test

27. A patient calls to make an appointment for a routine pelvic exam which includes a Pap smear. What type of instructions does the nurse give the patient about preparing for the exam?
    a. "Do not douche for at least 24 hours before the exam."
    b. "Do not eat or drink anything after midnight."
    c. "Clean genitals with mild soap and water before the exam."
    d. "Do not wear a tampon if you are menstruating."

28. A 79-year-old man is being seen for difficulty voiding and some blood in the urine. Which is the first screening test likely to be done?
    a. Cytologic cultures
    b. Prostate-specific antigen testing
    c. Serum levels for testosterone
    d. Serologic studies

29. An African-American male patient has a prostate-specific antigen (PSA) level less than 2.5 ng/mL. Which information should the nurse give to the patient?
    a. African-American men typically have lower-than-normal PSA levels.
    b. Level indicates a need for follow-up for possible prostate cancer.
    c. PSA level of less than 2.5 ng/mL is generally considered normal.
    d. Test should be repeated on an annual basis to monitor the abnormality.

30. A patient received treatment for prostate cancer. Which test is most likely to be ordered to monitor the disease after treatment?
    a. Transrectal biopsy
    b. PSA test
    c. HPV test
    d. Routine prostate examination

31. The patient reports fatigue and low libido. Based on the patient's report of symptoms, which laboratory result would the nurse seek out first?
    a. Pap smear results
    b. Rubella titer
    c. Red blood cell count
    d. Luteinizing hormone level

32. Which patient is most likely to require an iron supplement?
    a. 53-year-old woman who is entering menopause and has a breast mass
    b. 32-year-old female with heavy menstrual bleeding and an intrauterine device
    c. 70-year-old male who is diagnosed with benign prostatic hyperplasia
    d. 23-year-old woman who has pelvic inflammatory disease

33. The health care provider tells the nurse that the patient is being evaluated for galactorrhea and to please call with the relevant laboratory results. Which laboratory result will the nurse look for?
    a. Prolactin level
    b. Endometrial biopsy results
    c. Follicle-stimulating hormone (FSH) level
    d. Progesterone level

34. A 23-year-old female has a decreased level of FSH. What may this finding indicate?
    a. Midcycle of menses
    b. Pregnancy
    c. Premature menopause
    d. Infertility

35. Which statement about PSA testing is true?
    a. It is used to screen for prostate cancer.
    b. PSA levels above 25 ng/mL are associated with prostate cancer.
    c. Older men often have a lower-normal PSA level.
    d. It is done on patients over 60 years of age.

36. The nurse is teaching a patient about the contraindications for hysteroscopy. What does the nurse tell the patient?
    a. "During the procedure, normal or abnormal cells can be pushed through the fallopian tubes and into your pelvic cavity; therefore pregnancy is contraindicated."
    b. "The procedure causes irritation and can be very painful if your vaginal tissue is dry or fragile; therefore, the procedure is not recommended for postmenopausal women."
    c. "The procedure can cause a lot of bleeding so a recent prescription of an anticoagulant is a contraindication."
    d. "During the procedure, an iodine-based dye is used, so allergies to shellfish or iodine are contraindications."

37. What test is used to assess tubal anatomy and patency, and uterine problems?
    a. Computed tomography
    b. Laparoscopy
    c. Colposcopy
    d. Hysterosalpingography

38. The nurse is caring for a patient who had a laparoscopy. What is included in the postoperative care for this patient? *(Select all that apply.)*
    a. Administer oral analgesics for incisional pain.
    b. Notify the health care provider of postoperative shoulder pain.
    c. Reassure the patient that most painful sensations disappear within 4 to 6 weeks.
    d. Instruct the patient to change the small adhesive bandage as needed.
    e. Teach the patient to observe the incision for signs of infection or hematoma.
    f. Remind the patient to avoid strenuous activity for 4 to 6 weeks after the procedure.

39. The nurse is helping a patient schedule an appointment for a hysteroscopy. When does the nurse advise the patient that the procedure should be done?
    a. 5 days after menses have ceased
    b. 5 days before the beginning of menses
    c. During the menstrual period
    d. Whenever she can take 3 to 4 days off of work

40. A patient has just been informed by the health care provider that she has specific BRCA1 and BRCA2 gene mutations. Which brochure would the nurse prepare for the patient?
    a. "Role of Nutrition Therapy in Reproductive Health"
    b. "Risk Factors and Treatments for Infertility"
    c. "Risk Factors and Treatments for Breast Cancer"
    d. "Colposcopy and Other Tests for Cervical Cancer"

41. Which man has the greatest risk for developing prostate cancer?
    a. Patient's grandfather, age 82 years, has benign prostatic hyperplasia.
    b. Patient's father was diagnosed and treated for prostate cancer at age 50.
    c. Patient's mother took diethylstilbestrol (DES) to control bleeding during pregnancy.
    d. Patient's brother had delayed development of sexual characteristics.

42. The nurse is assisting a patient who needs a pelvic examination. Which action will the nurse perform?
    a. Clean perineum with antiseptic solution.
    b. Administer a mild analgesic.
    c. Assess for allergies to iodine.
    d. Instruct to empty the urinary bladder.

43. A patient has just been informed that she has an abnormal Pap smear and a positive HPV test. The nurse should be prepared to provide information about which topic?
    a. Increased risk for cervical cancer
    b. Increased risk for endometrial cancer
    c. Increased risk for herpes simplex virus type 2
    d. Increased risk for human immunodeficiency virus

44. The nurse is talking to a patient who is about to undergo a hysterosalpingogram. The patient discloses information that may not have been available to the health care provider when the test was initially scheduled. Which disclosure could cause the provider to cancel or reschedule the test?
    a. Took an over-the-counter acetaminophen 1 hour ago
    b. Has fever with malodorous vaginal discharge
    c. Has a previous history of uterine fibroids
    d. Is on day 10 of the menstrual cycle

45. What preprocedural instructions would the nurse give the patient about a mammogram?
    a. Do not eat or drink anything 6 to 7 hours before the test.
    b. Abstain from sexual relations prior to test to avoid pregnancy.
    c. Do not use lotions, creams, or powder on breasts before the study.
    d. Wear a supportive bra and bring a breast pad for use after testing.

46. What postprocedure instructions would the nurse give to a patient who just had a colposcopy?
    a. Do not drive or operate heavy machinery while taking prescribed pain medication.
    b. Do not use tampons and abstain from sexual intercourse for at least 1 week.
    c. Wear a perineal pad and expect bleeding with small clots for the first 24 hours.
    d. Perform breast self-examination every month and report changes to provider.

47. The patient needs to be scheduled for an endometrial biopsy to assess unusually heavy menstrual bleeding. Which question is the most important to ask, in relation to scheduling the examination?
    a. "Have you ever had a spontaneous miscarriage or an elective abortion?"
    b. "How many pads per day are you using during the heaviest flow?"
    c. "What was the date of your last menstrual period and are you regular?"
    d. "Do any unexpected symptoms accompany the heavy menstrual flow?"

48. What postprocedure instructions would the nurse give to a patient who had a prostate biopsy?
    a. Light rectal bleeding and blood in the urine or stools is expected for a few days.
    b. Swelling of the biopsy area and difficulty urinating are expected for 1 week.
    c. Low-grade fever and bright-red penile discharge are normal for several days.
    d. Return to see the health care provider in 1 week for recheck of biopsy site.

70 CHAPTER

Care of Patients with Breast Disorders

1. For a patient with mild discomfort from fibro-cystic breast condition (FBC), what will the nurse teach the patient about self-care measures?
   a. Avoid or limit reaching upwards or lifting objects above the head.
   b. Avoid wearing a bra to decrease the pressure on the breast tissue.
   c. Take analgesics and limit salt before menses to help decrease swelling.
   d. Take selective estrogen receptor modulator as prescribed.

2. A 22-year-old woman is being seen for a self-detected mass in her right breast. Clinical examination reveals an oval-shaped, freely mobile, and rubbery lesion measuring 1 cm × 2.5 cm. What type of tumor is this most likely to be?
   a. Ductal ectasia
   b. Papilloma
   c. Fibroadenoma
   d. Macrocyst

3. A 33-year-old woman reports that the skin over her left breast is reddened, warm, and has swelling. These characteristics are typically found in which type of breast disorder?
   a. Intraductal papilloma
   b. Fibroadenoma
   c. Inflammatory breast cancer
   d. Lobular carcinoma in situ

4. The medical record of a patient indicates small, nonpalpable cysts inside the breast glands that were discovered 3 months ago. Which breast disorder is this most likely to be?
   a. Papilloma
   b. Microcysts
   c. Ductal ectasia
   d. Fibroadenoma

5. The nurse is preparing an information packet about reconstructive breast surgery. What information does the nurse include about health risks for large-breasted women?
   a. Increased risk for fungal infections and backaches
   b. Increased difficulty in nursing a baby
   c. Likelihood of foul discharge from the nipples
   d. Increased risk for fibrocystic disease

6. A patient with FBC has just undergone fine needle aspiration to drain the cyst fluid and reduce pressure and pain. At what points does the nurse prepare patient education material about breast biopsy? *(Select all that apply.)*
   a. If hormonal replacement therapy is prescribed
   b. If fluid is not aspirated
   c. If the mammogram shows suspicious findings
   d. If fluid buildup recurs
   e. If the mass remains palpable after aspiration
   f. If aspirated fluid reveals cancer cells

7. A patient with FBC is prescribed drug therapy to manage symptoms. The nurse prepares teaching materials for which group of medications?
   a. Antiandrogen agents, calcium supplements, opioids
   b. Monoclonal antibody agents, corticosteroids
   c. Aromatase inhibitors, potassium supplements, nonsteroidal antiinflammatory drugs (NSAIDs)
   d. Oral contraceptives, vitamin therapy, diuretics

8. A 54-year-old woman has identified a hard breast mass with irregular borders, redness, and edema. She reports a greenish-brown nipple discharge and enlarged axillary nodes. Based on the patient's age and description of the symptoms, what does the nurse suspect?
   a. Fibroadenoma
   b. Fibrocystic breast condition
   c. Ductal ectasia
   d. Intraductal papilloma

9. The nurse notes in the electronic medical record that the patient has a round, firm, non-tender, mobile breast mass not attached to breast tissue or the chest wall. What does this describe?
   a. Fibroadenoma
   b. Fibrocystic disease
   c. Breast cysts
   d. Ductal ectasia

10. The nurse is reviewing discharge instructions for a patient who had breast augmentation surgery. What does the nurse include in these instructions? *(Select all that apply.)*
    a. Expect soreness in chest and arms for several months.
    b. Breasts will feel tight and sensitive; the breast skin may feel warm or itchy.
    c. Anticipate having difficulty raising the arms over the head.
    d. Perform lifting, pushing, and pulling exercises several times a day.
    e. Walk every few hours to prevent deep vein thrombosis.
    f. Expect some swelling for 3 to 4 weeks after surgery.

11. What is the most common breast dysfunction found in the male breast?
    a. Nipple discharge
    b. Nipple retraction
    c. Gynecomastia
    d. Disseminated breast cancer

12. What does the nurse instruct the patient to do before a scheduled breast augmentation surgery? *(Select all that apply.)*
    a. Stop oral contraceptives.
    b. Stop smoking.
    c. Avoid taking NSAIDs.
    d. Avoid taking *Ginkgo biloba*.
    e. Wear a supportive bra.

13. After surgery, a female patient has been told her breast tumor contains estrogen receptors (ER positive). How will this type of cancer be treated?
    a. Additional surgery
    b. Hormonal therapy
    c. Radiation therapy
    d. Targeted therapy

14. Based on risk factors and personal history, which woman has the greatest risk of developing breast cancer?
    a. Physician, age 56, who had her first child at age 38
    b. Ballet dancer, age 20, who has a 5-year-old son
    c. Radiation technician, age 24, who had her menarche at age 13
    d. Housewife, age 42, who had breast reduction surgery at age 26

15. The nurse is counseling a woman recently diagnosed with breast cancer. Which factor has the most influence on the choice for treatment?
    a. Age at the time of diagnosis
    b. Overall health status
    c. Personal choice and type of insurance
    d. Extent and location of metastasis of the breast mass

16. A young patient is suspected of having invasive breast cancer. Based on the types and frequencies of breast cancer, what is the patient most likely to be diagnosed with?
    a. Fibrocystic breast condition
    b. Infiltrating ductal carcinoma
    c. Lobular carcinoma in situ
    d. Ductal carcinoma in situ

17. Which factor is the incidence of breast disease most closely related to?
    a. Lifestyle choices
    b. Aging
    c. Ethnic background
    d. Socioeconomic status

18. Which combination of screening techniques is best for early detection of breast cancer? *(Select all that apply.)*
    a. Mammogram
    b. Clinical breast exam
    c. Needle aspiration of breast tissue
    d. Breast self-awareness
    e. Computed tomography

19. Cancer surveillance for high-risk women is used to detect cancer in its early stages and is referred to as what kind of prevention?
    a. Primary
    b. Secondary
    c. Tertiary
    d. Prophylactic

20. According to the American Cancer Society, what are the recommendations for early detection by screening for breast masses?
    a. Women aged 40 years and older should have an annual mammogram.
    b. High-risk women should begin annual mammograms at age 40 years.
    c. High-risk women should begin annual magnetic resonance imaging at age 40 years.
    d. Women aged 40 years or older should have a mammogram every 3 years.

21. The nurse is teaching a 24-year-old patient about breast self-examination (BSE). What does the nurse tell the patient about the time to perform BSE?
    a. The day before her menstrual flow is due
    b. On the third day after her menstrual flow starts
    c. When ovulation occurs
    d. One week after her menstrual period

22. Which factor makes the mammogram a more sensitive screening tool than other tests?
    a. Higher compliance rate than BSE because it is done annually
    b. Less expensive than other tests that identify tumor markers
    c. Able to reveal masses too small to be palpated manually
    d. Able to differentiate between fluid and solid masses

23. A patient stopped having menses about a year ago. When does the nurse advise the patient to perform BSE?
    a. The first day of every other month
    b. After menopause, BSE does not detect masses
    c. The last day of each month
    d. Any day of the month, but follow a consistent schedule

24. The nurse is teaching the patient about BSE. Which actions are correct parts of the procedure? *(Select all that apply.)*
    a. "Lie down on your back and place your right arm behind your head."
    b. "Use the palm of your left hand to feel for lumps in the right breast."
    c. "Use three different levels of pressure to feel all the breast tissue."
    d. "Move around the breast in an up and down pattern."
    e. "Stand in front of a mirror, press your hands firmly down on your hips and observe breasts."

25. During clinical breast exam (CBE), the examiner observes a small mass in the breast. What is the most important item to include in the documentation of this finding?
    a. "Face of the clock" location of the mass
    b. Amount of pressure required to detect the mass
    c. Patient's self-awareness of the location
    d. Method used to examine the breast

26. Which sign/symptom detected during CBE suggests advanced breast disease?
    a. Gynecomastia
    b. Oval-shaped, mobile, rubbery mass
    c. Thin, milky discharge from the nipple
    d. Skin change of peau d'orange

27. Women who have a personal history of breast cancer are at high risk for developing a recurrence or new breast cancer with the presence of which factors? *(Select all that apply.)*
    a. BRCA3 genetic mutation
    b. Strong family history
    c. BRCA2 genetic mutation
    d. BRCA1 genetic mutation
    e. History of breast reduction

28. The nurse is instructing a patient with ductal ectasia about her risk for breast cancer. What does the nurse tell the patient?
    a. It is considered a precancerous condition.
    b. There is no increased risk of developing breast cancer.
    c. Features of the condition automatically rule out cancer.
    d. Lifestyle changes are recommended to reduce risk.

29. A patient had breast reconstruction surgery two days ago. A Jackson-Pratt drain was placed to collect serosanguineous fluid. The nurse notices at 7:00 AM that the drainage container contains 150 mL. It was last emptied at 6:00 AM. What is the priority nursing intervention?
    a. Notify the health care provider about the amount and type of drainage for the past hour.
    b. Empty the drain every 2 hours so the suction will be more effective.
    c. Chart the type and amount of drainage and continue to monitor.
    d. Reinforce the drainage site with a sterile bulky dressing.

30. A patient had a partial mastectomy yesterday and the nurse notes that the patient is very anxious because of removal of breast tissue. What is the nurse's priority intervention?
    a. Use distraction until the patient improves and is able to think more clearly.
    b. Encourage the patient to have a positive attitude so she will heal faster.
    c. Ensure that the patient takes prn anxiolytic medication every 4 to 6 hours.
    d. Encourage the patient to discuss her fears and ask questions about her concerns.

31. A patient had a partial mastectomy. When teaching about care of the arm on the affected side, what does the nurse tell the patient?
    a. Start arm exercises as soon as the drains are removed from the incision.
    b. Keep the arm elevated so the elbow is above the shoulder and the wrist is above the elbow.
    c. Do not take blood pressure in the arm on the affected side for the first 6 months after surgery.
    d. Do push-ups and arm circles on a routine basis for a full recovery.

32. A patient has just been diagnosed with breast cancer and informed that surgery is likely to be needed. The patient seems anxious and upset. What is the priority nursing care for this patient?
    a. Provide patient education about treatment options.
    b. Assist the patient to make independent decisions.
    c. Provide reassurance about long-term outcomes.
    d. Allow patient to talk openly about feelings.

33. Which intervention would be used for a patient after a modified radical mastectomy?
    a. Position the patient on the affected side to aid flow of drainage from the incision site.
    b. Arm on the affected side should be in a dependent position postoperatively.
    c. Give pain medication so that arm exercises can begin as soon as possible.
    d. Teach signs and symptoms of infection and how to monitor for altered wound healing.

34. A patient who had surgery for breast cancer appears in need of continued community support. The nurse refers the patient to which organization?
    a. Reach to Recovery
    b. Empty Arms
    c. Resolve to Reach
    d. National Alliance on Mental Illness

35. The nurse is counseling a woman who has had several discussions with the health care provider about her risk for breast cancer. The nurse reinforces that prophylactic mastectomy would have what effect on her risk for developing breast cancer?
    a. Has no impact on the overall risk
    b. Eliminates the risk completely
    c. Reduces the risk for breast cancer
    d. Decreases risk for uterine cancers

36. Which woman has the highest risk for developing breast cancer?
    a. 68-year-old who takes hormone replacement therapy
    b. 35-year-old who has three children and had one miscarriage
    c. 23-year-old who started menstruating at age 12
    d. 40-year-old who has two cousins who had breast cancer

37. A patient found a mass in her breast 6 months ago. What question does the nurse ask related to possible metastases of a potential cancer?
    a. "Why did you wait 6 months before seeking medical attention?"
    b. "Have you noticed any joint or bone pain or other changes in your body?"
    c. "Have you ever had any exposure to radiation or toxic chemicals?"
    d. "Has your sister or mother ever been diagnosed with breast cancer?"

38. A patient has just been diagnosed with advanced breast cancer. Which behavior by the patient is the strongest indicator of readiness for additional patient teaching and information?
    a. Cheerfully talking about her family and the vacation they will take to Europe
    b. Being active and angrily throwing her belongings into her suitcase
    c. Crying and being upset, asking the nurse to call a spiritual counselor
    d. Being quiet and thoughtfully fingering the lace on her new bra

39. A patient in the medical-surgical unit says to the nurse, "My doctor told me I have advanced breast cancer and I want to give you this bracelet, because you have been so sweet to me today." What does the nurse do next?
    a. Contact the health care provider because the comment signals suicide intent.
    b. Sit with the patient and allow her to take the lead in the conversation.
    c. Contact the charge nurse because the news is overwhelming.
    d. Explain to the patient that it is unethical for nurses to accept expensive gifts.

40. The nurse is reviewing the laboratory results from a postmenopausal woman being evaluated for a breast mass. What type of metastasis does the increased serum calcium and alkaline phosphatase levels suggest?
    a. Brain
    b. Bone
    c. Lung
    d. Liver

41. The nurse is talking to a woman recently diagnosed with breast cancer who confides, "I am going to use nutritional and herbal therapy instead of taking drugs and radiation that would make my hair fall out." What is the nurse's best response?
    a. "Research shows complementary therapy can replace conventional medicine."
    b. "Have you reviewed all treatment options with your health care provider?"
    c. "Alternative nutritional therapies would interfere with conventional therapies."
    d. "Where did you hear about this nutritional and herbal treatment?"

42. The nurse is caring for a patient who had a right-sided modified radical mastectomy. Which task does the nurse delegate to the unlicensed assist personnel (UAP)?
    a. Observe the drainage in the Jackson-Pratt drain.
    b. Take blood pressure on the right arm only.
    c. Assist the patient to ambulate the day after surgery.
    d. Instruct the patient about arm positioning.

43. A patient is lying in bed after a mastectomy. How does the nurse position the patient?
    a. Head of the bed up at least 30 degrees with the affected arm elevated on a pillow
    b. Supine body position with the affected arm positioned straight by the side
    c. Any position that is the most comfortable to the patient
    d. Side-lying position with the unaffected side down towards mattress

44. A patient is one day postsurgery after a mastectomy and is anxious to begin the prescribed exercises. Which exercise is appropriate for the patient's first efforts?
    a. Flex the fingers so that the hands slowly "walk" up the wall.
    b. Squeeze the affected hand around a soft, round object.
    c. Swing the rope in small circles and gradually increase to larger circles.
    d. Grab the ends of the rope, and extend the arms until they are straight.

45. A patient is being discharged with a prescription for tamoxifen to decrease the chance of breast cancer recurrence. Because of the common side effect, what does the nurse suggest to the patient in taking this drug?
    a. Have soda crackers and ginger ale on hand.
    b. Install a handrail around the bathtub.
    c. Purchase a scale to monitor body weight.
    d. Buy a soft-bristle toothbrush.

46. A patient is prescribed trastuzumab (Herceptin) for breast cancer. What is the priority nursing intervention for this patient?
    a. Obtain an order for baseline electrocardiography (ECG).
    b. Assess for signs of bleeding.
    c. Premedicate with an antiemetic.
    d. Rotate injection sites.

47. The nurse is caring for a patient who is diagnosed with ductal ectasia. What is the primary goal of the nursing care?
    a. Reduce the anxiety associated with the threat of breast cancer.
    b. Review side effects of radiation and chemotherapy treatments.
    c. Give support for decision-making about prophylactic mastectomy.
    d. Assess for readiness and willingness to seek a support group.

48. The nurse is assessing a woman with very large breasts. In addition to the routine assessment of the breasts, what specific assessment will the nurse perform on this patient?
    a. Pay special attention to the size and shape of the nipples.
    b. Observe underneath the breasts for fungal infection.
    c. Ask if the patient has considered reduction mammoplasty.
    d. Assess for pain in the joints or bones.

49. What is important information regarding breast cancer surveillance for a patient who had breast augmentation surgery?
    a. The prosthesis interferes with lump detection by BSE or CBE.
    b. Mammograms are not useful because implant material is artificial.
    c. Implant displacement x-rays allow more complete examination.
    d. Breast augmentation increases the risk for breast cancer.

50. For women with genetic risk factors for breast cancer, which intervention would address one of the modifiable risk factors?
    a. Discuss strategies to avoid weight gain and obesity.
    b. Encourage frequent genetic testing for tumors.
    c. Have testing for BRCA1 and BRCA2 gene mutations.
    d. Consider hormone replacement therapy.

51. The nurse hears in shift report that a 32-year-old patient had a prophylactic oophorectomy. What subjective symptom(s) does the nurse anticipate that the patient would report?
    a. Swelling of upper arms
    b. Tenderness of breasts
    c. Menopausal symptoms
    d. Nausea related to medications

52. Which diagnostic test is considered the most definitive for diagnosing breast cancer?
    a. Magnetic resonance imaging
    b. Mammography
    c. Breast tomosynthesis
    d. Breast biopsy

53. The patient with breast cancer is considering acupuncture as an adjunctive therapy. The nurse would advise the patient to avoid acupuncture because of which laboratory result?
    a. Low red blood cell count
    b. Low serum glucose level
    c. Low white blood cell count
    d. Low serum calcium level

54. What is the major advantage of neoadjuvant therapy?
    a. Newest chemotherapy for several different types of breast cancer
    b. Has fewer and milder side effects than conventional chemotherapy
    c. Shrinkage of tumor allows lumpectomy rather than mastectomy
    d. Tumor frequently resolves spontaneously without surgical intervention

55. The nurse must assign a UAP to assist a patient who is undergoing brachytherapy for breast cancer treatment. What is the most important question that the nurse will ask the UAP prior to making the assignment?
    a. "Do you know how to dispose of radioactive body fluids?"
    b. "Is there any chance that you could be pregnant?"
    c. "Have you ever cared for a patient during brachytherapy?"
    d. "Have you ever had any radiation exposure?"

56. The nurse is designing a teaching plan for a patient who had surgery for breast cancer. What information does the nurse include in the plan? *(Select all that apply.)*
    a. Do not use lotions or ointments on the area.
    b. Delay using deodorant under the affected arm until healing is complete.
    c. Swelling and redness of the scar itself are considered normal and permanent.
    d. Report any increased heat and tenderness of the area to the surgeon.
    e. Wear loose pajamas at home for 6 to 8 weeks.
    f. Begin active range-of-motion exercises 1 week after surgery.

71 CHAPTER

Care of Patients with Gynecologic Problems

1. For a patient with endometriosis, which supplement might offer relief of the muscle cramping?
   a. Vitamin C
   b. Vitamin D
   c. Potassium
   d. Magnesium

2. A 20-year-old woman is being evaluated for possible toxic shock syndrome. What question would the nurse ask?
   a. "How many pads do you use on heavy flow days?"
   b. "Have you ever used intravaginal estrogen therapy?"
   c. "Do you have a history of multiple sexual partners?"
   d. "Do you use internal contraceptives?"

3. A patient tells the nurse that she was told that she had a "chocolate" cyst. Which assessment is the nurse mostly likely to perform?
   a. Ask for description of the vaginal discharge.
   b. Assess onset and description of pain.
   c. Assess for family history of cervical cancer.
   d. Ask about personal or family history of renal disease.

4. A 22-year-old patient reports abdominal pain that seems to start several days before her menstrual period. What questions does the nurse ask in order to obtain a thorough menstrual history? *(Select all that apply.)*
   a. "How old were you when you started menstruation?"
   b. "Typically, how long does your period last?"
   c. "How would you describe your menstrual flow?"
   d. "When did you last have sexual intercourse?"
   e. "Would you like information about contraception?"

5. What self-management strategy would the nurse recommend to a patient to prevent vulvovaginitis?
   a. Wear nylon underwear.
   b. Douche daily to remove vaginal secretions.
   c. Apply antiseptic cream daily to perineal area.
   d. Avoid wearing tight-fitting clothing.

6. A current treatment of nonemergent dysfunctional uterine bleeding includes which medication?
   a. Oral or patch contraceptives
   b. Tamoxifen (Nolvadex)
   c. Magnesium supplement
   d. Cisplatin (Platinol)

7. The nurse is teaching self-care management to a 39-year-old woman who had an abdominal hysterectomy. Which point would be emphasized to avoid complications of this surgery?
   a. Bathe and douche daily to prevent infection.
   b. Take temperature twice a day for the first 3 days after surgery.
   c. Resume typical exercise routines as soon as possible.
   d. Gently massage calves if tenderness or swelling occurs.

8. What types of examinations are done to reveal the presence of uterine enlargement related to fibroids? *(Select all that apply.)*
   a. Abdominal examination
   b. Vaginal examination
   c. Rectal examination
   d. Excretory urography
   e. Transvaginal ultrasound with saline infusion

9. Which woman is at greatest risk for developing pelvic organ prolapse?
   a. 16-year-old adolescent caring for her first child
   b. 25-year-old who became sexually active at age 15
   c. 34-year-old who has a history of endometriosis
   d. 48-year-old obese mother of four children

10. Which woman is at greatest risk for dysfunctional uterine bleeding?
    a. 20-year-old housewife who has one child
    b. 45-year-old attorney with a stressful life
    c. 30-year-old nurse who smoked for 10 years
    d. 25-year-old teacher who rarely exercises

11. Following a uterine embolization using a vascular closure device, what patient care would the nurse provide? *(Select all that apply.)*
    a. Assist the patient to ambulate 2 hours after the procedure.
    b. Keep the patient on bedrest with the leg immobilized for 4 hours before ambulating.
    c. Encourage the patient to drink a lot of fluids.
    d. Assess the patient's pain level and administer analgesics as needed.
    e. Raise the head of the bed.

12. An obese 57-year-old patient describes excessive menstrual bleeding that occurs approximately every 10 days. The nurse educates the patient for which diagnostic test that is used to evaluate for endometrial cancer?
    a. Bimanual pelvic examination
    b. Transvaginal ultrasound
    c. Sonohysterography
    d. Endometrial biopsy

13. A 36-year-old patient is diagnosed with dysfunctional uterine bleeding. During the pelvic exam, the health care provider determines that the bleeding is acute and heavy. What is the nurse's priority action?
    a. Prepare the patient for immediate transport to the operating room.
    b. Prepare to administer combination hormonal therapy.
    c. Anticipate an order for a hormonal contraceptive patch.
    d. Prepare to administer injectable medroxyprogesterone acetate (Depo-Provera).

14. A patient who is very upset asks the nurse, "My doctor says I have endometriosis. What does it mean?" What is the nurse's best response?
    a. "It is an early warning sign of endometrial cancer, but you still need more testing."
    b. "A special type of tissue, called *endometrial tissue*, is outside of your uterus."
    c. "It's a special tissue which grows rapidly, but it is not dangerous."
    d. "It is a type of infection and inflammation of the endometrial tissue."

15. What signs/symptoms does the nurse assess in a patient with dysfunctional uterine bleeding? *(Select all that apply.)*
    a. Male hair pattern
    b. Gastric ulcers
    c. Thyroid enlargement
    d. Abdominal pain
    e. Abdominal masses

16. What is the primary treatment for dysfunctional uterine bleeding in perimenopausal women?
    a. Intravaginal estrogen therapy
    b. Progestin or combination hormone therapy
    c. Laparoscopic myomectomy
    d. Magnetic resonance-guided focused ultrasound

17. A patient has excessive bleeding from uterine fibroids. Which therapy stops the blood flow to the fibroids?
    a. An infusion of conjugated estrogens
    b. Dilation and curettage
    c. Topical vaginal estrogen therapy
    d. Endometrial ablation

18. A patient has undergone a total hysterectomy with vaginal repair. The nurse advises her about careful intercourse and which over-the-counter product to decrease sexual discomfort related to intercourse?
    a. Hydrocortisone cream
    b. Water-based lubricants
    c. Petroleum jelly
    d. Vitamin A and D ointment

19. The nurse is caring for a patient who had hysteroscopic surgery. The patient reports severe lower abdominal pain, she appears pale, and has trouble focusing on the nurse's questions about the pain. Vital signs show: T 98.6° F, P 120/min, R 24/min, BP 103/60. Which complication does the nurse suspect?
    a. Hemorrhage
    b. Embolism
    c. Fluid overload
    d. Incomplete suppression of menstruation

20. The patient reports itching, change in vaginal discharge, and an odor. The nurse suspects that the patient has vulvovaginitis. Based on knowledge about the common causes of vulvovaginitis, which question would the nurse ask?
    a. "Have you recently been taking antibiotics?"
    b. "Have you been swimming in a lake or pond?"
    c. "Do you consistently wipe from front to back?"
    d. "Do you use tampons or menstrual pads?"

21. The nurse sees that a patient has been advised by the health care provider to apply lindane (Kwell) to the affected area. What is a self-care measure for this patient to ensure that the symptoms do not return after using the medication?
    a. Wash the area daily with hydrogen peroxide.
    b. Take a sitz bath for 30 minutes several times a day.
    c. Wash clothes, linens, and disinfect the home environment.
    d. Remove any irritants or allergens (e.g., change detergents).

22. A patient with a fever, myalgia, sore throat, and sunburn-like rash is admitted with the diagnosis of toxic shock syndrome. What additional clinical manifestation should the nurse assess for?
    a. Hypotension
    b. Vaginal bleeding
    c. Bradycardia
    d. Polyuria

23. The nurse is teaching a group of women about prevention of toxic shock syndrome. What preventive measures does the nurse include? *(Select all that apply.)*
    a. "Avoid the use of superabsorbent tampons."
    b. "Use sanitary napkins at night."
    c. "Avoid using internal contraceptives."
    d. "Void immediately after intercourse."
    e. "Change your tampon every 8 hours."

24. A patient is admitted with toxic shock syndrome. What organism is frequently associated with this syndrome when it occurs as a menstrually related infection?
    a. *Escherichia coli*
    b. *Staphylococcus aureus*
    c. *Haemophilus influenzae*
    d. Beta-hemolytic streptococcus

25. A patient reports the sensation of feeling as if "something is falling out" along with painful intercourse, backache, and a feeling of heaviness or pressure in the pelvis. Which question does the nurse ask to assess for a cystocele?
    a. "Are you having urinary frequency or urgency?"
    b. "Do you feel constipated?"
    c. "Have you had problems with hemorrhoids?"
    d. "Have you had any heavy vaginal bleeding?"

26. A patient had an anterior colporrhaphy and is returning to the clinic for the follow-up appointment. Which patient statement indicates that the procedure has achieved the desired therapeutic outcome?
    a. "The abdominal pain is almost gone."
    b. "I have good control over my urination."
    c. "I am no longer having that constipated feeling."
    d. "My vaginal bleeding has resolved."

27. A patient has had a posterior colporrhaphy. What is included in the nursing care of this patient? *(Select all that apply.)*
    a. Administer pain medication before a bowel movement.
    b. Instruct to avoid straining during a bowel movement.
    c. Resume regular activities after discharge from the hospital.
    d. Provide sitz baths.
    e. Promote a low-residue (low-fiber) diet.

28. The nurse is giving discharge teaching to a patient who had a transvaginal repair for pelvic organ prolapse using a surgical mesh. What does the nurse include?
    a. Avoid cigarette smoking for at least one month.
    b. Abstain from sexual intercourse for 6 weeks.
    c. Reduce calories to lose 2 pounds a month.
    d. Avoid tub baths to prevent soaking the mesh.

29. A patient is diagnosed with uterine leiomyomas. What does the nurse expect to see in the documentation for this patient as the chief presenting symptom?
    a. Foul-smelling vaginal discharge
    b. Heavy vaginal bleeding
    c. Intermittent abdominal pain
    d. Urinary incontinence

30. A patient with uterine leiomyomas reports a feeling of pelvic pressure, constipation, and urinary retention. She says, "I can't button my pants anymore." What does the nurse assess for to further evaluate the patient's symptoms?
    a. Check the lower extremities for fluid retention.
    b. Assess the abdomen for distention or enlargement.
    c. Measure the fluid intake and urine output.
    d. Inspect the perineal area for bleeding or discharge.

31. A patient has had a pelvic examination and needs an additional diagnostic test for possible uterine leiomyomas. The nurse prepares the patient for which first-choice diagnostic test?
    a. Transvaginal ultrasound
    b. Laparoscopy
    c. Hysteroscopy
    d. Endometrial biopsy

32. What is the priority nursing care most commonly seen preoperatively and postoperatively in a patient with leiomyomas?
    a. Preventing infection
    b. Managing severe pain
    c. Monitoring for bleeding
    d. Assessing for and managing anxiety

33. What disease is strongly associated with prolonged exposure to estrogen without the protective effects of progesterone?
    a. Endometriosis
    b. Uterine cancer
    c. Leiomyomas
    d. Endometrial cancer

34. A patient with cancer has also been diagnosed with uterine leiomyomas. Which procedure does the nurse prepare the patient for?
    a. Myomectomy
    b. Hysterectomy
    c. Endometrial ablation
    d. Magnetic resonance-guided focused ultrasound surgery

35. A patient who had a total abdominal hysterectomy is anxious to resume her activities because she has young children at home. What postprocedure information does the nurse provide to the patient? *(Select all that apply.)*
    a. Climb stairs to build strength and endurance.
    b. Avoid sitting for prolonged periods.
    c. Do not lift anything heavier than 5 to 10 lbs.
    d. Walk or jog at least 1-2 miles every day.
    e. When sitting, do not cross the legs.

36. The nurse is caring for several patients who had total abdominal hysterectomies. All patients are coming to the clinic for their 6-week follow-up appointment. Which patient demeanor is the strongest indicator that there is a need for psychological referral?
    a. Quiet and withdrawn but asks appropriate questions
    b. Tense and impatient but answers questions correctly
    c. Disheveled and lackluster and displays a lack of interest in questions
    d. Cheerful and distractible and answers questions with excessive detail

37. The nurse is giving discharge teaching to a woman who had a local cervical ablation. What information would be included? *(Select all that apply.)*
    a. Sexual activity may be resumed usually in 1 week.
    b. Change tampons every 4 hours
    c. Report heavy vaginal bleeding or foul-smelling drainage.
    d. Showering is permitted, but no tub baths.
    e. Avoid lifting heavy objects for 3 weeks.

38. A patient with swelling in the perineal area is diagnosed with a Bartholin cyst. Nonsurgical management is recommended. What does the nurse instruct the patient to do?
    a. Apply moist heat (e.g., sitz baths or hot wet packs) to the vulva.
    b. Return immediately to the clinic if the cyst ruptures.
    c. Contact all sexual partners about the need for treatment.
    d. Change the dressing at least three times a day.

39. Which diagnostic tests are considered the gold standard tests for determining the presence of endometrial thickening and cancer? *(Select all that apply.)*
    a. Transvaginal ultrasound
    b. Abdominal ultrasound
    c. Magnetic resonance imaging (MRI)
    d. Computed tomography (CT) of the pelvis
    e. Endometrial biopsy

40. The surgical procedure for stage I disease of endometrial cancer involves removal of which components? *(Select all that apply.)*
    a. Uterus
    b. Vagina
    c. Fallopian tubes
    d. Rectum
    e. Ovaries

41. The nurse is caring for a patient with a radioactive implant in the uterus. Which instruction will the nurse give to unlicensed assistive personnel (UAP)?
    a. Patient is on bedrest and excessive movement is restricted.
    b. Assist the patient to ambulate in the hall at least three times per shift.
    c. Assist the patient to get up to the toilet or the commode chair.
    d. Linens and patient gown should be frequently changed for drainage.

42. A patient is receiving external radiation therapy for treatment of endometrial cancer. What task does the nurse delegate to the UAP?
    a. Gently wash the markings outlining the treatment site.
    b. Monitor for signs of skin breakdown, especially in the perineal area.
    c. Assist the patient to ambulate if she feels fatigue or tiredness.
    d. Clean the urinary catheter and meatus with mild soap and water.

43. A patient receiving chemotherapy treatments reports fatigue, loss of energy, and experiencing an "emotional crisis every day and my hair is falling out." What does the nurse do first to help the patient adapt to body changes?
    a. Suggest participation in self-management.
    b. Encourage the patient to ventilate feelings.
    c. Help the patient to select a wig or scarf.
    d. Encourage the patient to talk to her family.

44. The nurse encourages a teenage patient to receive the human papillomavirus (HPV) vaccine (Gardasil) because it protects against which type of cancer?
    a. Endometrial cancer
    b. Cervical cancer
    c. Ovarian cancer
    d. Uterine cancer

45. What information would the nurse give to a sexually active 22-year-old woman about conventional Papanicolaou (Pap) smear testing?
    a. Every 2 to 3 years is sufficient.
    b. Annual screening is recommended.
    c. Testing can stop after three consecutive normal Pap smears.
    d. If there are no risk factors, testing is not necessary.

46. Which classic symptom is indicative of invasive gynecologic cancer in an older patient?
    a. Swelling of one leg
    b. Dark and foul-smelling discharge
    c. Painless vaginal bleeding
    d. Flank pain

47. The nurse is taking a history on a patient with probable gynecologic cancer. Which clinical manifestation is a sign of metastasis?
    a. Watery vaginal discharge
    b. Constipation
    c. Dyspareunia
    d. Dysuria

48. A patient had loop electrosurgical excision procedure (LEEP) for treatment and diagnosis of cervical cancer. In the discharge instructions, what does the nurse tell the patient to expect after the procedure?
    a. Spotting
    b. Menses-like vaginal bleeding
    c. Cramps lasting 24 hours
    d. Watery discharge

49. The nurse is teaching a patient who is being discharged after having a total abdominal hysterectomy. Which conditions does the nurse tell the patient to immediately report to the surgeon? (Select all that apply.)
    a. Vaginal drainage that becomes thicker or foul-smelling
    b. Hot flashes and night sweats
    c. Temperature over 100° F (38° C)
    d. Burning during urination
    e. Feeling more tired and sleeping longer

50. A patient had a total abdominal hysterectomy. Which patient behavior is the best indicator that she is coping and adapting successfully?
    a. Refuses to look at the wound, but encourages the nursing students to look
    b. Sits quietly and passively while the nurse performs wound care
    c. Asks questions about the wound care, but seems reluctant to do self-care
    d. Frequently stares at the wound site, but refuses to touch the area

51. The home health nurse is reviewing the patient's medication list and sees that the patient was given doxorubicin (Adriamycin) at the hospital. What gynecologic diagnosis would the nurse expect to see as part of the patient's history?
    a. Endometrial cancer
    b. Cervical polyps
    c. Endometriosis
    d. Bartholin cyst

52. The nurse is preparing patient teaching for several young women who will undergo surgical procedures for gynecologic problems. Which surgical procedure is most likely to induce menopausal symptoms?
    a. Bilateral salpingo-oophorectomy
    b. Endometrial ablation
    c. Uterine artery embolization
    d. Hysteroscopic myomectomy

53. The nurse is giving instructions to a patient who is undergoing brachytherapy for cervical cancer. What information does the nurse include? *(Select all that apply.)*
    a. "Limit interactions with others between treatments for their protection."
    b. "You are not radioactive between treatments."
    c. "Report any blood in the urine or severe diarrhea immediately."
    d. "Expect heavy vaginal bleeding during this time."
    e. "You will be on bedrest during the treatment session."

54. What is the primary factor for the low survival rates for patients who are diagnosed with ovarian cancer?
    a. Ovarian cancer develops in patients with underlying immunosuppression and poor health.
    b. Ovarian cancer does not respond well to conventional radiation and chemotherapy treatments.
    c. Symptoms are mild and vague, therefore the cancer is often not detected until its late stage.
    d. There are no specific diagnostic tests that can confirm or rule out ovarian cancer.

55. Young women who have intercourse as teenagers and/or have multiple sex partners are at high risk for which disease?
    a. Endometriosis
    b. Cervical cancer
    c. Amenorrhea
    d. Ovarian cancer

56. In recalling dietary intake for a recent 24-hour period, a female patient describes eating eggs, whole milk, and bacon for breakfast; fried chicken and French fries for lunch; three-cheese pizza and ice cream for dinner. This type of diet places her at increased risk for which disorder?
    a. Dysfunctional uterine bleeding
    b. Dyspareunia
    c. Early menopause
    d. Cancer of the ovaries

Care of Patients with Male Reproductive Problems

1. A patient tells the nurse that he was diagnosed with benign prostatic hyperplasia (BPH). Based on this medical diagnosis, which symptom is the patient most likely to report?
   a. Pain in the scrotum
   b. Trouble passing urine
   c. Erectile dysfunction (ED)
   d. Constipation

2. The nurse teaches a patient with BPH to follow which instructions? *(Select all that apply.)*
   a. Avoid diuretics.
   b. Avoid sexual intercourse.
   c. Avoid antihistamines.
   d. Avoid caffeine.
   e. Avoid drinking large amounts of fluid in a short time.

3. Which type of surgery is most commonly used to treat BPH?
   a. Contact laser prostatectomy
   b. Radical prostatectomy
   c. Open prostatectomy
   d. Transurethral resection of the prostate (TURP)

4. The nurse is preparing to assess an obese patient who reports subjective symptoms and urinary patterns associated with BPH. Which technique does the nurse use to perform the physical assessment?
   a. Instruct the patient to undress from the waist down, then inspect and palpate the bladder.
   b. Have the patient drink several large glasses of water and percuss the bladder.
   c. Apply gentle pressure to the bladder to elicit urgency; then instruct the patient to void.
   d. Instruct the patient to void and then use the bedside ultrasound bladder scanner.

5. The nurse is interviewing a patient to determine the presence of lower urinary tract symptoms (LUTS) associated with BPH. Which questions would the nurse ask? *(Select all that apply.)*
   a. "Do you have difficulty starting and continuing urination?"
   b. "Have you ever had a kidney infection?"
   c. "Do you have reduced force and size of the urinary stream?"
   d. "Have you noticed postvoid dribbling or leaking?"
   e. "How many times do you have to get up during the night to urinate?"
   f. "Have you noticed blood at the start or at the end of voiding?"

6. The advanced-practice nurse is preparing to examine a patient's prostate gland. Before the exam, what does the nurse tell the patient?
   a. He may feel the urge to defecate or faint as the prostate is palpated.
   b. He should lie supine with knees bent in a fully flexed position.
   c. The examination is very painful, but it lasts just a few seconds.
   d. The gland will be massaged to obtain a fluid sample for possible prostatitis.

7. The nurse is reviewing the laboratory results from a patient being evaluated for LUTS. What does an elevated prostate-specific antigen (PSA) level and serum acid phosphatase level in this patient indicate?
   a. Infection
   b. Prostate cancer
   c. BPH
   d. Infertility

8. The nurse sees that the patient is taking tamsulosin (Flomax). Which question would the nurse ask to determine if the medication is achieving the desired therapeutic effect?
   a. "Are you having any trouble passing urine?"
   b. "Does your urine have a strong odor or appear cloudy?"
   c. "Are you having any problems with achieving an erection?"
   d. "Have you had problems with fatigue or feeling sleepy?"

9. Which assessment tool is commonly used to ask patients about the effect of urinary symptoms on their quality of life?
   a. American Urological Assessment Scale
   b. International Urological Assessment Tool
   c. American Prostate Symptom Tool
   d. International Prostate Symptom Score

10. A patient has an enlarged prostate. Which procedure does the nurse anticipate that the health care provider will order to test for bladder obstruction?
    a. Urodynamic pressure-flow study
    b. Bladder scan
    c. Transrectal ultrasound
    d. Computer tomography scan

11. The nurse is designing a teaching plan for a patient with an enlarged prostate and obstructive symptoms. What does the nurse teach the patient to avoid?
    a. Sexual intercourse
    b. Diuretics
    c. Straining to urinate
    d. Masturbation

12. Patients with which condition meet the criteria for a having a TURP? *(Select all that apply.)*
    a. Acute urinary retention
    b. Hydronephrosis
    c. Acute urinary tract infection
    d. Kidney stone
    e. Hematuria

13. A patient had a TURP and has a three-way urinary catheter taped to the left thigh. What does the nurse instruct about the position of the left leg?
    a. Maintain slight abduction.
    b. Maintain slight flexion of the hip.
    c. Keep the leg elevated.
    d. Keep the leg straight.

14. An older patient is scheduled for an annual physical including a PSA and a digital rectal examination (DRE). How are these two tests scheduled for the patient?
    a. PSA is drawn before the DRE is performed.
    b. DRE is done several weeks before the PSA.
    c. PSA is reviewed first because DRE may be unnecessary.
    d. Both tests can be done at the convenience of the patient.

15. An older adult patient had a TURP at 8:00 AM. At 3:00 PM, the nurse assesses the patient. Which finding does the nurse report to the health care provider?
    a. Patient reports a continuous urge to void.
    b. Patient keeps attempting to void around catheter.
    c. Patient wants to get out of bed.
    d. Patient keeps moving and ketchup-like output is noted.

16. The nurse notes bright-red blood with numerous clots in the urinary drainage bag for a patient who had a TURP. After notifying the surgeon, what does the nurse do next?
    a. Irrigate the catheter with normal saline per protocol.
    b. Remove the urinary catheter and save the tip for culture.
    c. Start an IV infusion and draw blood for type and cross.
    d. Empty the drainage bag and record the appearance of output.

17. The nurse is giving discharge instructions to a patient who had a TURP. What does the nurse include in the instructions?
    a. Reassurance that loss of control of urination or dribbling of urine is temporary
    b. Instructions about how to apply a condom catheter and monitor for skin breakdown
    c. Advice about how to control bleeding and passage of blood clots
    d. Information about the side effects related to aminocaproic acid (Amicar)

18. The nurse is giving instructions to the unlicensed assistive personnel (UAP) about hygienic care for an older adult patient who is uncircumcised. What does the nurse instruct the UAP to do?
    a. Defer cleaning the penis because of patient embarrassment.
    b. Replace the foreskin over the penis after bathing.
    c. Observe the penis and the foreskin for redness or odor.
    d. Avoid touching the foreskin because of hypersensitivity.

19. An older patient reports that he has an enlarged prostate with chronic urinary retention, but declines to seek treatment because "it's been that way for a long time." The nurse would encourage a follow-up appointment to prevent which complication of this chronic condition?
    a. Prostate cancer
    b. ED
    c. Hydronephrosis
    d. Testicular cancer

20. The patient had several diagnostic tests to evaluate report of LUTS. Which finding suggests that the patient may have kidney disease?
    a. Elevated white blood cell count
    b. Elevated serum creatinine
    c. Elevated red blood cell count
    d. Elevated prostate-specific antigen

21. The nurse is teaching a patient who is taking finasteride (Proscar), an 5-alpha reductase inhibitor (5-ARI). What medication side effects does the nurse include in the teaching? *(Select all that apply.)*
    a. Urinary incontinence
    b. ED
    c. Dizziness
    d. Headaches
    e. Decreased libido

22. The nurse notes that the patient has just started taking an alpha blocker medication to treat BPH. What instruction, related to the medication side effects, will the nurse give to the UAP who will assist the patient with activities of daily living (ADLs)?
    a. Frequently offer the patient the urinal.
    b. Have him sit up slowly and pause before standing.
    c. Remind the patient to drink plenty of extra fluids.
    d. Frequently check the linens for soiling and moisture.

23. The nurse hears in shift report that the patient had a transurethral needle ablation. Which question would the nurse ask the patient to determine if the procedure achieved the intended therapeutic goal?
    a. "Did the pain resolve completely after the procedure?"
    b. "Are you able to achieve and sustain an erection?"
    c. "Have your problems with urination been resolved?"
    d. "Have you had a PSA level to see if the cancer is in remission?"

24. A patient is undergoing large-volume bladder irrigation. During and after the procedure, the nurse observes the patient for confusion, muscle weakness, and increased gastrointestinal motility related to which potentially adverse effect of large-volume irrigation?
    a. Hyponatremia
    b. Hypovolemia
    c. Hypokalemia
    d. Hypotension

25. The patient has an indwelling catheter in place following a TURP. What instructions will the nurse give to the UAP with regards to the catheter?
    a. Secure the catheter so there is no tension.
    b. Irrigate the catheter to prevent clotting.
    c. Maintain traction on the catheter.
    d. Defer catheter care until the patient is discharged.

26. A patient needs surgical intervention for an enlarged prostate, but also needs to maintain his anticoagulant therapy. Which brochure would be the most appropriate to prepare for the patient?
    a. "Talking to Your Doctor About Holmium Laser Enucleation of the Prostate (Ho-LEP)"
    b. "Transurethral Resection of the Prostate (TURP), the Gold Standard Treatment"
    c. "Is Laparoscopic Radical Prostatectomy (LRP) with Robotic Assistance Right for You?"
    d. "Common Questions About the Open Surgical Technique for Radical Prostatectomy."

27. The patient has a continuous bladder irrigation via a three-way urinary catheter. At 7:00 AM, the urine drainage bag was emptied and 1000 mL of irrigation fluid was started. At 11:00 AM, 350 mL of irrigation fluid was administered through the catheter. The urinary drainage bag contains 600 mL. How many mL of urine has the patient produced in the past 4 hours?
    _____ mL

28. The nurse is caring for an older patient who had a urinary catheter inserted after a TURP. The patient is intermittently confused, and picks at the IV tubing and the catheter. What should the nurse try first?
    a. Obtain an order to restrain the patient's hands and forearms.
    b. Sedate the patient until the IV tube and catheter can be removed.
    c. Inform the family that a family member will have to sit by the patient.
    d. Give the patient a familiar object to hold, such as a family picture.

29. The patient had a TURP several days ago and the urinary catheter was removed 6 hours ago. Which sign/symptom must be resolved before the patient is discharged?
    a. Patient has not voided since the catheter was removed.
    b. Patient reports a burning sensation with urination.
    c. Patient reports dribbling and leakage since catheter was removed.
    d. Patient reports anxiety related to sexual function because of TURP.

30. Which man has the highest risk for prostate cancer?
    a. A 65-year-old Asian-American man with a history of BPH
    b. A 45-year-old Caucasian-American man who has several cousins with prostate cancer
    c. A 55-year-old Hispanic-American man who has poor dietary practices
    d. A 75-year-old African-American man whose brother had prostate cancer

31. The nurse is reviewing PSA results for a patient who had a prostatectomy for prostate cancer several weeks ago. The PSA level is 40 ng/mL. How does the nurse interpret this data?
    a. At this stage, PSA level of 40 ng/mL is expected.
    b. The cancer was completely removed.
    c. The cancer is most likely recurring.
    d. Prostate irritation and infection are present.

32. What are common serum tumor markers that confirm a diagnosis of testicular cancer? (Select all that apply.)
    a. Lactate dehydrogenase (LDH)
    b. Early prostate cancer antigen (EPCA-2)
    c. Glutathione S-transferase (GST P1)
    d. Alpha-fetoprotein (AFP)
    e. Beta human chorionic gonadotropin (hCG)

33. The nurse is reviewing the laboratory results for a patient with prostate cancer. Which laboratory result suggests metastasis to the bone?
    a. Decreased alpha fetoprotein
    b. Increased blood urea nitrogen
    c. Elevated serum alkaline phosphatase
    d. Decreased serum creatinine

34. A patient had a transrectal ultrasound with biopsy earlier in the day. What urine characteristics does the nurse expect to see?
    a. Light pink urine
    b. Bright red urine
    c. Dark urine with small clots
    d. Very pale yellow urine

35. The nurse is teaching a patient diagnosed with ED about the common treatments and therapies. Which topics does the nurse include? *(Select all that apply.)*
    a. Phosphodiesterace-5 (PDE-5) inhibitors
    b. Intraurethral applications
    c. Vacuum devices
    d. Active surveillance
    e. Penile implants

36. During the first 24 hours after prostatectomy, what is the priority assessment in the nursing care plan?
    a. Hemorrhage
    b. Infection
    c. Hydronephrosis
    d. Confusion

37. The nurse is talking to a 35-year-old African-American man about PSA testing. The patient tells the nurse that his father and an older brother were diagnosed with prostate cancer in their 50s. What should the nurse tell the patient?
    a. "Although authorities do not always agree, PSA testing usually starts at age 50."
    b. "Your genetic and racial risk factors suggest testing should begin at age 40."
    c. "Because of your African-American heritage, you should start testing at age 45."
    d. "PSA testing can be started at any time for all males at any age."

38. The nurse is teaching a patient at risk for prostate cancer about food sources of omega-3 fatty acids. Which food does the nurse suggest?
    a. Red meat
    b. Fish
    c. Watermelon
    d. Oatmeal

39. Which sign or symptom is associated with advanced prostate cancer?
    a. Difficulty starting urination
    b. Swollen groin lymph nodes
    c. Frequent bladder infections
    d. ED

40. What are common sites of metastasis for prostate cancer? *(Select all that apply.)*
    a. Pancreas
    b. Bones of the pelvis
    c. Liver
    d. Bones of the lower extremities
    e. Lungs

41. A patient had a transrectal ultrasound with biopsy. After this procedure, what does the nurse instruct the patient to do? *(Select all that apply.)*
    a. Report fever, chills, bloody urine, and any difficulty voiding.
    b. Avoid strenuous physical activity.
    c. Limit fluid intake for several hours after the procedure.
    d. Expect decreased urine output for 24 hours after the procedure.
    e. Expect some mild perineal and abdominal pain.

42. An older patient's wife is very upset because "my husband was just told that he had prostate cancer. He feels fine now, but the doctor told him to watch and wait. Why are we just watching? What are we watching for?" What is the nurse's best response?
    a. "Prostate cancer is slow-growing. Your husband needs regular DRE and PSA testing and here is a list of symptoms to watch for."
    b. "This is very upsetting news. Let's sit down and talk about how you feel and then I will have the doctor talk to you again."
    c. "It's okay, don't be upset. This is a very common way to handle prostate cancer for men who are your husband's age."
    d. "I can get you some information about prostate cancer. This will help you understand why the doctor said this to your husband."

43. The nurse is caring for a patient who had an open radical prostatectomy. During the assessment, the nurse notes that the penis and scrotum are swollen. What does the nurse do next?
    a. Notify the health care provider and monitor for an inability to void or increasing pain.
    b. Elevate the scrotum and penis; intermittently apply ice to the area for 24 to 48 hours.
    c. Assist the patient to increase mobility, especially early ambulation.
    d. Observe the urethral meatus for redness and discharge and monitor urine output.

44. The nurse is teaching a patient who had an open radical prostatectomy about how to manage the common potential long-term complications. What does the nurse teach the patient?
    a. How to perform testicular self-examination
    b. How to manage a permanent suprapubic catheter
    c. How to perform Kegel perineal exercises
    d. How to use dietary modifications to acidify the urine

45. A patient has undergone external beam radiation therapy (EBRT) for palliative treatment of prostate cancer. What suggestions does the nurse make to help the patient manage acute radiation cystitis secondary to EBRT?
    a. Limit intake of water and other fluids.
    b. Avoid consumption of caffeinated drinks.
    c. Increase consumption of dairy products.
    d. Wash genitals with mild soap and water.

46. A patient is receiving internal radiation therapy (brachytherapy) and has had a low-dose radiation seed implanted directly into the prostate gland. What nursing implication is related to this therapy?
    a. Ensure that any staff member or visitor who is pregnant is not exposed to the patient.
    b. Organize the nursing care so that exposure to the patient is limited to a few minutes.
    c. Instruct UAP that all urine specimens should be immediately discarded.
    d. Teach the patient that fatigue is common, but should pass after several months.

47. A patient is prescribed the luteinizing hormone–releasing hormone (LH-RH) agonist leuprolide (Lupron) for treatment of a prostate tumor. What possible side effect of this medication does the nurse advise the patient about?
    a. Nipple discharge
    b. Scrotal enlargement
    c. Fragility of the skin
    d. ED

48. A patient reports having uncomfortable and unsettling episodes of "hot flashes" after receiving hormonal therapy for a prostate tumor. To alleviate this symptom, which prescription medication does the nurse assist the patient in obtaining?
    a. Biphosphonate drug such as pamidronate (Aredia)
    b. Antiandrogen drug such as bicalutamide (Casodex)
    c. Hormonal inhibitor drug such as megestrol acetate (Megace)
    d. Antimuscarinic agents such as tolterodine (Detrol)

49. The nurse is teaching a patient about self-care following a radical prostatectomy. What does the nurse include in the health teaching? *(Select all that apply.)*
    a. Teach how to care for the indwelling catheter and manifestations of infection.
    b. Walk short distances.
    c. PSA blood tests are taken 12 weeks after surgery and then once a year.
    d. Maintain an upright position and do not walk bent or flexed.
    e. Shower rather than soak in a bathtub for the first 2 to 3 weeks.

50. A patient is diagnosed with prostatitis. Which intervention does the nurse use to alleviate the discomfort associated with this condition?
    a. Apply ice packs intermittently to reduce swelling.
    b. Restrict fluid intake, especially in the late evening.
    c. Assist with comfort measures such as sitz baths for pain.
    d. Suggest scrotal support during the day and elevating testes at night.

51. The patient is diagnosed with acute bacterial prostatitis. What assessment findings does the nurse expect to find? *(Select all that apply.)*
    a. Fever
    b. Chills
    c. Dysuria
    d. Urinary incontinence
    e. Urethral discharge

52. The patient is prescribed trimethoprim/sulfamethoxazole (Bactrim, Septra) for prostatitis. Which laboratory result indicates that the medication is having the desired therapeutic effect?
    a. Normalization of white cell count
    b. Decreased blood urea nitrogen level
    c. Increased red blood cell count
    d. Prostate-specific antigen within normal limits

53. The nurse is performing an assessment on a patient with organic ED. What are possible causes of this condition? *(Select all that apply.)*
    a. Medications for hypertension
    b. Obesity
    c. Thyroid disorders
    d. Diabetes mellitus
    e. Diverticulitis

54. A patient reports having ED and is seeking a prescription for sildenafil (Viagra). Because of the potential for dangerous drug-drug interactions, the nurse asks the patient specifically if he takes which type of drug?
    a. Nonsteroidal antiinflammatory drugs (NSAIDs)
    b. Nitrates
    c. Opioids
    d. Antilipemics

55. A patient who has testicular cancer is likely to have which common problem?
    a. Priapism
    b. ED
    c. Azoospermia
    d. Cryptorchidism

56. The advanced-practice nurse is performing a testicular exam on a young Caucasian male patient. The practitioner finds a lump, which the patient reports is painless. This finding is considered the most common manifestation of which disease or disorder?
    a. Testicular cancer
    b. ED
    c. Prostate cancer
    d. Epididymitis

57. A young patient has been diagnosed with testicular cancer. He and his wife had been trying to conceive a child for several months. What information does the nurse give the couple about sperm storage?
    a. Arrangements for sperm storage should be made as soon as possible after diagnosis.
    b. Sperm collection should be completed after radiation therapy or chemotherapy.
    c. Two or three samples should be collected 6 days apart.
    d. Saving sperm prevents fears related to ED.

58. The nurse is caring for a patient who had minimally invasive surgery (MIS) for testicular cancer. The nurse is also caring for a patient who had an open radical retroperitoneal lymph node dissection for testicular cancer. The nurse anticipates that the second patient has more of a risk for which condition?
    a. Paralytic ileus
    b. Urinary incontinence
    c. Metastatic disease
    d. Fluid overload

59. The nurse is teaching a patient who had an open retroperitoneal lymph node dissection. What instructions does the nurse give to the patient? *(Select all that apply.)*
    a. Do not lift anything over 45 lbs.
    b. Limit intake of fluids to 1000 mL per day.
    c. Do not drive a car for several weeks.
    d. Perform monthly testicular self-examination on the remaining testis.
    e. Have follow-up diagnostic testing for at least 3 years after the surgery.

60. The nurse is explaining the diagnosis of hydrocele to the patient. Which figure will the nurse select to help the patient understand the condition? _____

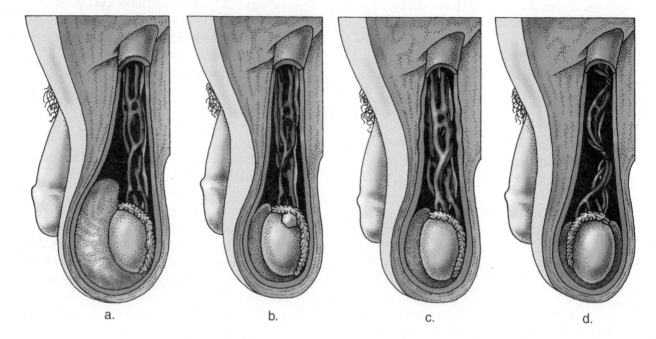

a.   b.   c.   d.

73 CHAPTER

Care of Transgender Patients

1. Which patient statement most accurately describes identifying oneself as transgender?
   a. "I enjoy wearing women's clothes. Women's fashions are pretty and interesting."
   b. "I think men are more powerful and influential, so I would rather be viewed as male."
   c. "Since childhood, I have always felt like I was born into the wrong body."
   d. "I have always been sexually attracted to other males and other men often reciprocate."

2. According to the American Psychiatric Association, which circumstance best describes gender identity?
   a. At birth, midwife informs parents that they have a healthy baby girl.
   b. Biologically, the person has obvious male sexual organs.
   c. The person takes on the social roles of mother, wife, and sister.
   d. Family, friends, and others treat the child as a little boy.

3. The nurse reads in the patient's medical record that the patient has gender dysphoria. Which question is the nurse most likely to first ask the patient?
   a. "Are you seeking interventions for sex reassignment?"
   b. "How do you prefer to be addressed?"
   c. "Do you think of yourself as female or male?"
   d. "What issues of sexuality would you like to discuss?"

4. A male patient with gender dysphoria confides in the nurse that he notices that his 4-year-old son shows a preference for playing with dolls and other traditional girls' toys. What is the nurse's best response?
   a. "Let him choose his own toys and he will be happier."
   b. "It's normal for children to explore different gender behaviors."
   c. "When you see him playing with dolls, how does that make you feel?"
   d. "Did you play with dolls and other girls' toys when you were a child?"

5. The nursing student is writing a report about caring for a 56-year-old patient with diabetes mellitus who identified himself as transgender. Which sentence reflects proper use of terminology?
   a. "Today, I learned how to properly care for a transvestite who has diabetes."
   b. "I developed a therapeutic relationship with a 56-year-old tranny with diabetes."
   c. "A 56-year-old transgender had complications related to his diabetes."
   d. "A 56-year-old transgender patient was admitted for complications due to diabetes."

6. Which comment from a family member would be most strongly associated with the term "natal sex"?
   a. "My little girl likes to play with her brother's toys and she admires her brother."
   b. "My brother just called me. His wife delivered a healthy baby girl this morning."
   c. "My brother seems a bit effeminate, but I wouldn't call him transgender."
   d. "My sister is unsure if she is sexually attracted to men or to women."

7. The acronym LGBTQ—(lesbian, gay, bisexual, transgender, and queer/questioning) is used to describe a group of people of minority sexual and gender identities under one population category. Which of these terms refer specifically to sexual orientation? *(Select all that apply.)*
   a. Lesbian
   b. Gay
   c. Bisexual
   d. Transgender
   e. Queer/questioning

8. A patient identifies self as genderqueer. How does the nurse interpret this?
   a. Patient's significant other will be the same gender.
   b. Patient prefers to have male sexual partners.
   c. Patient's gender identity does not conform to male or female.
   d. Patient identifies self as female, but natal sex is identified as male.

9. A transwoman patient of color comes to the clinic for treatment because she was physically assaulted and beaten. As the nurse begins the interview, the patient becomes angry and defensive and accuses the nurse of discrimination. How does the nurse interpret the patient's behavior?
   a. Recognizes that own verbal and/or non-verbal behavior has offend the patient.
   b. Suspects that the patient is likely to be unstable because of gender dysphoria.
   c. Realizes that the patient is reacting to bias-related violence and emotional distress.
   d. Acknowledges a personal lack of understanding of transgender issues.

10. The nurse is interviewing a transgender patient who reports depression related to continuous verbal harassment, threats, and intimidation. Which patient statement is the greatest concern for failure to cope with stressors?
    a. "I smoke three packs of cigarettes every day."
    b. "I have tried to commit suicide several times."
    c. "When I get really down, I drink and use recreational drugs."
    d. "Last night I went to a bar and picked up a stranger for sex."

11. The nurse is assisting a health care provider perform a genital examination on a transgender patient. During the exam, the provider is respectful and professional towards the patient. Later, the nurse hears the provider making jokes within earshot of the patient. What should the nurse do first?
    a. Apologize to the patient and reassure that the provider is caring and trustworthy.
    b. Report the provider to the appropriate licensing board for discipline.
    c. Take the provider aside and inform him that the patient heard what was said.
    d. Remind the provider about ethical responsibilities to treat patients with dignity.

12. In caring for transgender patients, under which circumstance would the nurse make a clinical judgment and decide to forego extensive questioning about gender identity?
    a. Needs treatment for a sprained ankle sustained during a soccer game
    b. Has recurrent urinary tract infections despite medication compliance
    c. Appears to be a male, but requests a pelvic examination by a female provider
    d. Is dressed as a man and wants information about hormones that feminize the body

13. The nurse sees that John Smith, natal sex: male, needs insertion of an indwelling urinary catheter for hourly measurements of urine output. However, when the nurse enters the room, the patient appears to be female. What should the nurse do first?
    a. Introduce self, verify patient's identity by checking name band, and explain the procedure for catheterization.
    b. Inspect the genitalia and adapt catheter insertion as appropriate while avoiding use of gender-specific language.
    c. Respectfully address the patient as Mr. Smith, and perform catheter insertion for a male patient.
    d. Politely excuse self and obtain advice from the charge nurse about whether to treat the patient as a male or a female.

14. The nurse is working in an inner-city clinic that serves a diverse population. While all patients are apt to ask for directions to restrooms, the staff is continuously debating about how to direct LGBTQ patients to public restrooms. What should the nursing staff do?
    a. Agree to give general directions to both male and female restrooms to everyone.
    b. Ask administration to post more signs so that directions to restrooms are explicit.
    c. Advocate for creation of designated unisex or single-stall restrooms.
    d. Directly ask patients if they would like directions to the male or female restrooms.

15. A new nurse has been conscientious about asking all transgender patients about preferred use of pronouns and names, but inadvertently makes an error while caring for a patient. What should the new nurse do?
    a. Apologize and explain that working with transgender patients is a new experience.
    b. Assume that the patient is used to this type of error and continue care.
    c. Watch the patient's nonverbal behavior to gauge if the error was noticed.
    d. Self-correct and continue with care rather than making a prolonged apology.

16. The nurse is taking a health history and inquiring about any interventions that the patient has had for gender reassignment. Which questions would the nurse include? *(Select all that apply.)*
    a. "Have you made any changes in gender expression, such as clothes or hairstyle?"
    b. "Have you ever had psychotherapy for body image or to strengthen coping mechanisms?"
    c. "Are you currently taking any hormonal therapy to feminize or masculinize your body?"
    d. "How have your parents and other people responded to changes in your appearance?"
    e. "Have you had or considered having surgery to change sexual characteristics?"

17. For a patient who is taking estrogen therapy, which vital sign is most important to assess for the detection of a health risk that can be caused by this therapy?
    a. Temperature
    b. Pulse
    c. Respiration
    d. Blood pressure

18. The nurse is caring for an older transgender adult who transitioned years ago from male to female (MtF). Which question is the nurse most likely to ask?
    a. "Have you had any hot flashes or vaginal dryness?"
    b. "Do you experience urinary retention or dribbling?"
    c. "How old were you when you went through menopause?"
    d. "Did you have any problems after your hysterectomy?"

19. The nurse must insert a urinary catheter in a transgender patient who is in early transition from female to male (FtM). The patient appears to be a male and identifies self as male. Why would the nurse assess the genitalia prior to opening the sterile catheter kit?
    a. The nurse would expect to see a larger-than-average–sized male penis which may require a larger catheter.
    b. The presence of hormonal-enhanced clitoral tissue makes catheterization very difficult and a smaller catheter may be needed.
    c. Genitals may not match physical appearance, so technique and equipment must be modified accordingly.
    d. There is a high risk for necrosis of the neopenis, which should be reported to the provider before catheterization.

20. According to the World Professional Association for Transgender Health, which patient(s) would not meet the criteria for hormone therapy? *(Select all that apply.)*
    a. A 16-year-old who has had gender dysphoria since early childhood.
    b. A 35-year-old lesbian with history of suicide attempts.
    c. A 62-year-old with known gender dysphoria who has symptoms of dementia.
    d. A 30-year-old with gender dysphoria and no physical or mental health problems.
    e. A 22-year-old who has bisexual relationships, but calls self queer/questioning.

21. A patient is considering estrogen therapy for MtF transition. What is an expected physical change that will occur with this therapy?
    a. Weight loss
    b. Thicker, longer hair
    c. Decreased testicular size
    d. Feminization of vocalization

22. A patient is taking estrogen therapy. Which patient report is cause for greatest concern?
    a. Breast tenderness
    b. Tenderness and swelling in the calf
    c. Nausea with vomiting
    d. Decreased erectile function

23. The nurse sees that in addition to estrogen therapy, the patient is also taking spironolactone (Aldactone). Which laboratory result will the nurse assess to ensure the patient does not suffer adverse effects due to the medication?
    a. Blood glucose level
    b. White blood cell count
    c. Serum potassium level
    d. Platelet count

24. The FtM patient reports that he has been taking testosterone therapy. What is an indication that the medication is having the desired effect?
    a. Patient reports a decreased libido.
    b. Nurse observes increased body hair.
    c. Nurse observes average male penis.
    d. Patient reports breast tenderness.

25. The nurse is doing the preoperative care for an MtF patient who will undergo a vaginoplasty. What is included in the care for this patient? *(Select all that apply.)*
    a. Administer a Fleet enema and laxatives as ordered.
    b. Give nothing by mouth (NPO) for 24 hours prior to surgery.
    c. Monitor and report hemoglobin and hematocrit results.
    d. Administer preoperative antimicrobials to minimize infection.
    e. Monitor and record the drainage from Jackson-Pratt drain.

26. The nurse is providing the first 12 hours of postoperative care for a MtF patient who underwent a vaginoplasty with epidural anesthesia. What is an expected assessment finding?
    a. Patient is unable to move legs.
    b. The pedal pulses are diminished.
    c. Feet and ankles are cold to the touch.
    d. Patient has a decreased level of conscientiousness.

27. Which patient report indicates that the patient is experiencing the most serious complication of vaginoplasty?
    a. Reports burning sensation during urination
    b. Reports leakage of stool from the vagina
    c. Reports urinary incontinence when sneezing
    d. Reports tenderness and bruising on labia

28. A FtM patient is seeking information about sex reassignment surgery. Which reconstructive surgery is the most difficult and the least likely to yield patient satisfaction?
    a. Bilateral mastectomy
    b. Hysterectomy and bilateral salpingo-oophorectomy
    c. Pectoral muscle implants
    d. Phalloplasty

Care of Patients with Sexually Transmitted Disease

1. What is the first symptom of primary syphilis?
   a. Small painless, indurated, smooth, weeping lesion
   b. Urinary frequency, burning incontinence, and dribbling
   c. Malaise, low-grade fever, and general muscular aches and pains
   d. Rash that changes from papules to squamous papules to pustules

2. A patient phones the clinic because of a one-time exposure to syphilis that occurred about 6 weeks ago. He reports being asymptomatic and abstinent since the incident. What is the nurse's best response?
   a. "The first sign is a chancre which will usually develop by the third week."
   b. "Continue abstinence for up to 90 days and observe the genitalia for painless sores."
   c. "Use a latex or polyurethane condom for genital and anal intercourse."
   d. "The chancre can appear and then disappear, so you must come in for testing."

3. A patient is admitted for emergency surgery after an accident. In addition, the patient has a pustular rash related to secondary syphilis. What instructions does the nurse give to the unlicensed assistive personnel (UAP)?
   a. Gloves should be worn at all times when touching the patient.
   b. The lesions are highly contagious, so the patient should do own hygienic care.
   c. No instructions are given to the UAP because patient confidentiality is essential.
   d. If the skin is open and draining pus or fluid, use gloves during patient care.

4. A patient is diagnosed with primary syphilis. The nurse prepares to administer and educate the patient about which treatment regimen?
   a. Benzathine penicillin G given intramuscularly as a single 2.4 million unit dose, and follow-up evaluation at 6, 12, and 24 months
   b. Benzathine penicillin G given intramuscularly for 7 days, and follow-up evaluation at 6, 12, and 24 months
   c. Ceftriaxone (Rocephin) 125 mg intramuscularly in a single dose, plus azithromycin (Zithromax) 1 g orally in a single dose, and follow-up evaluation at 6, 12, and 24 months
   d. Metronidazole (Flagyl) 500 mg orally twice daily for 14 days, and follow-up evaluation at 6, 12, and 24 months

5. A patient has no reaction to a penicillin skin test, so the health care provider orders benzathine penicillin G intramuscularly. What does the nurse do immediately after the injection?
   a. Ask the patient to give contact information for all sexual partners.
   b. Instruct the patient to go home to rest for 2 to 4 hours.
   c. Observe the patient for 2 hours to detect any allergic reaction.
   d. Observe the patient for at least 30 minutes to detect any allergic reaction.

6. The health care provider tells the nurse that a patient has Jarisch-Herxheimer reaction. Which interventions does the nurse anticipate?
   a. Oxygen, epinephrine, and antihistamines
   b. Emergency IV fluid resuscitation
   c. Analgesics and antipyretics
   d. Monitoring for symptom resolution

7. A patient is diagnosed with late tertiary syphilis. In addition to benign lesions of the skin and mucous membranes, what other findings does the nurse expect to see documented in the patient's record?
   a. Chronic renal failure
   b. Arthritis and arthralgias
   c. Cardiovascular syphilis
   d. Contagious chancroid lesions

8. A patient is diagnosed with early latent syphilis. Which assessment will the nurse make related to the medication that is likely to be prescribed for the patient?
   a. Assess for allergies to penicillin.
   b. Check results of coagulation studies.
   c. Assess for history of noncompliance.
   d. Ask if the patient takes nitrates.

9. A patient reports a possible exposure to syphilis. Which screening tests are typically done first?
   a. Serology testing, such as glycoprotein G antibody-based, to identify either type 1 or 2
   b. Venereal Disease Research Laboratory (VDRL) serum test and the more sensitive rapid plasma reagin (RPR)
   c. Fluorescent treponemal antibody absorption (FTA-ABS) test or the microhemagglutination assay for *T. pallidum* (MHA-TP)
   d. Viral cell culture or polymerase chain reaction (PCR) assays of the lesions

10. Which sexually transmitted diseases (STDs) are reportable to the local health authorities in every state? *(Select all that apply.)*
    a. Chlamydia
    b. Genital herpes
    c. Gonorrhea
    d. Syphilis
    e. Chancroid
    f. Human immunodeficiency virus (HIV)

11. What is the causative organism of syphilis?
    a. *Neisseria gonorrhoeae*
    b. *Chlamydia trachomatis*
    c. *Treponema pallidum*
    d. Cytomegalovirus

12. What sexually transmitted organisms are most often responsible for pelvic inflammatory disease (PID)?
    a. *Chlamydia trachomatis* and *Neisseria gonorrhoeae*
    b. Herpes simplex virus and *Escherichia coli*
    c. *Haemophilus influenzae* and staphylococcus
    d. *Treponema pallidum* and *Gardnerella vaginalis*

13. What are the goals of the medication therapy used for treating genital herpes? *(Select all that apply.)*
    a. Reduce symptoms
    b. Reduce the risk of transmission
    c. Reduce discomfort
    d. Prevent recurrence
    e. Cure

14. Based on evidence from the U.S. Preventive Task Force, which teaching strategy is most likely to yield a change in individual sexual behavior?
    a. Annual community presentation about risks factors for STDs
    b. Review of personal behaviors during annual Pap testing
    c. Frequent high-intensity education and counseling
    d. Ready access to STD statistics via Internet or email

15. The nurse is teaching a patient being discharged after treatment for genital herpes. Which patient statement indicates a need for further teaching?
    a. "I can be contagious even when I do not have any lesions."
    b. "If I get pregnant, I need to tell my nurse midwife that I have genital herpes."
    c. "After taking acyclovir (Zovirax), I will never have to worry about exposing my partner."
    d. "I need an annual Pap smear because of my increased risk for cervical cancer."

16. A female patient is prescribed azithromycin (Zithromax) 1 g orally in a single dose for the treatment of *Chlamydia trachomatis*. What additional information does the nurse give the patient about treatment issues?
    a. Abstinence from sex is required until 7 days from the date of treatment.
    b. Even with treatment, there is a risk for meningitis and endocarditis.
    c. There is no need for rescreening unless there is a new exposure.
    d. Watch for and report headache, malaise, arthralgia, and anorexia.

17. Why do women develop complications more often than men when being treated for gonorrhea?
    a. Treatment for the disease can leave women infertile.
    b. Men are more likely to have symptoms and will seek curative treatment.
    c. Estrogen leaves the woman more resistant to antibiotic therapy.
    d. The disease is much more difficult to cure in women.

18. The patient tells the nurse that he had unprotected sexual intercourse 1 week ago and just found out that the person might have gonorrhea. The patient reports that he has been watching for symptoms, but has not noticed anything, so he is hoping that he is okay. What is the nurse's best response?
    a. "Symptoms usually develop in 3 to 10 days, but you should be tested even if there are no symptoms."
    b. "Abstain from sex for 7 more days, then come in for testing. Meanwhile, watch for symptoms."
    c. "If you are not having any symptoms after one week, it is unlikely that you were infected."
    d. "We can give you a prescription for antibiotics, but you must avoid sex for 2 to 3 months."

19. The nurse is performing a history and physical on the male patient who suspects exposure to an STD. Which symptom is the most common in the male with chlamydia?
    a. Painful intercourse
    b. Urethritis
    c. Dark yellow urine
    d. Thick, green discharge

20. When obtaining a complete obstetric-gynecologic history, the nurse also takes a sexual history from the patient. Which approach is the most therapeutic to elicit information from the patient?
    a. Use a checklist to ask "yes" and "no" questions.
    b. Ask the patient to detail her sexual history.
    c. Ask directly if the patient has ever had an STD.
    d. Ask open-ended questions.

21. For the nurse to be an effective clinician when working with patients who have issues with sexuality, STDs, or other sexual concerns, what must the nurse do first?
    a. Take a course on sexual relations and counseling.
    b. Know all about his or her patient's concerns, problems, or needs.
    c. Be aware of his or her own sexual values, attitudes, and sexuality.
    d. Set up a meeting with the patient's sexual partner.

22. A female patient reporting a troublesome vaginal discharge is diagnosed with trichomoniasis and is given medication to treat the infection. What does the nurse teach the patient about the diagnosis?
    a. *Trichomonas vaginalis* is self-limiting, but medicine is needed to treat the vaginal itching.
    b. The patient's sexual partner must be treated if the problem is to be resolved.
    c. The medication should be applied liberally to the external genitalia once a day.
    d. The vaginal infection can cause infertility in childbearing women.

23. Women with PID are at an increased risk for which condition?
    a. Amenorrhea
    b. Appendicitis
    c. Infertility
    d. Cardiac disease

24. What is the most common chief complaint that leads a patient with PID to seek medical health care?
    a. Vaginal itching
    b. Lower abdominal pain
    c. Malaise with fever
    d. Abnormal menstrual flow

25. A patient with PID is on bedrest with bathroom privileges. What position is best for the patient while on bedrest?
    a. Prone
    b. Supine
    c. Side-lying
    d. Semi-Fowler's

26. A patient with PID is discharged home on oral antibiotics. What are the important measures for the nurse to include in patient teaching? *(Select all that apply.)*
    a. "Douche 3 times a week to aid healing."
    b. "Report an increase in temperature right away."
    c. "Continue taking the antibiotics until the medication is gone."
    d. "Do not have intercourse until after the follow-up appointment."
    e. "Take antacids if the antibiotics upset your stomach."

27. When performing discharge teaching about resuming sexual relations to a female patient diagnosed with an STD, what does the nurse teach the patient?
    a. Douche within 24 hours after vaginal intercourse.
    b. Sexual relations are prohibited for 3 months.
    c. Intercourse should be postponed until the treatment regimen is completed.
    d. Intercourse is permitted unless there is an increase in abdominal pain.

28. What does the nurse tell a patient with PID about the practice of vaginal douching?
    a. It increases a woman's risk for developing PID.
    b. It should be done daily to reduce vaginal secretions.
    c. Vinegar is the only safe solution to use.
    d. Use only disposable equipment.

29. Which infection describes an STD that is limited to the vagina, is very irritating, but has no long-term sequelae?
    a. Chlamydia
    b. Herpes simplex type 2
    c. Candida
    d. Granuloma inguinale

30. A patient with human papillomavirus will commonly develop which disease?
    a. Human immunodeficiency virus
    b. Genital warts
    c. Granuloma inguinale
    d. Chancroid

31. The nurse is preparing an information packet about women's health considerations for STDs. What information does the nurse include? *(Select all that apply.)*
    a. Young women generally have excellent knowledge about the risk of STDs.
    b. Young women frequently believe that they are vulnerable to STDs.
    c. Young women mistakenly believe that contraceptives protect them from STDs.
    d. Mucosal tears in postmenopausal women may also place them at greater risk for STDs.
    e. Women have more asymptomatic infections that may delay diagnosis and treatment.

32. A young female patient requires hospitalization for a severe case of genital herpes. What information is given to the patient regarding the long-term consequences?
    a. There is an increased risk of central nervous system complications.
    b. There is a risk of neonatal transmission and an increased risk for acquiring HIV infection.
    c. There is an increased risk for scars and adhesions of the fallopian tubes.
    d. There is an increased risk for multiple types of reproductive cancers at a young age.

33. The nurse is counseling a patient who is experiencing recurrent outbreaks of genital herpes. What suggestions for symptomatic treatment does the nurse include?
    a. Oral analgesics, sitz baths, and increased oral fluid intake
    b. Topical anesthetics, nutritional therapy, and warm compresses
    c. Abstinence, frequent bathing, and fluid restriction
    d. Bedrest and application of podofilox (Condylox) 0.5% solution

34. A patient is diagnosed with *Condylomata acuminata*. What are the desired outcomes of management for this patient?
    a. Reduce pain and prevent recurrence
    b. Prevent long-term complications to the cardiac system
    c. Remove the warts and treat the symptoms
    d. Prevent infertility and systemic infection

35. A patient requires treatment for genital warts. Which treatment is done by the patient at home if given the proper instructions?
    a. Imiquimod (Aldara) 5% cream
    b. Cryotherapy with liquid nitrogen
    c. Podophyllin resin 10% in a compound of tincture of benzoin
    d. Trichloroacetic acid (TCA) or bichloroacetic acid (BCA)

36. What is the incubation period for genital warts?
    a. 3 to 7 days
    b. 2 to 20 days
    c. 10 to 90 days
    d. 2 to 3 months

37. A patient has had podophyllin treatment for *Condylomata acuminata*. For which sign/symptom does the nurse tell the patient to return for further treatment?
    a. Discomfort at the site
    b. Bleeding from the site
    c. Infection at the site
    d. Sloughing of parts of warts

38. A male patient reports that a female sexual partner just told him that she was treated for gonorrhea. What symptoms does the nurse ask him about, because they are the most likely to occur with gonorrhea in a male?
    a. Small, painless lump that occurred on the penis, but spontaneously disappeared
    b. Numerous small, painless, papillary growths in the genital area
    c. Painful intercourse because of scrotal swelling and epididymitis
    d. Dysuria and a profuse yellowish green or scant clear penile discharge

39. A patient is being treated for gonorrhea. The nurse would question the use of which medication for this patient?
    a. Ceftriaxone (Rocephin)
    b. Benzathine penicillin (Bicillin LA)
    c. Azithromycin (Zithromax)
    d. Ciprofloxacin (Cipro)

40. A female patient is tested for and diagnosed with gonorrhea. The nurse advocates that the choice of drug therapy include medications that concurrently treat which condition?
    a. Genital herpes
    b. Chlamydia
    c. Syphilis
    d. Genital warts

41. A young woman discovers she has chlamydia after going to her health care provider for a routine Pap smear and pelvic exam. She is reluctant to accept the diagnosis, because she is asymptomatic and "does not have any money for unnecessary treatment right now." What is the nurse's best response?
    a. Explain that there is a single-dose of medication which has a one-time cost.
    b. Talk to the woman about her financial situation and help her find resources.
    c. Encourage the patient to express her reluctance and disbelief.
    d. Tell her that it is possible to have chlamydia without having any symptoms.

42. A patient with an STD freely admits to being a commercial sex worker. In talking to this patient, the nurse recognizes that she has not disclosed a true name, address, or partner contact information. What is the best treatment strategy to use with this patient?
    a. Reassure her that all health data are confidential and will be handled with discretion.
    b. Spend extra time with the patient to elicit trust so that she will give correct information.
    c. Administer a one-dose course of treatment and dispense a box of condoms.
    d. Give her all medications for a 7-day treatment and convey a nonjudgmental attitude.

43. Which factors increase the risk for PID? *(Select all that apply.)*
    a. Age younger than 26 years
    b. Multiple sexual partners
    c. Smoking
    d. Caffeine use
    e. History of chlamydia or gonococcal infection
    f. History of gastrointestinal infections

44. A young female patient with a history of previous STDs has a hunched-over gait and has difficulty getting on the examination table. On observing this behavior, what does the nurse first assess for?
    a. Lower abdominal pain
    b. Lower back pain
    c. Musculoskeletal weakness
    d. Vaginal bleeding

45. The nurse is reviewing laboratory results for a patient with PID. Which lab results does the nurse expect to see? *(Select all that apply.)*
    a. Elevation in white blood cell (WBC) count
    b. Elevation in erythrocyte sedimentation rate (ESR)
    c. Decreased level of C-reactive protein
    d. Presence of human chorionic gonadotropin (hCG) in urine
    e. Presence of more than 10 WBCs per high-power field for vaginal discharge

46. In the emergency department, a patient is diagnosed with PID and there is an order to discharge the patient home with a prescription for antibiotics. What circumstance causes the nurse to question the order for discharge to home?
    a. The patient is several months postpartum, but had very mild symptoms.
    b. The patient is nauseated, but able to tolerate small amounts of oral fluids.
    c. The patient is pregnant, but willing to attempt self-care if properly instructed.
    d. The patient is afraid to go home, but the sister and husband are available to help.

47. The nurse is caring for a patient admitted for PID. Which task does the nurse delegate to the UAP?
    a. Apply a heating pad to the lower abdomen or back.
    b. Place the patient in semi-Fowler's position.
    c. Ask the patient if the pain is a 2 to 3 on a pain scale of 0 to 10.
    d. Report to the nurse if the patient is anxious about infertility.

48. A patient reports an itching or tingling sensation felt in the skin 1 to 2 days followed by a blister on the penis which ruptured spontaneously with painful erosion. These symptoms are consistent with which condition?
    a. Syphilis
    b. Genital warts
    c. Genital herpes
    d. Gonorrhea

49. The nurse is teaching a group of high-school students about the use of condoms. What information does the nurse include? *(Select all that apply.)*
    a. Use spermicide (nonoxynol-9) with condoms.
    b. Female condoms are too difficult to use for inexperienced partners.
    c. Keep condoms (especially latex) in a cool, dry place out of direct sunlight.
    d. Do not use condoms that are in damaged packages or that are brittle or discolored.
    e. Put condoms on the penis before foreplay or arousal.
    f. If you use a lubricant, make sure that the lubricant is water-based.

50. Which STD is associated with an increased risk for cervical cancer?
    a. Syphilis
    b. *Condylomata acuminata*: HPV type 16
    c. *Condylomata acuminata*: HPV type 6
    d. PID

51. Which group has the greatest risk for contracting primary and secondary syphilis?
    a. Adolescent boys
    b. Postmenopausal women
    c. Women who have sex with women
    d. Men who have sex with men

52. The nurse has just finished teaching an 18-year-old male patient about STDs and safe sex practices. Which patient statement most indicates that the patient will succeed in making a behavior change?
    a. "I don't intend to have sex anymore until I get married."
    b. "You have given me a lot to think about. I know I am taking risks."
    c. "I am going directly to the pharmacy and buy a supply of condoms."
    d. "Wearing gloves during foreplay seems weird, but I guess I could try it."

53. Which patient circumstance is most appropriate for expedited partner treatment (EPT)?
    a. Partner is afraid to come to health care facility.
    b. Partners are clients of a commercial sex worker.
    c. Patient and partner are both HIV-positive.
    d. Patient and partner have multiple other partners.

54. The nurse sees that the patient was prescribed valacyclovir (Valtrex). Which patient statement indicates that the goal of therapy is being met?
    a. "The rash is still present, but I hardly notice it."
    b. "Pain in my joints is much less than before treatment."
    c. "Abdominal pain is no longer interfering with movement."
    d. "The sores are not as painful as they were before."

55. How should the nurse respond to a patient with altered sexuality as a result of STD? *(Select all that apply.)*
    a. Report and document all findings.
    b. Provide pain control measures.
    c. Teach about prescribed antibiotic or antiviral therapy.
    d. Emphasize avoidance of sexual intercourse.
    e. Emphasize importance of treating all sexual partners.

56. In performing a genital exam on a teen-
     age patient, the examiner sees multiple large
     cauliflower-like growths in the perineal area.
     The patient reports these appeared about 3
     months after her first sexual experience. What
     does the examiner suspect?
     a. *Condylomata acuminata*
     b. Genital herpes
     c. Salpingitis
     d. Gonorrhea

Answer Key

CHAPTER 1

1. d
2. b
3. a, b, c, f
4. a, b, c, e
5. b
6. d
7. b
8. b
9. a, b, d, e
10. c
11. a
12. c
13. a, c, d, e
14. c

CHAPTER 2

1. a, b, c, d
2. a, b, d, e
3. a, c, d, e, g
4. c
5. a, d, e, f
6. b, c, e
7. a, c, d, e
8. a, d
9. a
10. a, b, c, e
11. b, c, d
12. a, e
13. a, b, e
14. c
15. a, c, d
16. b
17. a
18. c
19. a, d, e
20. a, b, c, e

CHAPTER 3

1. b
2. a, b, c, d, e
3. c
4. b
5. c
6. c
7. d
8. a
9. a
10. c
11. d
12. a
13. c
14. b
15. a
16. c
17. b
18. d
19. a, b
20. b
21. d
22. a
23. b
24. a, c
25. d
26. d
27. a, b, e
28. b
29. c
30. a
31. b
32. a, b, c, d
33. c
34. a
35. c, e
36. d
37. b
38. c
39. b, c, e
40. d
41. c, e
42. d
43. b
44. a
45. b
46. c
47. d
48. a
49. a, c, d, e
50. b
51. d
52. a
53. c
54. d
55. b
56. c
57. c
58. b
59. b
60. d

CHAPTER 4

1. a
2. d
3. a, c, d
4. a, c, e, f
5. d
6. c
7. a
8. b
9. a, c, d
10. d
11. b, c, d
12. d
13. b
14. c
15. a
16. b
17. b
18. a, c, d

CHAPTER 5

1. c
2. a, b, c, d
3. a, b, c, e
4. c
5. b
6. c
7. a, b, d, e
8. c
9. a, b, e

CHAPTER 6

1. d
2. c
3. a, b, c, e
4. d
5. c
6. a, c, d, e
7. a, b, d, e
8. a
9. a
10. d
11. a
12. a, c, d, e
13. a, c, d, e, f
14. a, c, d
15. a
16. b
17. c
18. d
19. a, b, c, e
20. a
21. a, b, c, e
22. c
23. c
24. b
25. b
26. c
27. a, b, c
28. c
29. d
30. a, b
31. a
32. c
33. a
34. a, c, e
35. c
36. c

CHAPTER 7

1. b, c, d
2. c
3. d
4. c
5. c
6. a, c, d, e
7. b, c, e
8. c, e, f
9. c
10. a
11. a, b, d
12. d
13. b, c, d, e
14. b

15. a
16. c
17. c
18. a, c, e
19. a, c
20. d
21. a, b, d, e

CHAPTER 8

1. b
2. a, b, d, e, f
3. c
4. b
5. d
6. b
7. d
8. b, d, e
9. d
10. d
11. b, c, e
12. c
13. a, c, e, f
14. b, c, e
15. c
16. b, c, e
17. c
18. a
19. c
20. c
21. d
22. b
23. a
24. b
25. a
26. b
27. b
28. a
29. a
30. c
31. b, c
32. b
33. d
34. b
35. b
36. a. 2; b. 1; c. 3; d. 4
37. d
38. c
39. b
40. d
41. a. 3; b. 2; c. 1; d. 4; e. 5
42. c
43. b
44. a
45. c
46. d
47. b
48. b
49. a
50. c
51. c

52. d
53. c
54. a
55. c
56. b

CHAPTER 9

1. a, b, c, e, f
2. b, d, e
3. c
4. c, d, e
5. b
6. c
7. c
8. a
9. d
10. b, c, e
11. a
12. b, c
13. a, c, d, e
14. c
15. c
16. c
17. a
18. a, c, d
19. a
20. d
21. b
22. a
23. c
24. c
25. c
26. c
27. c
28. c
29. c
30. a
31. a, c, d, e
32. b
33. b, c, d, a
34. a
35. d
36. a, b, e
37. c
38. b
39. c
40. a
41. c, d, e
42. c
43. b
44. a
45. b, d, e
46. c
47. b
48. c
49. a, c, d
50. b
51. c
52. b
53. c

54. d
55. c
56. d
57. a, c, d, e, f
58. c
59. c
60. b, c, d
61. a, b, e
62. a, b, d, e
63. a
64. a
65. c
66. a, b, e
67. b
68. b, d, e, f
69. a
70. b
71. d
72. b
73. b
74. a
75. a, b, e
76. b, d
77. b
78. c
79. d
80. c, e
81. b, e, c, a, d
82. b
83. c
84. c
85. a
86. b
87. a, b, d
88. a, b, c, e
89. a, b, d, e
90. a, b, d, e

CHAPTER 10

1. d
2. a
3. c
4. b
5. a, c, d, f
6. b
7. d
8. c
9. c
10. a
11. a
12. a, c, d, e
13. c
14. d
15. c
16. a
17. a
18. a
19. d, e
20. d
21. a, c, d

22. a, c, e
23. a
24. c
25. b
26. a
27. b
28. c
29. c
30. d
31. c
32. d
33. c, e
34. d
35. b

CHAPTER 11

1. a, b, d, f, h
2. b
3. b
4. d
5. a, d, e
6. b
7. a, b, c, e, f
8. a
9. d
10. b, c, e
11. c
12. a
13. a
14. c
15. b
16. d
17. c
18. c
19. b
20. a
21. c
22. b
23. b, d, e
24. b, c, d
25. a, d, e
26. b, d, e
27. b, c, e
28. c
29. a
30. a, d, e
31. b, d, e
32. a, c, d, f
33. d
34. c
35. c, d, e
36. a
37. a
38. d
39. a
40. b
41. a, e
42. d
43. b, e
44. c

45. a
46. a, b, d
47. a, d, f
48. b
49. b, c, d
50. d
51. b, c, e
52. a
53. d
54. d
55. a, c, e
56. b
57. a
58. b
59. b
60. d
61. b, c, d
62. a, c, d
63. b
64. b, c, d
65. a
66. c
67. b
68. b, d, e
69. c
70. b
71. b
72. b
73. a
74. b, c, e
75. a, e, f, g
76. a, c, e
77. b
78. a
79. a, b, c, d
80. c
81. d
82. b
83. c
84. a
85. a
86. a
87. a, c, d
88. d
89. b
90. b, e
91. a
92. a, c, e
93. b, c, d
94. c
95. a
96. b
97. a, d, e
98. a, c, d
99. b, d, e
100. d
101. d
102. a
103. c
104. d

105. a
106. c
107. a, b, c

CHAPTER 12

1. a, b, d
2. b
3. a
4. a, c
5. b
6. b, c, d
7. a, b, e
8. a
9. b
10. a, b, c
11. b
12. a, b, e
13. b
14. c
15. a
16. b
17. d
18. c
19. a
20. c
21. b
22. b, c
23. c
24. b, d, e
25. b
26. a
27. c
28. a, c, f
29. a, b, c, f
30. c
31. b
32. c
33. d
34. d
35. d
36. b
37. c
38. b
39. c
40. a
41. b, d, e
42. a, c
43. b, d
44. a
45. d
46. c
47. b, e
48. b
49. b
50. b
51. c
52. c
53. c
54. b, c, e

CHAPTER 13

1. a
2. b, d, e
3. b
4. a, b, c, d, f
5. a, b, c
6. c
7. b, d, e, g
8. d
9. a, c, e
10. d
11. b
12. a
13. d
14. a
15. d
16. b
17. c
18. b
19. c
20. c
21. a
22. a
23. b, c
24. c
25. c
26. a
27. b, e, f
28. c
29. a
30. c, d, e
31. d
32. d
33. b
34. d
35. b, c, d
36. b
37. a, c, d
38. a, b, c, e
39. c
40. d
41. a, c, e
42. d
43. a, b, e
44. d
45. a
46. a, c, d, e, f
47. c
48. b
49. b, c, e
50. c
51. a, b, c, f
52. c
53. a
54. a, b, c, e
55. d
56. c
57. d
58. c
59. a

60. d
61. a
62. c

CHAPTER 14

1. c
2. b, d, e
3. a, c, d
4. d
5. b
6. a
7. c
8. a
9. b
10. c
11. d
12. b, c, e
13. b
14. a, b, c
15. a, b, d, e
16. a
17. b
18. b, c, e, f
19. a
20. c
21. a, b, d, e
22. a, b, d, e
23. a, d, e

CHAPTER 15

1. a
2. a, c, d
3. b, c
4. a, c, d, e, f
5. a
6. d
7. a, c, d, f
8. b
9. b
10. a, b, c, e, g
11. d
12. b, c, e
13. d
14. a, d, e
15. b
16. b, c, d, e
17. d
18. c
19. c
20. c
21. a, c, d, g
22. b
23. c
24. d
25. c

CHAPTER 16

1. d
2. b

3. d
4. c, d, e
5. c
6. b, c, e
7. b
8. c
9. a, b, e
10. a, b, e
11. b, c, d, e
12. b, d, f
13. a
14. d
15. b
16. d
17. a
18. d
19. b
20. c
21. a, b, d, e
22. b, c, e
23. b, d
24. a
25. c
26. a, b, d, e
27. c
28. a, c, d
29. a, c, e

CHAPTER 17

1. a, b, c, e
2. a, b, c, e
3. a, c, e
4. d
5. b
6. a, b, e
7. a, b, d, e
8. a, b, d, e
9. b
10. a, b, d, e
11. b
12. c
13. b, c, e
14. a, c, d
15. a, b, c, e, f
16. b
17. c, d, e
18. a
19. a
20. a
21. b
22. a, c, d
23. c
24. c
25. a, b, d
26. a
27. b
28. b
29. a
30. a
31. a, b, c

32. c
33. b
34. a
35. c, d
36. c
37. c
38. a
39. a, b, e
40. a, d
41. b, d, e
42. a
43. a
44. a, b, d
45. a
46. c
47. a, b
48. a
49. b

CHAPTER 18

1. d
2. a, c, d
3. a, b, c, e
4. b, e, f
5. c
6. a, c, e
7. b
8. a, b, d, e
9. c
10. b
11. d, e
12. b, c, d
13. b
14. c
15. a, b, d, e
16. c
17. a, b, c, d
18. a, c, d
19. a, b, d, e
20. a, c, d
21. a, b, c, e
22. a, b, d
23. b, c, e
24. b
25. a, b, d, e
26. c
27. b
28. a
29. b, c, e
30. a, c, d
31. d
32. c, e
33. b, c, d
34. b, c, e, f
35. a, e
36. c
37. b
38. a, b, d, e
39. a, b, c
40. b

41. d
42. a
43. a, c, d, g
44. a, c, d, e
45. a
46. c
47. a, b, c
48. c
49. a, b
50. a, b, c, d
51. d
52. a, b, d, e
53. a, b, c
54. b, e
55. c
56. b
57. a, c
58. c
59. b
60. d
61. d
62. a, b, e
63. a, b, c, d
64. b, d
65. c
66. a
67. a, b, c
68. a
69. a, c, e
70. d, e
71. a, b
72. a, c, d
73. c

CHAPTER 19

1. b, c, e
2. b
3. b, d, e
4. b, e
5. c
6. d, e
7. a, b, d
8. b, c
9. a, c, d
10. d
11. b
12. b, c, e
13. b
14. c
15. a
16. a, e
17. a, b, d
18. d
19. a
20. a, c, d, e
21. a
22. a, c, d, e
23. d
24. c
25. b, c, d

26. a, c, d
27. b
28. b, c, d
29. c
30. d
31. d
32. b
33. a, b, c
34. a, b, d
35. a, b, d
36. a, b, d, e
37. a, c, d
38. a
39. a, c, d
40. a, c
41. b
42. a, c, d
43. d

CHAPTER 20

1. b
2. a, b, c
3. a
4. b, d, f
5. a
6. d
7. c
8. a, b, e
9. b, d
10. a, c, d, e
11. b
12. b, d
13. a, b, e
14. a, b, e, f
15. d
16. c
17. b
18. a
19. a, e
20. a, b, d
21. a, d, e
22. b
23. c, e
24. a, b, d, e
25. c
26. b
27. a, b, c, d
28. a, b
29. a, b, d
30. c
31. a, d, f
32. c
33. b, d
34. c
35. a
36. d
37. a
38. a, b, d, e

CHAPTER 21

1. b
2. a
3. b
4. c
5. a
6. c
7. b, d, e
8. c
9. d
10. a. 4; b. 1; c. 3; d. 2
11. b
12. a, b, c, d
13. d
14. a
15. b, c, d
16. a
17. b
18. b
19. c
20. a
21. a
22. c
23. a, b, c, d
24. Step 2
25. a
26. c
27. d
28. c
29. a
30. a
31. d
32. a, b, c
33. b
34. b
35. a
36. c

CHAPTER 22

1. b
2. b, c, e
3. a, c, e
4. b
5. a
6. a, b, c, d
7. a
8. c
9. b
10. b
11. b
12. d
13. d
14. a, b, c
15. d
16. a
17. c
18. c
19. a
20. a, b, e

21. a, b, c, d
22. c
23. d
24. c
25. a
26. a, c
27. d
28. b
29. b
30. a
31. b, c
32. c
33. c
34. b
35. c
36. d
37. c
38. a, c, d
39. a
40. b
41. c
42. b
43. c
44. c
45. a
46. a, d
47. a
48. a
49. a, b, c, e
50. c
51. c
52. d
53. c

CHAPTER 23

1. c
2. a
3. a
4. b, c, e
5. d
6. a, b, c, f
7. a
8. b, c, d
9. b, c, d
10. a, c
11. d
12. c
13. b
14. d
15. a, b, d
16. b
17. b
18. d
19. a
20. d
21. a
22. d
23. b, d, e
24. d
25. b

26. a, b, d, e
27. b
28. b
29. c
30. a
31. c
32. b
33. d
34. a, c, d
35. b, c, e

CHAPTER 24

1. b
2. c
3. a
4. c
5. a
6. a
7. b, c, e, f
8. d
9. b
10. a
11. a, b, c, e
12. c
13. d
14. b
15. a
16. b
17. d
18. d
19. a, b, d, f
20. a
21. c
22. c
23. b
24. c
25. d
26. a
27. c
28. a
29. b
30. c
31. a
32. a, b, c, d, f
33. d
34. b
35. c
36. d
37. c
38. a
39. a
40. c
41. a
42. b
43. d
44. b
45. c
46. c
47. b
48. b

49. c
50. b
51. a
52. b
53. d
54. a
55. d
56. b
57. c
58. a
59. c
60. d
61. b
62. b
63. a
64. b
65. a

CHAPTER 25

1. a
2. 1500-1750
3. c
4. a
5. b, c, d, f
6. d
7. b
8. b
9. c
10. c
11. b
12. d
13. a
14. a, b, e
15. c
16. a
17. b
18. b
19. d
20. c
21. d
22. a, b, d
23. a
24. d
25. d
26. a
27. a, b, c, e
28. b
29. a, d, e
30. a, b, c, e
31. b
32. b
33. a
34. a
35. c
36. d
37. a
38. c
39. c
40. d
41. c

42. b
43. b
44. a. 1; b. 5; c. 3; d. 4; e. 2
45. c
46. a, c, d
47. b
48. c
49. a
50. c
51. c
52. d
53. b
54. b
55. c
56. a
57. d
58. a
59. b
60. b
61. a
62. 118 grams
63. a
64. d
65. b
66. d
67. b
68. c
69. a
70. a

CHAPTER 26

1. a
2. c
3. b, c, d, e
4. d
5. a
6. c
7. d
8. c
9. b
10. b
11. b
12. a, c, d, e
13. b
14. a
15. b
16. c
17. b
18. b, c, d
19. a, b, c
20. b
21. d
22. c
23. d
24. c
25. d
26. b
27. d
28. b
29. b

30. a, b, c, e
31. c
32. b
33. a
34. c
35. b
36. a
37. c
38. a
39. c
40. c
41. b
42. c
43. b
44. a
45. c
46. b
47. a, c, e
48. c
49. c, d, e
50. d
51. a, c, e
52. a
53. b
54. a, b, c, e
55. a
56. b
57. c
58. d
59. a, b, d, e
60. b
61. a, d
62. b
63. a, b, d, f
64. c
65. a
66. a
67. a
68. b, c, d
69. a
70. a
71. a
72. a
73. a
74. c
75. c
76. b
77. b
78. b, c, d
79. c
80. c
81. d
82. b, d, f
83. a
84. a
85. d

CHAPTER 27

1. a
2. a

3. b, c, d
4. b
5. b
6. c
7. a, b, d, e
8. d
9. b
10. b, c, e
11. a
12. b
13. b
14. a, b, c, e
15. c
16. a
17. b
18. d
19. c
20. b
21. b, c, e
22. b
23. b
24. c
25. b
26. c
27. a
28. a, b, e
29. a, b, c, d, f
30. d
31. c
32. a
33. c
34. c
35. c
36. a
37. a, e
38. b
39. c
40. a, b, e
41. a
42. d
43. b
44. c
45. a
46. a
47. c
48. b, d
49. d
50. d
51. b
52. b
53. a, b, c, d
54. d
55. b
56. a

CHAPTER 28

1. a, c, e
2. b, d, e
3. b, c, e
4. a, d, e

5. a, b, d
6. c
7. b, c, e
8. b
9. b
10. b
11. c
12. a
13. c
14. c
15. a, b, c, d
16. c
17. a, c, d, e
18. a
19. d
20. a
21. a, b, d, e
22. c
23. c
24. a
25. a, b, d, e
26. a
27. a
28. c
29. d
30. c
31. a, b, d, e
32. b
33. a, c, d, e
34. d
35. a
36. b
37. a, b, c
38. a, c, d, e, f
39. a
40. b
41. d
42. a
43. d
44. d
45. d
46. a, b, e
47. c
48. d
49. a, d, e
50. c
51. b
52. c
53. b
54. c

CHAPTER 29

1. d
2. b
3. c
4. a
5. a, b, e
6. c
7. a
8. a

9. a, c, d
10. c, e
11. d
12. c
13. c
14. b
15. a
16. a
17. b
18. c
19. a
20. a
21. c
22. a, c, d, e
23. b
24. a
25. a
26. c
27. b
28. c
29. d
30. d
31. a, c, d, e
32. d
33. d
34. a, c, e, f
35. a
36. c
37. b
38. a, b, d
39. a
40. a
41. a, c, d
42. d
43. c
44. c
45. a
46. d
47. a
48. a
49. b
50. c
51. d
52. d
53. c
54. a
55. c
56. a
57. b
58. d
59. a, d, e
60. c
61. a, c, e

CHAPTER 30

1. a, d, e
2. a, b, d, f
3. a, c, d, f
4. c
5. b

6. a, b, d, e
7. a
8. d
9. b
10. a, d
11. d
12. b, c, e
13. c
14. b
15. b
16. b
17. a, d, e
18. c
19. c
20. b
21. d
22. c
23. a, b, c, e
24. b
25. b
26. c
27. d
28. b
29. a
30. d
31. a, c, d
32. c
33. a
34. a, b, d, e
35. b
36. c
37. d
38. b
39. c
40. c
41. c
42. a
43. b
44. c
45. a
46. c
47. a
48. b, c, e
49. a, c, d, f
50. d
51. b
52. c
53. c
54. a
55. b, c, e
56. a, c, e
57. c
58. d
59. a
60. d
61. c
62. c
63. b
64. b
65. c

66. c
67. d
68. b
69. a
70. a
71. a, c, e
72. a
73. c
74. a

CHAPTER 31

1. c
2. d
3. a, c, d, e
4. a, b, d, e
5. a, c, e
6. a
7. b
8. b
9. a, c, d, e
10. c
11. d
12. a
13. a, c, e
14. c, d
15. c
16. a
17. b
18. b
19. b, c, d
20. c
21. a
22. b
23. c
24. a, b, c, e
25. c
26. b
27. b
28. a, d, e
29. a, e
30. d
31. a
32. c
33. a
34. c
35. a
36. c
37. c
38. d
39. d
40. a
41. b
42. c
43. a
44. a
45. b
46. a
47. a, b, d, e
48. a, b, d, e
49. b

50. c
51. b, c, d, f
52. c
53. b
54. b, c, d
55. a, c, e
56. a, c, e
57. a
58. d
59. c
60. d
61. d
62. b
63. a
64. b
65. a, b, d
66. b
67. c
68. c
69. b, c, e
70. b

CHAPTER 32

1. a, c, e
2. b
3. c
4. a, c, e
5. c
6. c
7. a, b, c, f
8. b
9. b
10. d
11. b
12. b, c, e
13. d
14. a, d, e
15. a, b, e
16. b
17. c
18. d
19. b
20. d
21. b, c, d, f
22. c
23. c
24. b
25. a
26. c
27. b, c, d, e
28. a, b, d, e
29. b
30. a, c, d, f
31. c
32. a
33. b
34. d
35. b, c, e, f
36. a
37. c

38. b
39. d
40. b
41. b
42. a, c, d, e
43. b, c, e
44. b
45. c
46. a, b, c, e, f
47. b
48. c
49. a, c, e
50. b
51. c
52. c
53. a
54. b, c, d, e, f
55. c
56. c
57. a
58. a
59. b
60. b
61. a
62. a
63. a, b, c, e, f
64. b, c, e
65. a, b, c, d
66. a, c, e
67. d
68. a, d, e
69. c
70. d
71. d
72. b
73. a
74. d
75. d
76. d
77. a, b, d
78. b, d, e, f
79. c
80. d
81. b
82. a
83. a
84. b
85. a
86. a, d

CHAPTER 33

1. b
2. a, c, d
3. a, d, e, f
4. a
5. a
6. a, b, d, f
7. a, b, e
8. b
9. c

10. a
11. b, d, e
12. a, c, d
13. b, d, f
14. b
15. b
16. b
17. d
18. c
19. a
20. c
21. d
22. b
23. b
24. a
25. a
26. b
27. a
28. a
29. c
30. d
31. b, d
32. c
33. d
34. a
35. a
36. d
37. a, c, d
38. b
39. a, c, d, e, f
40. a, c, d
41. c
42. c
43. b, c, e
44. a
45. b
46. a
47. c
48. d
49. b
50. a
51. a, d, e
52. a
53. a
54. a, b, d
55. b
56. c
57. d
58. a, b, d
59. a, b, d
60. a
61. b
62. a
63. c
64. d
65. b, e
66. b, d, e
67. c, d, e
68. b
69. a, b, d

70. a

CHAPTER 34

1. b
2. b
3. c
4. c
5. a
6. c
7. a
8. a
9. d
10. a
11. c
12. d
13. c
14. a
15. c
16. a, c, e
17. d
18. b
19. a
20. b
21. a, b, e, f
22. d
23. b, c, e
24. b
25. d
26. b
27. a
28. d
29. b
30. c
31. b
32. b
33. a, c, e
34. c
35. b
36. b
37. c
38. a, b, c, d
39. d
40. c
41. d
42. b, c, e
43. a
44. b, d, e
45. a
46. b
47. b
48. a
49. d
50. a
51. b
52. a, c, d, e
53. a
54. a
55. b, c, e
56. c
57. b

58. b
59. b
60. d
61. b
62. c
63. b
64. c
65. a
66. a, b, c, d
67. a, b, d, f
68. c
69. b
70. d
71. c
72. b
73. b
74. c
75. c
76. a, b, d
77. b, c, e
78. a, d, e
79. a
80. a
81. c
82. b, c, d, f
83. b
84. b, c, e
85. c
86. a, c, d, f
87. *Rate:* Atrial rate: Approx. 300 beats/min
Ventricular rate: 75 beats/min
Rhythm: Irregular (due to PACs)
P waves: 2 flutter waves per QRS complex; no P waves present
PR interval: None
QRS duration: 0.08 seconds
Interpretation: 2:1 atrial flutter with occasional PACs
88. *Rate:* About 50 beats/min
Rhythm: Regular
P waves: Regular; 1 per QRS
PR interval: 0.20 seconds
QRS duration: 0.08 seconds
Interpretation: Sinus bradycardia with PAC
89. *Rate:* 150 beats/min
Rhythm: Regular
P waves: Regular; notched 1 per QRS
PR interval: 0.12 seconds
QRS duration: 0.08 seconds
Interpretation: Atrial tachycardia
90. *Rate:* Beat-to-beat variability approx. 130 beats/min
Rhythm: Irregular, irregular
P waves: Fibrillation waves

PR interval: None
QRS duration: 0.08 seconds
Interpretation: Atrial fibrillation with rapid ventricular response
91. *Rate:* 83 beats/min
Rhythm: Regular
P waves: 1 per QRS
PR interval: 0.16 seconds
QRS duration: 0.08 seconds
Interpretation: Sinus rhythm with 2.3-second pause/sinus arrest
92. *Rate:* 150 beats/min
Rhythm: Regular
P waves: Regular; 1 per QRS
PR interval: 0.12 seconds
QRS duration: 0.04 seconds
Interpretation: Sinus tachycardia
93. *Rate:* Cannot be determined
Rhythm: Chaotic
P waves: None
PR interval: None
QRS duration: None
Interpretation: Ventricular fibrillation
94. *Rate:* 78 beats/min
Rhythm: Regular
P waves: Regular; 1 per QRS
PR interval: 0.20 seconds
QRS duration: 0.04 seconds
Interpretation: Sinus rhythm with PVC
95. *Rate:* Cannot be determined
Rhythm: Chaotic
P waves: None
PR interval: None
QRS duration: None
Interpretation: Ventricular fibrillation
96. *Rate:* Approx. 200 beats/min
Rhythm: Regular with wide-complex QRS
P waves: None
PR interval: None
QRS duration: Wide—0.28 seconds
Interpretation: Monomorphic ventricular tachycardia
97. *Rate:* None
Rhythm: None
P waves: None
PR interval: None
QRS duration: None
Interpretation: Asystole
98. *Rate:* 107 beats/min

Rhythm: Irregular, irregular
P waves: Fibrillation waves
PR interval: None
QRS duration: 0.08 seconds
Interpretation: Atrial fibrillation
99. *Rate:* Ventricular rate: Varies—starts at 42 beats/min, speeds up to 83 beats/min
Atrial rate: Approx. 350 beats/min
Rhythm: Regular
P waves: Flutter waves present
PR interval: None—not measured in this rhythm
QRS duration: 0.08 seconds
Interpretation: Atrial flutter (latter half looks like 3:1 flutter)
100. *Rate:* 75 beats/min
Rhythm: Regular
P waves: Regular; 1 per QRS
PR interval: 0.20 seconds
QRS duration: 0.08 seconds
Interpretation: Sinus rhythm with PJC
101. *Rate:* Ventricular: 35 beats/min
Atrial: 100 beats/min
Rhythm: Regular wide complex
P waves: Do not correspond with QRS complex
PR interval: None
QRS duration: 0.20 seconds
Interpretation: Third-degree AV block with underlying ventricular escape rhythm

CHAPTER 35

1. c
2. d
3. a
4. b
5. c
6. c
7. a, c, e
8. a, b, c, e, f
9. d
10. d
11. d
12. b
13. a, b, d, e
14. c
15. d
16. d
17. b
18. b
19. a
20. a

21. a, b, c, e
22. a, d, e
23. a
24. d
25. c
26. b
27. c
28. a
29. d
30. c
31. a
32. d
33. a
34. b
35. a
36. c
37. b
38. a, b, c, e
39. b
40. c, d, e, f
41. b
42. a
43. b, d
44. b, c, d
45. a, b, c, e
46. b
47. a
48. a
49. c
50. c
51. a
52. a
53. b
54. b
55. c
56. b
57. a
58. c
59. a
60. b, c, d, e, f
61. c
62. c
63. b, c, d
64. a, c, d, e
65. b
66. c
67. a
68. b
69. b
70. b
71. d
72. a, c, e
73. b
74. c
75. b
76. a
77. c
78. b
79. a
80. b

81. a, b, c, e
82. c
83. b
84. d
85. a, c, d, e
86. a, b, e
87. a
88. b
89. a, d, e, f

CHAPTER 36

1. a, b, c, e
2. a, b, d, e
3. b, c, d
4. a, b, d
5. a, d
6. d
7. b
8. d
9. b
10. d
11. b
12. a
13. b, c, d
14. b, c, d
15. a
16. b
17. b
18. b, c, d, e
19. d
20. a
21. d
22. c
23. a
24. b
25. d
26. a
27. c
28. a
29. b
30. a, b, c, f
31. b
32. a, c, d, e
33. b
34. b
35. d
36. a, b, c, f
37. a
38. b
39. c
40. d
41. b
42. b
43. a
44. c
45. a, b, d, f
46. c
47. a, d, e
48. a, c, d
49. a, c, e

50. b
51. a, b, c, e
52. b
53. a
54. d
55. a
56. b
57. d
58. a
59. a
60. b
61. a, b, e
62. b
63. a
64. c
65. a
66. b, c,
67. a, b, e
68. a
69. b, d, e, f
70. a
71. c
72. b
73. b
74. d
75. b
76. a
77. b
78. a, b, e
79. b, c, e, f
80. c
81. c
82. d
83. c
84. c
85. a, b, e
86. b
87. a
88. d
89. b
90. c, d, e
91. a
92. d
93. a
94. c
95. a
96. c
97. d
98. d
99. c, d, e
100. c
101. c
102. a, b, c
103. a
104. a, b, c, d, f
105. b
106. c
107. d
108. a
109. a, b, c, e

110. a
111. c
112. c
113. a, c, e
114. b, c, e
115. b
116. a
117. a, b, d, e
118. a
119. a, b, c, d
120. a
121. c
122. a, b, d, e
123. c
124. c
125. b
126. b
127. c

CHAPTER 37

1. a, b, d
2. b, c, d, e
3. a, c, e
4. d
5. b, c, d, f
6. a, b, d, e
7. b, d
8. c
9. c
10. d
11. d
12. a, b, c, d
13. c
14. a, c, e
15. c, e
16. a
17. c
18. b, e
19. c
20. a, b, d, e, f
21. b
22. a
23. c
24. a
25. a, b, c
26. b
27. a, b, c, d
28. b
29. d
30. c
31. a
32. b
33. b
34. b
35. c
36. c
37. a
38. c
39. d
40. d

41. c
42. d
43. b
44. c
45. a, b, d, e
46. a
47. d
48. c
49. c
50. a, c, d, f
51. d
52. a, b, c, e
53. b
54. d
55. b
56. a
57. a, c, e
58. c
59. a, c, d
60. a

CHAPTER 38

1. a, e
2. c, d, e
3. b
4. d
5. b, c, f
6. c
7. a
8. c
9. a
10. a, d, f
11. b
12. a, c
13. b
14. b, c, d, e
15. b
16. a
17. d, e
18. c
19. a
20. a
21. d
22. a, c, d, e
23. d
24. c
25. b
26. a, b, c, e, f
27. a, c, d, f
28. a
29. b
30. d, e
31. b
32. c
33. b, e
34. a, b, c, d
35. c
36. b
37. b
38. a, b, c, e, f

39. b
40. a, b, d
41. b
42. a, c, e, f
43. b
44. a, b, d, e, f
45. b, c, d
46. a
47. b
48. a
49. b
50. b
51. a
52. b
53. c
54. a
55. a
56. c
57. a
58. a, b, d, e, f
59. c
60. b
61. a
62. c
63. a
64. c
65. a
66. b
67. a
68. a, c, d, f
69. b
70. b
71. b, c, d, e
72. a, b, d, e, f
73. b
74. b
75. d
76. a
77. b
78. d
79. b
80. a
81. c
82. a, b, c, e
83. b
84. b, c, d
85. c
86. a
87. b
88. a
89. a, b, d, e, f
90. b
91. c
92. a, c

CHAPTER 39

1. a, b, c, d
2. d
3. b
4. a

5. d
6. b
7. a, c, e
8. b
9. a
10. d
11. c
12. c
13. b
14. b
15. d
16. a, b, e
17. d
18. c
19. a, b, c, d
20. a
21. c
22. b
23. d
24. c
25. d

CHAPTER 40

1. a, d, e, f
2. a, c, d, e
3. d
4. a
5. c
6. a
7. a, c, e
8. c
9. b
10. a
11. b, c, e
12. d
13. a, b, c, d, e
14. a
15. b
16. a, b, c, e
17. a
18. a
19. c
20. a, b, d, e, f
21. a
22. a, b
23. a, b, c, d, e
24. a
25. c
26. b
27. a, b, c, e, f
28. a, b, c, e
29. c
30. a, c, d, e
31. b
32. c
33. b
34. b
35. a
36. a
37. c

38. c
39. a
40. c
41. a
42. b
43. c
44. b
45. c

CHAPTER 41

1. b, f
2. a
3. d
4. b
5. a, c, d, f
6. d
7. b, e
8. d
9. a, b, d
10. a
11. b
12. a, b, d, e
13. c
14. a
15. a
16. c
17. d
18. c
19. a
20. a
21. c
22. a
23. a
24. b
25. b
26. b
27. a
28. b
29. b
30. c
31. c
32. d
33. b
34. c
35. d
36. a
37. d
38. d
39. a
40. d
41. a, b, c
42. a
43. a, b, d
44. d
45. d

CHAPTER 42

1. a, c, e
2. b, d, f

3. a, b, e, f
4. d
5. d
6. a
7. b
8. a
9. c
10. d
11. a
12. a, c, d, f
13. a
14. c
15. a
16. b
17. d
18. b
19. a
20. d
21. a, d
22. c
23. b
24. c
25. b
26. c
27. d
28. b
29. a, b, e, f
30. c
31. b
32. c
33. a
34. b
35. a, b, c, e
36. a
37. c
38. d
39. b
40. b
41. c
42. b
43. b
44. b, c, e, f
45. b

CHAPTER 43

1. b
2. b
3. a
4. d
5. a, b, c, e
6. b
7. a, b, c, e
8. b
9. c, e
10. a
11. a
12. d
13. b
14. a, b, d
15. c

16. b
17. a
18. a
19. b
20. b, d, e
21. b
22. c, e
23. b
24. b, c, e
25. c
26. a
27. b
28. b
29. d
30. a, e, f
31. c
32. a, b, c
33. c
34. b, e
35. d
36. a
37. c
38. b, c, e
39. b
40. d
41. a, c, e
42. b
43. c
44. a, b, e
45. b

CHAPTER 44

1. b, e, f
2. c
3. c, e
4. d
5. c, e
6. a
7. c
8. a, b, d
9. a, b, d, e
10. c
11. a
12. b
13. b, c, d, e, f
14. a
15. b
16. a
17. a
18. c
19. a, b, d
20. a, c, e, f
21. b
22. b
23. c
24. a
25. d
26. c
27. b
28. a

29. c
30. a
31. c
32. b
33. c
34. b
35. d, e, f
36. b
37. b
38. a
39. a
40. c
41. a
42. b
43. d
44. d
45. b
46. a, c, e
47. a
48. c, e
49. c
50. d
51. b, c, e
52. a, b, e, f
53. d
54. c
55. c
56. c
57. b
58. d
59. a
60. a, b, c, f
61. c
62. a
63. b
64. a
65. b, c, d
66. a, c, e
67. c

CHAPTER 45

1. b
2. a, b, d, e
3. a, c, d, e
4. a, b, d, e
5. d
6. c
7. a
8. b

9. b
10. b
11. b
12. c
13. b
14. a
15. a
16. a, c, d, e
17. d
18. b
19. b
20. c
21. a, b, d, e, f
22. a, b, c, e
23. a, b, d, f
24. a
25. b, c, d, f
26. a
27. d
28. c
29. b
30. a
31. d
32. b
33. a
34. d
35. b
36. a
37. d
38. c
39. c
40. b
41. c
42. b
43. a
44. d
45. c
46. a
47. c
48. c
49. c
50. b
51. a, c, d, e
52. a
53. b
54. a
55. b, c, e, f
56. a
57. b

58. c
59. d
60. a, c, d, f
61. b
62. a
63. d
64. c
65. b
66. d
67. c
68. d
69. d
70. b
71. a
72. a, c, e, f

CHAPTER 46

1. a. 4; b. 2; c. 3; d. 1; e. 5
2. b, d
3. a
4. d
5. d
6. a, b, c
7. d
8. c
9. c
10. c
11. a
12. c
13. a, d, e
14. a, c, d
15. b
16. d
17. c
18. a, c, d, f
19. d
20. b
21. a
22. b, c, e
23. a, c, d
24. b
25. a
26. c
27. b
28. d
29. b
30. c
31. c

32. b
33. d
34. b
35. c

CHAPTER 47

1. b
2. c
3. a, c, e
4. c
5. c
6. b
7. b
8. a
9. c
10. d
11. d
12. a
13. a
14. b
15. a, b, d, e
16. b
17. b
18. c
19. b
20. d
21. c
22. d
23. b
24. d
25. d
26. b
27. c
28. a
29. d
30. a, b, e

CHAPTER 48

1. a
2. c
3. b, d
4. b, c, d, e
5. a. 2; b. 3; c. 4; d. 5; e. 1; f. 6
6. d
7. c
8. a, c
9. b

10. Normal tympanic membrane appears shiny, transparent, or opaque and pearly/gray.

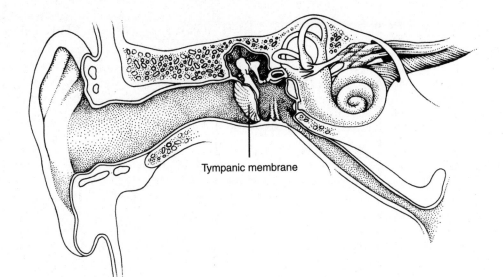

Tympanic membrane

11. a	47. b	21. a	10. b
12. b, d, e	48. b	22. a, c, d, e	11. a
13. d	49. d	23. c	12. c
14. c	50. a, b, c, e	24. d	13. a
15. c	51. c	25. a	14. c
16. a	52. b, c, d, e	26. b	15. d
17. d	53. c	27. a, c, d, e	16. b, d
18. c	54. c	28. d	17. a
19. c	55. b	29. b, c, d	18. a, c, e
20. c	56. c	30. b, c, e	19. a
21. b	57. a, b, c, e	31. a	20. b
22. c	58. c	32. b	21. b
23. a	59. a, b, d, e	33. c	22. a
24. c		34. d	23. b
25. a	**CHAPTER 49**	35. a	24. a
26. c		36. a, b, d, e	25. b
27. d	1. a	37. a, b	26. d
28. d	2. b, c	38. c	27. a
29. a	3. d	39. a, b, d	28. b
30. a	4. a	40. c	29. d
31. c	5. b	41. b	30. a
32. a, b, c, e	6. b	42. b	31. c
33. d	7. c	43. a	32. a
34. b	8. a	44. a, c, e	33. b
35. c	9. b		34. a, c, d
36. b, c, d, e	10. a, c, e	**CHAPTER 50**	35. d
37. a	11. a		36. a, b, d
38. a	12. d	1. b	37. b
39. b	13. b	2. a, c, f	38. c
40. c	14. d	3. c	39. a, c, d
41. b	15. c	4. b, c, d	40. d
42. a	16. c	5. a, c, e	41. c
43. a, b, e	17. d	6. b, c	42. a, b, f
44. b	18. b	7. b	43. a
45. d	19. b, c, e	8. a	44. a
46. b, c, d, e	20. d	9. a, c, f	45. c

46. b
47. a
48. c
49. b
50. a
51. c
52. a, d, e
53. b, d
54. a
55. d
56. a, b, d, e

CHAPTER 51

1. d
2. a, b, d, f
3. d
4. b
5. a
6. b
7. c
8. a
9. c
10. d
11. b, c, d
12. c
13. a
14. b
15. b
16. d
17. c
18. b
19. b
20. d
21. a
22. a
23. c
24. a
25. b, c
26. a, b, d, e
27. d
28. c
29. a
30. b, d
31. a, d, e
32. b
33. c
34. d
35. c
36. a
37. d
38. d
39. a
40. d
41. b
42. b
43. b
44. c
45. a
46. c
47. b

48. b, e
49. d
50. b
51. d
52. c
53. d
54. c
55. a
56. c
57. c
58. a, b, c, e
59. b
60. a, b
61. a, b, c
62. b, c, d
63. a, b, c, d
64. b
65. c
66. a, c, d, e
67. c
68. c
69. d
70. a, b, d, f
71. b
72. a
73. a, b, e

CHAPTER 52

1. c
2. d
3. b, d, e
4. a, c, e
5. b, c, e
6. a, b, c
7. d
8. a, c
9. a, b, d, e
10. d
11. d
12. c
13. a
14. b
15. a, b, e
16. c, e
17. c
18. c
19. a, b, d, e
20. d
21. a, c, d, e, f
22. c
23. b
24. b
25. d
26. c
27. a
28. a, b, e, f
29. b, c, e
30. a, c, d, f
31. b
32. a

33. c
34. a, c, d, e

CHAPTER 53

1. d
2. a
3. a
4. b
5. c
6. a
7. a
8. c
9. a, d, e
10. b
11. c
12. c
13. d
14. d
15. a, c, d, f
16. c
17. b, c, e, f
18. c
19. b, d, e
20. a
21. c
22. a, b, d, f
23. a
24. a, c, d
25. a, b, d

CHAPTER 54

1. b
2. a
3. a, e
4. a, d
5. c
6. b
7. d
8. b
9. a
10. d
11. d
12. b
13. a, b, c, e, f
14. d
15. a, c, d, e
16. b
17. a
18. a, b, c, e
19. a
20. a, b, c, d
21. d
22. b
23. c
24. a, b, c, e, f
25. b
26. a
27. c
28. b

29. b
30. a, b, d, e

CHAPTER 55

1. a, b, c, d
2. a, c, d, e
3. b, d, e
4. a, c, d
5. a
6. b
7. d
8. a
9. b
10. d
11. a
12. d
13. b, d, e
14. a
15. d
16. d
17. c
18. a
19. a, c, d, e
20. d
21. d
22. a, b, c, d
23. b
24. c
25. a, b, c, e
26. a, b, d, e, f
27. a
28. c
29. a, c
30. c
31. a, c, d, e
32. c
33. a, c, d, e
34. a
35. a
36. a
37. a, c, d, e

CHAPTER 56

1. a, b, d, e
2. c
3. d
4. a
5. a
6. b, c
7. d
8. c
9. c
10. c, e
11. c
12. b
13. a, c, e
14. a, d, e
15. c
16. b

17. a
18. a, b, e
19. a, c, e
20. a
21. c
22. d
23. b
24. a
25. b, c, e
26. d
27. c
28. a
29. a
30. b, c, d, e
31. a
32. b
33. d
34. a
35. c
36. a
37. b, e
38. a, b, d
39. b, c, d, e
40. a
41. b
42. c
43. a, c, e
44. a, c, d
45. a
46. b
47. d
48. a, f
49. b
50. a, c

CHAPTER 57

1. c
2. a, b
3. b
4. b, c, e
5. d
6. a, b, d
7. c
8. a
9. b
10. c
11. a
12. c
13. b
14. a, b, d
15. d
16. b
17. b, c, e
18. d
19. c
20. b, c, f
21. a
22. a
23. b
24. a, b, e

25. c
26. d
27. a, b, c, d
28. d
29. d
30. a
31. d
32. d
33. a
34. c
35. c
36. b, c, d, e
37. a
38. b
39. c
40. a, b, c, d
41. a

CHAPTER 58

1. a, b, c, e, f
2. d
3. c
4. a
5. d
6. a, c, d, e
7. b
8. a, b, d
9. b
10. a
11. a, b, c, f
12. b
13. b
14. a, c, d, e, f
15. a
16. a
17. d
18. a, b, d, e
19. a
20. d
21. b, c, e
22. b, c, f
23. a, b, c, e
24. a, b, d, e
25. b
26. c
27. a, b, d, e
28. a
29. a, b, c, e
30. b, c, d, e
31. a, c, e
32. b
33. d
34. c
35. a
36. d
37. c
38. d
39. a, c, e
40. a, c, d, e

CHAPTER 59

1. a
2. c
3. c
4. a
5. a, c, e, f
6. c
7. d
8. b
9. d
10. a
11. b
12. a
13. a, c, d
14. d
15. c
16. d
17. b
18. b
19. d
20. a
21. c
22. b
23. c
24. d
25. c
26. c
27. a, b, d, f
28. b
29. a, b, d, e
30. c
31. b, c, d, e, f
32. b
33. b
34. a, c, d
35. a, b, d

CHAPTER 60

1. a, c, e
2. a, b, c, e
3. b
4. a
5. c
6. a, b, d, e, f
7. a, c, d, e
8. a
9. b
10. a, b, c, d, f
11. b
12. c
13. a
14. b
15. b, c
16. d
17. b, c, d
18. c, d, e
19. a
20. b, c, e
21. a, c, d, e

22. d
23. d
24. a
25. b
26. d
27. a
28. b
29. a, b, c, e
30. b
31. a
32. a, c, d, e
33. b
34. a
35. d
36. d
37. a, b, c, d
38. b
39. a
40. b, e
41. b, c, d, e
42. a, c, d, e
43. a, b, d
44. d
45. a, c, e
46. d
47. a
48. a, b, d, e, f
49. a, c, d, e
50. d

CHAPTER 61

1. a, c, d, e
2. c
3. b
4. b, d
5. a, d, f
6. b
7. d
8. a, b, e
9. a
10. c
11. a
12. b
13. a, b, e
14. a
15. b
16. d
17. a, e
18. b
19. b, c, e
20. a, b, c, e
21. b, c, d
22. a
23. d
24. a, b, c, e
25. b, c, d
26. d
27. d
28. a, c, e
29. b

30. d
31. b
32. b, c, d, e
33. b
34. a
35. a
36. b
37. b
38. a, b, c, d
39. b
40. c, d, e, f
41. a, b, d, e
42. b
43. d
44. b

CHAPTER 62

1. d
2. c, e
3. a, b, d, e
4. c
5. a
6. a, e
7. d
8. b
9. a
10. a, b, c, e, f
11. d, e
12. a, b, c, d
13. c
14. d
15. c
16. a, d, e, f
17. a, b, c, d
18. b, c, d, e, f
19. b
20. b
21. a
22. c
23. b
24. a, c, d
25. b, c, e
26. a, b
27. a
28. a
29. c
30. b
31. c
32. a, c, d
33. a
34. c
35. a, c, e
36. a, d
37. b
38. b
39. d
40. b
41. b
42. d
43. d

44. d
45. d
46. a, c, e, f
47. b, c, e
48. a
49. a
50. b
51. b
52. d
53. b
54. a
55. a
56. a, c, d
57. b
58. d
59. d
60. a, b, c

CHAPTER 63

1. d
2. a, c, d, f
3. b
4. c
5. b
6. b
7. d
8. b
9. a
10. b
11. d
12. b
13. c
14. c
15. a, b, e
16. c
17. b
18. a
19. b
20. a, b, c, d
21. a, b, d, e
22. a, b
23. d
24. c
25. a
26. b
27. c
28. a, c, d
29. a
30. b
31. a, c, d, e
32. a, b, c, e
33. b, c, d, e
34. a, b, d, e, f
35. d
36. c, d
37. c
38. b
39. a, b, d, e
40. a, b, e
41. b

42. d
43. a
44. a
45. c
46. b
47. b, e, f
48. c
49. a, b, d
50. a
51. a, b
52. a, b, c, e
53. a, c
54. b
55. d
56. a, c, d

CHAPTER 64

1. b, d
2. c
3. b
4. b
5. a, b, d
6. c
7. d
8. d
9. c
10. c
11. a, b, d
12. b, c, d, e
13. a, b
14. a
15. c
16. d
17. c
18. a, c, e
19. b
20. a, c, d
21. a, b, d, e
22. d, e
23. a
24. b, c, e
25. b, e
26. a
27. b
28. d
29. c
30. c
31. a
32. a, c, e
33. b
34. c
35. b
36. a
37. a
38. c
39. d
40. a
41. b, d, e
42. d
43. b, c

44. b
45. d
46. a
47. a, b, c, d
48. c, d, e
49. a, b, d, e, f
50. c
51. a, b, d, e
52. d
53. b
54. c
55. b
56. a
57. c, e, f
58. d
59. a, c, d, e, f
60. c
61. b
62. c
63. c
64. a
65. b
66. b, c, d, e
67. a, b, d
68. b, c, e
69. d
70. b
71. c
72. a
73. b
74. d
75. c
76. b
77. b, d
78. a, c, d, e
79. d
80. a
81. b

CHAPTER 65

1. b
2. d
3. b
4. b
5. a, b, c
6. b
7. b
8. b
9. d
10. b
11. b
12. b
13. a
14. a
15. a
16. b
17. a
18. a
19. b
20. a, b, e

21. c
22. b
23. b
24. b
25. c
26. d
27. c
28. b
29. d
30. b
31. d
32. a
33. b, d, e
34. b
35. d
36. b
37. a
38. d
39. b
40. d
41. c
42. c
43. b
44. a
45. c, d, e
46. b
47. a
48. a
49. c
50. c
51. b
52. a
53. c
54. a
55. c
56. b
57. c
58. a. 2; b. 5; c. 4; d. 1; e. 3;
    f. 6
59. a
60. c
61. b
62. c
63. a
64. b
65. b
66. b
67. a
68. d
69. b
70. b
71. c
72. a, d, e, f
73. a
74. d

CHAPTER 66

1. c
2. b
3. b

4. c
5. a
6. a
7. d
8. b
9. b
10. c
11. a
12. d
13. a
14. a
15. d
16. c
17. a
18. c
19. a
20. b
21. b
22. d
23. c, d, e
24. a
25. b
26. a
27. c
28. b
29. d
30. d
31. d
32. a, d, e
33. c
34. a
35. d
36. c
37. a
38. c
39. d
40. a
41. a, b, c, d, f
42. b
43. a
44. c
45. b
46. b
47. c
48. a
49. b
50. d
51. a
52. a
53. d
54. c
55. d
56. b
57. a
58. d
59. b
60. c
61. d
62. d
63. a

64. a, b, c, e
65. d
66. b
67. a
68. a, c, d, e, f
69. c
70. c
71. d
72. c
73. d
74. b
75. d

CHAPTER 67

1. c
2. c
3. c
4. a, c, d, e
5. d
6. c
7. a
8. a, b, d
9. b
10. c
11. c
12. c
13. c
14. d
15. a
16. a
17. a
18. b
19. d
20. a
21. b, c, d
22. b
23. d
24. c
25. a
26. a
27. a
28. b
29. b
30. a
31. b
32. a
33. b, c, d, e
34. b
35. b
36. c
37. c
38. c
39. c
40. a
41. a
42. b
43. c
44. d
45. d
46. a, c, e

47. b
48. a
49. b
50. a
51. a
52. d
53. b
54. d
55. a
56. d
57. a, b, c
58. b
59. b, c, d
60. b
61. c
62. c
63. c, d
64. b
65. b
66. c
67. a
68. a
69. b, c, d, e
70. c
71. a
72. a
73. d
74. a
75. b
76. b, c, d, f
77. a
78. b
79. c
80. b
81. c
82. d
83. a, b, c, d, f
84. c
85. c
86. b, c, d, e
87. a, b, e

CHAPTER 68

1. a, b, c, e
2. a
3. b, d, e
4. a, b, d
5. b, c, e, f
6. a, b, e
7. b
8. c
9. a
10. b
11. c
12. a
13. c
14. a
15. a, b, c
16. a
17. d

18. b
19. b
20. a
21. b
22. a
23. a, c, d, f
24. a
25. d
26. a
27. a, c, d
28. d
29. a
30. b
31. a, c, d
32. a
33. 35
34. b, c, d
35. a, b, d, e
36. d
37. d
38. c
39. b
40. a
41. c
42. c
43. a
44. d
45. a
46. b
47. c
48. a
49. d
50. c
51. a, b, c, e
52. b
53. a
54. a, d, e, f
55. b
56. a
57. a, b, d, e, f
58. b
59. a
60. a
61. c
62. b
63. c
64. b
65. c
66. a, b, c
67. b
68. a, b, c, d, e
69. a, c, d, e

70. a
71. d
72. b
73. a
74. d
75. b
76. a
77. d
78. b, c, e
79. a
80. a
81. d
82. a. 3; b. 2; c. 4; d. 1
83. c
84. a
85. a
86. b
87. b, c, d, e
88. c
89. a
90. c
91. b, c
92. b, c, d, e, f
93. d
94. c
95. b
96. a, b, e

CHAPTER 69

1. a
2. b
3. a
4. a
5. d
6. a, c, e
7. c
8. d
9. a
10. a
11. a, c, e
12. a
13. d
14. a, b, d, e
15. b
16. b
17. c
18. a, c, d
19. b
20. d
21. a
22. a, b, e
23. c

24.

Fallopian tube
(oviduct)

25. b
26. c
27. a
28. b
29. c
30. b
31. c
32. b
33. a
34. d
35. a
36. a
37. d
38. a, d, e
39. a
40. c
41. b
42. d
43. a
44. b
45. c
46. b
47. c
48. a

CHAPTER 70

1. c
2. c

3. c
4. b
5. a
6. b, c, e, f
7. d
8. c
9. a
10. b, c, e, f
11. c
12. b, c, d
13. b
14. a
15. d
16. b
17. b
18. a, b, d
19. b
20. a
21. d
22. c
23. d
24. a, c, d, e
25. a
26. d
27. b, c, d
28. b
29. a
30. d
31. b

32. d
33. d
34. a
35. c
36. a
37. b
38. d
39. b
40. b
41. b
42. c
43. a
44. b
45. c
46. a
47. a
48. b
49. c
50. a
51. c
52. d
53. c
54. c
55. b
56. a, b, d, f

CHAPTER 71

1. d
2. d
3. b
4. a, b, c
5. d
6. a
7. b
8. a, b, c, e
9. d
10. b
11. a, d, e
12. d
13. b
14. b
15. a, c, d, e
16. b
17. d
18. b
19. a
20. a
21. c
22. a
23. a, b, c
24. b
25. a
26. b
27. a, b, d, e
28. b
29. b
30. b
31. a

32. c
33. d
34. b
35. b, c, e
36. c
37. c, d, e
38. a
39. a, e
40. a, c, e
41. a
42. c
43. b
44. b
45. b
46. c
47. d
48. a
49. a, c, d
50. c
51. a
52. a
53. b, c, e
54. c
55. b
56. d

CHAPTER 72

1. b
2. a, c, d, e
3. d
4. d
5. a, c, d, e, f
6. d
7. b
8. a
9. d
10. a
11. b
12. a, b, e
13. d
14. a
15. d
16. a
17. a
18. b
19. c
20. b
21. b, c, e
22. b
23. c
24. a
25. c
26. a
27. 250
28. d
29. a
30. d
31. c

32. a, d, e
33. c
34. a
35. a, b, c, e
36. a
37. b
38. b
39. b
40. b, c, e
41. a, b
42. a
43. b
44. c
45. b
46. d
47. d
48. c
49. a, b, d, e
50. c
51. a, b, c, e
52. a
53. a, c, d
54. b
55. c
56. a
57. a
58. a
59. c, d, e
60. a

CHAPTER 73

1. c
2. c
3. b
4. c
5. d
6. b
7. a, b, c
8. c
9. c
10. b
11. c
12. a
13. a
14. c
15. d
16. a, b, c, e
17. d
18. b
19. c
20. a, b, c, e
21. c
22. b
23. c
24. b
25. a, c, d
26. a
27. b
28. d

CHAPTER 74

1. a
2. d
3. a
4. a
5. d
6. c
7. c
8. a
9. b
10. a, c, d, e, f
11. c
12. a
13. a, b, c
14. c
15. c
16. a
17. b
18. a
19. b
20. d
21. c
22. b
23. c
24. b
25. d
26. b, c
27. c
28. a
29. c
30. b
31. c, d, e
32. b
33. a
34. c
35. a
36. d
37. c
38. d
39. d
40. b
41. b
42. c
43. a, b, c, e
44. a
45. a, b, e
46. c
47. b
48. c
49. c, d, f
50. b
51. d
52. c
53. a
54. d
55. a, b, c, e
56. a

Notes

Notes

Notes

Notes

Notes